Muscle Imaging
in Health and Disease

Springer

*New York
Berlin
Heidelberg
Barcelona
Budapest
Hong Kong
London
Milan
Paris
Santa Clara
Singapore
Tokyo*

James L. Fleckenstein, MD
University of Texas Southwestern Medical
Center at Dallas

John V. Crues III, MD
RadNet, Inc., Los Angeles

Carl D. Reimers, MD
Universität Göttingen, Germany

Editors

Muscle Imaging in Health and Disease

With 426 Illustrations

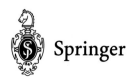

Springer

James L. Fleckenstein, MD
Department of Radiology
University of Texas Southwestern
    Medical Center at Dallas
Dallas, TX 75235-9071, USA

John V. Crues III, MD
RadNet, Inc.
Los Angeles, CA 90025-3303, USA

Carl D. Reimers, MD
Abteilung für Klinische Neurophysiologie
Universität Göttingen
37075 Göttingen
Germany

Library of Congress Cataloging-in-Publication Data
Muscle imaging in health and disease / James L. Fleckenstein, John
    V. Crues III, Carl D. Reimers, editors.
        p.   cm.
    Includes bibliographical references and index.
    ISBN 0-387-94231-9 (hardcover : alk. paper)
    1. Muscles—Imaging.   I. Fleckenstein, James L.   II. Crues, John
    V.   III. Reimers, Carl D.
    [DNLM: 1. Muscular Diseases—diagnosis.   2. Muscles—physiology.
3. Muscles—physiopathology.   4. Diagnostic Imaging.   WE 550 M9843
1996]
RC925.7.M8   1996
616.7′40754—dc20
DNLM/DLC
for Library of Congress   95-36652

Printed on acid-free paper

Production coordinated by Chernow Editorial Services, Inc. and managed by Karen Phillips; manufacturing supervised by Rhea Talbert.
Typeset by Best-set Typesetter Ltd., Hong Kong.
Printed and bound by Maple Vail Book Manufacturing Group, York, PA.
Printed in the United States of America.

9 8 7 6 5 4 3 2 1

ISBN 0-387-94231-9   Springer-Verlag New York Berlin Heidelberg
ISBN 3-540-94231-9   Springer-Verlag Berlin Heidelberg New York   SPIN 10424442

This book is dedicated to my parents,
William R. Fleckenstein and Shirley A. Fleckenstein.

Preface

Skeletal muscle is a subject of intense interest to a great many individuals ranging from the construction laborer with occupational-related myalgia to the elite body builder in search of better biceps definition; from the endurance athlete stretching for greater mileage gains to the aging healthy; and from the weak and infirmed to the fittest astronaut. With educational backgrounds as diverse as those who would like to know more about the latest technological advances in probing the mysteries of muscle in health and disease, it was challenging to attempt to summarize, for all interested parties, the tremendous strides made in diagnostic imaging of an organ system as complex anatomically and functionally as skeletal muscle. Although targeted to a medical audience, the book is hoped to find use as an aid to many in the study of anatomy, physiology, and the fitness sciences.

From a medical perspective, the book attempts to provide a broad background to aid in the evaluation of two types of patient who might be seen in the examination rooms of a range of physicians. The first is the patient with muscle weakness, the second is the patient with muscle pain. Either of these might be seen by a generalist, neurologist, rheumatologist, orthopaedic surgeon, emergency medicine specialist, or all of them! The clinical aspects of the topic are divided roughly along these two patient types, assuming the overly simplistic position that the weak patient may most often be afflicted with a neurological disease and the patient with muscle pain with an orthopaedic condition. In either patient, muscle disease is difficult to objectify. As a result, muscle as the source of patients' complaints is usually a diagnosis of exclusion, without an objective means of verifying the belief. Fortunately, the advent of noninvasive radiological tools provides clinicians with renewed abilities to evaluate the integrity and quality of muscle. In the current era of "managed" medical care, the ability to objectify deficient muscle quality by imaging studies may simplify the triage system by which patients are referred to specialists.

For radiologists, the book is hoped to be an introduction to the variety of disorders that may be uncovered by the powerful tools with which radiologists examine patients. Encountered either incidentally or as a primary directive, muscle abnormalities need to be dutifully reported with appropriate differential diagnoses so that subsequent evaluations and treatments are efficacious. Although specific diagnoses are rarely possible based on imaging findings alone, attention directed to a specific muscle or type of parenchymal process may be pivotal in patient management.

James L. Fleckenstein, MD

Acknowledgments

I thank the many referring physicians and technologists who provided patient material and technical expertise to make this as complete a work as possible. I would especially like to thank Mark Daugherty, George MacDonald, PhD, and Jennifer Layman for exceeding all reasonable bounds of duty to assist me in many aspects of this work. Also, the ever-discriminating eye and patient attitude of a superb photographer, Ms. Alison Russell, accounts for a large measure of whatever success this book attains. My secretary, Ms. Kathy Norman, was one of the main reasons the book is now in front of you—without her constant vigilance over the many chapters, deadlines, edits, international mailings, and FAXs, the project would never have been completed. Thanks are critically due to my many mentors who aided me along my circuitous pathway to this point, notably including Robert W. Parkey, MD, Ronald M. Peshock, MD, Peter A. Simkin, MD, and Cornelius Rosse, MD, PhD. I also thank Kevin Baker, Jerri Payne, P.A.C., Cindy Miller, Maria Morgan, Christie Ward, William Ennen, Reza Sadoogh, Rhonda Church, George Jacob, Jacob George, Don Harvey, Tommie Hall, Joe Reyes, Eddie Washington, Kay Thomas, Dorothy Gutekunst, and Virginia Reed Vaughn for their technical expertise. Last, but not least, thanks are due to the members of the Neuroradiology faculty at the University of Texas Southwestern Medical Center at Dallas, particularly Dianne Mendelsohn, MD, David P. Chason, MD, and Phillip Purdy, MD, for their critical support.

James L. Fleckenstein, MD

Contents

Contributors

WILLIAM BANK, MD
Department of Neurology, University of Pennsylvania, Philadelphia, PA 19104, USA

LOREN A. BERTOCCI, PhD
Institute for Exercise and Environmental Medicine, Presbyterian Hospital of Dallas, Dallas, TX 75231, USA

FREDERICK J. BONTE, MD
Department of Radiology, University of Texas Southwestern Medical Center at Dallas, Dallas, TX 75235-9071, USA

DENNIS K. BURNS, MD
Department of Pathology, University of Texas Southwestern Medical Center at Dallas, Dallas, TX 75235-9072, USA

IAN J. BUTLER, MD
Department of Neurology, University of Texas Medical School of Houston, Houston, TX 77030, USA

R. CEULEMANS, MD
University of Antwerp, B-2610 Antwerp, Belgium

DAVID P. CHASON, MD
Department of Radiology, University of Texas Southwestern Medical Center at Dallas, Dallas, TX 75235-8896, USA

GEOFFREY D. CLARKE, PhD
Department of Radiology, University of Texas Southwestern Medical Center at Dallas, Dallas, TX 75235-9071, USA

JOHN V. CRUES III, MD
Medical Director, RADNET, Inc., Los Angeles, CA 90025, USA

LUC S. DeCLERCK, MD, PhD
Department of Immunology, Allergy and Rheumatology, University of Antwerp, B-2610 Antwerp, Belgium

A.M. DE SCHEPPER, MD, PhD
University of Antwerp, B-2610 Antwerp, Belgium

MARIANNE DE VISSER, MD
Department of Neurology (H2-216), Academic Medical Center, 1105 AZ
Amsterdam, The Netherlands

MARYBETH EZAKI, MD
Texas Scottish-Rite Hospital for Children, Dallas, TX 75219, USA

ASMA Q. FISCHER, MD
University Hospital, Medical Staff Office, Augusta, GA 30901, USA

PETRA FISCHER, MD
Friedrich-Baur-Institut bei der Medizinischen Klinik und Neurologischen
Klinik, Klinikum Innenstadt, Ludwig-Maximilians-Universität, D80336
Munich, Germany

JAMES L. FLECKENSTEIN, MD
Department of Radiology, University of Texas Southwestern Medical Center
at Dallas, Dallas, TX 75235-8896, USA

BARRY D. FLETCHER, MD
Department of Diagnostic Imaging, St. Jude Children's Research Hospital,
Memphis, TN 38105, USA

RUSSELL C. FRITZ, MD
University of California School of Medicine, San Francisco, CA 94122, USA

ALINA GRECO, MD
Department of Magnetic Resonance Imaging, Princess Grace Hospital,
Monte Carlo, Principality of Monaco 98000

RONALD G. HALLER, MD
Institute for Exercise and Environmental Medicine, Presbyterian Hospital of
Dallas, Dallas, TX 75231, USA

MICHAELA HAMANN, MD
Department of Radiology, University of Bonn, 53127 Bonn, Germany

SOHEIL L. HANNA, MD
Department of Diagnostic Imaging, St. Jude Children's Research Hospital,
Memphis, TN 38105, USA

JOHN HECKMATT, MD
Department of Pediatrics and Neonatal Medicine, Hammersmith Hospital,
University of London, London W12 0NN, United Kingdom

ERICH HOFMANN, MD
Department of Neuroradiology, University of Würzburg, D-97080
Würzburg, Germany

JOHN L. HUNT, MD
Department of Surgery, University of Texas Southwestern Medical Center
at Dallas, Dallas, TX 75235-9031, USA

EDWARD F. JACKSON, PhD
Department of Radiology, University of Texas Southwestern Medical
School at Houston, Houston, TX 77030, USA

WERNER KAISER, MD
Department of Radiology, Friedrich-Schiller-University at Jena, D-07743
Jena, Germany

PIERRE KAMINSKY, MD
Service de Médecine, Centre Hospitalier Universitaire de Nancy, Hôpitaux
de Brabois, Vandoeuvre-les-Nancy, France

HERBERT KELLNER, MD
Medizinische Poliklinik, Klinikum Innenstadt, Ludwig-Maximilians-
Universität, D80336 Munich, Germany

WALTER F. KOCH, MD
Department of Orthopedic Surgery, St. Josef-Hospital, 53840 Troisdorf,
Germany

ANTTI LAMMINEN, MD
Department of Radiology, University Central Hospital, 00290 Helsinki,
Finland

ELWOOD LONGENECKER, BS
The Medical College of Georgia, Augusta, GA 30901, USA

CHRISTIAN J. LUKOSCH
Hôlderlinstrasse 7c, 35415 Pohlheim, Germany

GERHARD E. MAALE, MD
8230 Walnut Hill Lane, Dallas, TX 75231, USA

KEVIN McCULLY, MD
Center for Continuing Health, Monroe Office Center, Philadelphia, PA
19131, USA

MICHAEL T. McNAMARA, MD
Department of Magnetic Resonance Imaging, Princess Grace Hospital,
Monte Carlo, Principality of Monaco 98000

MATTHIAS NÄGELE, MD
Im Hagedorn 6, 77933 Lahr, Germany

PONNADA A. NARAYANA, PhD
Department of Radiology, University of Texas Health Science Center at
Houston, Houston, TX 77030, USA

ROBERT W. PARKEY, MD
Department of Radiology, University of Texas Southwestern Medical
Center at Dallas, Dallas, TX 75235-9071, USA

HELENA PIHKO, MD
Department of Diagnostic Radiology, University Central Hospital, 00290
Helsinki, Finland

DIETER E. PONGRATZ, MD
Friedrich-Baur-Institut bei der Neurologischen und Medizinischen Klinik,
Klinikum Innenstadt, Ludwig-Maximilians-Universität München, 8000
Munich 2, Germany

GARY F. PURDUE, MD
Department of Surgery, University of Texas Southwestern Medical Center
at Dallas, Dallas, TX 75235-9031, USA

CARL D. REIMERS, MD
Abteilung für Klinische Neurophysiologie, Universität Göttingen, 37075 Göttingen, Germany

KARLHEINZ REINERS, MD
Department of Neurology, University of Würzburg, D-97080 Würzburg, Germany

MARGA B. ROMINGER, MD
Hôlderlinstrasse 7c, 35415 Pohlheim, Germany

BERTHOLD C.G. SCHALKE, MD
Department of Neurology, University of Regensburg, D-93042 Regensburg, Germany

RAIMO E. SEPPONEN, D.Sc
Picker Nordstar, Inc., RIN-00510 Helsinki, Finland

FRANK G. SHELLOCK, PhD
Future Diagnostic, Inc., Los Angeles, CA 90048, USA

W.J. STEVENS, MD
Department of Immunology, Allergy and Rheumatology, University of Antwerp, B-2610 Antwerp, Belgium

JUKKA TANTTU, MD
Imaging Division, Instrumentarium Corporation, SF-00101 Helsinki, Finland

LESIA L. TYSON, MD
Dpartment of Radiology, University of Utah School of Medicine, Salt Lake City, UT 84132, USA

KRISTA VANDENBORNE, PhD, PT
Department of Rehabilitation Medicine, University of Pennsylvania, Philadelphia, PA 19104, USA

THOMAS J. VOGL, MD
Leitender Oberarzi, Freie Universität Berlin, Universitätsklinikum Rudolf Virchow, Standort Wedding–Strahlenklinik, Diagnostik, 1000 Berlin 65, Germany

PAUL M. WALKER, MD
Service de Médecine, Centre Hospitalier Universitaire de Nancy, Hôpitaux de Brabois, Vandoeuvre-les-Nancy, France

GLENN WALTER, BS
Department of Radiology, University of Pennsylvania, Philadelphia, PA 19104, USA

PAUL T. WEATHERALL, MD
Department of Radiology, University of Texas Southwestern Medical Center at Dallas, Dallas, TX 75235-9071, USA

Part I
Radiology Techniques

1
Ionizing Radiation Imaging Techniques in the Evaluation of Muscle Disorders

Geoffrey D. Clarke, Frederick J. Bonte, and James L. Fleckenstein

Ionizing radiation imaging techniques can be employed to reveal important structural and/or functional information about skeletal muscle and the development of such techniques has been a critical step forward in the evolution of noninvasive approaches in the understanding of skeletal muscle biology and pathology.[1] Unfortunately, health risks due to the radiation employed in these techniques inhibit widespread use of them in evaluating muscle in healthy persons. In addition, relatively low spatial and/or contrast resolution of the techniques are important factors that limit application in patient groups. However, the techniques remain useful tools in radiological practices that may not have access to, or availability of, the more optimal technique of magnetic resonance imaging or the degree of experience needed for routine ultrasound evaluation of muscle. Hence, a review of modalities employing ionizing radiation is warranted.

Soft Tissue Radiography

To large extent, radiographic contrast is determined by the ability of the different tissues to absorb x-ray photons. The absorption coefficients of various tissues depends on their chemical composition and the energy distribution of the x-rays. The absorption coefficients for three types of tissue important in imaging skeletal muscles and their absorption coefficients for five values of x-ray tube potential (kVp) are shown in Table 1.1. Note that the greatest relative differences between the absorption coefficients of these three tissues occurs at the lower energies, but for this energy range the dose load is prohibitive unless special imaging equipment and radiographic techniques are employed, such as used in film-screen mammography.

The small relative differences in x-ray absorption between various soft tissues limit detailed examination of muscular tissue. The projected shadows of the muscles are usually poorly outlined, homogeneous, and give no information about internal structure. Initial attempts at employing high-energy x-rays to examine skeletal muscles attempted to improve image detail by adding filtering screens, altering focusing distances and exposure times, changing films, and modifying development and reproduction procedures.[2–5] The results of these experiments were very limited but adequate to aid in evaluating a few pathological conditions in which muscular calcium accumulation or ossification were present. By using lower energy x-rays and fine-grain film, improvements were made so that skin, subcutaneous tissue, muscular fascia, and vessels could be recognized.[6–8]

Frantzell and Ingelmark examined 222 healthy persons of different ages and emphasized that fat is the constituent on which soft tissue radiography should concentrate.[7] They described the four essential locations of fat tissue as subcutaneous, interfascicular or perimysial, subfascicular or endomysial, and interstitial. They demonstrated that linear striations of the perimysial fat may become visible in pathological cases, and maintained that this compartment was the only one of particular interest in neuromuscular disease. Age-related increases of intramuscular fat, from nearly absent in 20-year-old males to up to 85% in 65-year-old females, was found mainly in other compartments.

Years later, DiChiro and Nelson used a similar approach to study histopathological correlation of the radiological findings of soft tissues of the extremities in a number of neuromuscular diseases.[9] They emphasized the importance of optimized photographic reproduction of soft x-rays. They also described disappointing results in the use of water-soluble contrast media to enhance muscular contrast. They observed that in healthy young persons the normal musculature is compact and homogeneous. Age, obesity, castration,[10] and immobilization were found to increase the subcutaneous, intermuscular, and subfascial fat, which increased the delineation of the individual muscles, whereas interstitial fat remained

TABLE 1.1. Radiological properties of musculoskeletal tissues.*

Tissue	Linear Absorption Coefficient (cm^{-1})				
	40 kVp	60 kVp	80 kVp	100 kVp	150 kVp
Muscle	0.25	0.21	0.19	0.18	0.16
Fat	0.27	0.18	0.16	0.15	0.14
Bone	0.84	0.45	0.34	0.30	0.25

*Johns HE, Cunningham JR. The physics of radiology, 4th ed. Springfield, IL: Charles Thomas, 1983.

normal under these conditions. They reported that in patients over 40 years old, a less orderly fat infiltration was found that was roentgenologically distinct from, and more frequent than, the linear streaks seen in patients with progressive muscular dystrophy. The linear fat streaks were reportedly always abnormal in patients below the age of 30. No significant difference was found between the fat striation observed in various forms of spinal muscular atrophy and myopathy. Although they observed that the fat content increased with increasing severity of the disease, biopsy results correlated better with clinical involvement and the x-ray technique was totally unreliable below the age of 5 or 6 years, particularly in a group of floppy babies. They concluded that only a progressive pattern of fine parallel striations, resembling "fish flesh," might be of diagnostic significance.

Palvolgyi made a new study of the basic radiological findings on soft tissue radiography of the limb muscles in healthy persons and in different neuromuscular disease.[11] He, too, found that in unhealthy young persons individual muscles could never be delineated, except for those of the forearm, and that other structural elements such as fascia, nerves, and blood vessels could be seen. Normal muscles were smooth, rounded, and homogeneous, and very symmetrical in appearance and size. Even a few millimeters of difference in size was considered abnormal. Muscular atrophy was found to be characterized by linear streaks of fat within the muscles. This was determined to be abnormal below the age of 30 but very frequent above 65 years. The author confirmed the inability to distinguish between neurogenic atrophy and primary myopathy with his x-ray technique.

Two years later, Palvolgyi and Gallai drew attention to the peculiar selectivity of muscular atrophy in various diseases, a feature that remains inexplicable today.[12] They observed selective areas of atrophy within individual muscles, selective atrophy of specific muscles and muscle groups, and asymmetry between two identical but contralateral muscles. Other studies by the same author have described soft tissue x-ray findings in muscular pseudohypertrophy,[13] anterior horn cell lesions,[14] closed muscle and tendon injuries of the upper arm,[15] and lacerations in tendons and muscles in the Ehlers-Danlos syndrome.[16]

Xeroradiography

Xeroradiography is a technique specifically geared towards the examination of soft tissues. The theoretical background and applicability of xeroradiography has been worked out in several articles.[17–20] Xeroradiography combines the use of less penetrating, "soft" x-rays and an aluminum plate receptor coated with a positively charged layer of selenium that is exposed instead of x-ray film. The x-rays pass through the soft tissue and strike the positively charged selenium layer, thereby discharging it and producing positive and negative charges in proportion to the characteristics of the penetrating x-rays. A cloud of negatively charged ink powder is then sprayed into the developing chamber, producing a pattern induced by the charged selenium. The powder is then transferred to paper by an electrostatic process and fixed by heat. The technique gives a weak overall contrast but a sharp and characteristic intensity of borders.

The use of xeroradiography for the study of the normal and pathological muscle tissue has been relatively limited. In 1977, Palvolgyi and Pentek presented a series of xerograms of the normal musculature of arms and legs.[21] In the same year a small study of 30 patients was published in which xeroradiographic and normal soft tissue radiograms were compared.[22] Xeroradiography of muscles was found to give more "harmonious pictures" with a better outline of fatty degenerations, muscle contours, calcifications, and edema. According to Osterman et al., the quality of the images can be further enhanced by using negative-mode imaging.[23] However, the xeroradiographic technique is clearly limited and is of mainly historical importance because commercial production of the necessary equipment ceased in 1990.

Computed Radiography

Direct digitization of radiographic images can be accomplished by replacing the traditional film-screen combination with a photostimulable phosphor plate in the imaging cassette. The exposed phosphor plate stores the image data, which is subsequently read out by scanning the plate with a laser beam that produces photostimulable luminescence. The luminescence is detected using a photomultiplier tube and the analog electronic data is then digitized. The image data is presented as a matrix of gray-scale values; each element of the matrix is called a picture element or pixel.

Directly digitized plain x-ray images promise several benefits over conventional film-screen systems.[24] The detector response is linear over a range of exposures, 100 times larger than that of x-ray film. This means that at the low and high ends of the sensitivity curve of the detectors, the measured value is still directly proportional to the exposure. This feature is in contrast to the sensitivity curves of film that have characteristic nonlinear "toe" and "shoulder" regions. Thus, in digital radiography images have a greater latitude (dynamic range).

In addition to the greater range of measurable exposures, the operator can improve image contrast by defining a "window" or range of gray-scale values to be displayed and adjusting the mean gray-scale value or "level" to the appropriate size. With digital imaging there is the capability for imaging regions of the body having a large range of subject contrast in a single exposure, which mitigates the need for two exposures taken with bone and soft tissue techniques. The improved linearity also allows a significant reduction of repeated exposures for difficult exams, such as some portable x-ray studies.

Improved visualization of soft tissue calcifications similar to that obtained using xeroradiography has been shown using computed radiography in the coronary arteries.[25] The results of at least one study suggested that the identification of soft tissue changes is more accurately observed using photostimulable phosphor technology.[26]

Phosphor plate detectors can utilize x-ray photons four to five times more efficiently than the fastest rare earth screen-film combinations presently in general use. The linear response and improved detector efficiency make it likely that radiation doses for computed radiographic examinations will be reduced by 25% to 50% compared to the same study performed with film-screen technology.

Although photostimulable phosphor technology has been available since the late 1980s, diffusion of these devices into general radiological practice has been slow. Slow acceptance of digital radiography has been attributed to differences in image format from conventional film radiography, the relatively high capital cost of computed radiography, decreased spatial resolution, restricted throughput of the laser scanning device, and new artifacts that must be understood and recognized.[26] Clearly, the full range of application for computed radiography has not yet been explored for the depiction of muscle tissue. The relatively low radiation dose of this technology may allow new, low kVp radiographic techniques to be developed for high-contrast soft tissue studies.

Computed Tomography Applied to Human Striated Skeletal Muscles

It is beyond the scope of this work to elaborate in detail upon the technicalities of computed tomography (CT) scanning and image processing. Descriptions of the different CT scanner types and geometric configurations used in clinical practice are available.[27,28] CT imaging is based on the principle of using digital processing to produce image reconstructions from projections. Projections are obtained by scanning a pencil-thin x-ray beam through the patient and measuring the amount of x-ray attenuation using gas ionization chambers or scintillation crystal detectors. The x-ray beam is scanned in a circular arc centered on the patient with each data accumulation occurring at a different angle. The data obtained from the attenuated x-ray beam being projected onto the detector at every angle are compiled, reconstructed, and filtered in order to produce the CT image. Each rotation about the patient can generate sufficient data from enough angles to produce an image of one transaxial slice. Images from multiple slices can be obtained by moving the patient table parallel to the axis of the scanner.[29]

In practice, the output of the x-ray tube is collimated to produce a fan of pencil-thin beams. The fan beam is used with x-ray detector arrays composed of up to 2000 elements, allowing single slice CT scans to be carried out in as little as one second. CT scanners allow the user to define a variety of slice thicknesses, pixel sizes, and field of view sizes.

Radiation doses depend on the choice of these imaging parameters, with higher resolution studies generally leading to greater exposures. Surface dose also increases with increasing body part thickness because greater x-ray exposures are generally required to penetrate the thicker body part and the surface of the body is closer to the x-ray tube. Typical surface doses range from 1 to 2 cGy for head studies and 3 to 5 cGy for body studies.[30,31] According to a recent study of conventional CT devices, the radiation dose to the bone marrow during a CT scan of the pelvis is 5 to 8 mGy.[1] This likely represents a higher dose than would be delivered in a survey of the total body, as outlined below, because in such a survey, fewer slices are obtained than in a conventional pelvis study and only a portion of the muscle survey would be through the axial skeleton, with the remainder being in the long bones, which, in adults, would contain little if any hematopoetic marrow.

The image pixel values obtained from the filtered back-projection process are directly related to the linear attenuation coefficient (Table 1.1) of the material being imaged. Numerical output data are expressed in Hounsfield Units (HU). The HU is defined as the attenuation value at a matrix point relative to the attenuation value for water and is calculated as follows:

$$HU = 1000(\mu/\mu_w - 1),$$

where μ is the average attenuation coefficient of the volume element (voxel) and μ_w is the linear attenuation coefficient of water. Thus, water has a CT number of zero and a region with a CT number of 100 HU has a linear attenuation coefficient that is 10% greater than that of water. CT scanners can typically produce 4096 gray-scale values, which are used to represent CT numbers from −1000 to +3095. Normal HU values for the various soft tissues, as reported by Grindrod et al., using currently outdated equipment, was 54 HU for normal muscle, −106 HU for fat, and 75 HU for fibrous tissue.[32] These values agree approximately with those from an example case done recently at our institution (Figure 1.1).

Significant artifacts arise in CT images.[27,28] The most prolific are errors in attenuation measurement due to a change in the spectral character of the x-ray beam as it traverses the patient. These "beam-hardening" artifacts present as streaks across the image and are most noticeable in images of body regions containing a large quantity of bone, such as the pelvis and spine (Figures 1.1 and 1.2). Partial volume artifacts arise from tissue with several different attenuation coefficients being present in the volume from which an image pixel is produced (voxel). If one small, highly attenuating object projects into the imaged voxel, then the entire CT number of the resulting pixel can be significantly in error. Partial volume artifacts in the slice thickness direction are particularly common because the voxel dimensions of the slice thickness are typically an order of magnitude

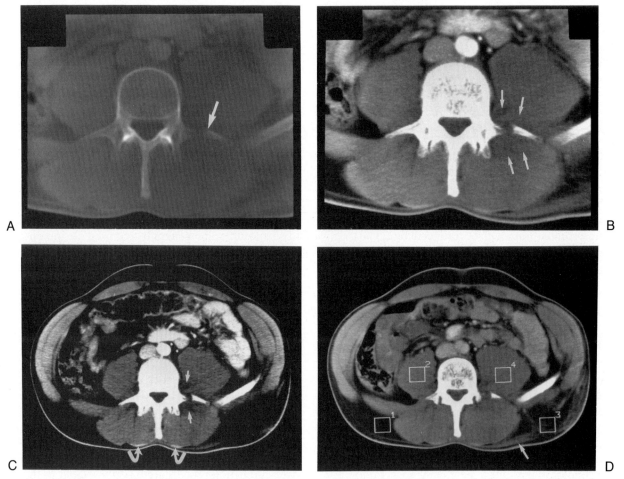

FIGURE 1.1. Computed tomograms of a trauma victim at the level of the umbilicus show the kind of information that can be highlighted by adjusting the window and level of the constructed image and by measuring densities in Hounsfield units (HUs). (A) The "bone window" evaluates objects of high density, such as the fractured lumbar transverse process (arrow), but is poorly sensitive to soft tissue pathology. (B) The "soft tissue window" better evaluates objects of lesser density such as muscle and fat. The muscle surrounding the fracture shows subtle low density (arrows). (C) The muscle edema can be made more conspicuous by narrowing the window width and decreasing the level, as shown in an unmagnified view. (D) The edematous changes in the subcutaneous fat are made more conspicuous (arrow) by widening the window width, as shown on image obtained slightly caudal to (C). Regions of interest (boxes numbered 1 through 4) can be used to quantitate tissue densities: 1 = fat, −85 HU; 2 = normal muscle, 65 HU; 3 = edematous fat, −45 HU; 4 = slightly edematous muscle, 60 HU. Note in these images the presence of a thin layer of blood, denoted by high density posteriorly along the midline fasciae (best seen in C, curved arrows).

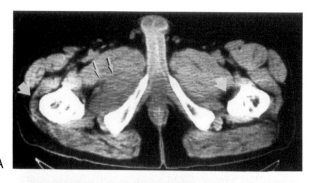

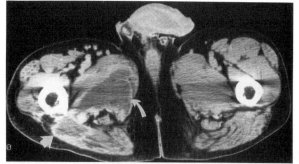

FIGURE 1.2. Limitations of CT in muscle disease. (A) Non-contrast axial image through the distal pelvis in a patient shows typical beam-hardening artifacts causing dark areas adjacent to femora (arrowheads). Edematous changes in right adductors are subtle and obscured by beam hardening (arrows). (B) Upon contrast infusion, the necrotic areas in the adductors (curved arrow) and gluteus maximus (arrowhead) are easier to detect, although beam hardening artifacts remain severe. (C) Short tau inversion recovery (STIR) magnetic resonance imaging shows the edematous adductors (curved arrow) and gluteus maximus (arrowhead) with superior sensitivity and without the need for intravenous injection.

greater than the in-plane pixel dimensions. Errors in detector calibration can be caused by changes in room temperature and atmospheric pressure. It is good practice to routinely perform an "air calibration" to account for these effects from study to study. Some scanners can even check the detector calibration during the scanning procedure. The faster CT scanning technology, mentioned above, has been developed in order to reduce the artifacts due to patient motion during the scan.

When the CT scan takes several seconds per slice there is a potential for streaking artifacts if the patient moves significantly.

Common electrical voltages applied to CT x-ray tubes are around 120 to 130 kVp regardless of the thickness or composition of the body part under study. The mean CT numbers of normal muscular tissue vary between 30 and 80 HU, depending mainly upon the muscle group measured.[33,34] However, it is important to remember that absolute numerical values obtained are highly dependent upon apparatus characteristics. A series of engineering trade-offs are made in the design of each model of CT system. Thus, beam hardening, nonlinearities, scattered radiation, and various approaches to filtering contribute differently to the final image depending on the design of the scanner. The complexity of these problems is accentuated by the great variability in patient body size, habitus, and centering.

As is the case with computed radiography, the contrast within a given range of CT values can be improved through the process of adjusting the window and level (Figure 1.1). The measurement of relative x-ray attenuation is performed by adjusting and determining a region of interest (ROI), the contours of which are under user control. Statistical output from the selected ROIs include mean, maximum, minimum, and standard deviation of the included CT pixel values. The data can also be displayed as a histogram that presents the CT numbers as a function of distance across an edge or other structure.

One Recommended Standard CT Survey of Skeletal Muscles in Patients

Because the radiation dose and time required for an exhaustive CT of the entire body would be prohibitive as a routine procedure in the examination of myopathies, a limited CT examination consisting of six well-selected scan levels was devised.[35] The original selection of standard CT levels for evaluation of neuromuscular disease was originally guided by a few well-defined objectives. First, the fact that certain muscle groups are affected more frequently and earlier than others in many myopathies was taken into account. Next, regions were chosen that maximized the number of muscles studied and the ratio of cross-sectional area of muscular shadows to area of bony and other reliable structural landmarks. Finally, several levels were excluded because of beam-hardening artifacts that were particularly severe, such as in the forearms.

In this scheme, transverse scans are obtained at six different levels, encompassing a great variety of muscles including those of (1) the neck, (2) the shoulder, (3) the trunk and spine, (4) the pelvis, (5) the thighs, and (6) the legs. This procedure allows inspection of approximately 70 muscles per side of the body. This is a considerable sampling of the total number of skeletal muscles and also represents a wide range of motor nerves and motor neuron pools. The standard examination procedure is therefore a suitable instrument for the investigation of myopathies, peripheral neuropathies, and medullary lesions.

Radioisotope Uptake in Skeletal Muscle

Nuclear medicine imaging methods employ radiation-emitting isotopes attached to metabolites or metabolite analogues in order to study physiological function of specific organs. These radiopharmaceuticals are injected into the patient and travel through the circulation to the organs targeted for imaging, where they emit gamma radiation. The gamma camera (or Anger camera) is composed of an array of radiation detectors coupled through photomultiplier tubes to a computer and serves as the passive imaging device. A collimation device, consisting of a matrix of pinhole septae, manufactured into a radiation opaque metal (usually lead), is placed between the patient and the gamma camera to improve spatial localization of the injected radioisotopes and reduces the contribution of scattered radiation to the image. Other methods, such as digital filtering and the rejection of gamma rays detected at inappropriate energies (energy windowing), are used to improve image quality.

Cross-sectional images may be obtained using two nuclear medicine methods. Single photon emission computed tomography (SPECT) uses a rotating gamma camera that collects radiation counts from angles all around the patient. A back-projection algorithm, similar to those used in x-ray CT, discussed above, produces an image matrix of a plane of the body. SPECT produces a three-dimensional data set and improves diagnostic accuracy by allowing views of multiple orientations and enhancing object-to-background contrast. Two or more Anger cameras may be coupled together to acquire counts from several directions at the same time and reduce the total scan duration.

The second method for cross-sectional nuclear medicine imaging, positron emission tomography (PET), relies on the detection of two 511-keV gamma rays produced by the mutual annihilation of an electron and a positron. This method is very expensive and not in widespread use, so it will not be discussed further.

Radioisotope techniques have been used for many years to study the composition of the human body and the sizes of its different compartments. Body potassium is an especially interesting parameter for studying the skeletal muscular compartment because of its selective association with muscle proteins. Of total body potassium, 95% is intracellular, a large proportion being intramuscular as well. Investigators have described marked decreases in total body potassium in cases of muscular atrophy of various kinds.[36,37] Delwaide et al. demonstrated a lowered body potassium in three types of neuromuscular disease: muscular dystrophy, neurogenic amyotrophy, and myasthenia gravis.[38]

The element thallium, as the thallous ion, has many of the properties of potassium and can serve as a potassium substitute for imaging purposes, not only in the myocardium but in peripheral muscle. Imaging muscle uptake of thallium-201 (^{201}Tl), injected intravenously as thallous chloride, has been used to evaluate the peripheral circulation.[39,40] Disease of peripheral arteries, especially in the legs, will produce defects in the pattern of thallium localization within muscles.

Chevreaud et al. studied 30 patients suffering from stages of arterial occlusive disease retrospectively using ^{201}Tl (20 mCi administered IV) in the skull, thigh, and calf.[41] An index, designed to express the microcirculatory effects of arterial lesions, was taken from the scintigraphic measurements on the various body parts before treatment. Angiography was also performed to determine the location and number of arterial stenoses and the results were graded as to the observed degree of arterial occlusions.

Calcification of muscle occurs in a great variety of conditions in which muscle necrosis is a feature, although the calcium is typically insufficient quantitatively to be visible on radiographs or CT scans. In these cases, radiopharmaceutical agents, such as technetium-99m stannous pyrophosphate (^{99m}Tc-PYP), are frequently used. Although ^{99m}Tc-PYP imaging has a role in the clinical evaluation of muscle necrosis, recall that not all muscle calcification signifies muscle necrosis. Metastatic calcification of muscle, for example, occurs in hyperparathyroidism when precipitation of calcium phosphate salts occurs. In such instances, ^{99m}Tc-PYP scintigraphy can be used to identify the regions of calcification (Figure 1.3).

The pathophysiology of muscle calcification in conditions in which muscle necrosis is a prominent feature deserves brief elaboration. In Duchenne's muscular dystrophy, for example, focal defects in the muscle cell membrane are an early morphologic abnormality.[42,43] This structural defect permits not only the outflow of muscle enzymes, such as creatine kinase, but also the flow of calcium-rich extracellular fluid into the cell. Regardless of the mechanism by which this disruption in calcium homeostasis develops, when intracellular calcium concentrations exceed critical levels, protein synthesis stalls, hypercontraction occurs, and calcium-sensitive proteases are activated, thereby promoting cell necrosis.[44-46]

The first important application of a radiopharmaceutical to study muscle necrosis was when Bonte et al. observed the uptake of ^{99m}Tc-PYP in myocardial infarctions.[47] Buja et al. attributed this phenomenon to increased cell membrane permeability resulting from anoxia produced by the ischemia of coronary occlusion.[48] Permeability leads to the influx of both pyrophosphate and calcium ions. The latter bind ^{99m}Tc-PYP, causing infarcted myocardium to appear as a "hot spot" on planar SPECT images of the chest, and is termed infarct-avid imaging. Because ^{99m}Tc-PYP offers the best differential between blood clearance, lesion uptake, and tracer skeletal localization, it remains the preferred radiopharmaceutical for this purpose.

Trauma to skeletal muscles may be associated with myofiber necrosis, which may effectively be identified using ^{99m}Tc-PYP, based on results with ^{99m}Tc-PYP in imaging necrotic myocardium. Increased ^{99m}Tc-PYP uptake has been used to identify muscle rendered necrotic as a result of electrical injuries and burns.[49,50] Because it is advisable to identify and debride necrotic muscular tissue to promote healing in these injuries, ^{99m}Tc-PYP imaging is still used for this purpose in a number of institutions (see Chapter 30).

Technetium-99m PYP imaging has been used to evaluate skeletal muscle athletic injuries.[51] Localization of ^{99m}Tc-PYP in leg muscles due to rhabdomyolysis produced by extreme exercise in "ultramarathon" runners was reported. As with injured myocardium, abnormal uptake appears in skeletal muscle within 24 to 48 h following injury, and gradually disappears on follow-up studies made up to 8 days later.

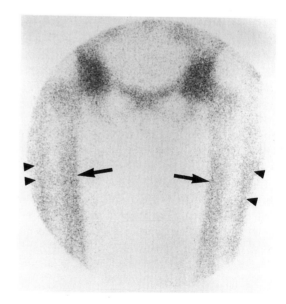

FIGURE 1.3. Hyperparathyroidism-associated mineralization of muscles: depiction using ^{99m}Tc-PYP. When the serum calcium and phosphate ion concentrations exceed critical levels, their salts precipitate in soft tissues, including muscles. After intravenous injection, ^{99m}Tc-PYP may participate in this process. This allows relatively noninvasive detection of muscles that undergo this so-called "metastatic" calcification. Posteroanterior planar view of the proximal thighs and lower pelvis of a patient with hyperparathyroidism shows normal uptake in the femurs (arrows). The uptake in the vastus lateralis (arrowheads) is abnormal and indicative of muscle mineralization.

Muscle inflammation is another area where radionuclides are helpful in patients. Muscle may be incorporated into an inflammatory process that involves other soft tissues and bone. Muscle involvement may be evaluated by means of skeletal scintigraphy, which is primarily performed to identify possible bone infection. The initial radionuclide tracer employed is often technetium-99m methylene diphosphonate (^{99m}Tc-MDP), a radiopharmaceutical that provides a satisfactory relationship between blood clearance and bone and soft tissue localization. This tracer is used in a procedure known as the "three-phase" bone scan.[52]

In this test, ^{99m}Tc-MDP is injected intravenously and scintillation camera views are made of the involved body part; in the case of extremities, both are imaged in each view to provide comparison. The first phase of the three-phase study consists of a series of views consisting of 1 to 2 seconds duration each, made during the period of a minute, in order to evaluate local blood flow. At the conclusion of the series, longer-duration views are obtained to evaluate the quantity of labeled blood pool in the region of interest. These images comprise the second phase. The third phase consists of views obtained at 2 to 4 h following tracer injection. At this time the tracer has assumed a stable distribution in bone, and its concentration is maximal with respect to soft tissues.

In the case of muscle infection, blood flow is usually augmented, and more than normal activity is seen on blood pool views. With most soft tissue infections the increased activity seen in the first two phases will have cleared on the third phase images (see Chapter 22). Residual increased tracer activity in bone is evidence of osteomyelitis.[53]

Karl et al. reported on the abnormal ^{99m}Tc-MDP scintigraphic appearance in the soft tissues of the pelvis in the distribution of the piriformis muscle for a case of piriformis muscle syndrome in which radiographic findings were normal.[54] They suggested that nuclear medicine studies could be used in addition to clinical criteria to improve the diagnosis of piriformis muscle syndrome.

When large areas of muscular necrosis accumulate calcium, they can be demonstrated by ^{99m}Tc-MDP ^{99m}Tc-PYP. This has been extensively corroborated.[55] In the case of complex infectious processes that may involve both bone and soft tissue in which a satisfactory diagnosis cannot be made with the use of radiographs and ^{99m}Tc-MDP bone imaging, supplementary imaging tests are often employed.

Gallium-67 (^{67}Ga), administered intravenously as the citrate, is rapidly bound to the plasma protein transferrin,[56] and secondarily to circulating leukocytes. It is thought to accumulate at the site of infections by diffusing into the extravascular space through loose intercellular junctions, and there becoming bound to lactoferrin, which is ingested by leukocytes.[57,58] Imaging with a scintillation camera is carried out at 6, 24, and, if necessary, 48 and 72 h following administration. Localization will occur in tissues that are the site of infection, including both bone and muscle.

An alternative secondary test may be performed using Indium-111 (^{111}In)-labeled leukocytes. In this test, the patient's own leukocytes are labeled in vitro with ^{111}In-oxine and returned to the patient.[59] The labeled cells accumulate at the site of either bone or soft tissue infection, with optimal images obtained at 24 h after administration of the radiopharmaceutical. Imaging with ^{111}In-labeled leukocytes is thought to be slightly more sensitive and specific for early acute infections, but ^{67}Ga imaging appears to be slightly superior in the case of chronic infections, and when the patient has been receiving a course of antibiotic therapy that may be more than 2 weeks in duration.[60,61]

Bowen et al. reported an abnormal pattern of localization of ^{67}Ga in Duchenne and some other types of dystrophy associated with pseudohypertrophy.[62] Based on results obtained in 27 subjects, Brown et al. suggested that ^{67}Ga scanning may assist in the detection of carriers of Duchenne muscular dystrophy carriers by combining quantitative nuclear medicine results with those derived from serum measurements of creatine kinase, lactate dehydrogenase, phosphokinase, and hemopexin in a logistic discrimination analysis.[63]

The inert gas, Xenon-133 (^{133}Xe), can be used to study tissue blood flow because it maintains good equilibrium between tissue and venous blood. The isotope, in saline, is injected intramuscularly and clearance of the isotope recorded in serial measurements. Chung et al. used ^{133}Xe measurements before and during submaximal bicycle exercise to determine blood flow in the quadriceps.[64] Results were similar to those reported by other groups using conventional probes.

Summary

Radiographic contrast in the imaging of soft tissues is not adequate for general diagnostic utility. Digital methods, such as x-ray CT and computed radiography, offer the possibility of improving soft tissue contrast by employing windowing and level functions. These methods may be used to improve evaluation of the relative involvement of muscle and bone in pathological processes. However, the underlying physics of radiography makes it difficult to accomplish much more than to discriminate between muscle, bone, and fat.

Nuclear medicine techniques can provide information on muscle function. Various nuclear medicine techniques have been used to obtain images depicting muscle viability, necrosis, infection, and blood flow. In general, however, none of the methods using ionizing radiation can produce images with soft tissue contrast at the levels obtainable using ultrasound and magnetic resonance imaging.

References

1. Rothenberg LN, Pentlow KS. Radiation dose in CT. Radiographics 1992;12:1225–1243.
2. Allen EP, Calder HW. Soft tissue radiography. Br J Radiol 1940;13:422–427.
3. Melot GJ. Roentgenologic examinations of the soft tissues; technical considerations; study of the axillary region. AJR 1941;46:189–196.
4. Pons H. Exploration radiologique des tissues mous. Ann Radiol (Paris) 1958;1:671–678.
5. Nemours-Auguste S. Radiographie des parties molles à voltage élevé. J Radiol Electrol Med Nucl 1959;40:319.
6. Frantzell A. Soft tissue radiography. Acta Radiol [Suppl] (Stockh), 1951:85.
7. Frantzell A, Ingelmark BE. Occurrence and distribution of fat in human muscles at various age levels. A morphologic and roentgenologic examination. Ups Lakaref Forh 1951;56:59–87.
8. Frantzell A, Hagberg B, Söderhjelm L. Werdnig-Hoffmann's progressive muscular atrophy. Creatine excretion following vitamin E treatment and muscle radiography. Ups Lakaref Forh 1952;56:209–223.
9. Di Chiro G, Nelson KB. Soft tissue radiography of the extremities in neuromuscular disease with histological correlations. Acta Radiol [Diagn] (Stockh) 1965;3:65–88.
10. Ingelmark BE, Helander E. The action of castration and inactivity on the fat content of striated muscle. Ups Lakaref Forh 1951;56:95–99.
11. Pálvölgyi R. Über die Röntgenmorphologie der Veränderungen der Extremitätenmusculatur. Radiologie 1978;18:469–474.
12. Pálvölgyi R, Gallai R. Use of X-ray techniques to demonstrate selectively increased damage to certain muscles in patients suffering from muscular diseases. ROFO 1980;133:58–62.
13. Pálvölgyi R, Gallai M. Roentgenmorphological aspects of muscular psuedohypertrophy. J Neurol Sci 1979;43:83–94.
14. Pálvölgyi R. Roentgenmorphological muscle changes in anterior horn cell lesions. ROFO 1979;130:338–341.
15. Pálvölgyi R, Bálint BJ, Radiographic diagnosis of closed muscle and tendon injuries of the upper arm. Arch Orthop Trauma Surg 1979;95:177–180.
16. Pálvölgyi R, Bálint BJ, Jozsa L. The Ehlers-Danlos syndrome causing lacerations in tendons and muscles. Arch Orthop Trauma Surg 1979;95:173–176.
17. Oliphant WD. Xeroradiography. 1. Apparatus and method of use. Br J Radiol 1955;28:543.
18. Roach JF, Hilleboe HE. Xeroradiography. AJR 1955;73:5–9.
19. Boag JW. Xeroradiography. Phys Med Biol 1973;18:3–37.
20. Wolfe JN. Xeroradiography: image content and comparison with film roentgenograms. AJR 1973;117:690–695.
21. Pálvölgyi R, Pentek Z. Xeroradiographic demonstration of soft tissues of the extremities. Acta Morphol Acad Sci Hung 1977;25:189–195.
22. Pálvölgyi R, Péntek Z, Csanaky A. Xeroradiographie in der röntgendiagnostik von extremitätenweichteilen. Fortschr Geb Roentgenstr Nuklearmed 1977;127:54–58.
23. Osterman FA Jr, Zeman GH, Rao GUV, Gayler BW, Kirk BG, James AE Jr. Negative-mode soft-tissue xeroradiography. Radiology 1977;124:689.
24. Murphey MD, Quale JL, Martin NL, Bramble JM, Cook LT, Dwyer SM. III. Computed radiography in musculoskeletal imaging: state of the art. AJR 1992;158:19–27.
25. Sakuma H, Takedo K, Hirano T, et al. Plain chest radiography with computed radiography: improved sensitivity for the detection of coronary artery calcification. AJR 1988;151:27–30.
26. Milos NJ, Aberle DR, Baraff LJ, Gold RH, Scanlan RL, Bassett LW. Initial clinical experience with computed radiography in an emergency department. Appl Radiol 1989;18:32–37.
27. Barnes GT, Lakshminarayanan AV. Computed tomography: physical principles and image quality considerations. In: Lee JKT, Sagel SS, Stanley RJ, eds. Computed body tomography with MRI correlation, 2nd ed. New York: Raven Press, 1989:1–21.
28. Pelc NJ, Closher JG. Principles of x-ray computed tomography, vol. 1. In: Taveras JT, Ferrucci JB, eds. Radiology: diagnosis-imaging-intervention, revised edition. Philadelphia: J.B. Lippincott Co., 1987:1–11.
29. Closher JG, Pelc NJ. Computerized tomography systems and performance, vol. 1. In: Taveras JT, Ferrucci JB, eds. Radiology: diagnosis-imaging-intervention, revised edition. Philadelphia: J.B. Lippincott Co., 1987:1–13.
30. Shope TB, Morgan TJ, Showalter CK, et al. Radiation dosimetry survey of computed tomography systems from ten manufacturers. Br J Radiol 1982;55:60–69.
31. Wagner LK, Archer BR, Zeck OF. Conceptus dose from two state-of-the-art CT scanners. Radiology 1986;159:787–792.
32. Grindrod S, Tofts P, Edwards R. Investigation of human skeletal muscle structure and composition by X-ray computerised tomography. Eur J Clin Invest 1983;13:465–468.
33. Bulcke JA, Termote J-L, Palmers Y, Crolla D. Computed tomography of the human skeletal muscular system. Neuroradiology 1979;17:127–136.
34. Mategrano VC, Petasnik JP, Clark J, Bin AC, Weinstein R. Attenuation values in computed tomography of the abdomen. Radiology 1977;125:135.
35. Bulcke JAL, Baert AL. Clinical and radiological aspects of myopathies. Heidelberg: Springer-Verlag, 1982:1–187.
36. Blahd WD, Lederer M, Casses B. The significance of decreased body potassium concentration in patients with muscular dystrophy and nondystrophic relatives. N Engl J Med 1967;276:1349–1352.
37. Kossmann RJ, Peterson DC, Andrews HL. Studies in neuro-muscular disease: total body potassium in muscular dystrophy and related diseases. Neurology (Minneap) 1965;15:855–865.

38. Delwaide PA, Delwaide PJ, Penders CA. Isotope studies of body composition in neuromuscular diseases. J Neurol Sci 1972;15:339–349.
39. Seder JS, Botvinick EH, Rahimtoola SH, Goldstone J, Price DC. Detecting and localizing peripheral arterial disease: Assessment of Tl-201 scintigraphy. AJR 1981;137:373.
40. Burt RW, Mullinix FM, Schauwecker DS, Richmond BD. Leg perfusion evaluated by delayed administration of thallium-201. Radiology 1984;151:219.
41. Chevreaud C, Thouvenot P, Lapeyre G, Laurens M-H, Renard C. Thallium 201 muscle scintigraphy: application to the management of patients with arterial occlusive disease. Angiology 1987;38:309–314.
42. Karpati G. A review of the morphologic features and consequences of muscle cell necrosis in Duchenne disease; clues to the pathogenesis. Excerpta Med Int Congr Ser 1977;343:117–131.
43. Schotland DL, Borrilla E, Wakayama Y. Pathogenesis of muscle cell damage in dystrophies: morphologic aspects including freeze fracture studies. In: Aguayo AJ, Karpati G, eds. Current topics in nerve and muscle research. Int Cong Ser 1979;455:29–38.
44. Busch WA, Stromer MH, Goll DE, Suzuki A. Ca^{2+}-specific removal of Z lines from rabbit skeletal muscle. J Cell Biol 1972;52:367–381.
45. Mokri B, Engel AG. Duchenne dystrophy: electron microscopic findings pointing to a basic or early abnormality in the plasma membrane of the muscle fiber. Neurology (Minneap) 1975;25:1111–1120.
46. Wrogeman K, Pena SDJ. Mitochondrial calcium overload: a general mechanism for cell necrosis in muscle diseases. Lancet 1976;1:672–674.
47. Bonte FJ, Parkey RW, Graham KD, Moore JG, Stokely EM. A new method for radionuclide imaging of myocardial infarcts. Radiology 1974;110:473.
48. Buja LM, Parkey RW, Bonte FJ, Stokely EM, Harris RA, Willerson JT. Morphological correlates of technetium-99m stannous pyrophosphate imaging of acute myocardial infarcts in dogs. Circulation 1975;52:592.
49. Hunt J, Lewis S, Parkey R, Baxter C. The use of technetium-99m stannous pyrophosphate scintigraphy to identify muscle damage in acute electrical burns. J Trauma 1979;19:409.
50. Spencer RR, Williams AG, Mettler FA, Christie JH, Rosenberg RD, Weaver WD. Tc-99m PYP scanning following low-voltage electrical injury. Clin Nucl Med 1983;8:591.
51. Matin P, Lang G, Carreta R, Simon G. Scintigraphic evaluation of muscle damage following extreme exercise: concise communication. J Nucl Med 1983;24:308.
52. Maurer AH, Chen DCP, Camargo EE, Wong DF, Wagner HN Jr, Alderson PO. Utility of three-phase skeletal scintigraphy in suspected osteomyelitis: concise communication. J Nucl Med 1981;22:941.
53. O'Mara RE. Benign bone disease. In: Gottschalk A, Hoffer PB, Potchen ET, eds. Diagnostic Nuclear Medicine, Second Edition, Baltimore: Williams & Wilkins, 1988.
54. Karl, RD Jr, Yedinak MA, Hartshorne MF, et al. Scintigraphic appearance of the piriformis muscle syndrome. J Nucl Med 1985;10:361–363.
55. Siegel ME, Stewart CA. Thallium-201 peripheral perfusion scans: feasibility of single-dose, single-day, rest and stress study. AJR 1981;136:1179.
56. Vallabhajosula SR, Harwig JF, Siemsen JK, Wolf W. Radiogallium localization in tumors: blood binding and transport and the role of transferrin. J Nucl Med 1970;21:650.
57. Baggiolini M, DeDube C, Masson PL, Meremans JF. Association of lactoferrin with specific granules in rabbit heterophil leukocytes. J Exp Med 1970;131:559.
58. Weiner RE, Hoffer PB, Thakur ML. Lactoferrin: its role as a Ga-67 binding protein in polymorphonuclear leukocytes. J Nucl Med 1981;22:32.
59. McAfee JC, Thakur M. Survey of radioactive agents for in vitro labeling of phagocytic leukocytes, I: Soluble agents. J Nucl Med 1976;17:480.
60. Coleman RE, Welch D. Possible pitfalls with clinical imaging of indium-111 leukocytes: concise communication. J Nucl Med 1980;21:122.
61. Coleman RE, Welch DM, Baker WJ, Beightol RW. Clinical experience using indium-111 labeled leukocytes. In: Thakur ML, Gottschalk A, eds. Indium-11 labeled neutrophils, platelets, and lymphocytes. New York: Trivirum, 1981.
62. Bowen P, Lentle BC, Jackson FI, Percy IS, Rigal WM. Abnormal localization of gallium-67 citrate in pseudohypertrophic muscular dystrophy. Lancet 1977;i:1072–1073.
63. Brown RG, Ash JM, Verellen-Dumoulin Ch, et al. Gallium-67 citrate localization in carriers of Duchenne muscular dystrophy. Int J Nucl Med Biol 1981;8:379–388.
64. Chung SY, Kim I, Ryo UY, Maskin C, Pinsky S. Blood flow measurement in muscle with Xe-133. Radiology 1987;165:571–572.

2
Muscle Ultrasound

Carl D. Reimers and Herbert Kellner

Ultrasound is a form of energy consisting of mechanically produced longitudinal waves with frequencies above the range of human hearing [i.e., above 15 to 20 cycles per second (Hertz, Hz)].[1] Medical imaging most commonly uses frequencies from 2 to 12 MHz.

Fundamental Principles of Ultrasound

Fundamental principles of ultrasound, which are important to understand sonographic imaging in medicine, are briefly described; exhaustive details on diagnostic ultrasound are reviewed elsewhere.[2] (Ultra)sound needs matter for transmission. Acoustic waves through matter are characterized by their wavelength, frequency, and amplitude. The velocity (i.e., the product of the wavelength and frequency of the sound beam) depends on the material through which it is passed (Table 2.1). The intensity is defined as the energy that passes through a specified area within 1 second (mW per cm^{-2}). The energy generated by ultrasound sources is extremely small. A piezoelectric crystal in an ultrasound transducer converts only milliwatts of electrical energy into ultrasound pulses. Sound interacts with material through which it passes. The sound intensity is reduced during the flow through the medium and is converted to heat (attenuation). The term Bel [or decibel (dB), $\frac{1}{10}$ of a Bel] describes the degree of sound attenuation or the opposite, called amplification. Decibel is a unit used to compare the intensities of two ultrasound beams: dB = 10 log I/I_0 (I = actual intensity; I_0 = initial intensity of the ultrasound beam). The degree of ultrasound attenuation also depends on the type of medium (Table 2.2). Attenuation increases in proportion to the path length and the ultrasound frequency. Attenuation is due to six different interactions between the ultrasound beam and the medium: absorption, refraction, diffraction, scattering, interference, and reflection (Table 2.3). The interaction primarily responsible for ultrasound images is reflection. Two factors influence the reflectivity: the acoustic impedance of the two media and the angle of incidence of the sound beam. The acoustic impedance is the product of the density of the medium and the velocity of the sound beam in this medium (Table 2.4). The reflectivity at an interface between two materials can be calculated by the following equation:

$$R = [(Z_2 - Z_1)/(Z_1 + Z_2)]^2$$

where R = sound beam reflected and Z_1, Z_2 = acoustic impedances, assuming an angle of incidence of 90°.

Ultrasound Equipment

The ultrasound transducer is a device that converts electrical into mechanical energy, operating on the principle of the piezoelectrical effect. Piezoelectrical crystals such as quartz, lithium niobate and sulfate, zirconate- and barium-titanate, and lead metaniobate vibrate and can produce sound at specific resonance frequencies when a voltage pulse is applied. On the other hand, mechanical force applied on the crystal results in an electrical potential. Additional components of the transducer are damping material behind the crystal and a matching layer sandwiched to the face of the crystal, both usually a combination of epoxy resin and tungsten powder, filler material, and possibly an acoustic lens.

The returning echo can be depicted on a cathode ray tube as a series of blips. Their amplitude depends on the intensity of the reflected echo (A-mode or amplitude mode), and the distance between each of the blips is proportional to the distance between interfaces. The A-mode is of no interest in muscle ultrasound. If the vertical axis of an A-mode drives on a two-dimensional gray-scale display like a strip of paper in a strip graph recorder, motions of interfaces can be depicted (M-mode or motion mode). Regarding muscle ultrasound, this mode is of particular interest for the documentation of

TABLE 2.1. Velocity of ultrasound (m/s) in various biological material.[2]

Air	330
Fat	1450
Water	1540
Soft tissue	1540
Blood	1570
Muscle	1585
Bone	4080

TABLE 2.3. Interactions between the ultrasound beam and the medium.[2]

Absorption	Result of internal frictional forces that oppose the vibration of molecules in the tissue. It increases with the viscosity of the material, its relaxation time, temperature, and the sound frequency.
Refraction	Change in direction of ultrasound when it crosses a boundary between two materials.
Scattering	Dispersion of the ultrasound beam in all directions when the beam interacts with interfaces smaller than its wavelength (i.e., the ratio of the velocity and frequency of the beam).
Diffraction	Spreading of the ultrasound beam as it moves farther from the sound source.
Interference	Superposition of sound waves to each other resulting in complex waves of higher or lower amplitudes, called constructive and destructive interference, respectively.
Reflection	Return of sound waves incident to an interface between two materials of different acoustic impedance.

spontaneous movements. The most important mode of pulse-echo sonography for myosonographic purposes is the B- or brightness mode. In this case gray-scale images are composed of a matrix of many picture elements, called pixels. The location of each pixel is determined by the location of the transducer element and the time between the initiation of the sound pulse and its return to the transducer.

There are two different types of ultrasound beams: continuous waves employed for Doppler flow measurements, and pulsed ultrasound for imaging. Today nearly all ultrasound images are created using real-time transducers. According to their shape, transducers are called linear or curved array, or sector scanners. Sector scanners consist of one or a few oscillating or rotating transducers (mechanical real-time transducer). Sector probes are of little importance for muscle ultrasound because of their unfavorable contact with the skin. *Electronic* (curved or linear array) probes contain up to 256 individual transducer elements that are sequentially activated. They generally provide adequate contact between the transducer and the body surface. The quality of the ultrasound image increases with the number of transducer elements in the probe (line density = number of lines in an image). For objects in motion, the frame rate (i.e., the number of images created per second) is important. In the near field (Fresnel Zone) the ultrasound beam is highly collimated; in the far field (Fraunhofer Zone) the beam diverges. The best image quality is provided at the transition from the near to the far field. The length of the near field increases proportional to the wavelength of the beam. Furthermore, the image quality is characterized by its spatial resolution, the size of the smallest

high-contrast object that can be imaged, and the contrast resolution, the ability to differentiate anatomic structures of similar tissue characteristics. The spatial resolution is the ability to image closely spaced interfaces. Two types of spatial resolution are distinguished: the axial or longitudinal resolution on the axis of the ultrasound beam, and the lateral or transverse resolution perpendicular to the beam. The axial resolution depends on the spatial pulse length, which is usually constant at 3 to 5 cycles, the ultrasound frequency, and the damping of the pulse. The lateral resolution is determined by the beam width, which depends on the size of the transducer element, the focusing of the beam, and the operating frequency. The ultrasound beam can be focused by means of acoustic lenses and electronically by delaying the echo pulses of the individual transducer elements. Usually axial resolution is better than lateral resolution; 1-mm axial and 2-mm lateral resolution are adequate for high-quality muscle ultrasound.

The returning echoes are processed by the receiver. The ratio of the smallest to the largest input signal that does not exhibit distortion is called the dynamic range,

TABLE 2.2. Attenuation coefficients ($10^{-2}\,\text{dB}\,\text{m}^{-1}$) in various biological materials.[2]

Bone	20
Air	12
Soft tissue (average)	1.0
Fat	0.63
Blood	0.18
Water	0.0022

TABLE 2.4. Acoustic impedance ($10^{-6}\,\text{kg}\,\text{m}^{-2}\,\text{s}^{-1}$) in various biological materials.[2]

Air	0.0004
Fat	1.38
Water	1.48
Blood	1.61
Muscle	1.70
Bone	7.80

measured in dB. The dynamic range defines the sensitivity of the receiver. Large dynamic ranges cannot be depicted on the display. Therefore, the echo signals must be logarithmically compressed. Additionally, as the echoes lose energy with increasing depth of the imaged tissue due to attenuation, amplification is required of those returning echoes, which need a longer time for their return to the transducer. This correction is called time gain compensation.

Ultrasound Artifacts

Interpretation of ultrasound images must take into consideration specific artifacts. If the ultrasound beam hits the interface of materials with significantly different acoustic impedances almost all of its energy will be reflected. The result is an acoustic shadow. Such shadows are physiologically produced by bone structures (Figures 2.1, 2.2) or pathologically by inclusions of calcifications in the skin or muscle. However, very small echogenic foci (e.g., calcifications) that are smaller than the width of the ultrasound beam may lack an acoustic shadow due to the so-called "beam-width" artifact.

If the ultrasound beam obliquely hits an interface between two materials that transmit the sound at different velocities, structures in the deeper material, the beam is depicted in an incorrect location due to refraction (refraction artifact).

Another important artifact is enhanced through-transmission. As described above, time gain compensation implies that sound energy decreases with the depth of the tissue. Echoes returning to the transducer are amplified exponentially with the time of their pass through the tissue. If the attenuation is reduced (e.g., by inclusions of fluid in the tissue), the echoes returning from deep structures are particularly amplified, resulting in the false impression of high echointensities.

The interfaces between subcutaneous fat and muscle or between muscle and the bone are highly reflective. Parts of the ultrasound beam are reflected back and forth between these interfaces and thus return late in the transducer, resulting in phantom structures (reverberation artifact) localized behind the deeper of the two interfaces (Figure 2.3). The distance between this interface and the phantoms is the multiple of the distance between the reflecting interfaces.

Muscles contain many fibroadipose septa. These septa are echogenic if the ultrasound beam hits them perpendicularly. However, if the ultrasound beam hits them obliquely the beam becomes deflected and may miss the transducer, resulting in falsely hypoechoic muscle structures (deflection phenomenon).

Finally, movements of the patient can reduce spatial resolution of the ultrasound image (motion artifact).

Depiction of Skeletal Muscles by Ultrasound

History

Ultrasound of skeletal muscles was first performed by Ikai and Fukunaga in 1968 for measurement of muscle thickness and cross-sections. Kramer[3] as well as Young and coworkers[4] were the first to examine patients with muscle disorders by ultrasound. The first sonograms were performed with compound transducers, which are currently outdated, having been replaced by real-time probes.

Examination Technique

The probe used for muscle ultrasound must offer a compromise between sufficient tissue penetration (i.e., low frequency) and good spatial resolution (i.e., high frequency). The frequencies most often employed for muscle ultrasound are 5 to 7.5 MHz in childhood and 3.5 to 5 MHz in adults or obese children. The muscular echointensities depend on parameters such as frequency, gain, and focus (Figures 2.1, 2.2, 2.4, 2.5). Systematic studies on the optimal imaging frequency have yet to be reported in the literature. To avoid refraction artifacts and the deflection phenomenon, the probe should be put strictly perpendicular to the imaged skin and muscles. The imaged tissue must not be pressed because the skin and muscle thickness will then be measured falsely small. Additionally, the echointensites of the muscles will be increased. An appropriate focus and time gain compensation must be guaranteed. Occasionally, a water path is necessary, particularly for imaging of superficial structures such as the muscles of the hand and foot. A generous amount of contact gel should always be used to ensure optimal acoustic coupling.

Normal Skeletal Muscles

Under normal circumstances skeletal muscle bundles have little echogenicity (i.e., are echo-poor). Fibro-adipose septae between the bundles are depicted as echogenic lines on longitudinal scans and small spots on transverse sections, giving the muscle a speckled appearance (Figures 2.4, 2.5). The overall echogenicity of the muscle decreases during isometric contraction because the echo-poor bundles thicken. Thus, when assessing the muscle echogenicity and the muscle diameter or thickness, the contraction state must be taken into account (see below). The muscle may have more than one belly separated by fibrous echogenic intersections (e.g., the rectus abdominis muscle). In circumpennate muscles (e.g., the tibialis anterior muscle), the aponeurosis is depicted as an echogenic stripe. The

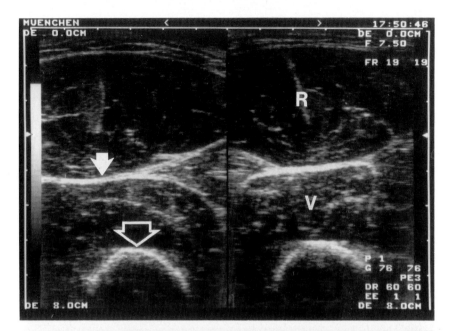

FIGURE 2.1. Normal ultrasound of the rectus femoris (R) and vastus intermedius (V) muscles (7.5 MHz, gain 76 dB; left side of the figure = right thigh and vice versa). Note low echo-intensities of the muscles, which are well delimited by echogenic fasciae (arrow). Open arrow = femur echo.

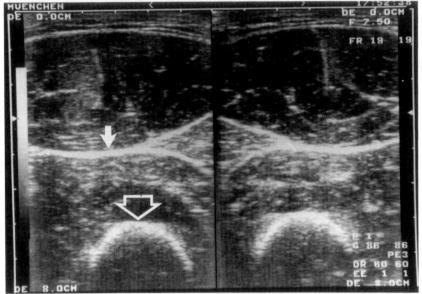

FIGURE 2.2. Same muscles of the same person as in Figure 2.1 (7.5 MHz, gain 86 dB). Echointensities are considerably higher due to higher gain.

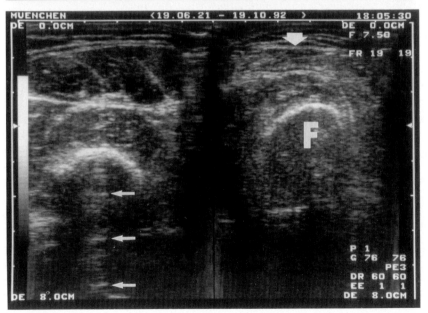

FIGURE 2.3. Lower motor neuron disease —transverse ultrasound scans of the rectus femoris and vastus intermedius muscles (7.5 MHz). Atrophy of the left-sided muscles (right side of the figure) is noted along with slightly elevated echo-intensities of the rectus femoris muscle (arrow). F = shadow of the femur, thin arrows = reverberation artifacts caused by (multiple) reflections between the echo of the femur and the fascia between the rectus femoris and vastus intermedius muscles.

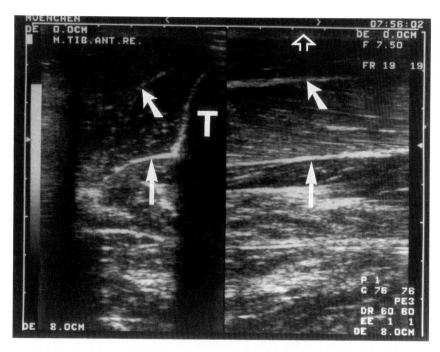

FIGURE 2.4. Normal ultrasound of the tibialis anterior muscle (7.5 MHz). Left side: transverse scan, right side: longitudinal scan. Fibroadipose septae are visualized by small echogenic points in the transverse scan and by thin echogenic lines on the longitudinal scan. T = tibial shadow, oblique arrow = aponeurosis, arrow = membrana interossea cruris between tibia and fibula, open arrow = very thin layer of subcutaneous fat.

fasciae are also readily visible as echogenic bands. The fascia of some muscles, such as the rectus femoris, consists of two layers separated by a film of fat tissue. Fornage[5] demonstrated that by employing appropriate equipment, nearly all muscles can be sonographically depicted. Nerves are represented by echogenic bands or spots, depending on the scan orientation relative to the nerve. Vessels are hypo- or anechoic. Bones are

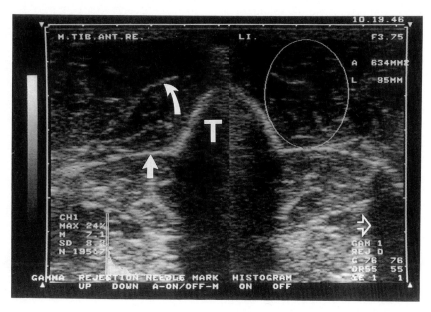

FIGURE 2.5. Normal transverse ultrasound scan of the same muscle of the same person as in Figure 2.4 (3.75 MHz) with gray-scale analysis of the echointensity of the left-sided muscle (ellipse; right side of the figure). T = tibial shadow, curved arrow = aponeurosis of the tibialis anterior muscle, arrow = membrana interossea cruris, open arrow = shadow of the fibula.

highly reflective, resulting in hyperechoic lines or curves depending on the scan orientation. The bone shadow is nearly anechoic. The subcutaneous fat is echo-poor. A few echogenic septae may be visible.

During isometric contraction the muscle mass increases whereas the overall echointensity of the muscle decreases.[1,6] Following exhaustive dynamic dorsiflexion exercise, Gershuni et al.[7] as well as van Holsbeeck and Introcaso[1] found an increase of the dimension of the anterior leg compartment by approximately 10% to 15% with a recovery of about 10 minutes (Figures 2.6, 2.7). However, Brahim and Zaccardelli did not find a significant change of muscle depth following treadmill running.[8] Reimers et al. found an increase of the thickness of the rectus femoris and vastus intermedius muscles after dynamic exercise and an increase in the echointensity of the vastus intermedius muscle.[6] Different results from various laboratories may represent differences in amount of water sequestered by active muscle in different exercises.

Pathological Skeletal Muscles

Table 2.5 summarizes the parameters that should be taken into account when diagnostic ultrasound is applied to patients with neuromuscular diseases. The subcutaneous fat layer may be thickened, and muscles may be atrophic, hypertrophic, or normal when imaged by ultrasound (Figure 2.8). Two types of hypertrophy can be distinguished: true hypertrophy (i.e., enlarged muscle size without mesenchymal abnormality), as in congenital myotonias, and pseudohypertrophy (i.e., enlarged muscle size accompanied by mesenchymal abnormality, usually lipomatosis), as in calf pseudohypertrophy in X-linked muscular dystrophies. In these diseases, the rectus femoris, sartorius, and gracilis muscles especially tend to be truly hypertrophic (Figure 2.8), whereas the calves tend to be pseudohypertrophic. For better objectivity, muscle thickness should be determined by means of an electronic caliper and compared to age- and sex-matched controls. The muscles' echogenicity may be increased or decreased. The objectivity of the assessment of echogenicity can be improved by quantitative measurement using computer-aided grayscale analysis[9–11] (Figure 2.5).

Dock et al. reported another technique of evaluating muscle echogenicity. They suggested counting the perimysial septae within 1 cm of muscle. They regarded 12 septae as an ideal cut-off value, with diseased muscles showing fewer septae.[12] Hyperechogenicity may be focal, multifocal, or homogeneous within a single muscle or within all muscles depicted. The fascial, septal, and bone echoes can be obscure and the bone "shadow" abnormally echogenic in the case of marked mesenchymal abnormaly of the muscle (Figure 2.9).

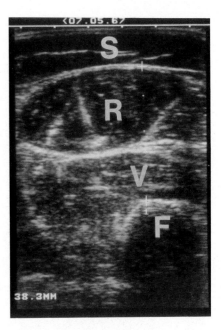

FIGURE 2.6. Normal transverse scan of the rectus femoris and vastus intermedius muscles in a relaxed state (7.5 MHz). Thickness of both muscles together = 38.3 mm. R = rectus femoris, V = vastus intermedius, S = subcutaneous fat, F = shadow of the femur.

Calcifications may be visible in the subcutaneous fat and within the muscle tissue (e.g., in myositis ossificans and childhood dermatomyositis). Ossifications adjacent to the bones result in irregularly shaped bone echoes.

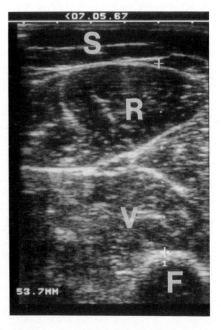

FIGURE 2.7. Transverse scan of the same muscles as in Figure 2.6 after exhaustive bicycle exercise. Thickness of the muscles has enlarged to 53.7 mm; echogenicity of the vastus intermedius is slightly increased.

TABLE 2.5. Ultrasound parameters interest in neuromuscular diseases.

Thickness of subcutaneous fat
Thickness of cross section of muscle (muscle atrophy, hypertrophy, aplasia)
Muscle echogenicity and its distribution (hypo- or hyperechoic)
Visibility of the fasciae, fibroadipose septae, and aponeuroses
Bone echo and "shadow"
Subcutaneous or intramuscular calcifications
Spontaneous movements (e.g., fasciculations)

Real-time ultrasound facilitates detection of spontaneous movements such as fasciculations,[13,14,15] as occur in lower motor neuron diseases (Figure 2.10). The B-mode permits easy detection of fasciculations in the whole muscle imaged. M-mode and video tapes are the appropriate imaging modes for their documentation. Fasciculations are demonstrated as twitchings of parts of muscles lasting about 0.2 to 0.5 s. Care must be taken that neither movements of the probe nor movements of the patient (e.g., due to being cold; patients with neuromuscular diseases often show an abnormal sensitivity to cold) imitate fasciculations. Fasciculations can easily be differentiated from pulses of vessels because of the irregular appearance of the former. Generally, fasciculations are most often seen in the quadriceps femoris and calf muscles.

In summary, muscle ultrasound is a widely available, very informative, and inexpensive method for detecting and documenting muscle atrophy or hypertrophy, mesenchymal abnormalities of the muscles, especially calcifications and fat, and involuntary muscle movements. The ability to differentiate soft tissue abnor-

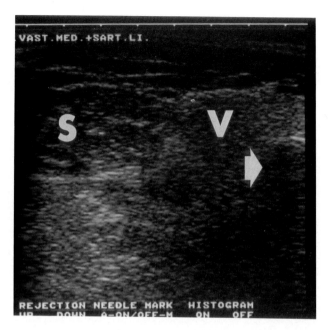

FIGURE 2.8. Progressive muscular dystrophy of Becker type. Transverse ultrasound scan of the sartorius (S) and vastus medialis (V) muscles (3.75 MHz). Visual assessment reveals true hypertrophy (hypertrophy without mesenchymal abnormalities) of the sartorius muscle and atrophy of the vastus medialis muscle. The echo of the femur is obscured (arrow).

malities, such as edema, fat, and fibrosis, is not as excellent as that of magnetic resonance imaging. Thus, in case of clinical suspicion of a neuromuscular disease, but normal ultrasound images, additional performing of magnetic resonance imaging may be necessary.

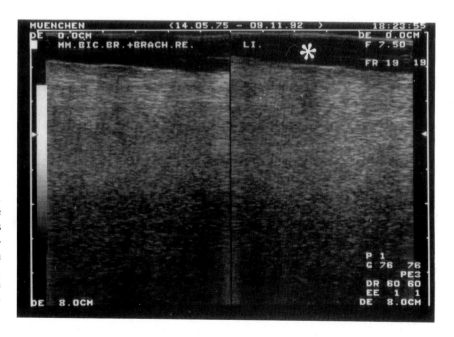

FIGURE 2.9. Centronuclear myopathy. Longitudinal ultrasound scan of the biceps brachii and brachialis muscles (7.5 MHz; left side of the figure = right-sided muscles and vice versa). Very high echointensities of the muscles, septae, and fasciae are visible whereas bone echoes are not visible. Asterisk = subcutaneous fat.

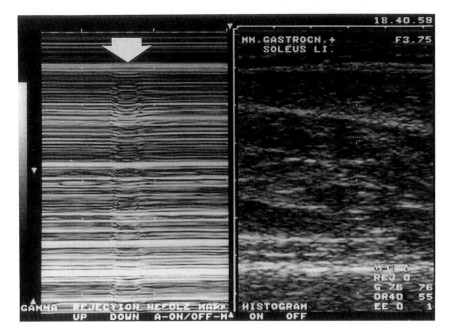

FIGURE 2.10. Lower motor neuron disease. Longitudinal scan of the left gastrocnemius and soleus muscles (3.75 MHz). Left side: M-mode documenting a fasciculation (arrow), right side: B-mode showing slightly atrophic muscles with normal echointensities.

References

1. van Holsbeeck M, Introcaso JH. Musculoskeletal ultrasound. St. Louis: Mosby Year Book, 1991.
2. Bushong SC, Archert BR. Diagnostic ultrasound. Physics, biology, and instrumentation. St. Louis: Mosby Year Book, 1991.
3. Kramer FL, Kurtz AB, Rubin C, Goldberg BB. Ultrasound appearance of myositis ossificans. Skeletal Radiol 1979;4: 19–20.
4. Young A, Hughes I, Russell P, Parker MJ. Measurement of quadriceps muscle wasting. Ann Rheum Dis 1979; 38:571.
5. Fornage BD. Ultrasonography of muscles and tendons. Examination technique and atlas of normal anatomy of the extremities. New York: Springer, 1989.
6. Reimers CD, Lochmüller H, Goebels N, et al. Der Einfluß von Muskelarbeit auf das Myosonogramm. Ultraschall Med 1995;16:79–83.
7. Gershuni DH, Gosink BB, Hargens AR, et al. Ultrasound evaluation of the anterior musculofascial compartment of the leg following exercise. Clin Orthop 1982;167:185–190.
8. Brahim F, Zaccardelli W. Ultrasound measurement of the anterior leg compartment. Am J Sports Med 1986;14: 300–302.
9. Forst R. Skelettmuskel-Sonographie bei neuromuskulären Erkrankungen. Stuttgart: Enke, 1986.
10. Heckmatt J, Rodillo E, Doherty M, et al. Quantitative sonography of muscle. J Child Neurol 1989;4(Suppl): S101–S106.
11. Schapira G, Laugier P, Rochette J, et al. Detection of Duchenne muscular dystrophy carriers: quantitative echography and creatine kinasemia. Hum Genet 1987;75: 19–23.
12. Dock W, Happak W, Grabenwöger F, et al. Neuromuscular diseases: evaluation with high-frequency sonography. Radiology 1990;177:825–828.
13. Reimers CD, Müller W, Schmidt-Achert M, et al. Sonographische Erfassung von Faszikulationen. Ultraschall 1988;9:237–239.
14. Rott H-D. Chorea Huntington: Objektivierung der extrapyramidalen Bewegungsunruhe mittels Ultraschall. Ultraschall 1986;7:193–194.
15. Walker FO, Donofrio PD, Harpold GJ, Ferrell WG. Sonographic imaging of muscle contraction and fasciculations: a correlation with electromyography. Muscle Nerve 1990;13:33–39.

3
Basic Principles of Magnetic Resonance Imaging

Jukka Tanttu and Raimo E. Sepponen

Basics of Nuclear Magnetic Resonance and Magnetic Resonance Imaging

Protons and neutrons have an inherent property called spin. Nuclei with an odd number of these elementary particles have a nonzero spin. These nuclei may be considered as small particles spinning around their own axis. Such nuclei include hydrogen (^{1}H), carbon (^{13}C), phosphorus (^{31}P), and sodium (^{23}Na).

The nucleus of a ^{1}H hydrogen atom consists of a single proton (Figure 3.1a). The proton may be considered as a spherical particle with a positive electric charge. Therefore, the spin of the proton generates an electrical current loop and hence a magnetic field (Figure 3.1b). The proton has a mass and a magnetic moment μ. Therefore, the spinning movement also generates an impulse moment I. These two moments are directed along the spinning axis.

When placed in a magnetic field B_0, μ tends to align with the direction of B_0. This tendency is resisted by I. These counteracting effects of μ and I lead to a precessional movement of the spinning axis around the direction of B_0 (Figure 3.1c). The angular velocity of the precession movement ω_0 is directly proportional to the strength of B_0 and to the gyromagnetic ratio of the nucleus γ. This relationship is expressed by the Larmor equation.

$$\omega_0 = 2\pi f_0 = \gamma B_0. \qquad (3.1)$$

The angular velocity ω_0 is called the Larmor angular velocity and the corresponding frequency f_0 the Larmor frequency. The gyromagnetic ratio γ is specific for each nuclear species. For hydrogen f_0 is approximately 42.6 MHz at a magnetic field of 1 tesla (T), and for phosphorous f_0 is about 17 MHz at 1 T.

In the absence of an external magnetic field nuclear magnetic moments are randomly oriented (Figure 3.2a). When a sample containing a large number of protons is placed in a magnetic field B_0, nuclear magnetic moments tend to align in the direction of B_0 (Figure 3.2b). How-ever, thermal movement prevents a complete alignment. Thus, the resulting net nuclear magnetization M_n is very weak. For the detection of nuclear magnetization, a nuclear magnetic resonance (NMR) experiment is performed. It can be shown that the precessing nuclear magnetic moments may be tilted by a weak magnetic field rotating at the Larmor velocity. Because the corresponding f_0 is in the radio frequency (RF) range (1 to 100 MHz), the perturbing field (B_1) is called an RF field.

For convenience, the concept of a rotating frame of reference $x'y'z'$ is introduced. In a laboratory frame of reference xyz, the z axis is parallel to B_0. The z' axis of the rotating frame of reference $x'y'z'$ is parallel to z but x' is fixed along the rotating B_1 field. In the $x'y'z'$ frame rotating at ω_0 one does not need to consider the precession of M_n around B_0. In the $x'y'z'$ frame M_n precesses around B_1 at the angular velocity $\omega_1 = \gamma B_1$ (Figure 3.3a). After the B_1 field is turned off the nuclear magnetization deviates from the z axis by a flip angle α. The value of α is determined by the amplitude and duration of the B_1 pulse. The B_1 pulses are usually called excitation or RF pulses. Specifically, if α is 90°, the corresponding B_1 pulse is called a 90° or $\pi/2$ pulse (Figure 3.3b).

In the laboratory frame of reference x,y,z, the tilted M_n may be divided in two orthogonal components: M_z parallel to z axis and M_{xy} rotating at ω_0 in the xy plane (Figure 3.4a). Specifically, if the tilt angle α is 90°, $M_z = 0$ and $M_{xy} = M_n$. The rotating M_{xy} induces a voltage in the signal coil of the measuring system (Figure 3.4b). The signal (S) is proportional to M_{xy}, which decays with time (Figure 3.4c). In a homogeneous B_0 field the decay is due to the effect of interactions between neighboring nuclei. This phenomenon is exponential and it is characterized by a time constant, T_2, called transverse or spin−spin relaxation time. The decay of M_{xy} after a 90° pulse is described in equation (3.2).

$$M_{xy} = M_n \sin \alpha \, e^{-t/T_2}. \qquad (3.2)$$

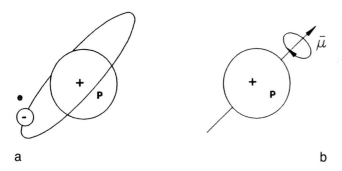

a

b

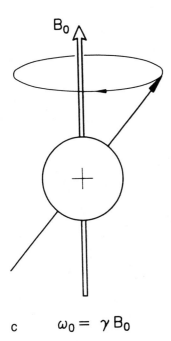

c $\omega_0 = \gamma B_0$

B_0, an NMR signal does not contain any information about the spatial distribution of nuclei. However, if the strength of the magnetic field varies spatially (i.e., there is a magnetic field gradient), one may use the frequency information of a signal to locate the nuclei.[2] The frequency information is extracted by applying a Fourier transformation to the signal. In magnetic resonance imaging (MRI), the main component of the external magnetic field is a homogeneous polarizing magnetic field B_0. The strength of B_0 in MRI equipment for routine clinical use varies from 0.02 to 2 T (1 T = 10,000 gauss). The spatial information is encoded in the phase and frequency of the precessional movement of the nuclei by using controlled magnetic field gradients. The presently used MRI methods utilize rapidly switching gradients that are generated as a result of three orthogonal gradients: G_x, G_y, G_z. The maximum gradient strength is typically below 20 mT/m.

Fourier Imaging

The Fourier imaging method[3] and its variants are the most widely utilized imaging methods in clinical MRI. In this technique the imaging volume is periodically excited

FIGURE 3.1. (a) The hydrogen atom consists of a proton and an electron. (b) A proton is spinning around its axis. The spinning movement generates a magnetic moment. (c) When placed in an external magnetic field, B_0, the magnetic moment precesses around the direction of B_0 with an angular speed. ω_0 the angular speed is proportional to the strength of B_0. The proportionality factor, γ, is the gyromagnetic ratio.

NMR-like resonance phenomena generally involves energy exchange at the resonance frequency. The energy is introduced to nuclear spins via the excitatory RF pulses. The nuclei give up the excitation energy as NMR signals and most of it is absorbed by surroundings ("lattice") and converted to thermal energy. After the B_1 pulse the return of the longitudinal magnetization M_z to its equilibrium value is a manifestation of this phenomenon. The process is characterized by relaxation time T_1, called longitudinal or spin–lattice relaxation time. Specifically, after a 90° pulse the recovery of M_z is described by equation (3.3) (Figure 3.5).[1]

$$M_z = M_n(1 - e^{-t/T_1}). \qquad (3.3)$$

When the sample is in a homogeneous magnetic field

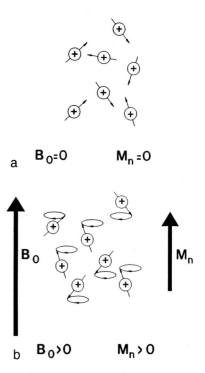

a $B_0 = 0$ $M_n = 0$

b $B_0 > 0$ $M_n > 0$

FIGURE 3.2. (a) When the external magnetic field B_0 is zero. The magnetic moments of nuclei are randomly oriented and the net magnetization M_n is zero. (b) When exposed to an external magnetic field, $B_0 > 0$, a majority of nuclear magnetic moments will align with the direction of B_0 and a net magnetization $M_n > 0$ will be generated.

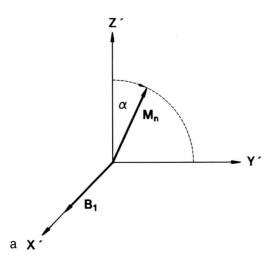

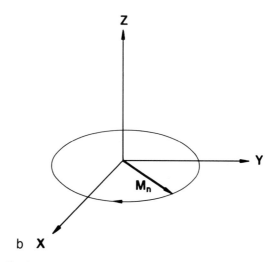

FIGURE 3.3. (a) The net magnetization M_n may be tilted away from the direction of B_0 with an application of a radio frequency field B_1. The flip angle is α. The x' axis of the rotating frame of reference, $x'y'z'$, is along the direction of B_1 field rotating at the angular speed. The z' axis is parallel to B_0. (b) The amplitude and duration of the B_1 field may be selected so that $\alpha = 90°$. In the laboratory frame of reference x, y, z, the tilted net magnetization M_n precesses with an angular speed around the direction of the z axis, which is parallel to B_0.

with short selective RF pulses. The selectivity is accomplished by switching on a magnetic field gradient, the slice selection gradient, prior to application of the excitation pulse. The orientation of the slice is orthogonal to the direction of the applied slice selection gradient. By a proper combination of the three orthogonal gradients, G_x, G_y, G_z, a selection gradient of any direction may be generated. The position of the slice in the direction of the slice selection gradient is defined by the frequency of the excitation pulse. The thickness of the slice is inversely proportional to the strength of the slice selection gradient and to the duration of the excitation pulse.

The ensuing NMR signals are collected with a so-called "read" gradient switched on and Fourier transformed. Each transformed signal is a projection of the spin density distribution of the object in the direction of the read gradient. In order to gain the necessary resolution in the orthogonal direction of the read gradient,

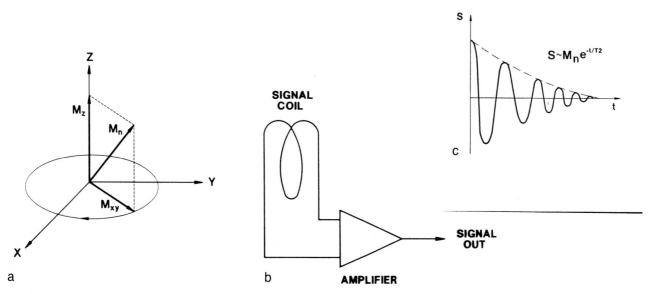

FIGURE 3.4. (a) The transverse component of M_n is M_{xy} and the longitudinal component is M_z. (b) The precessing M_{xy} induces a signal voltage in the signal coil. The signal voltage is amplified by the amplifier of the measuring system. (c) The signal S decays exponentially with a time constant T_2. T_2 is called a transverse relaxation time or spin–spin relaxation time. The signal amplitude is proportional to M_n.

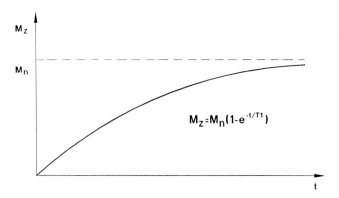

$$M_z = M_n(1 - e^{-t/T1})$$

FIGURE 3.5. The longitudinal component M_z is zero after M_n has been tilted 90°. M_z recovers exponentially towards the equilibrium value M_n with a time constant T_1. T_1 is called a longitudinal relaxation time or a spin–lattice relaxation time.

multiple signals with different amounts of phase encoding must be collected. The phase encoding is done by applying gradient pulses with different amplitudes prior to the signal collection. The encoding is possible also in the third, orthogonal dimension with an additional encoding gradient. The final image is reconstructed by applying two- or three-dimensional Fourier transformation to the set of collected signals.

The most widely used variant of the Fourier imaging method is the spin warp method.[4] In this technique the signal is collected as a gradient echo (field echo) or a pulse echo (Hahn's echo). The time period between the excitation signal and the center of the echo is called the time to echo (T_E). The period between successive excitation pulses is called the repetition period (T_R). Both T_R and T_E are important parameters for the contrast of the resulting image (Figure 3.6).

Contrast in MRI

The contrast in MRI is dependent on intrinsic parameters of tissues and extrinsic parameters that are dependent on the imaging equipment and sequence. The most important intrinsic muscle parameters are proton density, relaxation times, flow, and fat/water ratio. The important extrinsic parameters include the strength of B_0 and sequence parameters like T_R, type of echo, T_E, and flip angle α.[5]

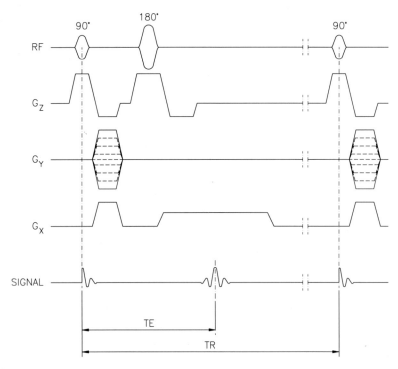

FIGURE 3.6. The pulse diagram of the spin warp imaging sequence utilizing the spin echo technique. The radio frequency (RF) excitation pulse (90°) and the refocusing pulse (180°) are slice selective. The slice selection gradient (G_z) is switched on during the RF pulses. The phase-encoding gradient (G_y) is switched on between the excitation and refocusing pulses. The readout gradient (G_x) is switched on before and after the refocusing RF pulse in order to generate the echo signal. The period between the successive excitation pulses is the repetition time (T_R) and the time between the excitation pulse and the center of the echo signal is time to echo (T_E).

Tissue Parameters

By the term "proton density" one refers to the number of protons that are visible in MRI. The visibility of nuclei depends mainly on their relaxation times. Protons that are constituents of highly mobile water and fat molecules have a relatively long T_2 (tens of milliseconds) and a relatively short T_1 (hundreds of milliseconds). This combination is favorable for the generation of strong NMR signals. Therefore, in MRI, proton density reflects water and fat concentrations in tissues. Generally, the contrast in MRI is due to relaxation differences between tissues. For example, the water content in a healthy muscle tissue is about 80%. In this respect muscle tissue is similar to spleen and brain tissues.[6] However, due to differences in relaxation properties, the intensity of muscle tissue is different from that of spleen or brain tissues in most MR images.

The longitudinal relaxation, characterized by T_1, results from excited nuclei returning to equilibrium. Energy transfer is induced by local magnetic field fluctuations at f_0. Magnetic fluctuations are generated by thermal molecular vibrations and motion. There is also a direct exchange of energy between nuclei. This is the major component of cross-relaxation between water and macromolecular protons and assumes close contacts between nuclei.

In tissue, a small amount of water is bound to macromolecules. The existence of the bound water compartment markedly increases the efficiency of crossrelaxation. The size of the bound water compartment is dependent on surface properties of macromolecules. Protons of macromolecules and bound water molecules may be considered to form a pool of protons with restricted mobility, H_r, and protons of mobile water molecules to form a pool of mobile protons, H_f. The relaxation in tissues is mainly due to the mutual interaction of these pools.[7]

The local magnetic fields due to magnetic moments of nuclei and electrons cause dephasing of precessing nuclear moments, which contributes to transverse relaxation, characterized by T_2. If nuclei move fast between different magnetic environments, the dephasing effect is averaged towards zero and the transverse relaxation rate is decreased.

The efficiency of cross-relaxation and the thermal motion of macromolecules as sources of relaxation are dependent on the resonance frequency f_0 (i.e., on B_0). In biological tissues with a significant concentration of macromolecules, T_1 decreases as B_0 decreases.[8] This field dependence of T_1 is usually called T_1 dispersion. The T_1 dispersion is tissue dependent. In muscle, the T_1 dispersion is among the strongest in body tissues. It has been demonstrated that T_1 dispersion at low field strength is sensitive to pathological changes in muscles.[9]

Generally, T_1 of muscle is approximately proportional to B_0. T_1 of muscle is about 250 ms at 0.1 T and 900 ms at 1.5 T. T_2 of muscle tissue is about 40 ms. T_2s of most tissues are weakly dependent on B_0.[10] T_2 of muscle has been reported to decrease about 10% when B_0 is increased from 0.064 to 2.94 T.[11]

In addition to the relaxation effects, the inhomogeneity of B_0 and the nonuniform magnetization of tissues cause signal decay after the excitation pulse. This decay is characterized by a time constant T_2^*. T_2^* is shorter than T_2 because it also includes the effects of magnetic inhomogeneity ΔB equation (3.4)

$$\frac{1}{T_2^*} = \frac{1}{T_2} + \frac{1}{\gamma \Delta B}. \tag{3.4}$$

Magnetic inhomogeneities are due to, for example, imperfections of B_0 and variations in magnetic properties (i.e., susceptibility of tissues).

Paramagnetic substances shorten the relaxation times. This effect may be noted in hematomas where the state of hemoglobin affects the relaxation times. In acute hematoma, hemoglobin is usually in the form of oxyhemoglobin, which is diamagnetic. Therefore, the longitudinal relaxation time of an acute hematoma is long compared to that of muscle tissue. Oxyhemoglobin changes by time to paramagnetic compounds like deoxyhemoglobin and methemoglobin. Therefore, the appearance of a hematoma (see Chapters 25 and 33) in MR images is dependent on the age of the hematoma. Due to the increased protein concentration in the clot and the presence of paramagnetic hemoglobin residuals, the visualization of a hematoma is dependent on B_0.[12]

Paramagnetic compounds are used as contrast agents in MRI. Contrast agents like Gd-DTPA are usually injected intravenously and distributed in the extracellular space. The subsequent increase in the relaxation rate is dependent on the tissue concentration of the introduced paramagnetic substance.[13] Contrast agent uptake varies significantly in different tissue and the altered relaxation properties may be used as contrast enhancement in MRI (see Chapter 30).

The protons in the methylene groups of fatty compounds have a rather short T_1 and a relatively long T_2. Due to this favorable combination, fatty tissues with a significant concentration of mobile methylene groups demonstrate a high intensity in most MR images. T_1 of fat is about 150 ms at 0.1 T and about 250 ms at 1.5 T. T_2 of fat is about 80 ms and does not demonstrate a significant dependence on B_0.[10]

Protons in fat molecules are surrounded by an electron cloud, which differs from the electron environment of protons of water molecules. The electron cloud shields the nucleus from external magnetic fields. The shielding effect is different for methylene protons and water

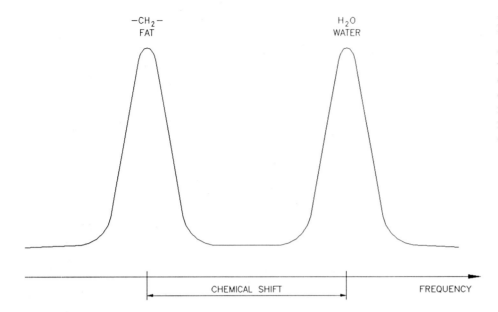

FIGURE 3.7. There is a difference between the resonance frequencies of fat ($-CH_2-$) and water (H_2O) protons due to the chemical shift effect. The frequency difference is approximately 3.5 ppm of the resonance frequency. At 1 T the frequency difference is about 150 Hz.

protons. This leads to a small difference between the resonance frequencies of fat and water protons. This difference is called the chemical shift, δ. The absolute frequency difference is proportional to B_0. Therefore, δ is reported in parts per million (ppm), which is a dimensionless unit. The chemical shift between methylene protons and water protons, δ_{fw}, is about 3.5 ppm (Figure 3.7). For example, at 1.5 T, δ_{fw} is about 225 Hz whereas at 0.1 T, δ_{fw} is 15 Hz. The resonance frequency difference of fat and water protons may be used to discriminate between tissues with different fat concentrations. It is also the source of the chemical shift misregistration artifact that is visible at fat/water interfaces on MR images.[14]

The timing and excitation parameters of an imaging sequence may be selected in such a manner that the resulting images are predominantly weighted by the selected tissue parameter.[5]

T_1-Weighted Images

T_1-weighted images are usually obtained by using progressive saturation or inversion recovery sequences. In the progressive saturation sequence the magnetization of tissues with a long T_1 is saturated by applying 90° pulses with a short T_R. The flip angle is 90° for maximal saturation and T_R is shorter than T_1 of the tissues under study. The T_2 contrast generated during T_E is antagonistic to the T_1 contrast; therefore, T_E should be short. Tissues with a long T_1, such as normal muscle tissue at a high magnetic field, and edematous tissue at all fields, will appear dark in the final image (Figure 3.8). Tissues with a high content of mobile protons and a short T_1, such as fat and some hemorrhagic lesions, will have high signal intensity.

The inversion recovery (IR) technique provides an improved T_1 contrast compared to progressive saturation

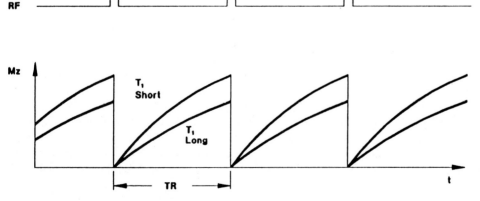

FIGURE 3.8. In the progressive saturation sequence the spins are excited with a series of 90° pulses with a short repetition time (T_R). The contrast is adjusted by a selection of T_R. The signals from tissues with a long T_1 are suppressed more than signals from tissues with a short T_1.

technique. In IR technique M_z is first inverted by a 180°
pulse and after the inversion time (T_I) the partially
recovered M_z is sampled with a conventional excitation-
signal collection sequence. If T_I is short compared to T_1
of tissues, the sequence is sometimes called STIR (short
tau inversion recovery) (Figure 3.9). STIR imaging is
often used to suppress fat signal. Another advantage is
the high sensitivity to pathologic tissue, which is due to
the synergistic T_1 and T_2 contrast.[15–17] These features
account for the preeminent role STIR has in muscle
MRI.

Because T_1 of muscle tissue is very dependent on B_0,
T_R and T_I should be adjusted differently for different
strengths of B_0 to achieve equivalent T_1 weighting on the
final images. An example of a T_1-weighted image of a leg
obtained at 1 T is presented in Figure 3.10.

Proton Density and T_2-Weighted Images

Practically all MR images are proton density (PD) and
T_2-weighted to a variable degree. The amount of T_2 contribution is determined by the length of T_E (Figure 3.11).
"Proton density" images are obtained using sequences
with long T_R and short T_E. These images reflect the
distribution of mobile protons in tissues. "T_2-weighted"
images are obtained with a spin echo sequence with long
T_R and long T_E. T_E should be long compared to T_2 of
tissues. In the sequences for proton density and T_2-

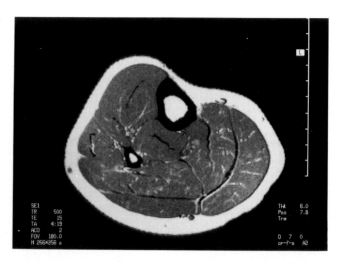

FIGURE 3.10. A T_1 weighted SE 500/15 image of a leg obtained
at 1 T. The intensity of fat is high due to the short T_1. The
magnetization of muscle tissue is suppressed due to incomplete
recovery between excitations. Thus, the signal intensity of
muscle tissue is low.

weighted images, T_R should be long enough to allow the
recovery of the tissue magnetization (i.e., $T_R \gg T_1$). If
T_R is short the resulting T_1 effect will, in general, reduce
the contrast of the final image.

In T_2-weighted images tissues with a long T_2 like fat
and edematous muscle appear bright. Normal muscle
tissue has a rather low intensity due to a short T_2. In
proton density images all these tissues have a high intensity. Examples of PD and T_2-weighted images of a leg
obtained at 1 T are presented in Figures 3.12 and 3.13,
respectively.

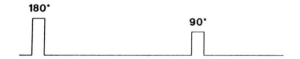

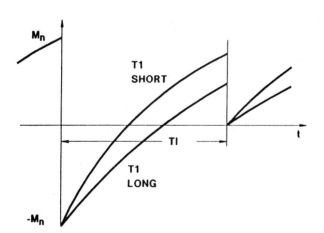

FIGURE 3.9. The inversion recovery (IR) sequence consists of
an 180° inversion pulse that is followed by the inversion time
(T_I). After T_I the conventional spin echo or gradient echo
signal collection sequence is performed. The contrast of the
final image may be adjusted by a selection of T_I.

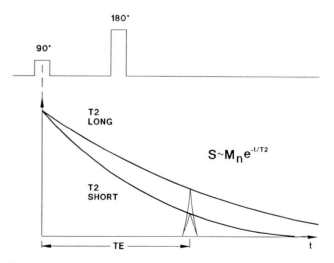

FIGURE 3.11. The amount of T_2 contrast on spin echo images
may be adjusted with the time to echo (T_E). An increase of T_E
will decrease the ratio of intensities of tissues with a short T_2
and a long T_2 on the final image.

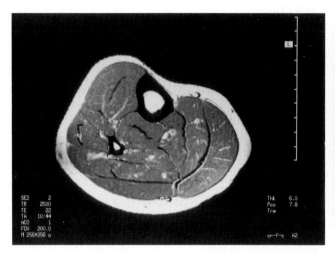

FIGURE 3.12. A "proton density" weighted SE 2500/22 image of a leg obtained at 0.1 T. Even with as short a T_E as 22 ms the intensity of muscle tissue is considerably lower than that of fat. This is due to the short T_2 of muscle tissue. The dark fat/muscle borderline on the right side of the image is a chemical shift artifact as described on page 26.

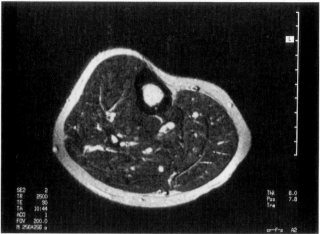

FIGURE 3.13. A T_2-weighted SE 2500/90 image of a leg obtained at 1 T. The intensity of fat is high due to the relatively long T_2. The signal intensity of muscle tissue is reduced due to the short T_2 of muscle.

Fast Imaging Techniques

Fast imaging techniques may be divided into two main categories: one strategy is to collect as many encoded echo signals after a single excitation pulse as possible. The techniques of this group include echo planar and fast spin echoes (FSE). The other group includes sequences in which the excitations are repeated with a short T_R. Examples of short T_R sequences are FLASH, GRASS, and FISP sequences. The contrast may be enhanced by an application of a magnetization preparation pulse before multiple excitation and signal collection sequence. Examples of these sequences are Turbo-FLASH and MP-RARE.[18]

The basic idea in the FSE technique is that one collects multiple spin echo signals, usually 4 to 64, with different phase encodings. Hence, multiple encoding steps are included in one excitation period. The echoes are generated with refocusing 180° pulses. Usually this technique is used for fast generation of T_2-weighted images.[18]

The echo planar method utilizes a gradient echo technique for the generation of a train of echoes with different phase encodings. A full image is obtained with a single excitation and echo generation sequence. The fastest imaging times are in the order of tens of milliseconds. The final images are T_2^*-weighted.

Recently, methods that include both gradient and pulse echoes have been introduced. The contrast of the

images may also be manipulated with preparation pulses (e.g., inversion and fat suppression pulses).

In the FLASH (Figure 3.14), GRASS, and FISP (Figure 3.15) techniques one utilizes gradient echo signals.[18-20] In the FLASH sequence the flip angle α is less than 90°, leaving a significant longitudinal magnetization. This avoids the saturation of the magnetization and

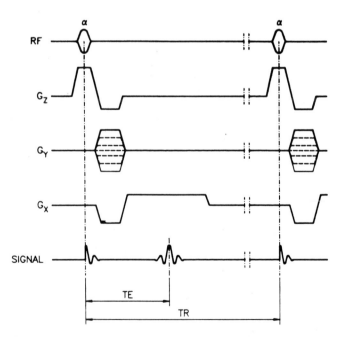

FIGURE 3.14. The FLASH sequence includes an excitation pulse with a small flip angle α and gradient echo signal collection. The contrast may be adjusted by a selection of α, T_R, and T_E. G_z: slice selection gradient, G_y: phase-encoding gradient, G_x: readout gradient, RF: radio frequency excitation pulses.

FIGURE 3.15. The pulse sequence for FISP (Fast Imaging with Steady-state Precession) technique. The net effect of gradients is balanced within each TR interval. Similar sequences are FAST, GRASS, and C-BASS.

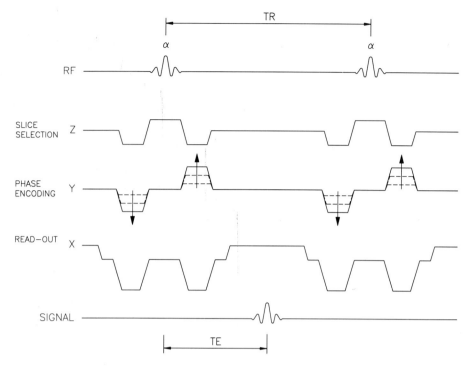

the excitation/data collection sequence may be repeated with a short T_R. The use of the gradient echo technique enables the use of a short T_E. The signal intensity is dependent on T_R, T_E, α, T_1, T_2^* and spin density $N(H)$

$$S = N(H)\frac{(1 - e^{-\frac{T_R}{T_1}})e^{-\frac{T_E}{T_2^*}}}{1 - e^{-\frac{T_R}{T_1}}\cos\alpha}\sin\alpha. \qquad (3.5)$$

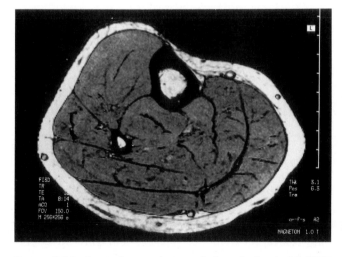

FIGURE 3.16. A steady-state image of a leg obtained with FISP 30/12 sequence at 1 T. The intensity of tissue on the image is proportional to the ratio T_2/T_1. Hence, muscle tissue appears darker than fat. Note the dark fat/water interfaces that are manifestations of the fat/water cancellation effect.

FLASH images obtained with a low α ($<30°$) have a PD weighted appearance. Fat is usually bright and tissues with a short T_2^* (e.g., hematomas) are dark.

When T_R is shorter than T_2 of tissues there is a significant transverse magnetization component before the next RF pulse. In steady-state sequences like FISP, the transverse magnetization and the z magnetization coexist all the time and they are interchanged by each RF pulse. The contrast in steady-state images is dependent on the ratio T_2/T_1. This ratio is large in tissues like CSF and fat, and therefore these tissues appear bright in steady-state images. An example of images obtained with the FISP sequence at 1 T is presented in Figure 3.16.

Chemical Shift Imaging

The chemical shift phenomenon may be used for discrimination of water and fatty components in tissues. Many chemical shift imaging (CSI) techniques have been developed. The frequency difference may be exploited utilizing selective excitation or selective saturation techniques.[21] In these the magnetization of either fat or water is selectively saturated or excited. Saturating the magnetization of fat protons enables one to generate a water image, and vice versa.

Another class of imaging sequences exploits the phase difference generated by the chemical shift effect after the excitation pulse. The chemical shift effect may be considered an inherent magnetic field gradient in tissues.

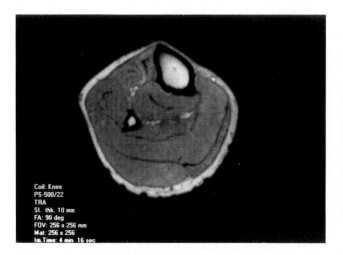

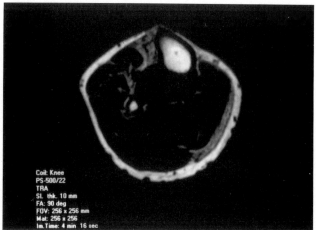

a

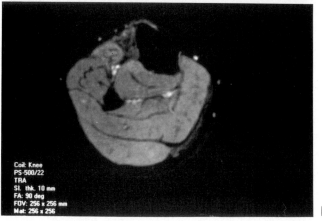

b

FIGURE 3.17. A gradient echo progressive saturation image (500/22) of a leg obtained at 0.1 T.

The phase difference is accumulated during the T_E in gradient echo techniques[22] and is proportional to the temporal asymmetry in spin echo sequences.[23,24] One may utilize phase imaging or Fourier techniques to generate separate fat and water images (Figures 3.17 and 3.18).

Magnetization Transfer

Protons in biological tissues are mostly bound to mobile water molecules. This pool of freely moving protons, H_f, has a long T_2, which enables the detection of NMR signals in MRI. There is also a relatively large pool of protons, H_r, which are bound to large macromolecules (e.g., proteins). NMR signals emitted by this pool have a very short T_2 and hence H_r is not directly visible in MR images. However, the interaction between H_f and H_r is important for the nuclear relaxation in biological tissues (Figure 3.19a). The magnetization transfer (MT), which happens mainly via cross-relaxation between these two pools, may be estimated or used as a new contrast parameter in MRI.[25]

The imaging techniques exploiting MT contrast include a preparation pulse that saturates the magnetization of H_r. This saturation is transferred to H_f. The reduction of the magnetization of the pool of free protons leads to a decrease in the NMR signal emitted by this pool. The observed decrease in the signal amplitude is significant in tissues with an effective interaction between the pools (Figure 3.19b). In muscle tissue, the macromolecule/water interaction is very effective and therefore the observed signal reduction due to MT is significant. In tissues such as subcutaneous, interstitial, and bone marrow fat, the MT effect is insignificant. The MT effect is also very small in fluids with a low

FIGURE 3.18. Fat (a) and water (b) images of the leg calculated from the magnitude and phase information of the gradient echo image in Figure 3.17. The fatty infiltration is visible as an increased signal on the image (a).

concentration of large macromolecules such as urine, CSF, and blood.[25,26] A demonstration of the added MT contrast on a conventional gradient echo image is presented in Figure 3.20.

Contrast Agents

The contrast in MR images may be changed by applying contrast agents, which alter relaxation times of tissues.[13] The most widely used contrast agent is gadolinium (Gd)-DTPA (Magnevist, Schering AG, Germany). Gadolinium has a strong paramagnetic moment, due to unpaired electrons, and therefore effectively decreases the relaxation times, especially T_1 (Figure 3.21). The shortening of T_1 may be exploited by T_1-weighted sequences with a short T_R, a short T_E, and a 90° flip angle. Tissues that have a significant concentration of paramagnetic contrast agent will show exhibit a high signal intensity. The contrast may be improved with the MT

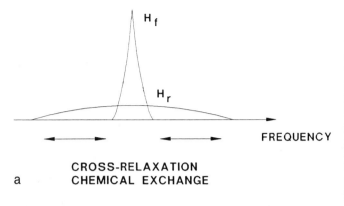

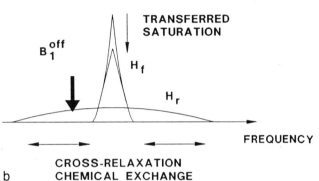

FIGURE 3.19. Interaction between protons of macromolecules and protons of water molecules. (a) The protons of H_r have a very short T_2. Therefore, the line width of the signal from H_r is broad (tens of kilohertz). The protons of H_f have a long T_2 and the line width is narrow (few hertz). There is a cross-relaxation between the pools. (b) When the magnetization of H_r is saturated with a saturation pulse B_1^{off} the saturation is transferred to H_f via the interaction. The amount of transferred saturation is observed as a decrease of the magnetization of H_f.

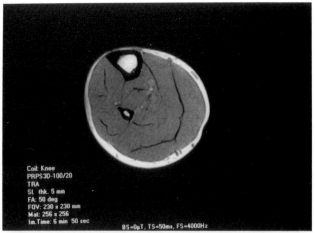

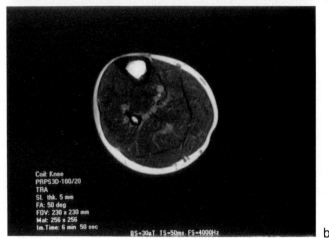

FIGURE 3.20. The effect of added magnetization transfer contrast on a gradient echo (100/20) image of a leg. (a) 100/20 image without the saturation pulse. (b) 100/20 image with an off-frequency saturation pulse. The frequency offset is 4 kHz, amplitude of the pulse is 30 μT, and the duration of the pulse is 50 ms. The signal from fat is not affected but the signal from muscle tissue is significantly reduced due to the transferred saturation.

technique: the signal emitted by tissues with predominantly macromolecular relaxation decreases whereas the signal emitted by tissues with paramagnetic relaxation is not affected as much.

Some contrast agents such as superparamagnetic particles decrease the relaxation time T_2^*. Tissues that have a significant concentration of superparamagnetic particles appear dark in T_2^*-weighted images. Typically, T_2^*-weighted images are generated with a gradient echo technique.

MR Angiography

MR angiography (MRA) methods may be divided into two main categories: time-of-flight (TOF) methods and phase contrast (PC) methods.[5]

Under the effect of a gradient field, protons in flowing blood gain a different phase compared to the protons in

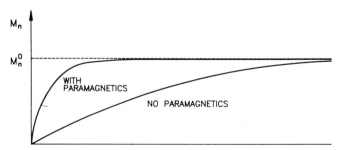

FIGURE 3.21. Paramagnetic substances, such as Gd-DTPA, increase the relaxation rates. The recovery of the nuclear magnetization M_n towards the equilibrium value M_n^0 is faster in tissues with paramagnetics than that in tissues without paramagnetics.

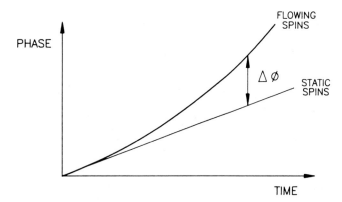

FIGURE 3.22. Phase contrast. Spins that are flowing in the direction of a magnetic field gradient gain different phase in their precessional movement than spins in static tissues. The gained phase difference, $\Delta\phi$, discriminates flowing and static spins.

static tissues (Figure 3.22). With proper gradient pulse waveforms, this phase difference may be minimized (e.g. flow compensation) or emphasized. In the PC methods the latter approach is utilized: special flow-encoding gradients are used to discriminate flowing fluid from static tissues.

TOF methods are based on the signal intensity difference between flowing blood and static tissues. Short T_R sequences usually with flow compensation are utilized. The signal of static tissue is suppressed due to the T_1 weighting. The blood flowing into the selected slice, however, has not been saturated and thus gives a high signal intensity (Figure 3.23). Several adjacent, thin slices are successively obtained using 3D or 2D sequences. The final angiographic image is obtained by stacking the collected slices and using the Maximum Intensity Projection (MIP) technique to eliminate the weak background signals.

The TOF method with a 3D imaging sequence is typically used to image fast flowing blood (e.g., in large arteries), whereas TOF method with a 2D imaging sequence and PC techniques are considered to be better in the cases where the velocity of flow is low (e.g., in veins and small arteries). MRA is a noninvasive method and does not require any contrast agents. It can easily be performed in addition to the conventional MR imaging sequences. The problems are related to turbulence of the flow and tortuous vessels. Further development of the methods is needed to obviate these problems.

Spectroscopy

Details of MR spectroscopy exceed the scope of this section, but extensive reviews are available elsewhere.[27-35] In brief, MR imaging uses ^1H as the target nuclei due to its high abundance in soft tissues and strong magnetic moment. However, ^{31}P, ^{13}C, ^{23}Na, potassium (^{39}K), and fluorine (^{19}F) are also biologically interesting nuclei. In addition to anatomical imaging, hydrogen may be used to observe metabolites such as lactate, which is increased in anaerobic conditions (see Chapter 8). The resonance frequency of lactate protons differs from that of water protons. However, the resonance signals from water protons are approximately 10,000 times stronger than those from lactate protons. Selective saturation techniques are necessary to suppress the signal from water and lipid protons.

Only a small part, about 1%, of carbon in the body consists of the ^{13}C isotope. The magnetic moment of ^{13}C is rather small. Hence, the detection of the carbon MR resonance is a very difficult task. A high B_0 field or special techniques are needed to improve the signal-to-noise ratio.[27]

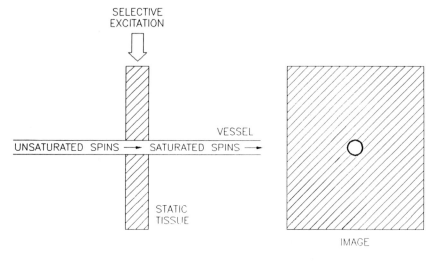

FIGURE 3.23. In the time of flight (TOF) angiography technique the spins of a static tissue are saturated by excitation pulses with a short repetition time. Because the excitation pulses are slice selective the spins that arrive in the slice between successive excitations have not been saturated. Therefore, the blood in the vessel appears bright on the final image.

Phosphorus (^{31}P) is interesting because of the relatively high concentration of phosphorus in muscle tissue (see Chapters 9 and 10). The amount of high-energy phosphates such as adenosine triphosphate, phosphocreatinine, and inorganic phosphates may be determined with MR spectroscopy. Especially the ratio of inorganic phosphate to phosphocreatine (Pi/PCr) is useful in evaluation of metabolic effects of exercise and diseases.[28] However, in MR spectroscopic studies of body organs accurate localization of the volume of interest (VOI) in tissue is a prerequisite for meaningful results.[29-31] The combination of localization and spectroscopic techniques is somewhat complicated. Special imaging and localization techniques are used for the collection of localized spectroscopic information.

There are many techniques that do not require switching gradients during the collection of NMR signals. B_0 may be shaped so that the resonance condition is met only in a limited volume.[30] Surface coil techniques have also been used.[31] The sensitive volume of the coil limits the tissue volume which contributes the signal. The resolution may be improved with the rotating frame zeugmatography technique which utilizes a gradient in the B_1 field. Selective excitation technique has been used quite extensively. In such methods multiple excitation pulses are used to limit the volume of interest.[32,33]

Spectroscopic imaging techniques have been developed. Basically the CSI methods described earlier are spectroscopic imaging techniques. The signal may be collected without any gradient switched on. The spatial information is encoded in the initial phase of the signal by gradient pulses with variable amplitudes.[34] If a priori information of the spectrum may be used, one may limit the spectroscopic resolution.[35] In this case one may encode the spectral information in the initial phase of the signal by using the asymmetry of the spin echo.[24]

Conclusion

MR imaging techniques have evolved during the past two decades. The improvements in the future include increased imaging speed and resolution. MRI is a very sensitive imaging method but its specificity is rather low. In the case of muscle tissue, fat/water discrimination, and magnetization transfer, the application of contrast agents may provide substantial additional information in many diagnostic situations. Muscle tissue has many specific properties, such as a good macromolecule/water interaction and a homogeneous structure. The freedom in the selection of the imaging plane and the variety of imaging and spectroscopic conditions give the user new possibilities to noninvasively study human skeletal muscles.

References

1. Farrar TC, Becker ED. Pulse and Fourier transform NMR. New York: Academic Press, 1971.
2. Lauterbur PC. Image formation by induced local interactions: examples employing nuclear magnetic resonance. Nature 1973;242:190–191.
3. Kumar A, Welti DE, Ernst RR. NMR Fourier zeugmatography. J Magn Reson 1975;18:69–83.
4. Edelstein WA, Hutchison JMS, Johnson G, Redpath T. Spin warp NMR imaging and its applications to human whole body imaging. Phys Med Biol 1980;25:751–756.
5. Stark DD, Bradley WG. Magnetic resonance imaging. 2nd ed. St Louis: Mosby Year Book, 1992.
6. Mathur-De Vré R. Biomedical implications of the relaxation behaviour of water related to NMR imaging. Br J Radiol 1984;57:955–976.
7. Koenig SH, Brown RD III, Ugolini R. A unified view of relaxation in protein solution and tissue, including hydration and magnetization transfer. Magn Reson Med 1993; 14:77–83.
8. Koenig SH, Brown RD III, Adams D, Emerson D, Harrison CG. Magnetic field dependence of 1/T1 of protons in tissue. Invest Radiol 1984;19:76–81.
9. Lamminen AE, Tanttu JI, Sepponen RE, Pihko H, Korhola OA. T1ρ dispersion imaging of diseased muscle tissue. Br J Radiol 1993;66:783–787.
10. Bottomley PA, Foster TH, Argersinger RE, Pfeifer LM, A review of normal tissue hydrogen NMR relaxation times and relaxation mechanisms from 1–100 MHz: dependence on tissue type, NMR frequency, temperature, species, excision, and age. Med Phys 1984;11:425–448.
11. Chen J-H, Avram HE, Crooks LE, Arakawa M, Kaufman L, Brito AC. In vivo relaxation times and hydrogen density at 0.064–4.85 T in rats with implanted mammary adenocarcinomas. Radiology 1992;184:427–434.
12. Brooks RA, Di Chiro G, Patronas N. MR imaging of cerebral hematomas at different field strengths: theory and applications. J Comput Assist Tomogr 1989;13:194–206.
13. Lauffer RB. Magnetic resonance contrast media: principles and progress. Magn Reson Q 1990;6:65–84.
14. Soila KP, Viamonte M, Starewicz PM. Chemical shift misregistration effect in magnetic resonance imaging. Radiology 1984;153:819–820.
15. Bydder GM, Young IR. MR imaging: clinical use of the inversion recovery sequence. J Comput Assist Tomogr 1985;9:659–675.
16. Dwyer AJ, Frank JA, Sank VJ, Reining JW, Hickey AM, Doppman JL. Short-TI inversion recovery pulse sequence: analysis and initial experience in cancer imaging. Radiology 1988;168:827–836.
17. Fleckenstein JL, Archer BT, Barker BA, Vaughan JT, Parkey RW, Peshock RM. Fast short-tau inversion recovery MR imaging. Radiology 1991;179:499–504.
18. Wehrli FW. Fast-scan magnetic resonance: principles and applications. New York: Raven Press, 1991.
19. Haase A, Frahm J, Matthaei D, et al. FLASH imaging. Rapid NMR imaging using low flip-angle pulses. J Magn Reson 1986;67:258–266.

20. Elster AD. Gradient-Echo MR imaging: techniques and acronyms. Radiology 1993;186:1–8.
21. Haase A, Frahm J. Multiple chemical-shift-selective NMR imaging using stimulated echoes. J Magn Res 1985;64:94–102.
22. Lamminen AE, Tanttu JI, Sepponen RE, Suramo JI, Pihko H. Magnetic resonance of diseased skeletal muscle: combined T1 measurement and chemical shift imaging. Br J Radiol 1990;63:591–596.
23. Dixon WT. Simple proton spectroscopic imaging. Radiology 1984;153:189–194.
24. Sepponen RE, Sepponen JT, Tanttu JI. A method for chemical shift imaging: demonstration of bone marrow involvement with proton chemical shift imaging. J Comput Assist Tomogr 1984;8:585–587.
25. Wolff SD, Balaban RS. Magnetization transfer contrast (MTC) and tissue water proton relaxation in vivo. Magn Reson Med 1989;10:135–144.
26. Swallow CE, Kahn CE, Halbach RE, Tanttu JI, Sepponen RE. Magnetization transfer contrast imaging of the human leg at 0.1 T: a preliminary study. Magn Reson Imaging 1992;10:361–364.
27. Bottomley PA, Hardy CJ, Roemer PB. Proton-decoupled Overhauser-enhanced, spatially localized carbon-13 spectroscopy in humans. J Magn Reson Med 1989;12:348–352.
28. McCully K, Shellock FG, Bank WJ, Posner JD. The use of nuclear magnetic resonance to evaluate muscle injury. Med Sci Sports Exerc 1992;24:537–542.
29. Fleckenstein JL, Bertocci LA, Nunnally RL, Parkey RW, Peshock RM. Exercise-enhanced MR imaging of variations in forearm muscle anatomy and use: importance in MR spectroscopy. AJR 1989;153:693–698.
30. Newman RJ, Bore PJ, Chan L, Gadian DG, Styles P, Taylor D, Radda GK. Nuclear magnetic resonance studies of forearm muscle in Duchenne dystrophy. Br Med J 1982;284:1072–1074.
31. Jeneson JAL, van Dobbenburgh JO, van Echteld CJA, Lekkerkerk C, Janssen WJM, Dorland L, Berger R, Brown TR. Experimental design of ^{31}P MRS assessment of human forearm muscle function: restrictions imposed by functional anatomy. Magn Reson Med 1993;30:634–640.
32. Frahm J, Merboldt K-D, Hänicke W. Localized proton spectroscopy using stimulated echoes. Magn Reson Med 1987;72:502–508.
33. Ordidge RJ, Connelly A, Lohman JAB. Image-selected in vivo spectroscopy (ISIS). A new technique for spatially selective NMR spectroscopy. Magn Reson Med 1986;66:283–284.
34. Brown TR, Kincaid BM, Ugurbil K. NMR chemical shift imaging in three dimensions. Proc Natl Acad Sci USA 1982;79:3523–3526.
35. Bendel P, Lai C, Lauterbur PC. ^{31}P spectroscopic zeugmatography of phosphorous metabolites. J Magn Reson 1980;38:343–356.

Part II
Human Muscular Anatomy

Introduction

James L. Fleckenstein

Many texbooks exist in which magnetic resonance imaging (MRI) demonstrates human anatomy. Most endeavor to highlight all anatomy in a given image, but frequently leave large gaps between slices. This is particularly true of musculoskeletal texts because the relatively large expanses of tissue that intervene between the anatomically complex joints *appear* to be relatively simple. In fact, this tissue, composed largely of skeletal muscle, is frequently highly complex. Also, because joints are a primary focus of many MRI practices, most previous musculoskeletal atlases primarily focused on joints. However, as the utility of muscle imaging becomes more and more recognized, and small complex regions of muscular anatomy are revealed to be abnormal by imaging studies, the need for a detailed understanding of muscular anatomy has become acute. In an effort to satisfy this need, a different emphasis was taken here to noninvasively dissect anatomy.

First, this part concentrates on the expanses of muscle between joints. Second, the axial plane with respect to the long axis of the body was exclusively selected for imaging. This was justified as the most economical approach because all muscles in an axial cross-section can usually be simultaneously related to all others in the limb. Third, bones, ligaments, tendons, nerves, and blood vessels are, for the most part, unlabeled. This is not because the images do not demonstrate them. In fact, image resolution is quite high, with pixel dimensions being on the order of 0.3 mm to 1.2 mm for small and large regions of interest, respectively. Such high resolution simply defies the ability of annotation schemes to identify all structures. Identification of all anatomical structures is quite easy for the interested student by cross-referencing this material with any of a wide variety of readily available textbooks.

A fourth departure from the customary approach of visualizing anatomy is by combining form and function in the MRI suite. Exercises were performed immediately prior to acquisition of most of the images, which is well documented to cause improved delineation of actively recruited muscle, especially using the STIR sequence (see Chapter 7). This was done in order to allow function (i.e., exercise), rather than arrows, to depict the margins of individual muscles. This obviates difficulties encountered in most other atlases in which poor distinction between adjacent muscles hinders their identification, particularly in complex regions such as the forearm. For this reason, some anatomical regions (e.g., forearm) are more exhaustively studied here than are more simple regions (e.g., thigh).

Using exercise to highlight anatomy brought certain costs, not the least of which was a tremendous amount of scanner time and the time of one very willing volunteer (who now has an improved physique)! Practical limitations included that some difficulty was encountered in precisely repositioning the subject, which resulted in imperfectly co-planar images. Employment of a longitudinal "scout" image to indicate the locations of the axial images was therefore problematic. Hence, verbal descriptions of slice locations are employed here. In all cases, a T_1-weighted image is shown first without annotation and subsequently, liberally annotated STIR images showing exercise-induced anatomy. It is possible in many cases to look back on the high resolution T_1-

weighted image to find the muscle so easily visible on the exercise-enhanced image, while in other cases, even with the aid of the STIR sequence, no definable margin can be found to separate anatomic compartments. This is due, at least in part, to occasional absence of fascial interfaces between functionally dissimilar pools of muscle fibers.

Another difficulty with the approach chosen here was that not all muscles could be effectively exercise-enhanced, particularly those of the head, feet and spine. Where successful, the results are shown. For others, the reader is referred to standard texts.[1,2] Finally, it would have been optimal to describe in detail the exercise performed in each case but this was minimized. Exercises employed commercially available equipment and the results were frequently not those expected based on the claims of the manufacturer. The only commercial vendor to support the project was Philips Medical Systems of North America, Shelton, CT, the manufacturer of the MRI device on which the studies were conducted.

The adage that "a picture is worth a thousand words" is fortunately true. The accompanying 300 images identify, with little need for text, a great many of the muscles of the human body, which amount to well over four hundred. Verbal description of relationships between muscles and other structures is therefore relegated to other books. Abbreviations of muscles are provided for each major anatomical section, along with a table describing innervation of the muscles. Occasionally, arrows without names attached are overlaid onto images to highlight fascial or functional borders between muscles that are annotated elsewhere. As in all images in this book, the subjects right side is to the reader's left.

APPENDIX Upper Extremity

Muscle	Root	Trunk	Division	Cord	Peripheral Nerve
Shoulder Girdle					
deltoid	C5,C6	upper	posterior	posterior	axillary
infraspinatus	C5,C6	upper			suprascapular
latissimus dorsi	C6,C7,C8	upper, middle, lower	posterior	posterior	thoracodorsal
levator scapulae	C3,C4				dorsal scapular
pectoralis major-clavicular portion	C5,C6	upper	anterior	lateral	lateral pectoral
pectoralis major-sternocostal portion	C7,C8,T1	middle, lower	anterior	medial	medial pectoral
pectoralis minor	C6,C7,C8	upper, middle, lower	anterior	medial, lateral	pectoral
rhomboideus major & minor	C5				dorsal scapular
serratus anterior	C5,C6,C7				long thoracic
supraspinatus	C5,C6	upper			suprascapular
teres major	C5,C6	upper	posterior	posterior	lower subscapular
teres minor	C5,C6	upper	posterior	posterior	axillary
supraspinatus	C5,C6	upper			suprascapular
trapezius	C3,C4				accessory
Arm					
biceps brachialis	C5,C6	upper	anterior	lateral	musculocutaneous
brachialis	C5,C6	upper	anterior	lateral	musculocutaneous
coracobrachialis	C6,C7	upper, middle	anterior	lateral	musculocutaneous
triceps	C7,C8,T1	middle, lower	posterior	posterior	radial
Forearm					
abductor pollicis longus	C7,C8	middle, lower	posterior	posterior	radial posterior interosseous
anconeus	C7,C8	middle, lower	posterior	posterior	radial
brachioradialis	C5,C6	upper	posterior	posterior	radial
extensor carpi radialis brevis	C6,C7	upper, middle	posterior	posterior	radial
extensor carpi radialis longus	C6,C7	upper, middle	posterior	posterior	radial
extensor carpi ulnaris	C6,C7,C8	upper, middle, lower	posterior	posterior	radial posterior interosseus
extensor digiti minimi	C7,C8	middle, lower	posterior	posterior	radial posterior interosseus
extensor digitorum communis	C7,C8	middle, lower	posterior	posterior	radial posterior interosseus
extensor indicis proprius	C7,C8	middle, lower	posterior	posterior	radial posterior interosseus
extensor pollicis brevis	C7,C8	middle, lower	posterior	posterior	radial posterior interosseus
extensor pollicis longus	C7,C8	middle, lower	posterior	posterior	radial posterior interosseus
flexor carpi radialis	C6,C7,C8	upper, middle, lower	anterior	lateral, medial	median
flexor carpi ulnaris	C8,T1	lower	anterior	medial	ulnar
flexor digitorum profundus index and long	C7,C8	middle, lower	anterior	medial	median anterior interosseus
flexor digitorum profundus ring and small	C8,T1	lower	anterior	medial	ulnar
flexor digitorum superficialis	C7,C8,T1	middle, lower	anterior	lateral, medial	median
flexor pollicis longus	C7,C8,T1	middle, lower	anterior	lateral, medial	median
palmaris longus	C7,C8,T1	middle, lower	anterior	lateral, medial	median
pronator quadratus	C7,C8,T1	middle, lower	anterior	lateral, medial	median anterior interosseus
pronator teres	C6,C7	upper, middle	anterior	lateral	median
supinator	C5,C6	upper	posterior	posterior	radial posterior interosseus
Hand					
abductor digiti minimi	C8,T1	lower	anterior	medial	ulnar
abductor pollicis brevis	C8,T1	lower	anterior	medial	median
adductor pollicis	C8,T1	lower	anterior	medial	ulnar
dorsal interossei	C8,T1	lower	anterior	medial	ulnar
flexor pollicis brevis deep head	C8,T1	lower	anterior	medial	ulnar
flexor pollicis brevis superficial head	C8,T1	lower	anterior	medial	median
1st & 2nd lumbricales	C8,T1	lower	anterior	medial	median
3rd & 4th lumbricales	C8,T1	lower	anterior	medial	ulnar
opponens digiti minimi	C8,T1	lower	anterior	medial	ulnar
opponens pollicis	C8,T1	lower	anterior	medial	median
volar interossei	C8,T1	lower	anterior	medial	ulnar

Lower Extremity

Muscle	Root	Division	Peripheral nerve
Pelvis and Hip			
gluteus maximus	L5,S1	sacral plexus	inferior gluteal
gluteus medius	L4,L5	sacral plexus	superior gluteal
gluteus minimus	L4,L5	sacral plexus	superior gluteal
inferior gemellus	L5,S1,S2	sacral plexus	inferior gluteal
obturator externus	L?-L4	lumbar plexus	obturator
obturator internus	L5,S1,S2	sacral plexus	
piriformis	S1,S2	sacral plexus	sciatic
quadratus femoris	L4-S2	sacral plexus	sciatic
superior gemellus	L5,S1,S2	sacral plexus	inferior gluteal
Thigh			
adductor brevis	L2,L3,L4	anterior	obturator
adductor longus	L2,L3,L4	anterior	obturator
adductor magnus	L2-L5	anterior	obturator, sciatic
adductor minimi	L2-L5	anterior	obturator
biceps femoris long head	L5,S1	anterior	sciatic
biceps femoris short head	L5,S1,S2	posterior	sciatic
gracilis	L2,L3,L4	anterior	obturator
iliopsoas	L2,L3,L4	posterior	femoral
pectineus	L2,L3,L4	posterior	femoral
quadriceps femoris	L2,L3,L4	posterior	femoral
vastus lateralis			
vastus medialis			
vastus intermedius			
rectus femoris			
sartorius	L2,L3,L4	posterior	femoral
semimembranosus	L5,S1,S2	anterior	sciatic
semitendinosus	L5,S1,S2	anterior	sciatic
tensor fascia lata	L4,L5,S1	sacral plexus	superior gluteal
Leg			
extensor digitorum longus	L5,S1	posterior	deep peroneal
extensor hallucis longus	L5,S1	posterior	deep peroneal
flexor digitorum longus	L5,S1,S2	ventral	tibial
flexor hallucis longus	L5,S1,S2	ventral	tibial
gastrocnemius	S1,S2	ventral	tibial
medial head			
lateral head			
peroneus brevis	L5,S1,S2	posterior	superficial peroneal
peroneus longus	L5,S1,S2	posterior	superficial peroneal
popliteus	L5,S1	anterior	tibial
soleus	L5,S1,S2	anterior	tibial
tibialis anterior	L4,L5	posterior	deep peroneal
tibialis posterior	L5,S1	anterior	tibial
Foot			
abductor digiti minimi	S1,S2	ventral	lateral plantar
abductor hallucis	S1,S2	ventral	medial plantar
adductor hallucis	S1,S2	ventral	lateral plantar
extensor digitorum brevis	L5,S1	dorsal	deep peroneal
flexor digiti minimi	S1,S2	ventral	lateral plantar
flexor digitorum brevis	S1,S2	ventral	medial plantar
flexor hallucis brevis	S1,S2	ventral	medial plantar
interossei	S1,S2		lateral plantar
quadratus plantae	S1,S2	ventral	lateral plantar

References

1. Schweitzer ME, Resnick D. Normal anatomy of the foot and ankle. In: Deutsch AL, Mink JH, Kerr R., eds. MRI of the foot and ankle. New York: Raven. 1992.

2. Eycleshymer AC, and Schoemaker DM. A cross-sectional anatomy. New York: Appleton-Century, 1938.

4
MRI of the Trunk and Spine

James L. Fleckenstein

The Spine and Trunk: Neck and Cervical Spine

TABLE 4.1. Abbreviations for Figures 4.1–4.5.

Digastric	D	Scalenus medius	m
Levator scapulae	Le	Scalenus posterior	p
Longissimus	Lo	Semispinalis capitis	Se
Longissimus capitis	Lp	Semispinalis cervicis	Sev
Longissimus cervicis	Lv	Serratus anterior	SA
Longus capitis and colli	L	Splenius capitis	Sp
Multifidus	M	Splenius cervicis	Spv
Obliquus capitis	OC	Sternocleidomastoid	Sm
Omohyoid	Oh	Sternohyoid	Sh
Platysma	Pl	Sternothyroid	St
Rectus capitis	R	Thyrohyoid	Th
Rhomboids	Rh	Trapezius	T
Scalenus anterior	a		

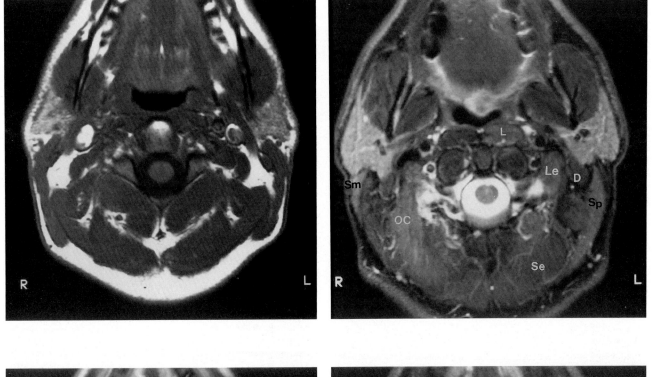

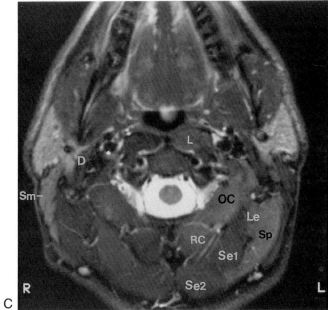

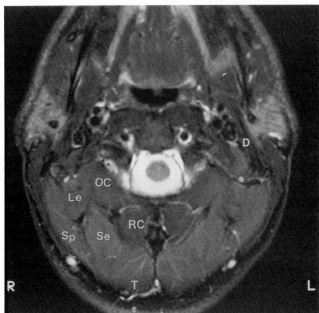

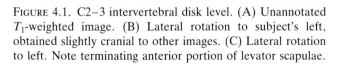

FIGURE 4.1. C2–3 intervertebral disk level. (A) Unannotated T_1-weighted image. (B) Lateral rotation to subject's left, obtained slightly cranial to other images. (C) Lateral rotation to left. Note terminating anterior portion of levator scapulae.

(D) Neck extension. Trapezius is very thin and difficult to appreciate. Digastric is a thin, unenhanced strap on these images. Se1 and Se2 are explained in Figure 4.20.

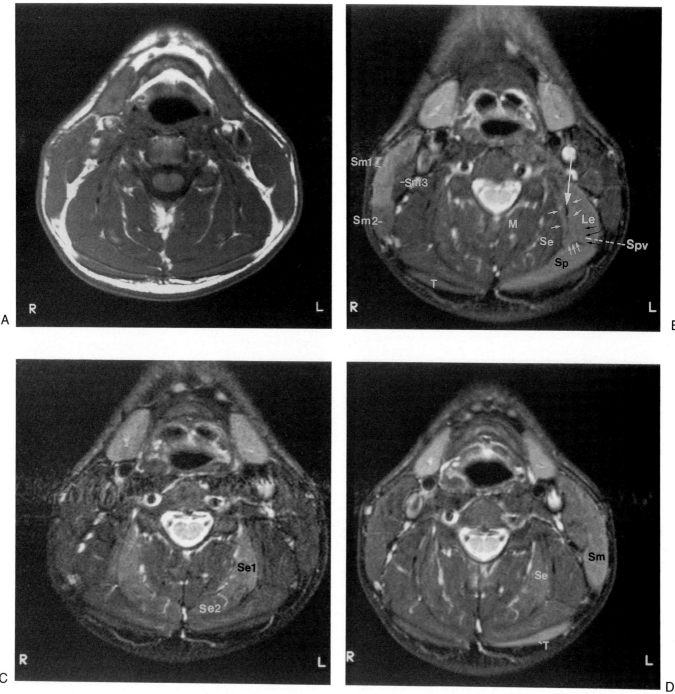

FIGURE 4.2. C5–6, hyoid level. (A) Unannotated T_1-weighted image. (B) Left lateral rotation. Note close proximity of longissimus (between small white arrows) and levator scapulae. Longissimus muscles are small and thin, being divisible in the anteroposterior direction (along plane of long arrow) into cervicis (lateral) and capitis (medial). Splenius muscles consist of the smaller cervicis (anterior) and the larger capitis (posterior). Note the close proximity of levator scapulae to the splenius capitis and intervening splenius cervicis (black arrows highlight faint fascia separating levator and splenius cervicis). In the deepest layer, multifidus is impossible to distinguish from spinalis cervicalis and cervicis capitis. Note three functionally different recruited portions of sternocleidomastoid including the most recruited portion (SM1) and less recruited portions (SM2 and SM3). These functionally disparate portions of sternocleidomastoid can be identified at other levels in other exercises (see below). (C) Limited neck extension. Note that the semispinalis capitis muscle is heterogeneously recruited into more anterior (Se1) and posterior (Se2) components. This functional effect can be seen on other images as well. (D) Left lateral neck flexion. Note homogeneous recruitment of sternocleidomastoid and trapezius.

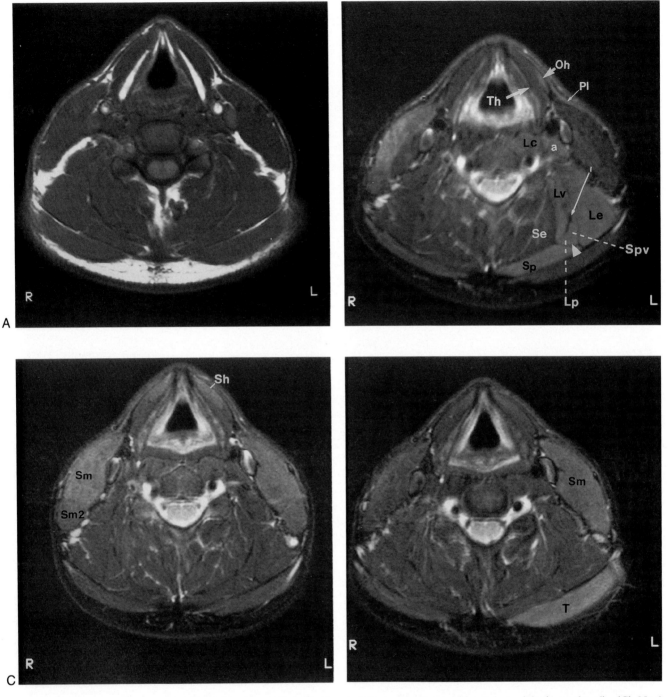

FIGURE 4.3. C6–7 intervertebral disk, thyroid cartilage level. (A) Unannotated T_1-weighted image. (B) Lateral rotation to left. Note recruitment of omohyoid and platysma on left. These muscles overlie thyrohyoid and sterno thyroid which could not be exercise-enhanced. Note bordering fasciae between longissimus cervicis and capitis (long arrow) as well as that between splenius capitis and cervicis (arrowhead). (C) Neck flexion. Note reduced recruitment of posterior portion of sternocleidomastoid (SM2). Note sternohyoid muscle recruited just anterior to omohyoid. (D) Left lateral neck flexion. Note homogeneous recruitment of sternocleidomastoid and trapezius.

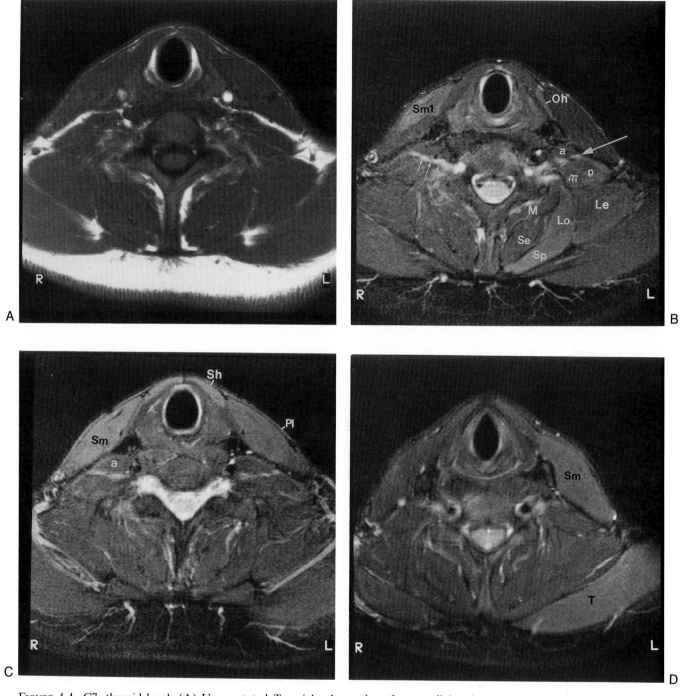

FIGURE 4.4. C7, thyroid level. (A) Unannotated T_1-weighted image. (B) Left lateral neck rotation. Note on these and other images how the brachial plexus (arrows) separates anterior scalene from medial and posterior scalenes. (C) Neck flexion. (D) Left lateral neck flexion.

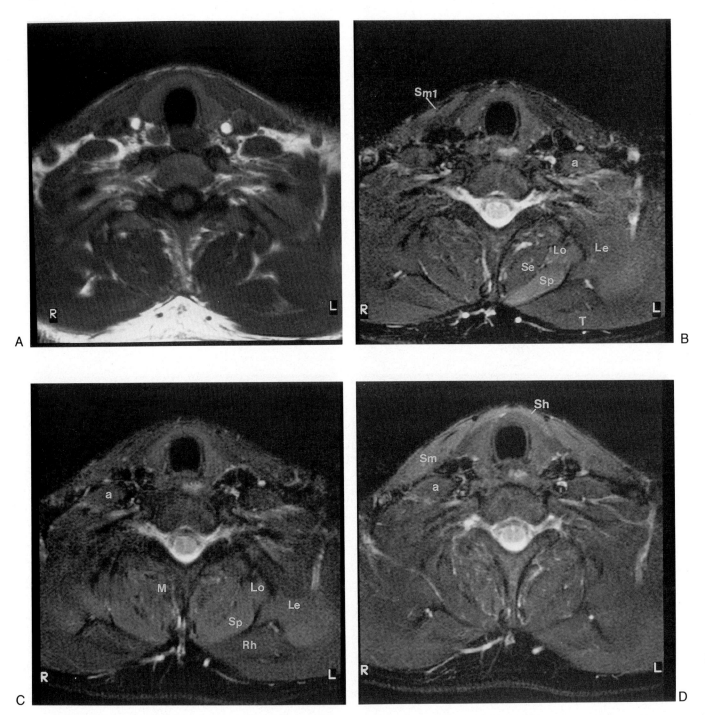

FIGURE 4.5. C8 neural foramen level. (A) Unannotated T_1-weighted image. (B) Left lateral neck rotation. (C) Neck extension. Note asymmetric recruitment of levator scapulae. (D) Neck flexion.

The Spine and Trunk: Chest and Shoulder Girdle

TABLE 4.2. Abbreviations for Figures 4.6–4.11.

Biceps brachialis	B	Multifidus	M
long head	Bl	Pectoralis major	Pj
short head	Bs	Pectoralis minor	Pi
Brachialis	Br	Rhomboideus major & minor	R
Coracobrachialis	C	Serratus anterior	SA
Deltoid	D	Spinalis dorsalis	SD
anterior slips	Da	Subscapularis	Sb
lateral slips	Dl	Supraspinatus	S
posterior slips	Dp	Teres major	Tj
Iliocostalis	Ic	Teres minor	Ti
Infraspinatus	I	Trapezius	Tp
Intercostalis internus and externus	IE	Triceps	T
Latissimus dorsi	LD	long head	To
Levator scapulae	Le	medial head	Tm
Longissimus dorsalis	LgD	lateral head	Tl

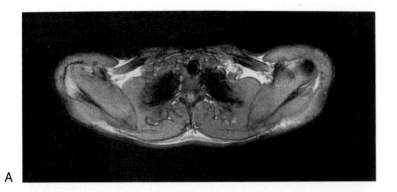

A

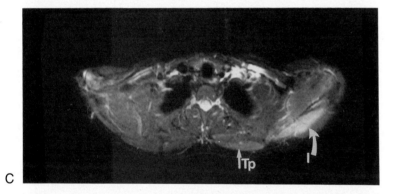

B

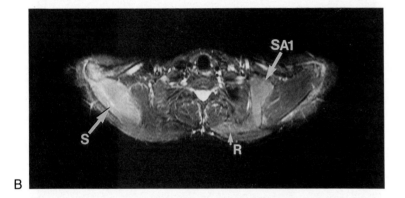

C

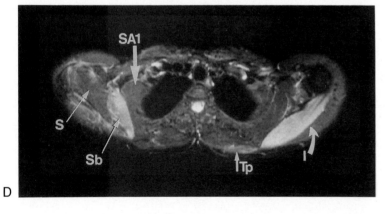

D

FIGURE 4.6. Clavicles, upper thoracic spine. (A) Un-annotated T_1-weighted image. (B) Right shoulder abduction, left shoulder adduction. The first digitation of serratus anterior is functionally isolated, (SA1) along with rhomboids. (C,D) Right arm internal rotation and left arm external rotation (4.6D obtained 2 cm caudal to 4.6C, with left shoulder caudal to the right). Note that external rotation isolates left infraspinatus and trapezius, while internal rotation distinguishes subscapularis from nearby muscles.

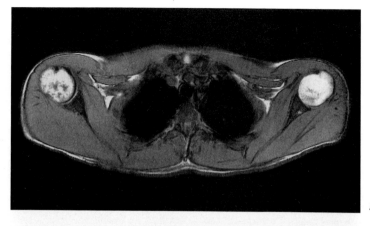

A

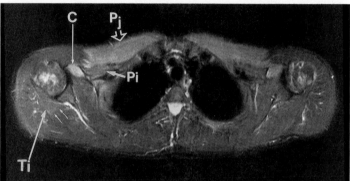

B

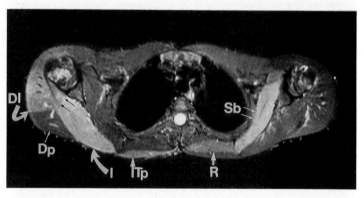

C

FIGURE 4.7. Humeral heads, bicipital grooves, gleno-humeral articulations. (A) Unannotated T_1-weighted image. (B) The "push-up." Note isolation of pectoralis major and coracobrachialis. (C) Right arm abduction ("golf swing") and left arm adduction. Note layered relationship of trapezius to rhomboid and infraspinatus to subscapularis. During abduction, deltoid is functionally divisible into separate portions with the posterior aspect (Dp) inactive relative to the lateral (Dl). Teres minor is difficult to identify on axial images but is shown here (lateral to small black arrows) adjacent to nearby infraspinatus. (D) Right arm internal rotation and left arm external rotation at level slightly caudal to Figure 4.7B and C. Note distinction of inactive right coracobrachialis and pectoralis minor. Note external rotation isolates left infraspinatus and trapezius, while internal rotation distinguishes subscapularis from nearby muscles and faintly isolates teres minor, similar to Figure 4.7B.

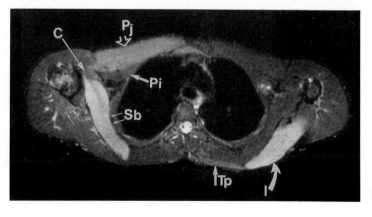

D

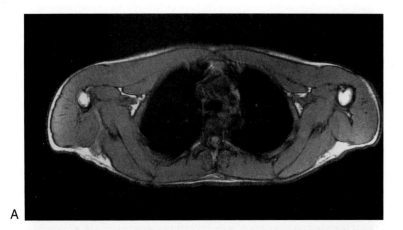

A

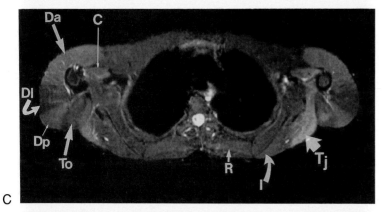

B

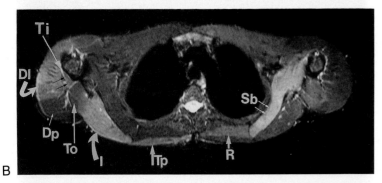

C

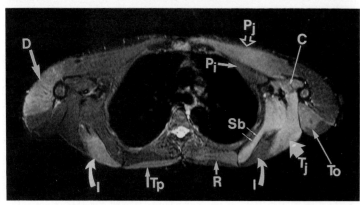

D

FIGURE 4.8. Second portion of axillary artery, denoted by the artery crossing behind pectoralis minor. (A) Unannotated T_1-weighted image. (B) Right arm abduction "golf swing" and left arm internal rotation. (C) "Lat pull down." Note the anterior portion of deltoid (Da) being functionally separated from lateral portion (Dl), which in turn is separable from the posterior portion (Dp). The long head of triceps is seen as it turns medial near its origin from the infra-glenoid tubercle of scapula. Note that exercise distinguishes teres major from infraspinatus muscle and that teres major inserts onto the humerus just posterior to coracobrachialis. Note on these and subsequent images that distinction between teres major and latissimus dorsi is not readily possible. (D) Right arm abduction "golf swing" and left arm internal rotation (4 cm inferior to 4.8B). On the right, exercise recruits lateral deltoid as well as infraspinatus and trapezius. Internal rotation of left humerus involves multiple muscles; note functional distinction between unnamed portions of the long head of triceps with the more superficial portion not being recruited in this exercise.

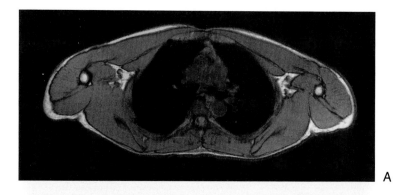

A

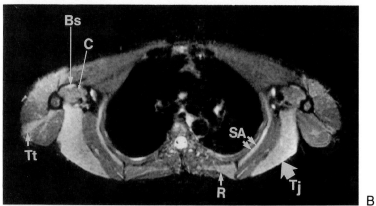

B

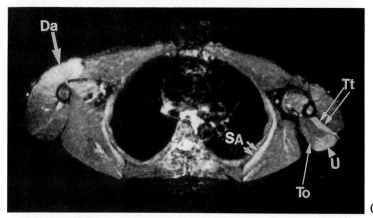

C

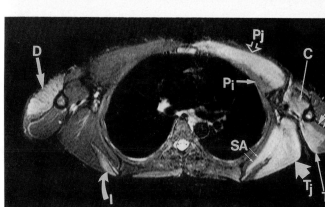

D

FIGURE 4.9. Tracheal bifurcation, apex of axilla. (A) Unannotated T_1-weighted image. (B) "Lat pull down." Despite the name of the exercise, multiple muscles are employed in addition to latissimus dorsi. Interestingly, the short head of biceps is isolated from long head and coracobrachialis upon which it lies. The lateral head of triceps is selectively recruited and its proximal origin from the humerus is demonstrated on the right. (C) Striking distinction on the left between the proximal origin of the lateral head of triceps and the long head of triceps is possible. An unnamed (U) superficial and functionally distinct portion of the long head is clearly demarcated. (D) Right arm abduction "golf swing" and left arm internal rotation. Note complex interaction of arm and chest wall muscles during relatively simple exercise.

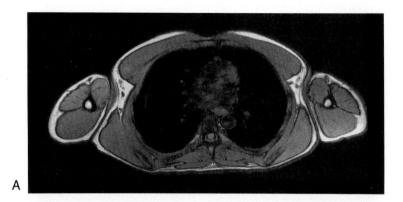

A

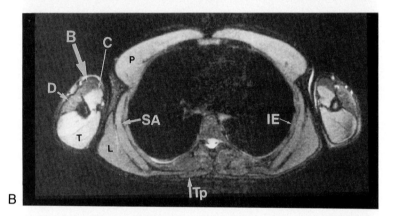

B

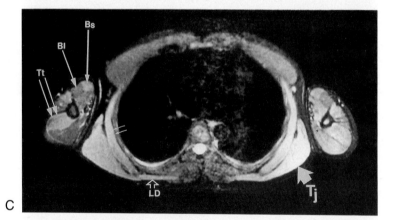

C

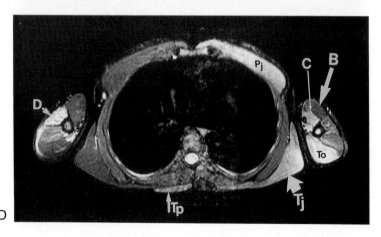

D

FIGURE 4.10. Level of cardiac atria and distal deltoid. (A) Unannotated T_1-weighted image. (B) "Push-ups." Many recruited muscles can be identified. In the arm, coracobrachialis is readily distinguished from biceps. (C) "Lat pull down." Distinction between short and long heads of biceps as well as lateral head of triceps is made readily. (D) Right arm abduction "golf swing" and left arm internal rotation. Marked distinction between serratus anterior and major portions of pectoralis and latissimus dorsi/teres major can be seen.

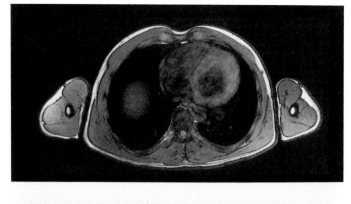

A

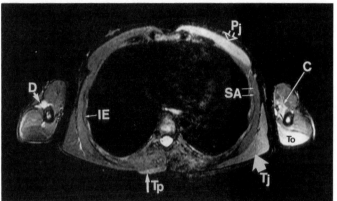

B

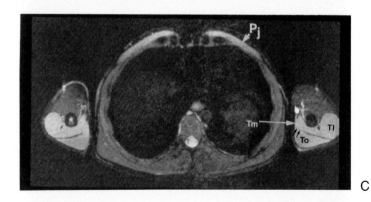

C

FIGURE 4.11. Midthoracic spine, midarm, cardiac ventricles. (A) Unannotated T_1-weighted image. (B) Right arm abduction "golf swing" and left arm internal rotation. The distal deltoid insertion occurs at approximately the same level as that of the distal coracobrachialis. Note in Chapter 5 that brachialis originates at approximately this level. (C) "Push-ups." Distinction between the three heads of triceps is not possible. (D) Trunk extension of midthoracic paraspinal muscles. Trapezius remains the most superficial muscle, overlying latissimus dorsi. These muscles overlie longissimus dorsalis medially and iliocostalis slightly laterally. The small deep muscles of the spine, spinalis dorsi, multifidus and rotatores are difficult to distinguish.

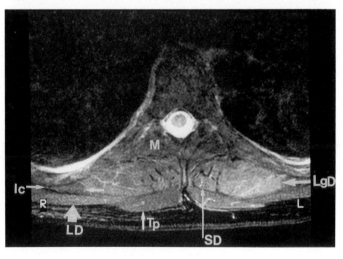

D

The Spine and Trunk:
Lower Trunk, Abdomen, and Pelvis

TABLE 4.3. Abbreviations for Figures 4.12–4.19.

Gluteus maximus	Ma	Obturator externus	ObE
medius	Me	internus	ObI
minimus	Mi	Pectineus	Pc
Iliacus	I	Piriformis	P
Iliocostalis	Ic	Psoas	Ps
Iliopsoas	Ip	Quadratus lumborum	QL
Latissimus dorsi	LD	Rectus abdominis	RA
Longissimus	Lg	Rectus femoris	RF
Multifidus	M	Sartorius	S
Obliquus abdominus internus	Oi	Superior gemelli	SG
externus	Oe	Tensor fasciae latae	TF

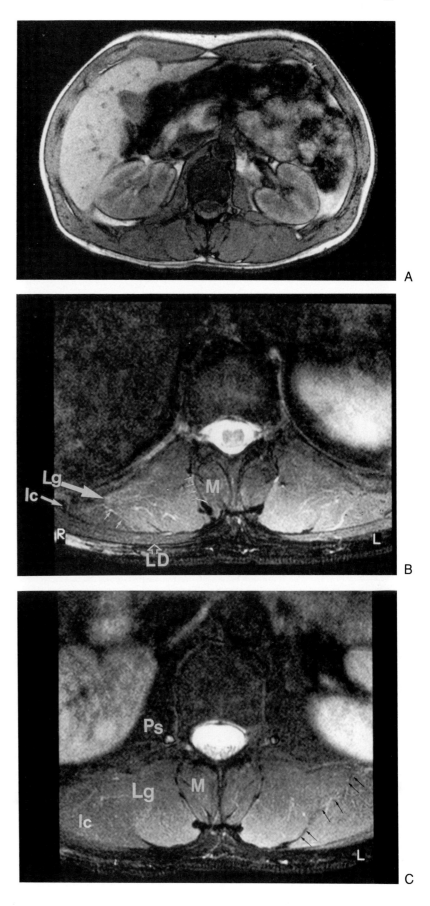

FIGURE 4.12. L1–2, kidneys. (A) Unannotated T_1-weighted image. (B) Trunk extension with left lateral rotation. Note that relative inactivity of right iliocostalis aids in distinction between that muscle and longissimus. (C) Trunk extension with left lateral rotation, 4 cm caudal to Figure 4.12B. Distinction between multifidus, longissimus and iliocostalis is somewhat difficult, however, note fascial interface between the latter two muscles on left (arrows). Psoas is not recruited.

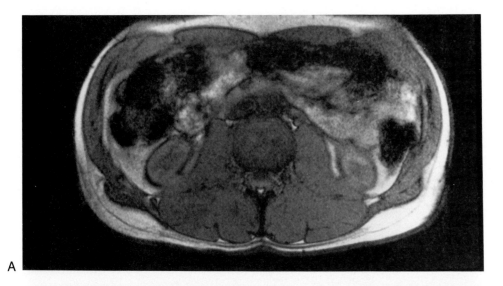

A

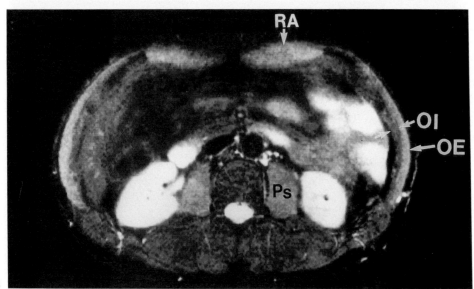

B

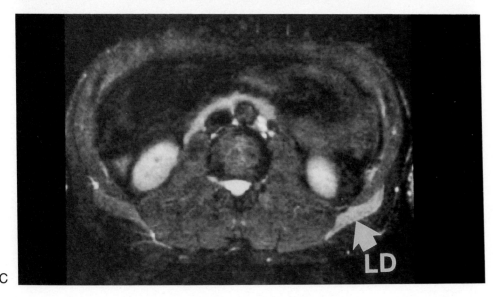

C

FIGURE 4.13. Inferior kidney, L-3. (A) Unannotated T_1-weighted image. (B) "Sit-ups." Rectus abdominis muscle is recruited as is external oblique, the latter evident particularly in comparison to the internal oblique. Psoas is also recruited. (C) "Lat pull down" confirms the location of distal-most latissimus dorsi.

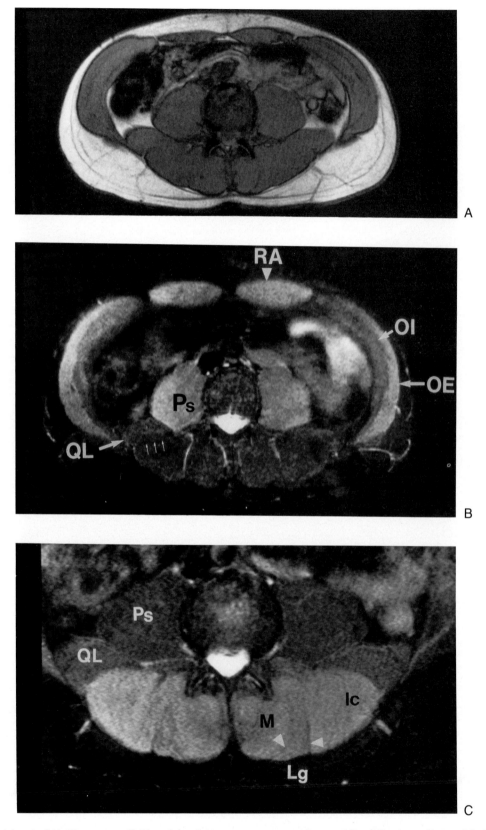

FIGURE 4.14. L4 level. (A) Unannotated T_1-weighted image. (B) "Sit-ups." While psoas is recruited, quadratus lumborum is not. (C) Trunk extension. The three muscles that comprise the erector spinae, while difficult to distinguish from each other, are easily distinguished from the trunk flexors, quadratus lumborum and psoas.

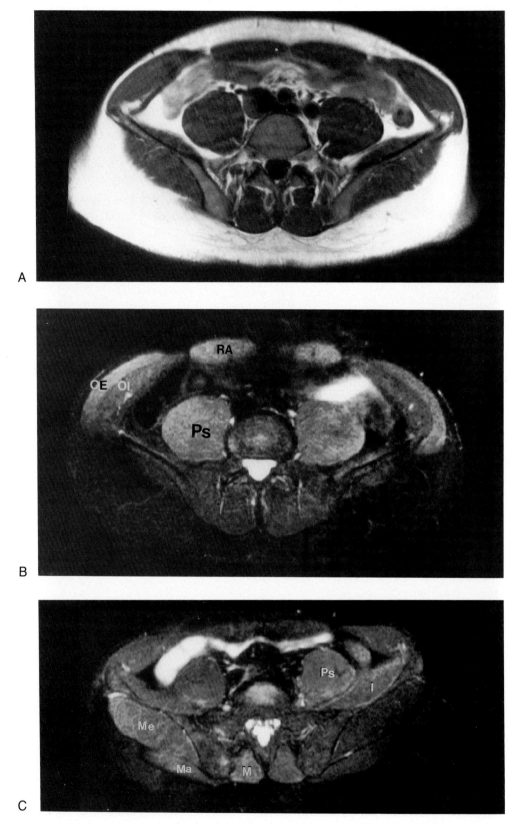

FIGURE 4.15. L-5 neural foramen level. (A) Unannotated T_1-weighted image. (B) "Sit-ups." (C) During left hip flexion, right-sided hip stabilizers, gluteus medius and maximus are also recruited.

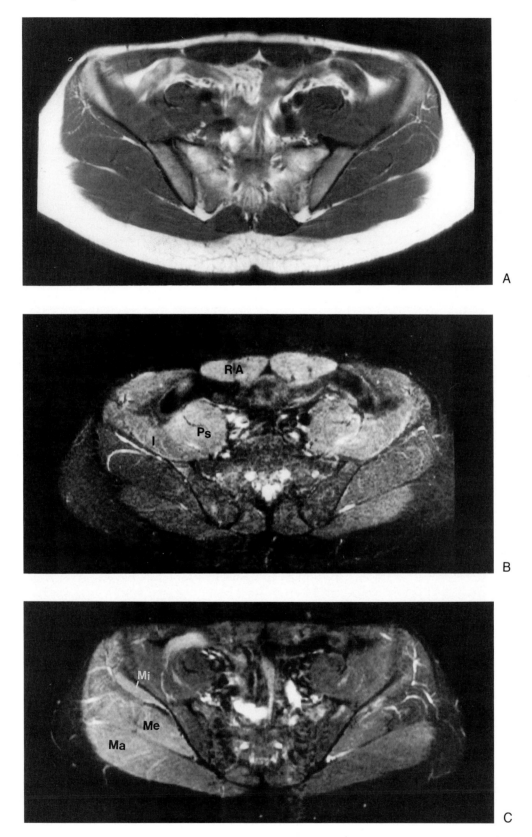

FIGURE 4.16. Sacroiliac joints. (A) Unannotated T_1-weighted image. (B) "Sit-ups" provides contrast between iliacus, psoas and gluteal muscles. (C) During left hip adduction, pelvic stabilization by right gluteals is apparent.

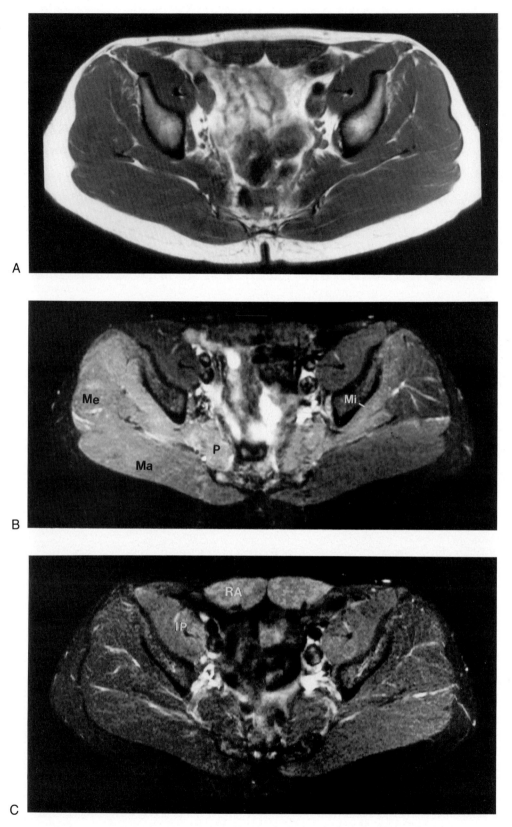

FIGURE 4.17. Superior anterior iliac spines. (A) Unannotated T_1-weighted image. (B) Left hip abduction recruits gluteus minimus and piriformis muscles but note prominent isolation of synergistically recruited gluteus muscles on the right. (C) "Sit-ups."

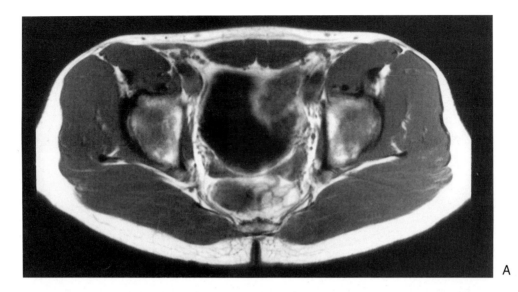

A

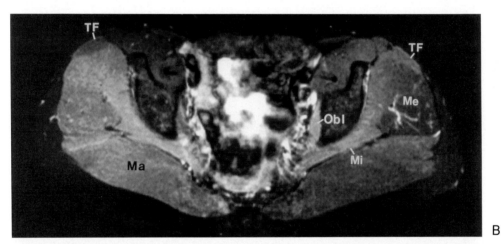

B

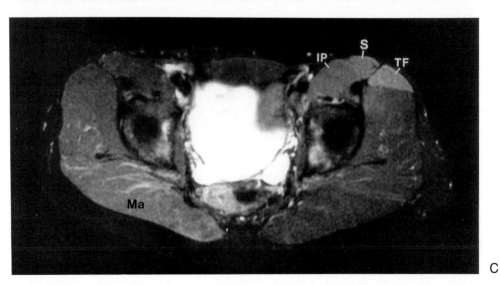

C

FIGURE 4.18. Proximal hip level, just superior to the femoral heads. (A) Unannotated T_1-weighted image. (B) Left hip abduction isolates tensor fascia lata, obturator internus and gluteus minimis. Note that synergistic recruitment of right-sided pelvic stabilizers isolates inactive tensor fascia lata from gluteus medius. (C) Left hip flexion and right hip extension isolates opposing muscle groups.

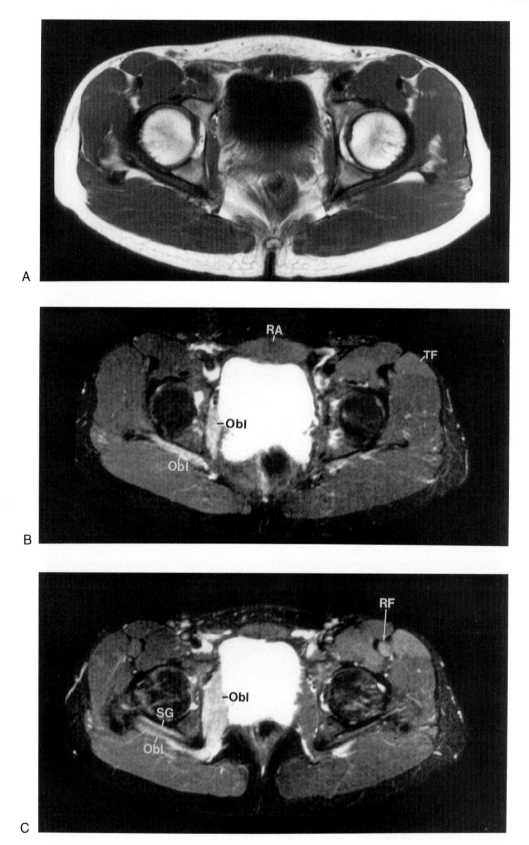

FIGURE 4.19. Hip joint level. (A) Unannotated T_1-weighted image. (B) External rotation of the right hip isolates obturator internus. (C) At level slightly distal to 4.19A, the same exercise identifies superior gemelli, although inferior gemelli could not be isolated. Left hip flexion resulted in recruitment of tensor fascia lata and proximal-most rectus femoris.

5
MRI of the Upper Extremity

James L. Fleckenstein

The Upper Extremity: The Arm

TABLE 5.1. Abbreviations for Figures 5.1–5.5.

Biceps brachialis	B	Pectoralis minor	Pi
long head	Bl	Rhomboideus major & minor	R
short head	Bs	Serratus anterior	SA
Brachialis	Br	Subscapularis	Sb
Coracobrachialis	C	Teres major	Tj
Deltoid	D	Triceps	T
Deltoid-posterior slips	Dp	long head	To
Infraspinatus	I	medial head	Tm
Pectoralis major	Pj	lateral head	Tl

Note: Some muscles of the arm were included in Chapter 4 (Figures 4.6–4.11).

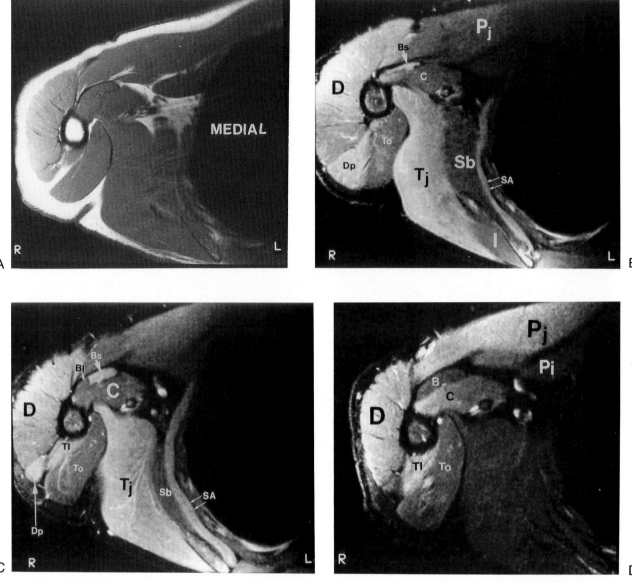

FIGURE 5.1. Apex of axilla at junction of second and third portions of axillary artery. (A) Unannotated T_1-weighted image. (B) "Lat pull down." Observe a posterior portion of deltoid (Dp) behaving functionally separate from laterally situated fibers. Also, note separation of long and short heads of biceps as they traverse the anterior surface of coracobrachialis. The long head of triceps is seen just distal to its origin from the infraglenoid tubercle of the scapula. (C) "Lat pull down."

Obtained 1 cm distal to Figure 5.1B. Note relationships between heads of biceps and triceps and deltoid. (D) "Push-ups." Note distinction between long and lateral heads of triceps at level of the origin of lateral head. Interesting from a recruitment point of view is that while pectoralis major is strongly recruited, pectoralis minor is not. Also, while coracobrachialis is recruited, biceps are not.

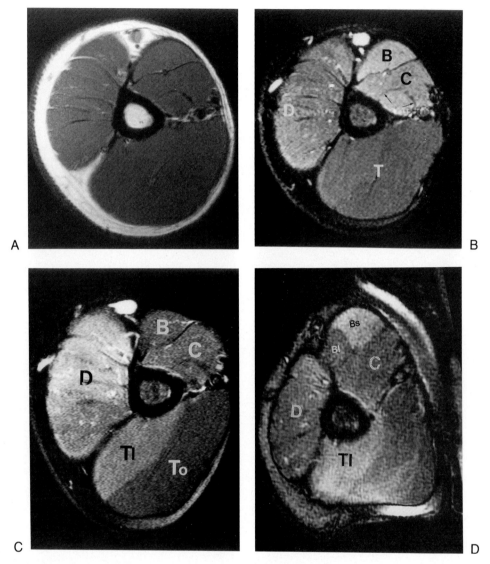

FIGURE 5.2. Proximal arm, distal deltoid level. (A) Unannotated T_1-weighted image. (B) "Biceps curl" exercise. Note homogeneous recruitment of biceps and coracobrachialis. Coracobrachialis in this subject has a distinct fascial subdivision within it. (C) "Reverse fly" exercise. (D) "Lat pull down" exercise.

J.L. Fleckenstein

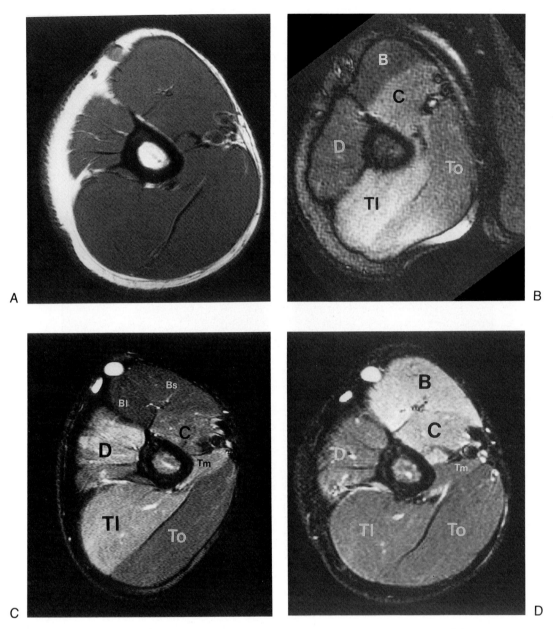

FIGURE 5.3. Proximal arm, 2 cm distal to Figure 5.2. (A) Unannotated T_1-weighted image. (B) "Push-ups" exercise. (C) "Reverse fly" exercise. (D) "Biceps curl" exercise.

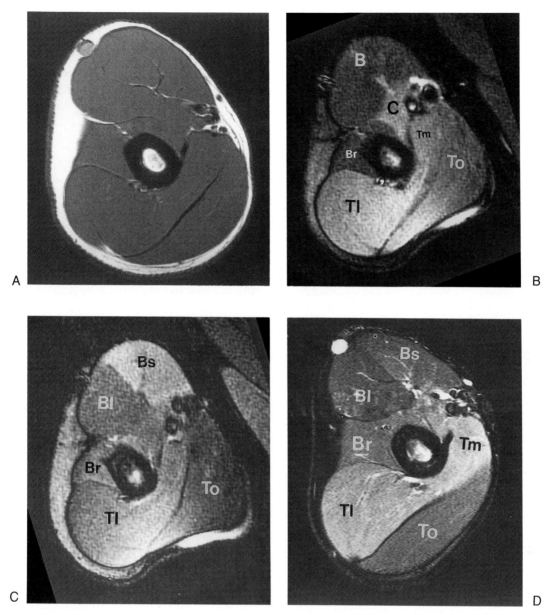

FIGURE 5.4. Midarm, proximal brachialis level. (A) Unannotated T_1-weighted image. (B) "Push-ups" exercise. (C) "Lat pull down" exercise. (D) "Reverse fly" exercise.

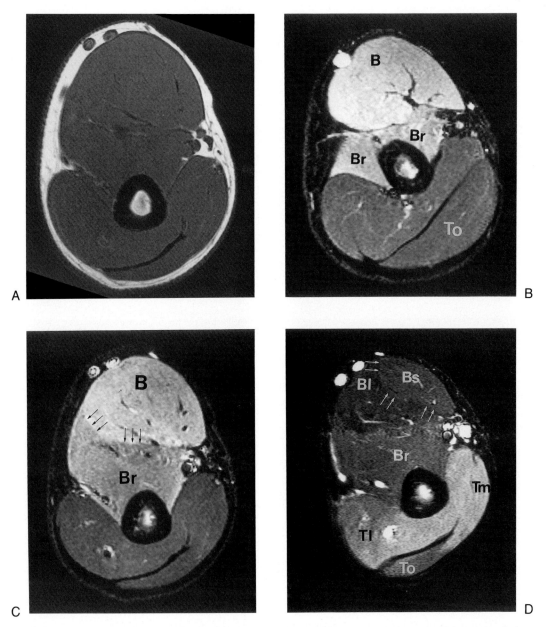

FIGURE 5.5. Junction of mid- and distal 1/3 of arm, 2 cm distal to Figure 5.4. (A) Unannotated T_1-weighted image. (B) "Biceps curls" exercise, slightly proximal to Figure 5.5A. (C) Same exercise as in Figure 5.5B, 2 cm more distally. Note faint distinction between brachialis and biceps. (D) "Reverse fly" exercise. Note lack of involvement of long head of triceps and slight distinction between brachialis and the short head and the long head of biceps.

The Upper Extremity: Forearm

TABLE 5.2. Abbreviations for Figures 5.6–5.23.

Abductor pollicis longus	APL	Flexor carpi radialis	FCR
Anconeus	A	Flexor carpi ulnaris	FCU
Biceps	B	Flexor digitorum profundus	FDP
Brachialis	Br	index portion	I
Brachioradialis	Brd	long portion	L
Extensor carpi radialis longus	ECRL	Flexor digitorum superficialis	FDS
Extensor carpi radialis brevis	ECRB	index portion	SI
Extensor carpi ulnaris	ECU	small portion	SS
Extensor digitorum communis	ED	Palmaris longus	PL
index portion	EDI	Pronator quadratus	PQ
Extensor digiti minimi	EDM	Pronator teres	PT
Extensor indicis proprius	EPI	Supinator	S
Extensor pollicis brevis	EPB	Triceps	T
Extensor pollicis longus	EPL		

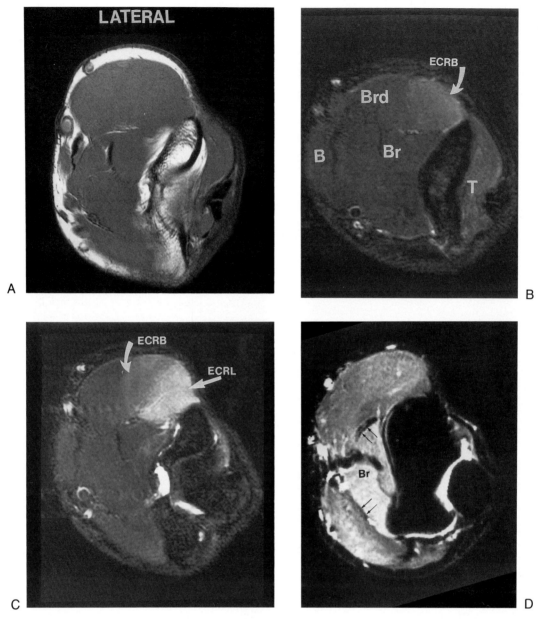

FIGURE 5.6. Distal-most arm, proximal elbow. Note that whereas the upper arm images (Figures 5.1–5.5) were obtained with the medial portion of the arm facing to the reader's right, images of elbow and forearm are displayed with the dorsal portions to the reader's right. In this way, the reader can view the images as if looking down along the length of their own extended right forearm (thumb pointing medial and slightly upwards). (A) Unannotated T_1-weighted image. (B) Wrist extension exercise. Level is approximately 1 cm proximal to that of Figure 5.6A. (C) Same exercise as Figure 5.6B. Ulna-humeral articulation, approximately 2 cm distal to Figure 5.6B. Note the volar relationship of extensor carpi radialis brevis to extensor carpi radialis longus. The overlying brachioradialis and medially located brachialis are more difficult to distinguish. (D) "Biceps curl" exercise. Note clear distinction of distal brachialis. Level is approximately 1 cm distal to Figure 5.6C.

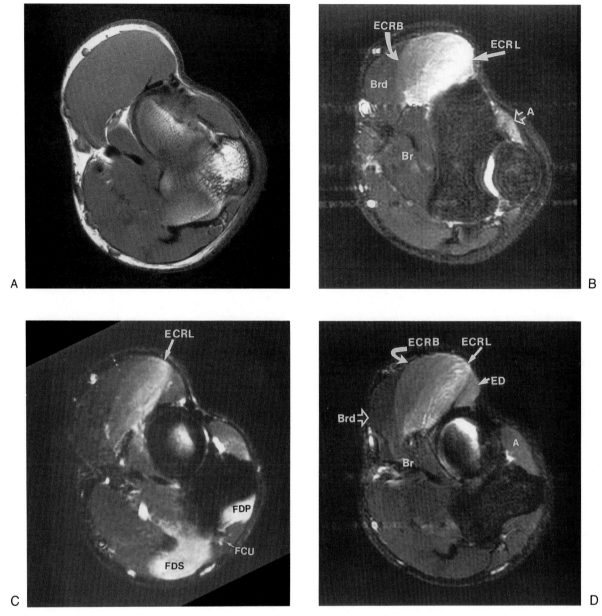

FIGURE 5.7. Humeral epicondyles, approximately 5 mm distal to Figure 5.6D. (A) Unannotated T_1-weighted image. (B) Wrist extension exercise, as in Figures 5.6B and 5.6C, imaged at level nearly identical to 5.6D. Note clearly revealed relationships of extensor carpi radialis brevis and extensor carpi radialis longus to brachialis and brachioradialis. (C) Handgrip exercise, imaged at level approximately 1 cm distal to Figure 5.7B. Note recruitment of extensor carpi radialis longus, as well as finger flexors. (D) Wrist extension exercise.

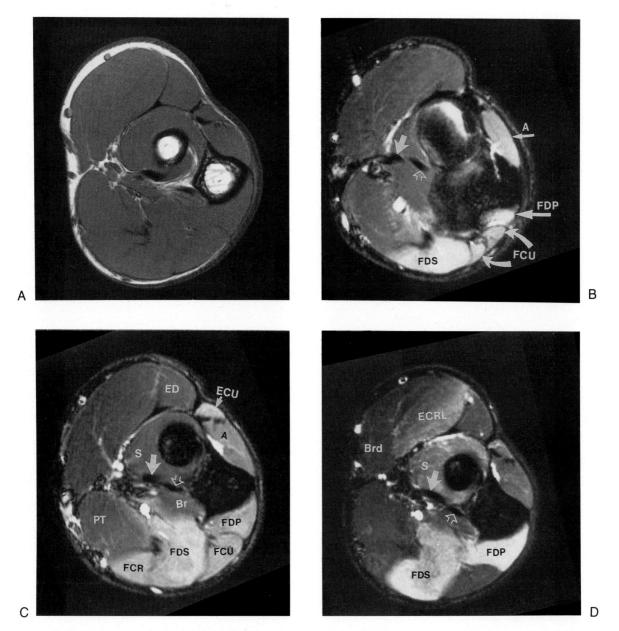

FIGURE 5.8. Level of insertions of biceps and brachialis tendons into the proximal radius and ulna, respectively. (A) Unannotated T_1-weighted image. (B) Wrist flexion exercise, with ulnar deviation. Approximately 1 cm proximal to Figure 5.8A, at level nearly identical to that of 5.7C, shows slightly more proximal aspects of biceps and brachialis tendons (closed and open arrowheads, respectively). Note that finger flexors as well as wrist flexors are recruited. The two heads of flexor carpi ulnaris can be discriminated near their origins (curved arrows). (C) Obtained slightly distal to Figure 5.8B, and following the same exercise. Note that extensor carpi ulnaris is also recruited. (D) Handgrip exercise. Note that extensor carpi radialis longus and supinator are recruited synergistically.

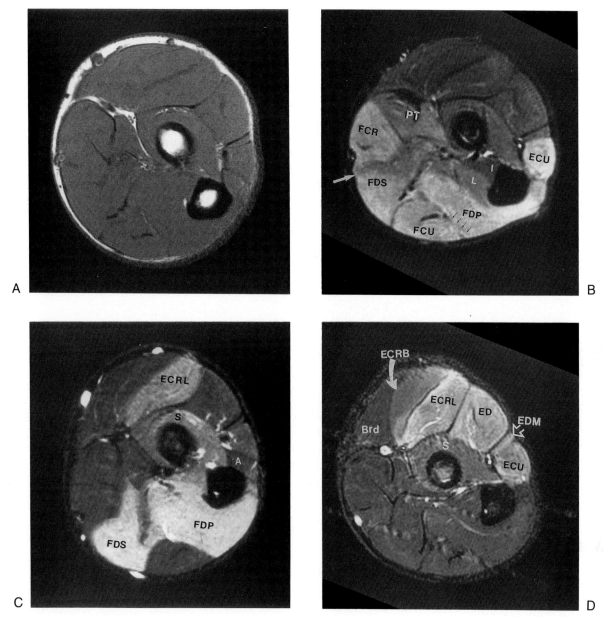

FIGURE 5.9. Proximal 1/3 of the forearm, midsupinator level. (A) Unannotated T_1-weighted image. (B) Wrist flexion combined with finger flexion with ulnar deviation. Note recruitment of pronator teres. The palmaris longus, a small and variable muscle occurring in the superficial forearm, is absent from this subject, but it would be expected to at approximate location of the arrow, just ulnar to flexor carpi radialis, overlying the radial portion of flexor digitorum superficialis. Observe that flexor digitorum profundus is heterogeneously recruited; the index (I) and long (L) finger portions are less intensely recruited than neighboring portions of finger flexors. For detailed finger-specific anatomy, see Figures 5.11–5.18. (C) Handgrip exercise. (D) Wrist extension exercise.

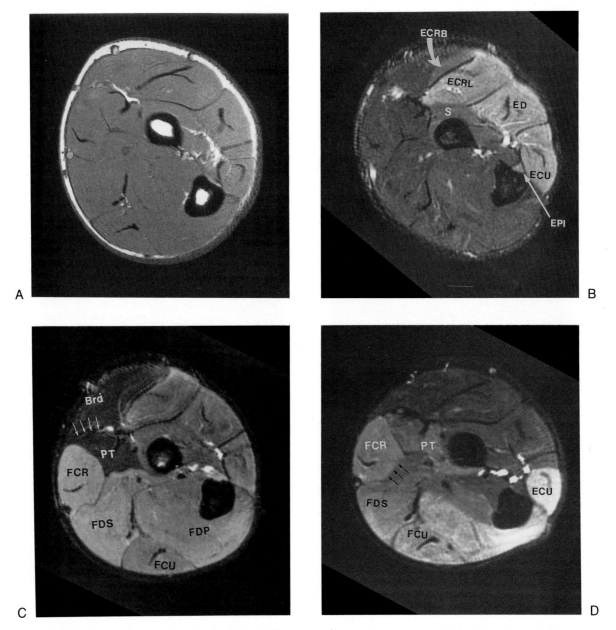

FIGURE 5.10. Distal supinator level, approximately 1 cm distal to Figure 5.9. (A) Unannotated T_1-weighted image. (B) Wrist extension exercise. Note recruitment of extensor indicis proprius. (C) Wrist flexion performed shortly after wrist exten-sion. Note isolated inactivity of brachioradialis and pronator teres, the fascial interface between which is annotated with arrows. (D) Wrist flexion with ulnar deviation.

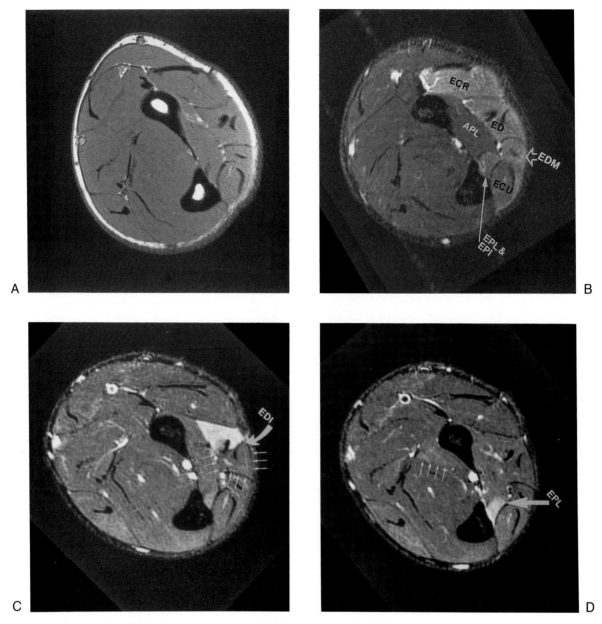

FIGURE 5.11. Midforearm level. (A) Unannotated T_1-weighted image. (B) Wrist extension exercise. The proximal aspects of extensor pollicis and extensor indicis proprius cannot be differentiated. (C) Extension of proximal interphalangeal joint of index finger. Note that the radial portion of extensor digitorum communis is recruited by this movement. The ulnar portion of muscle is devoted to long and ring finger extension. (D) Thumb interphalangeal joint extension. Note isolation of extensor pollicis and faint recruitment of antagonist, flexor pollicis longus (arrows).

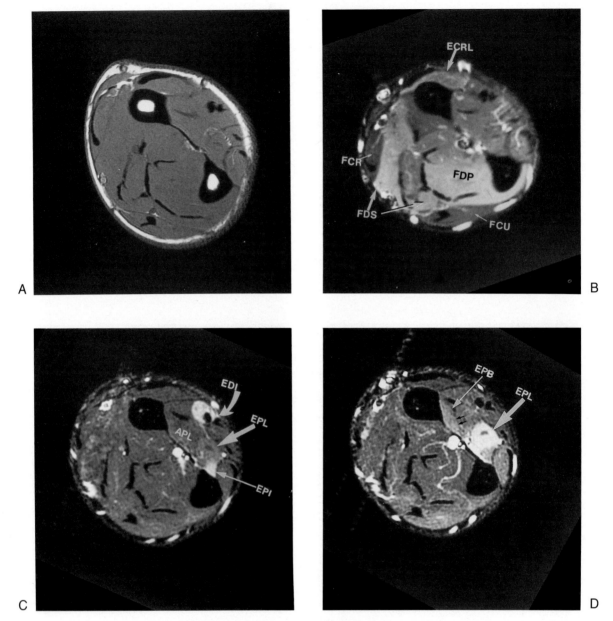

FIGURE 5.12. Midforearm level, 3 cm distal to Figure 5.11. (A) Unannotated T_1-weighted image. (B) Handgrip exercise. (C) Extension of proximal interphalangeal joint of index finger, as in Figure 5.11C. Note location of abductor pollicis longus radial extensor pollicis longus. (D) Thumb interphalangeal joint extension, as in Figure 5.11D. Note faint recruitment of origin of extensor pollicis brevis. Arrows denote boundary between extensor pollicis brevis and abductor pollicis longus, which intervenes between the two thumb extensors.

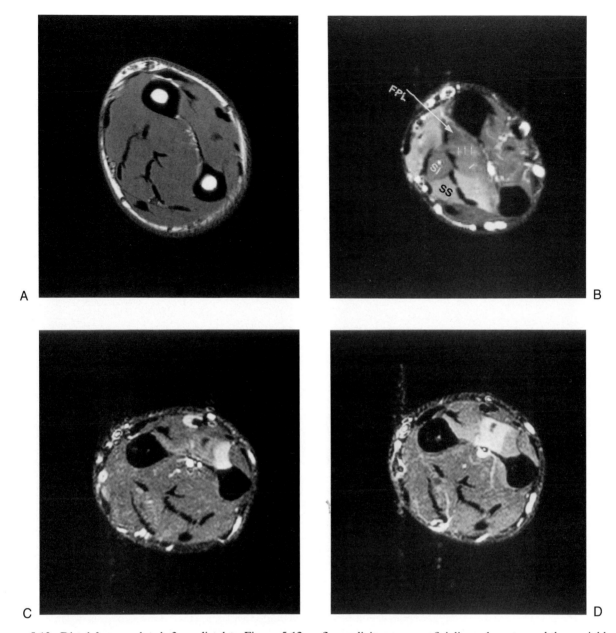

FIGURE 5.13. Distal forearm level, 3 cm distal to Figure 5.12. (A) Unannotated T_1-weighted image. (B) Handgrip exercise. Note that only a portion of flexor digitorum superficialis is recruited and flexor pollicis longus is not strongly exercise-enhanced. The index portion of flexor digitorum profundus and flexor digitorum superficialis are less stressed than neighboring portions of the same muscles, such as the small portion of flexor digitorum superficialis. (C) Extension of proximal interphalangeal joint of index finger. (D) Thumb interphalangeal joint extension.

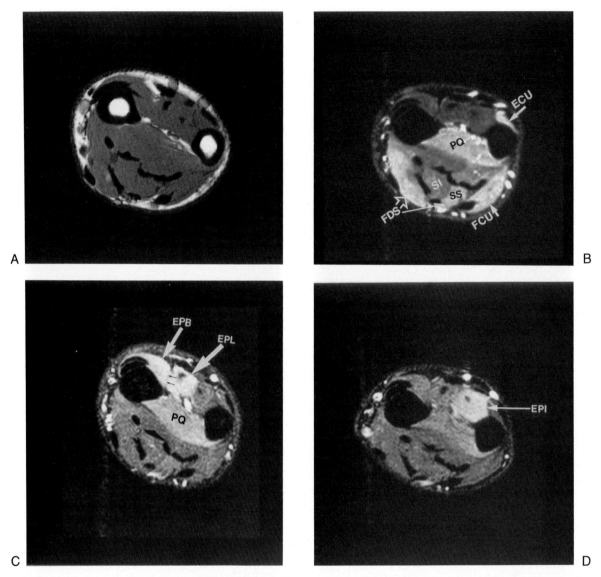

FIGURE 5.14. Distal forearm level, 3 cm distal to Figure 5.13. (A) Unannotated T_1-weighted image. (B) Wrist flexion with ulnar deviation. Flexor carpi radialis has tapered to a tendon and is no longer visible as a muscle. Differential recruitment of finger-specific portions of deep and superficial finger flexors is evident. (C) Exhaustive thumb extension. Note that both thumb extensors are recruited and abductor pollicis longus has tapered to a tendon. (D) Extension of proximal interphalangeal joint of index finger.

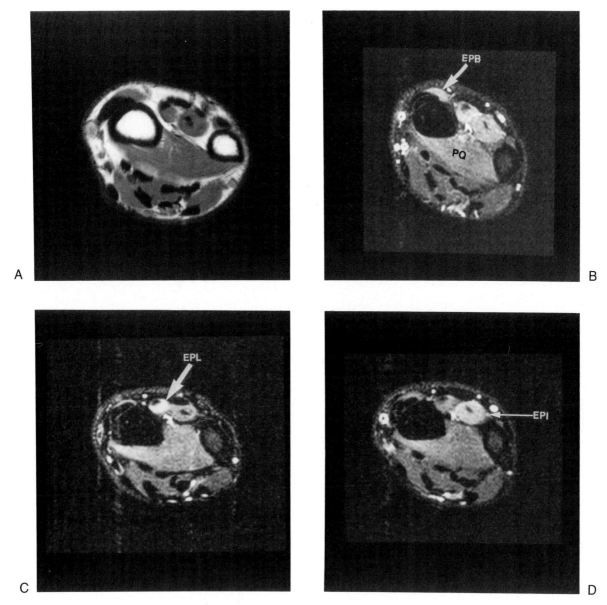

FIGURE 5.15. Distal forearm level, 2 cm distal to Figure 5.14. (A) Unannotated T_1-weighted image. (B) Thumb interphalangeal joint extension. (C) Thumb interphalangeal joint extension, 1 cm distal to Figure 5.15B. Extensor pollicis brevis has tapered to a tendon. (D) Extension of proximal interphalangeal joint of index finger.

The Upper Extremity: Finger-Specific Extrinsic Muscles of the Hand

The following eight sets of images were obtained using 9 mm sections every 13 mm from the midproximal forearm, near the distal brachialis, to the middistal forearm. Each set was acquired following isolated flexion of a single finger joint: the proximal interphalangeal joints for flexor digitorum superficialis and distal interphalangeal joints for flexor digitorum profundus.

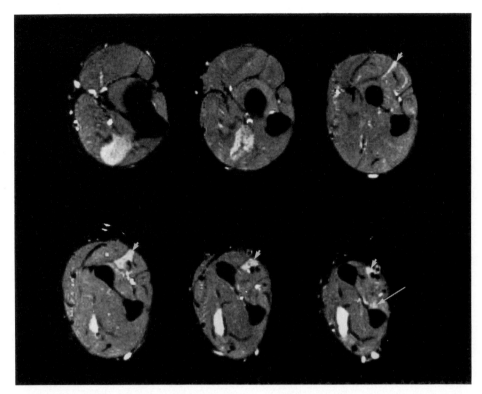

FIGURE 5.16. Index portion of flexor digitorum superficialis. Although flexion was the dominant action, recruitment of extensors of the index finger are also evident (short arrow = index portion of the digitorum communis, long arrow = extensor indicis proprius).

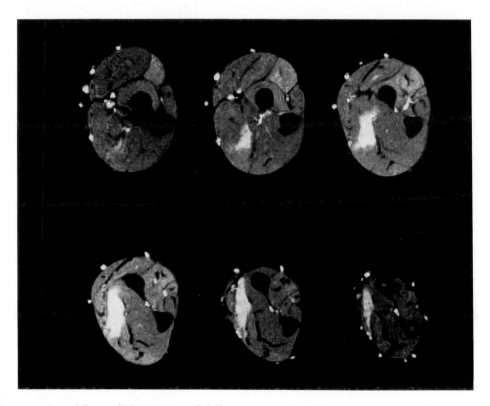

FIGURE 5.17. Long portion of flexor digitorum superficialis.

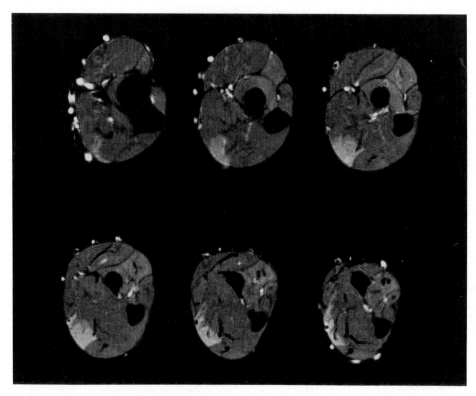

FIGURE 5.18. Ring portion of flexor digitorum superficialis.

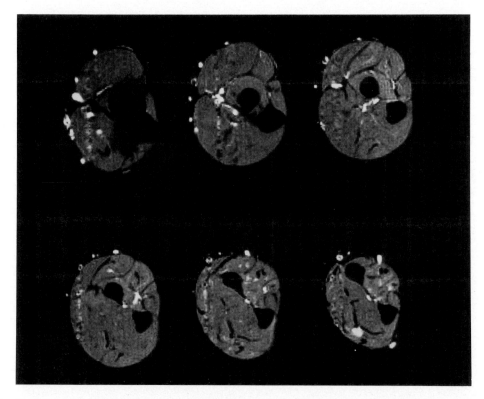

FIGURE 5.19. Small portion of flexor digitorum superficialis. Note that this finger's component does not even begin until the distal forearm.

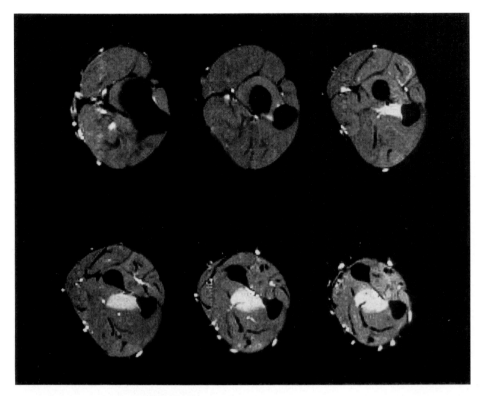

FIGURE 5.20. Index portion of flexor digitorum profundus.

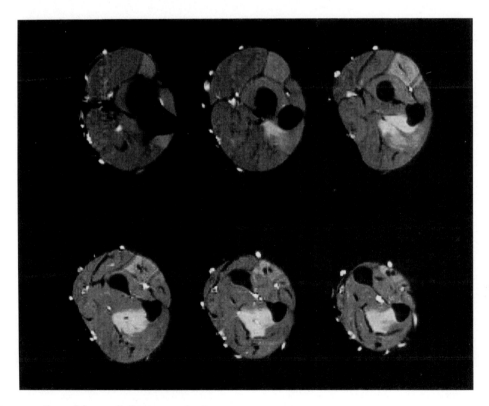

FIGURE 5.21. Long portion of flexor digitorum profundus.

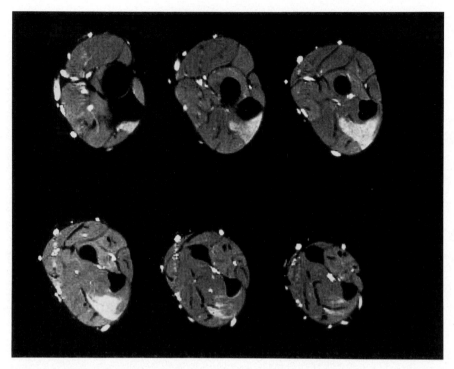

FIGURE 5.22. Ring portion of flexor digitorum profundus.

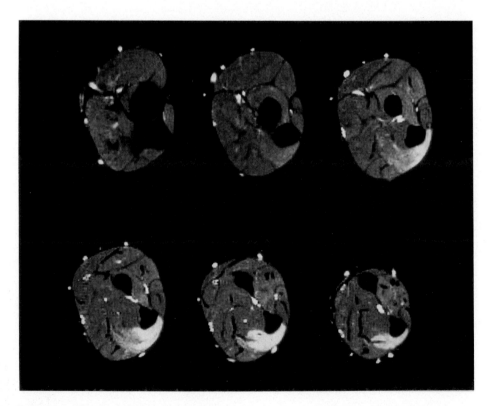

FIGURE 5.23. Small portion of flexor digitorum profundus.

The Upper Extremity: The Hand

TABLE 5.3. Abbreviations for Figures 5.24–5.27.

Abductor digiti quinti	ADQ	Interossei dorsal	DI
Abductor pollicis brevis	APB	palmar	PI
Adductor pollicis	AP	Lumbricales	L
Flexor digiti minimi	FDM	Opponens digiti minimi	ODM
Flexor pollicis brevis	FPB	Opponens pollicis	OP

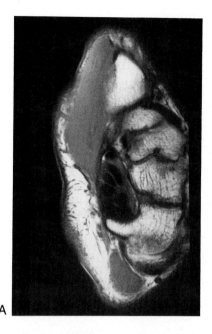

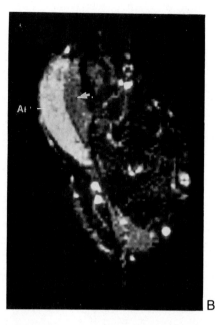

FIGURE 5.24. Proximal hand, thenar eminence, hook of hamate. (A) Unannotated T_1-weighted image. (B) Isolated abduction isolates abductor pollicis brevis in the proximal hand; however, the remaining, underlying thenar muscles, opponens pollicis and flexor pollicis brevis, cannot be distinguished.

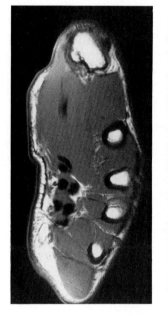

A

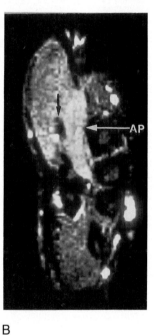

B

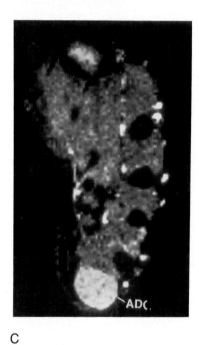

C

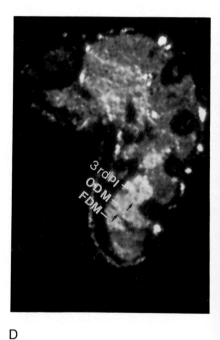

D

FIGURE 5.25. Proximal hand, mid-thenar and hypothenar eminences, proximal metacarpals. (A) Unannotated T_1-weighted image. (B) Isolated thumb adduction. The tendon of flexor pollicis longus (arrow) defines the plane between the more deeply located adductor pollicis and the superficially located thenar muscle group. (C) Isolated abduction of the small finger identifies abductor digiti quinti. (D) Opposition of the thumb and small finger against resistance further distinguishes the hypothenar muscles, including opponens digiti minimi.

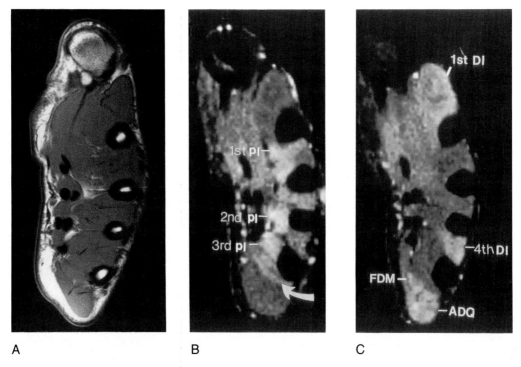

FIGURE 5.26. Mid-metacarpal level. (A) Unannotated T_1-weighted image. (B) Finger adduction toward midline of the hand primarily stresses palmar interossei. Note activation also of opponens digiti minimi (curved arrow). (C) Finger abduction away from midline.

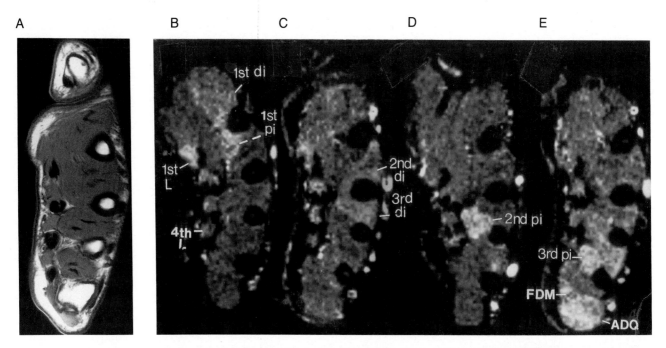

FIGURE 5.27. Distal metacarpal level. (A) Unannotated T_1-weighted image. Isolated flexion of the index (B), long (C), ring (D), and small (E) fingers recruits the relevant intrinsic hand muscles with variable isolation of lumbrical muscles.

6
MRI of the Lower Extremity

James L. Fleckenstein

The Lower Extremity: Hips and Thighs

TABLE 6.1. Abbreviations for Figures 6.1–6.12.

Adductor brevis	AB	Obturator externus	ObE
Adductor longus	AL	Pectineus	Pc
Adductor magnus	AM	Piriformis	P
Adductor minimus	Ami	Quadriceps femoris	QF
Biceps femoris-long head	BL	vastus lateralis	VL
short head	BS	vastus medialis	VM
Gastrocnemius-lateral head	Gl	vastus intermedius	VI
medial head	Gm	rectus femoris	RF
Gluteus maximus	Ma	Sartorius	S
Gracilis	G	Semimembranosus	Sm
Iliopsoas	IP	Semitendinosus	St
Levator ani	LA	Tensor fascia lata	TF

Note: Some hip muscles are included in images of trunk (Figure 4.15 through 4.19).

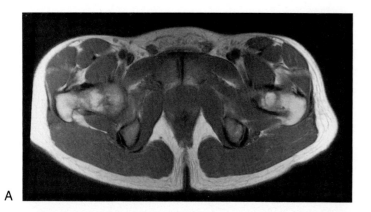

A

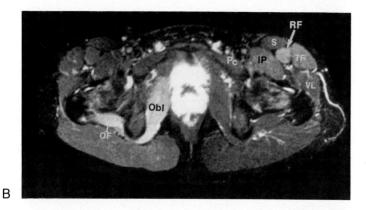

B

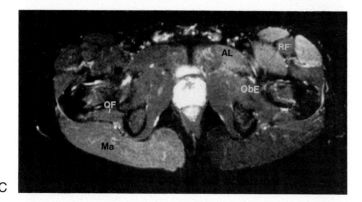

C

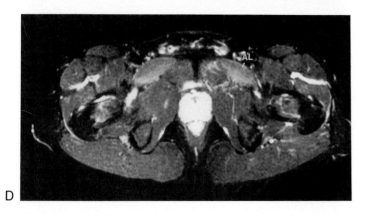

D

FIGURE 6.1. Pubic symphysis. (A) Unannotated T_1-weighted image. (B) Abduction of the flexed right hip isolates the obturator internus and quadratus femoris. During left knee extension, the rectus femoris is primarily recruited. (C) Right hip extension was performed, along with left hip flexion alternating with left thigh adduction. (D) Using a commercially available thigh adduction device popularized by television advertisements, isolated recruitment of the adductor longus is identified.

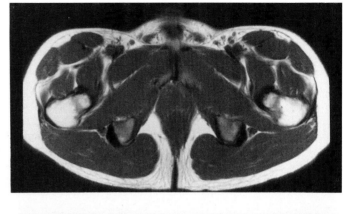

A

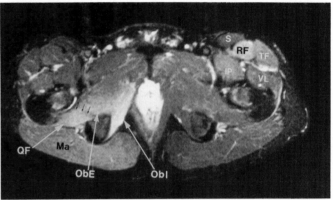

B

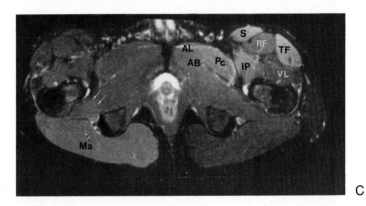

C

FIGURE 6.2. Lesser tuberosity of the femur. (A) Un-annotated T_1-weighted image. (B) Abduction of the flexed right hip isolates the obturator internus and externus and quadratus femoris. However, distinguishing them from each other is difficult. During left knee extension, the rectus femoris is primarily recruited. (C) Right hip extension results in faint distinction of quadratus femoris from obturator externus (arrows). Left hip flexion alternating with left thigh adduction. (D) Using the same device as in Figure 6.1D, separation of adductors from obturators is achieved. However, pectineus and adductor longus cannot be individually resolved.

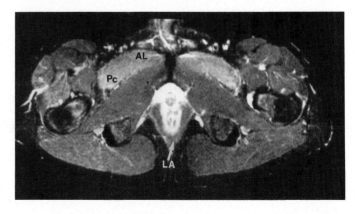

D

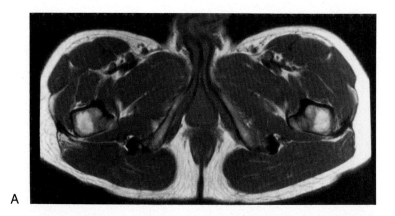

A

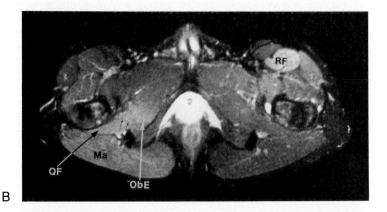

B

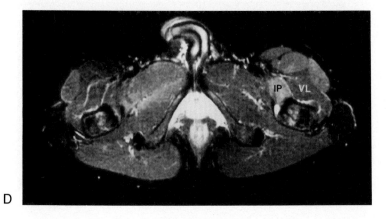

C

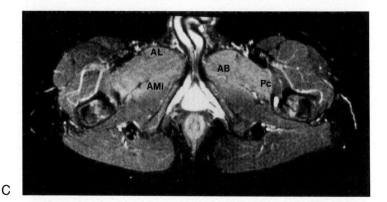

D

FIGURE 6.3. The ischia. (A) Unannotated T_1-weighted image. (B) Abduction of the flexed right hip. Note gluteus maximus is recruited relative to the same muscle on the left. During left knee extension, the rectus femoris is primarily recruited. (C) Thigh adduction. Note approximate locations of various adductors. (D) Right hip adduction. Left hip flexion shows the distal attachment of the iliopsoas onto the femur.

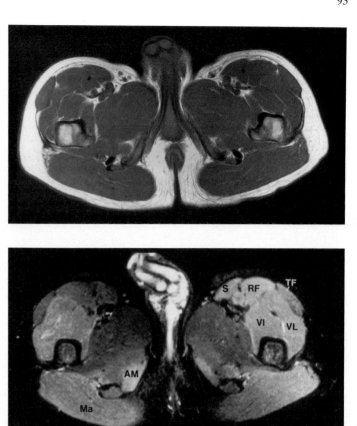

A

B

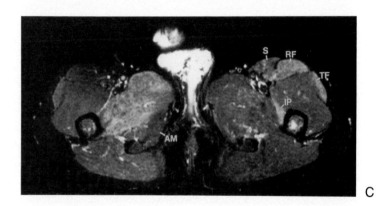

C

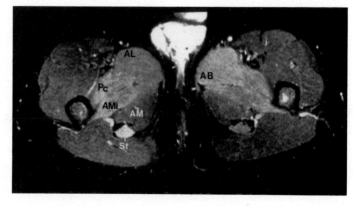

D

FIGURE 6.4. Ischial tuberosities. (A) Unannotated T_1-weighted image. (B) Cycling exercise. Note particularly little activity of the adductor muscles, with the exception of adductor magnus. (C) Left hip flexion, right thigh adduction. (D) Bilateral thigh adduction, alternating with right knee flexion and left hip extension.

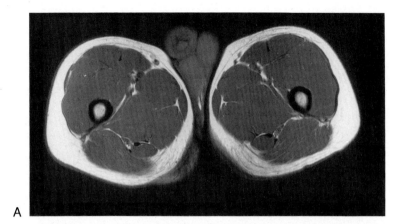

A

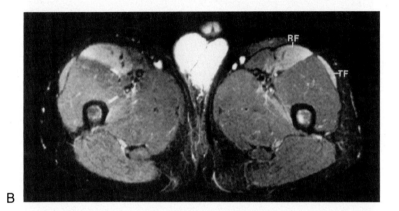

B

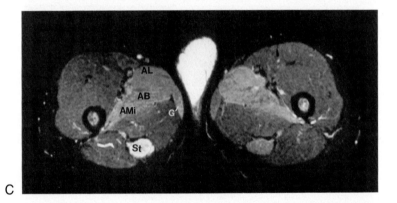

C

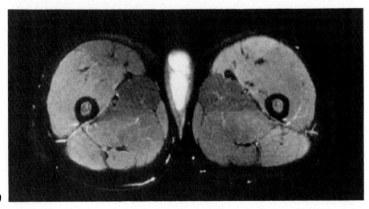

D

FIGURE 6.5. Proximal thigh, scrotum level. (A) Unannotated T_1-weighted image. (B) Quadriceps exercise? Although the manufacturer described this exercise as a "quad burner," fatigue in the anterior thigh was associated with apparent recruitment primarily of the rectus femoris and tensor fascia lata rather than the vasti. (C) Combined bilateral thigh adduction, left hip extension and right knee flexion. (D) Cycling exercise. Note recruitment pattern is analagous to an "inverse image" of that produced by thigh adduction, as in Figure 6.5C.

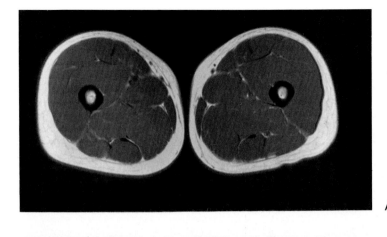

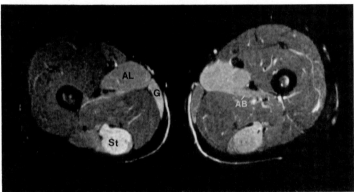

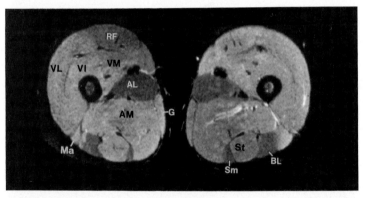

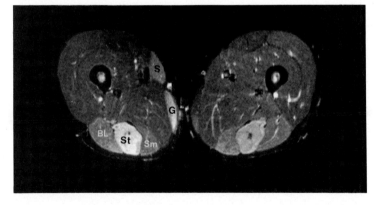

FIGURE 6.6. Proximal thigh, approximately 5 cm below Figure 6.5. (A) Unannotated T_1-weighted image. (B) Combined bilateral thigh adduction, left hip extension and right knee flexion. Note relatively clear separation of adductor longus from adductor brevis. (C) Cycling exercise. (D) Left hip extension and right knee flexion.

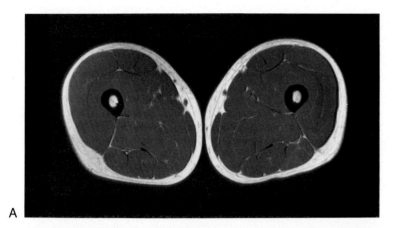

A

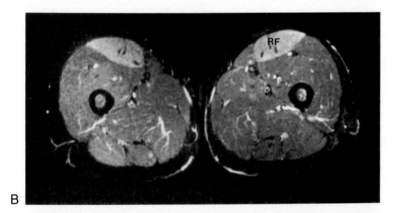

B

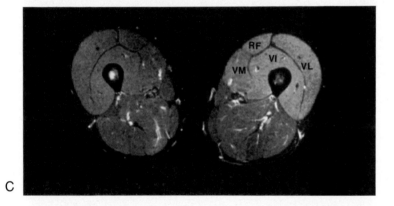

C

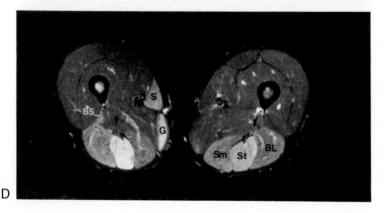

D

FIGURE 6.7. Proximal thigh, approximately 5 cm distal to Figure 6.6. (A) Unannotated T_1-weighted image. (B) "Quad burner" exercise. (C) A real "quad burner": this exercise was performed by sitting against a wall without the benefit of a chair with the knees and hips flexed for approximately 1 minute before the MRI. Note that all of the quadriceps muscles are recruited, particularly on the left. (D) Left hip extension, right knee flexion. Note the short head of the biceps femoris is recruited during knee flexion but not the hip extension.

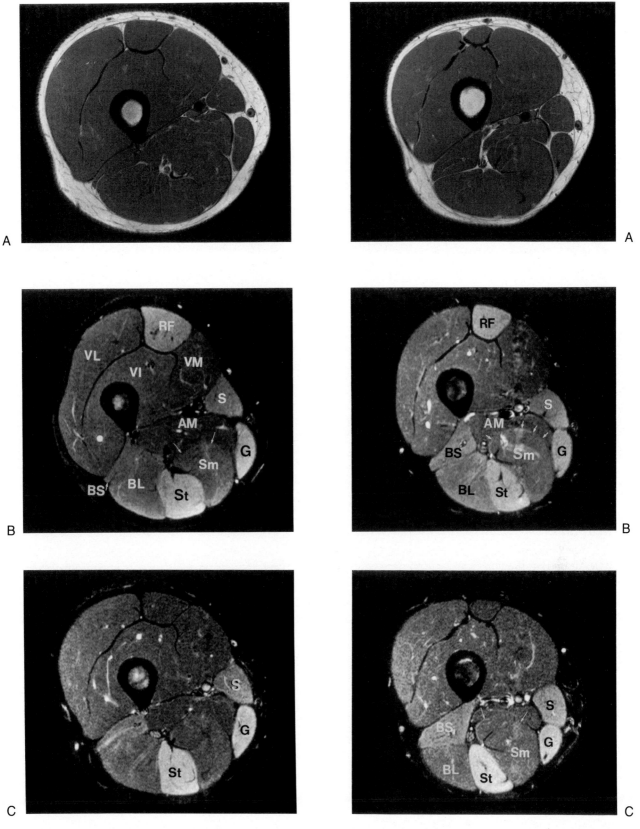

FIGURE 6.8. Mid-thigh level. (A) Unannotated T_1-weighted image. (B) Knee flexion combined with knee extension. Note subtle boundaries between the adductor magnus and the semi-membranosus. (C) Isolated knee flexion.

FIGURE 6.9. 3 cm distal to Figure 6.8. (A) Unannotated T_1-weighted image. (B) Combined knee flexion and extension. (C) Isolated knee flexion. Note distinction between the long and short heads of the biceps femoris and subtle distinction between the distal-most adductor magnus and semimembranosus.

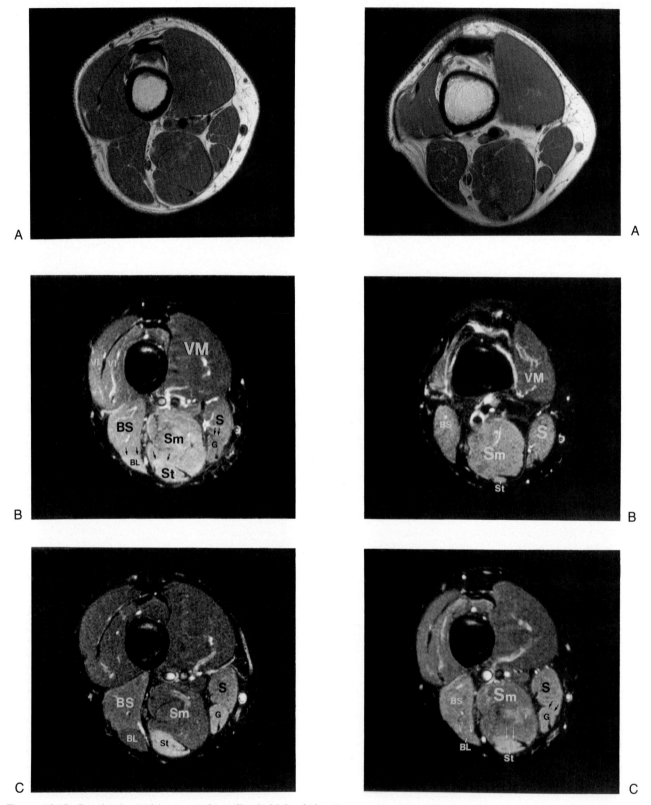

FIGURE 6.10. Proximal quadriceps tendon, distal thigh. (A) Unannotated T_1-weighted image. (B) Isolated hip extension. (C) Isolated knee flexion.

FIGURE 6.11. 3 cm distal to Figure 6.10. (A) Unannotated T_1-weighted image. (B) Hip extension. (C) Knee flexion.

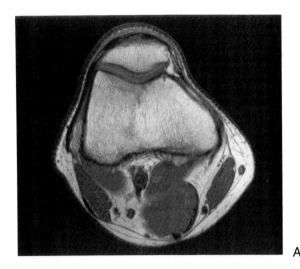

A

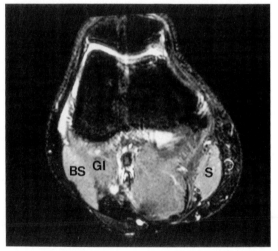

B

C

FIGURE 6.12. Patellofemoral articulation. (A) Unannotated T_1-weighted image. (B) Ankle plantar flexion. Note that the medial head of the gastrocnemius muscle is faintly differentiable from the semimembranosus. (C) Knee flexion. Note distinction of distal sartorius and short head of biceps femoris from gastrocnemius muscles. The lateral head of the gastrocnemius marks the approximate location of the origin of the plantaris muscle, when it is present. The plantaris, a variable muscle, is absent from this individual.

The Lower Extremity: The Leg

TABLE 6.2. Abbreviations for Figures 6.13–6.18.

Extensor digitorum longus	ED	Peroneal group (i.e., peroneal longus and brevis)	PG
Extensor hallucis longus	EHL	Peroneus longus	PL
Flexor digitorum longus	FD	Popliteus	Po
Flexor hallucis longus	FHL	Soleus	So
Gastrocnemius		Tibialis anterior	AT
medial head	Gm	Tibialis posterior	TP
lateral head	Gl		

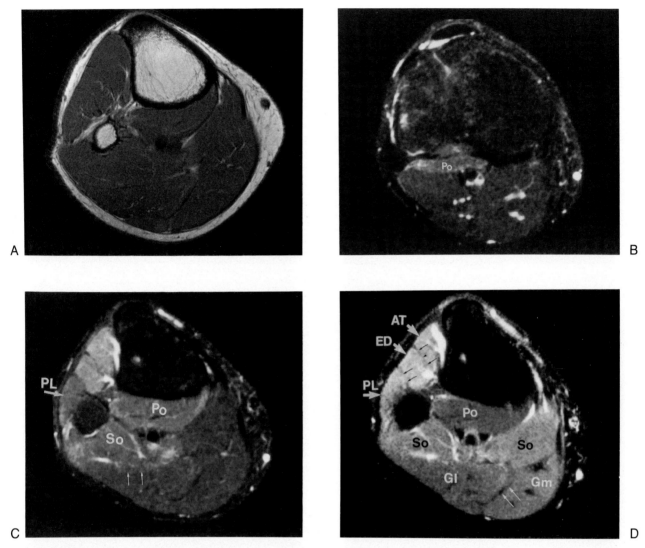

FIGURE 6.13. Proximal leg, 8 cm distal to patellofemoral articulation. (A) Unannotated T_1-weighted image. (B) External rotation of the leg. At a level 3 cm proximal to that shown in Figure 6.13A, isolated activation of the popliteus is observed. (C) Same exercise as in preceding image, but at same level as Figure 6.13A. At this proximal location of the leg, the peroneal longus is the only lateral compartment muscle present. On images obtained more distally, distinction between peroneal longus and brevis is not possible. On those images, the lateral compartment is denoted by "PG," indicating "peroneal group." (D) Ankle dorsiflexion exercise: Note lack of recruitment of the popliteus muscle and that soleus is thinner in the midline of the leg than in the more lateral and medial portions. Note also how far medial the lateral head extends; this medial extension is where the plantaris is usually found (small, thin arrows).

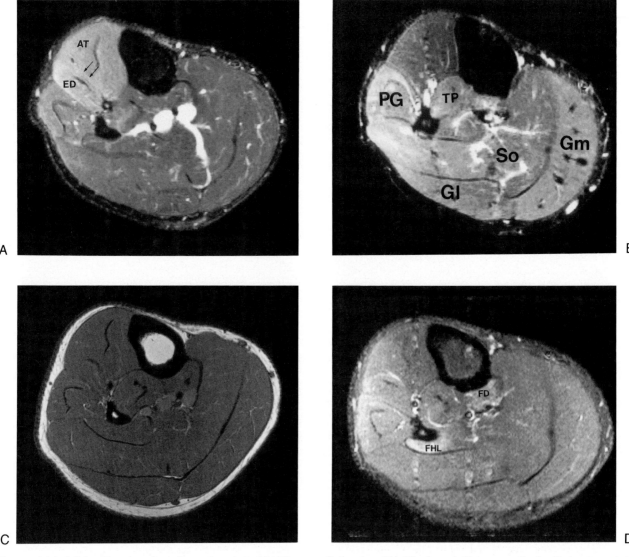

FIGURE 6.14. Mid-calf: point of maximum leg girth. (A) Unannotated T_1-weighted image. (B) Ankle plantarflexion with recruitment of most muscles excluding the anterior compartment. (C) Ankle dorsiflexion fails to discriminate muscles of the anterior compartment, i.e., tibialis anterior and extensor digitorum. (D) Flexion of all toes results in distinction of the great toe flexor, flexor hallucis longus, from that of the remaining toes, flexor digitorum longus. These muscles are shown near their origins here.

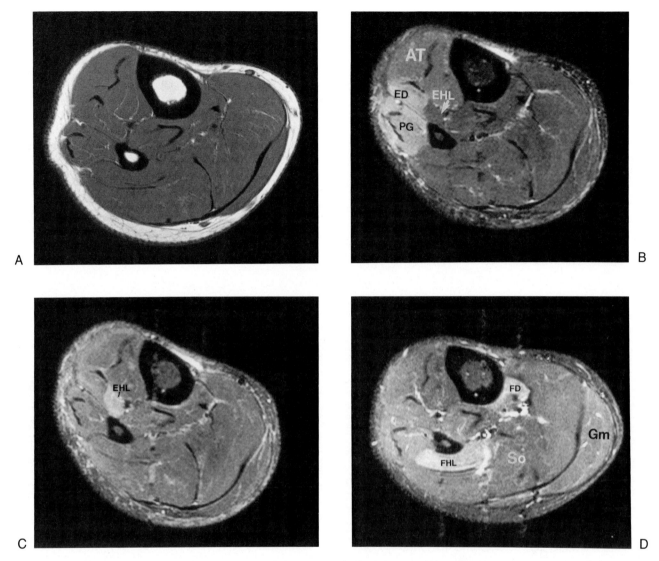

FIGURE 6.15. Distal aspect of the gastrocnemius. (A) Unannotated T_1-weighted image. (B) Ankle eversion, with great toe flexed so as to isolate the extensor digitorum from the extensor hallucis longus. (C) Isolated great toe extension. (D) Flexion of great and other toes, as in Figure 6.14D.

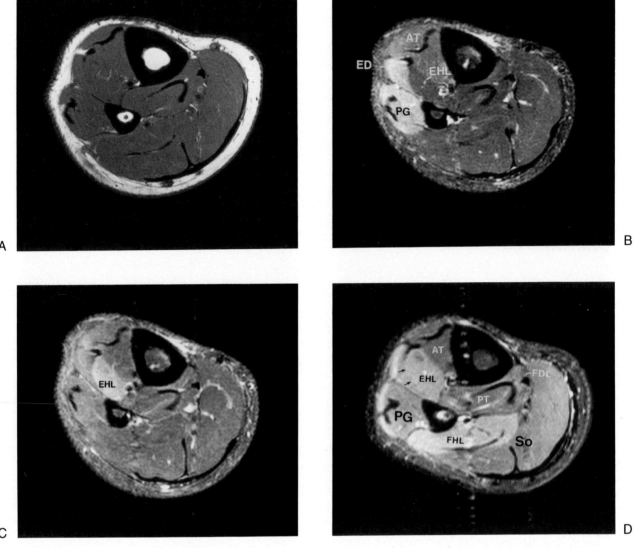

FIGURE 6.16. Mid-leg, 2 cm distal to Figure 6.15. (A) Unannotated T_1-weighted image. (B) Ankle eversion as in Figure 6.15B. (C) Isolated great toe extension as in Figure 6.15C. (D) Great toe exercise. Although flexion of the great toe was intended to be isolated, recruitment of the extensor could not be avoided.

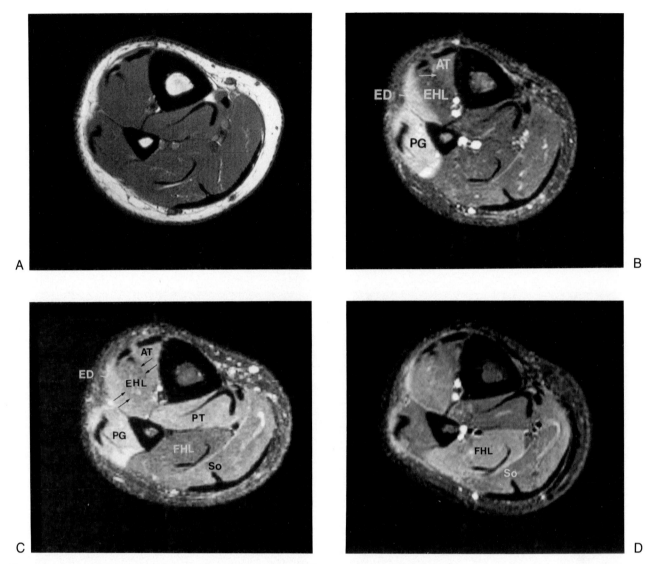

FIGURE 6.17. 2 cm distal to Figure 6.16. (A) Unannotated T_1-weighted image. (B) Ankle eversion, as in Figures 6.15B and 6.16B. (C) Although isolated ankle inversion was attempted so as to distinguish the tibialis posterior, recruitment of the peroneal group could not be avoided. (D) Great toe flexion.

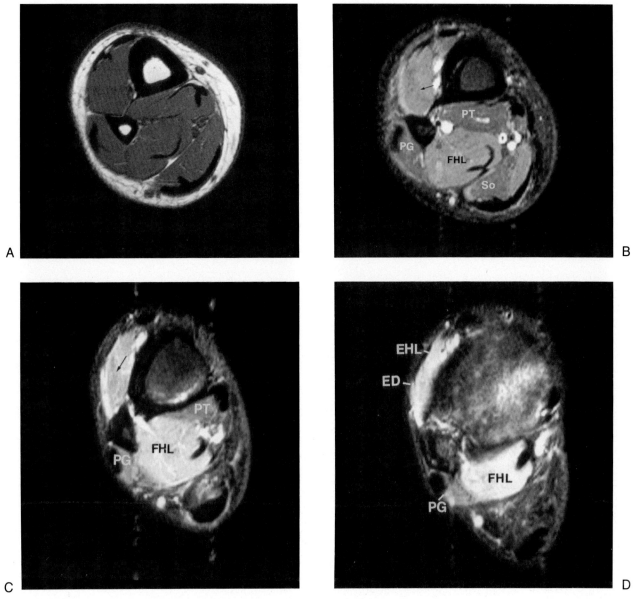

FIGURE 6.18. Distal soleus, 3 cm distal to Figure 6.17. (A) Unannotated T_1-weighted image. (B) Great toe flexion. (C) Great toe flexion 2 cm distal to Figure 6.18B. Recruitment of antagonistic toe extensors could not be avoided. (D) Great toe flexion 2 cm distal to Figure 6.18C.

The Lower Extremity: The Foot

TABLE 6.3. Abbreviations for Figures 6.19–6.22.

Abductor digiti minimi	ADM	Flexor digiti minimi	FDM
Abductor hallucis	AH	Flexor digitorum brevis	FDB
Adductor hallucis	ADH	Flexor hallucis brevis	FHB
transverse head	ADHt	lateral head	FHBl
oblique head	ADHo	medial head	FHBm
Extensor digitorum brevis	DB	Interossei (dorsal and plantar)	I
Extensor hallucis brevis	HB	Quadratus plantae	QP

Note: These images were obtained in the coronal plane with respect to the long axis of the foot.

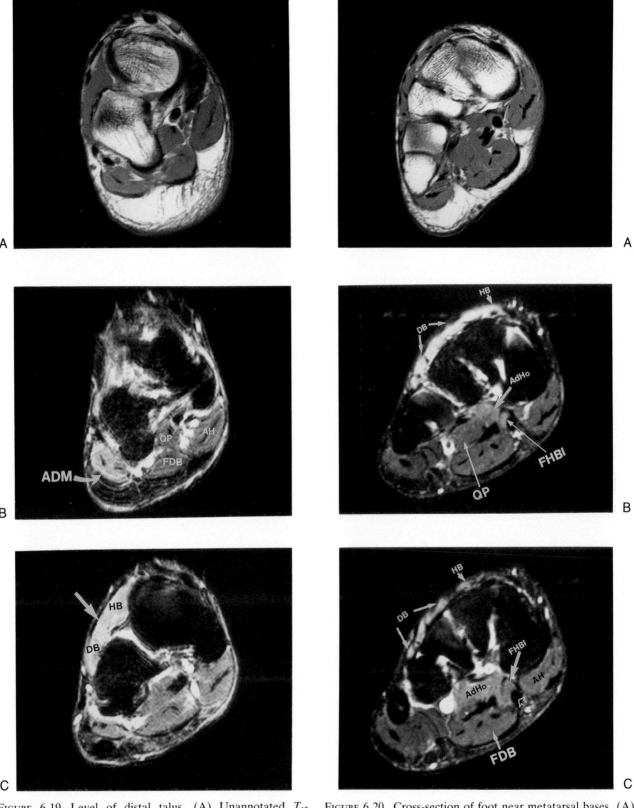

FIGURE 6.19. Level of distal talus. (A) Unannotated T_1-weighted image. (B) Abduction of small and great toes. At level 1 cm distal to Figure 6.19A, note that abductor digiti minimi is highlighted slightly. (C) Toe extension. Discrimination between toe extensors is difficult (arrow).

FIGURE 6.20. Cross-section of foot near metatarsal bases. (A) Unannotated T_1-weighted image. (B) Great toe flexion. (C) Great toe flexion, 1 cm distal to Figure 6.20B. Note close proximity of the lateral head of flexor hallicus brevis to the tendon of flexor hallicus longus (arrowhead). Note that adductor hallicus is recruited and that it replaces the position of quadratus plantae deep to toe flexors.

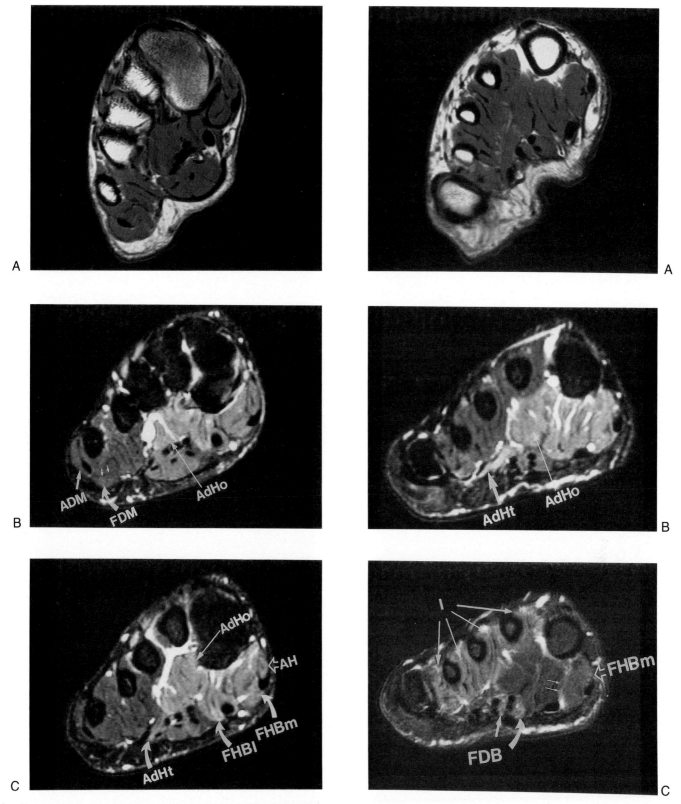

FIGURE 6.21. 2 cm distal to Figure 6.20. (A) Unannotated T_1-weighted image. (B) Great toe flexion. (C) Great toe flexion 1 cm distal to Figure 6.21B.

FIGURE 6.22. Level of fifth metatarsal head. (A) Unannotated T_1-weighted image. (B) Great toe flexion. Note the two heads of adductor hallucis. (C) Flexion of four toes with attempted exclusion of the great toe. Note recruitment of all visualized interossei and of medial head of flexor hallucis brevis.

Part III
Muscle Physiology and Pathophysiology

7
Diagnostic Imaging of Skeletal Muscle Exercise Physiology and Pathophysiology

Frank G. Shellock, Lesia L. Tyson, and James L. Fleckenstein

For many years, the study of skeletal muscle physiology and pathophysiology did not benefit significantly from radiological technology. This is because older technologies relied upon high-energy photons, such as x-rays and gamma rays, which are highly limited in their ability to detect the mesenchymal alterations that occur during exercise and sports injuries (Chapter 1). Moreover, the ionizing nature of these techniques prevented their use in healthy subjects for obvious ethical reasons.

The arrival of ultrasound enhanced the noninvasive study of muscle morphology. Because of the safety of the technique, it could theoretically enable the investigation of physiological aspects of muscle in normal volunteers. However, through the 1960s and 1970s, ultrasound was used primarily by industry to probe the composition of muscle to noninvasively assess the quality of meat in livestock.[1] Other than assessment of muscle size,[2-4] ultrasound was not applied to the study of human muscle physiology and pathophysiology. More recently, however, ultrasound was used to probe physiological issues related to muscular contraction.[5-7]

The ability to obtain cross-sectional images of human limbs using ultrasound and especially computed tomography (CT) allowed reliable quantitation of a critical determinant of human muscular performance: muscle size. CT enabled relatively simple digitization of muscle cross-sectional areas and so eliminated the dependence of physiologists upon anthropomorphic measurements of limb size. Although these modern techniques markedly improved the measurement of muscle size,[8-11] the requirement of ionizing radiation made direct measurement of muscle volume impractical and unethical, especially given that subjects in whom such measurements are of interest include primarily individuals who are healthy and in whom any health risk of imaging is prohibitive. This health issue was not trivial, because it prevented application of the technique of functional assessments of muscle during exercise, an application that has been exploited to a considerable extent by magnetic resonance imaging (MRI).

MRI is highly valuable as a tool in the study of skeletal muscle anatomy, exercise physiology, and exercise pathophysiology. Structural determinations of healthy skeletal muscle are now possible on any MRI device. These include cross-sectional area,[11-26] volume,[12-15] and inertial moment arm lengths.[27] Additional, more sophisticated techniques have been applied in preliminary studies to monitor electrical conductance through striated muscle[28,29] and measurements of muscle motion,[30-32] including velocity,[30] and related measurements of muscle displacement.[31] Less technically challenging, but still largely in development, include MR techniques of determining muscle fiber type,[33-35] perfusion,[36] and fiber architecture.[13,16,23,24] Perhaps the most intensively studied physiological phenomenon is that of changes in muscle water content during exercise.[36-64]

Just as the overlying skin hides skeletal muscle from direct evaluation in studies of muscle physiology, so has it hampered studies probing basic mechanisms that underlie muscle pathophysiology in patient groups. From the seemingly benign condition that all of us have experienced after indulging in an exercise activity to which we are unaccustomed [i.e., delayed onset muscle soreness (DOMS)], to the more burdensome problems of acute muscle injuries and their sequelae, and the life-threatening conditions of muscular dystrophy and rhabdomyolysis, MRI continues to develop as an important tool to unwrap the shroud of mystery that envelopes muscle by allowing the safe visualization of compositional changes that accompany these processes.[65-76]

This chapter will detail progress made in using MR imaging of skeletal muscle in studies of exercise physiology and pathophysiology.

MRI Technique

Although the physical processes involved in MR imaging are provided elsewhere (Chapter 3), a review of the sensitivity of available pulse sequences to physiological changes in muscle proton relaxation times is appropriate. It is important to recall that in its quiescent state, normal skeletal muscle has an intermediate-to-long T_1 relaxation time and a short T_2 relaxation time relative to other soft tissues.[39,47,65–67] During exercise, the transient increase in water content that occurs in muscle causes prolongation of the T_2 relaxation time, as well as an increase in proton density.[36–64] Reports on the change in T_1 relaxation time with exercise are more variable, ranging from large[39,45] to small[36,37,47] changes.

Part of the reason for the disparity in T_1 values likely results from the method of measurement. In a progressive saturation scheme, such as that used in most MRI studies, at least two separate pulse sequences with different repetition times (T_R) are applied during a time interval that the T_1, and especially T_2, is changing. This contrasts the situation whereby T_2 is measured, in which a single T_R is used and at least two echoes are selected to monitor transverse relaxation.

One of the coauthors (JLF) recalculated data originally indicating a large T_1 time.[39] When the order of serially acquired sequences used to calculate the T_1 was altered (from long T_R-short T_R to short T_R-long T_R), the exercise-induced change in T_1 was no longer significant (unpublished observations). This led to an experiment using many T_Rs applied during periods of vascular occlusion imposed in order to assure stability of the T_2 time during the measurement intervals. This experiment confirmed a significant increase in the T_1 time of exercised muscle.[36] However, the magnitude was much less than that of T_2, supporting Bratton's early observations[37] and those of subsequent investigators who used signal intensity of T_1 weighted (short T_E/short T_R) images to infer T_1 time changes.[47]

T_1-weighted images are not only poorly sensitive to acute changes in muscle fluid content during exercise, but are also poorly sensitive to the larger changes in muscle water that accompany exertion-related muscle injuries.[65] However, T_1-weighted spin echo pulse sequences are useful for the study of pathophysiology of sports injuries, for example, by revealing the presence of substances having short T_1 relaxation times, such as subacute hematoma and fatty infiltration of muscles.[65] In addition, because the signal-to-noise ratio is relatively high on T_1-weighted spin echo pulse sequences, they are useful for demonstrating anatomic relationships, such as between muscle and fascia (Figure 7.1).

T_2-weighted (long T_R, long T_E) spin echo pulse sequences are very useful in the study of muscle in health and disease because of their high sensitivity to increases

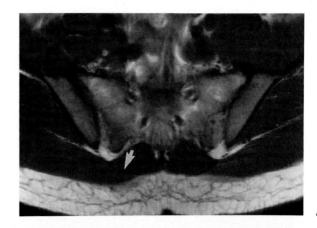

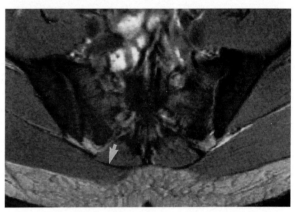

FIGURE 7.1. MRI sequence choices to study anatomy of muscle at rest. Comparing axial T_1-weighted spin echo image (500/15, A) of pelvis to T_1-weighted gradient echo image (500/15/90°, B) shows similar contrast between the tissues but note how fascial boundaries between muscles, such as between the multifidus and gluteus muscles (arrow), are more readily seen using the gradient echo sequence.

in muscle water content, as previously reviewed.[36] Hence, the typical appearance of edematous muscle is that of negligible change on T_1-weighted images and clearly increased signal change on T_2-weighted images. Although difficulties arise when one uses MRI to search for edematous changes in muscle that contains large amounts of fat (see Chapters 12 and 21), fatty infiltration is rare in individuals without neuromuscular disease.

Short tau (inversion time) inversion recovery (STIR) sequences are sensitive to the additive effects of the changes in muscle T_1, T_2, and proton density that occur with exercise or injury. Suppression of signal from fat is an added benefit of the STIR sequence because fat and edema may have similar appearances on T_2-weighted spin echo images. Hence, as a single sequence, it is highly attractive in the evaluation of physiological and pathophysiological edema. Thus, it is not surprising that STIR has been used with high frequency in published reports on MRI of sports medicine.[65,71–74]

A limitation of conventional STIR imaging is the relatively long acquisition time required for imaging. Decreased imaging times have been achieved with STIR sequences by decreasing the T_R, the number of excitations, and the number of phase encoding steps.[72] More recently, dramatic time savings have been achieved by performing phase encoding on successive echoes [i.e., fast spin echo (FSE) sequences]. Tissue contrast characteristics of FSE sequences are only slightly different from those obtained using conventional imaging.[76] Therefore, the STIR sequence has continued to dominate studies designed to identify changes in water content associated with exercise or signal intensity alterations related to exertional muscle injuries.

It is possible to generate images that are similar in contrast to the STIR sequence by use of T_2-weighted FSE sequences with frequency-selective pulses to suppress signal from fat. However, these are generally not as robust as STIR due to their stringent need for high magnetic field homogeneity; also, in order to have the same sensitivity to muscle edema as STIR, longer T_E times are needed (see Chapter 21).

Gradient echo pulse sequences have been used to study muscular anatomy, exercise-induced enhancement of skeletal muscle, and muscle injuries with relatively short scan times.[39,65,70] This is usually accomplished by T_2^*-weighted sequences, using a short flip angle to minimize the effects of T_1 differences on the image. Gradient echo pulse sequences may be used for anatomic depiction of muscle anatomy because they produce an outlining or "India ink" effect that accentuates interfaces between muscle and fascia (Figure 7.1). This facilitates the determination of individual muscle groups and is especially useful when examining complex anatomy. Gradient echo sequences with inclusion of a saturation pulse, applied off the resonance peak of free water protons, can be used to increase the information available regarding the physical state of water in the tissue. This has been applied in physiological studies of skeletal muscle to characterize acute effects of brief intense exercise on muscle water,[39-42] as well as in studies of pathological conditions, such as compartment syndromes (see Chapter 28).

An obvious advantage to using MRI for assessment of skeletal muscle is that multiple imaging planes are possible. The axial plane allows simultaneous visualization of all the muscles in a cross-section of an extremity, facilitating comparison of muscle signal intensities between adjacent functional groups. In certain regions, however, such as the shoulder and pelvic girdles, the long axes of some muscles run orthogonal to the axial plane. In these cases, sagittal, coronal, or oblique planes may optimize the anatomic depiction. In general, however, longitudinal planes are most useful to supplement the scan, allowing localization of bony landmarks and determination of the spatial extent of signal intensity changes.

MR Imaging of Skeletal Muscle at Rest

Obtaining morphometric measurements on human skeletal muscle is important for a variety of research and clinical applications. These include the assessment of muscle size as a primary determinant of muscular strength. Using MRI, one can simultaneously study muscle size as well as obtain detailed information about the other connective tissues, and hence arrive at data sets that provide comprehensive biophysical measures. For example, one can combine muscle size with bone lengths to calculate lever arm distances and moment arm lengths for biomechanical studies.[27] Such parameters can be used to assess efficacy of strength training in healthy individuals and of physical rehabilitation programs in neuromuscular and orthopedic disorders.[4,14,16]

Cross-Sectional Area, Architecture, and Volume Assessment of Skeletal Muscle

A decrease or increase in muscle fiber cross-sectional area is believed to be the major mechanism responsible for skeletal muscle atrophy or hypertrophy in athletes and/or patients. The clinical determination of atrophy or hypertrophy may be limited by overlying subcutaneous fat, by deep fat stores, and/or by normal muscles surrounding the focal changes that occur in some neuromuscular diseases.[65] Hypertrophic and atrophic muscles may be present simultaneously in some of these disorders, resulting in no clinically detectable change in overall muscle bulk. Furthermore, the presence of hypertrophied muscles may compensate functionally for atrophied muscles, complicating strength testing assessments of improvement or deterioration of specific muscle groups.

Because of its superior soft tissue contrast and the lack of ionizing radiation, MRI allows the safe quantitation of muscle cross-sectional areas and even total muscle volumes for intraindividual and interindividual analysis of muscle size. In addition, MRI has been shown to provide accurate information regarding in vivo muscle architecture, as described by Fukunaga et al.[13] and Narici et al.[23,24] This information is critical for complete evaluation of muscle function because the maximum force exerted by a muscle is related to the total cross-sectional area of all of the fibers in a group, and the maximum rate of shortening is related to the length of the longest fibers within the muscle.[13]

Previous human studies designed to examine and characterize muscle volume and fiber architecture relied upon data obtained from cadavers. However, there are major limitations of predicting functional properties of muscle from cadaveric studies. For example, spurious alterations in muscle volume and morphology can be introduced by fixation and other treatment-related artifacts of the sample. Also, cadaveric material is frequently obtained from elderly subjects in whom disuse atrophy likely preceded death.[13] Obviously, MRI studies performed in vivo have no similar limitations in assessing muscle morphology.

Changes in muscle cross-sectional area of human quadriceps seen on MRI were correlated with changes in force and neural activation by Narici et al.[16] Strength training produced hypertrophy, which accounted for a 40% increase in force, whereas the remaining 60% was attributed to an increase in neural drive and, possibly, to changes in muscle architecture.[16] Roman et al.[14] used MRI to assess the effects of resistance training on muscle mass in elderly men. In that study, a heavy resistance exercise program increased the volume of elbow flexors by 14%, as determined by MRI. Roman et al.[14] also showed that measuring muscle volume, as opposed to CSA, eliminated a source of potential intraindividual variation in muscle size determination because significant differences in CSA occurred when one slice level was compared to a contiguous level. This meant that slight differences in the precise location at which CSA was determined could adversely affect the accuracy of repeated determinations of muscle size.

The role of muscle size as a determinant of strength is best determined by quantitating the volume of muscle actually performing the activity.[14,20,21] In a related application, the volume of muscle damaged by exercise correlated well with the decrement in strength.[15] In a study of the effect of simulated weightlessness in human subjects during 5 wks of horizontal bed rest, LeBlanc et al.[18] used MRI to assess calf muscle area. Differential muscle losses occurred whereby there were significant decreases in the cross-sectional area of the ankle plantar flexors without any substantial alteration seen in the mass of the dorsiflexors. In addition, the affected muscles had significant decreases in muscular strength. Hather et al. reported a similar loss of lower limb muscle mass associated with another form of simulated weightlessness, lower limb suspension, which was documented using MRI measurements of muscle cross-sectional areas.[26] In a study having potential relevance to rehabilitation medicine, Kariya et al.[17] used MRI to evaluate the functional condition of atrophied thigh muscles after cruciate ligament injuries. Besides the presence of decreased muscle volume of the quadriceps, T_2 values were also prolonged in the vastus lateralis, vastus intermedius, and vastus medialis, presumably as a result of disuse. However, LeBlanc et al.[18,19,25,66] used MRI to investigate models of disuse [i.e., simulated weightlessness in humans (bed rest) and animals (tail

suspension)]. Despite the presence of atrophied muscle, there were no changes in T_1 or T_2 relaxation times to promote the likelihood of additional pathologic conditions.[19,66] Hence, compositional changes of muscle that occur as muscle size changes remains an area needing clarification from future MRI investigations.

Multiple cross-sectional images obtained using MRI can be reformatted using commercially available computer software to display in one image all the morphologic information acquired on multiple consecutive two-dimensional images[12,15] (Figures 7.2, 7.3). In this way, three-dimensional reconstruction of skeletal muscle from MRI can improve the delineation of pathological from normal muscles.

Muscle Fiber Typing

Skeletal muscle fiber composition is adapted by heredity and activity for the work that the fibers are required to perform. One classification scheme designates the type of muscle fibers based on how rapidly the fibers produce a twitch contraction in response to an electrical stimulus. These slow-twitch and fast-twitch fibers have unique qualities with respect to contractile speed, metabolism, and neural factors. Slow-twitch fibers possess high concentrations of oxidative enzymes whereas either oxidative or glycolytic enzymes dominate in fast-twitch fibers, with the majority being primarily glycolytic. Because of the importance of the specific muscle fiber type involved in neuromuscular disease and in exercise science, an invasive procedure, the muscle biopsy, is often performed to determine fiber types.

To date, MRI is the only imaging technique used to probe muscle fiber-type composition[33,77] (Figure 7.4). However, results and conclusions of these studies lack uniformity. Adzamli et al. first reported prolongation of proton T_2 and T_1 relaxation times in slow-, compared to fast-twitch rabbit muscles, a difference that was proportional to the greater extracellular water content of the slow-twitch fibers.[33] The importance of water compartmentation was substantiated by a higher concentration of infused gadolinium DTPA, a marker of the extracellular space, in slow-twitch fibers. Interestingly, data from one group studying humans reported opposite findings. There, muscle proton T_1 and T_2 relaxation times positively correlated with the percentage of fast-twitch fibers.[34,35] A subsequent study in humans found no correlation between T_2 and percentage of fast-twitch fibers.[77] Interestingly, that study found the correlation between muscle T_1 relaxation time and the percentage of fast twitch to be negative, not positive as Kuno et al.[35] reported. The negative correlation is more consistent with the findings from animal studies. The reason(s) for apparent discrepancies between studies is unknown. In summary,

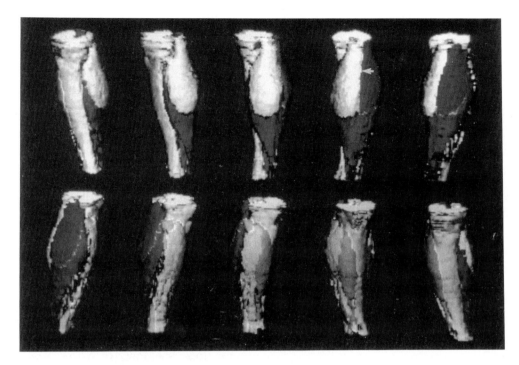

FIGURE 7.2. Three-dimensional rendering of multiple axial T_1-weighted images of lower leg shows muscle volume and morphology of individual muscle groups (note that three-dimensional model is rotated incrementally, 15°).

although additional work is required to define the role and accuracy of MRI in muscle fiber type analysis, results to date are promising.

Dynamic MRI of Skeletal Muscle

The effects of contraction on skeletal muscle are many, including physical, chemical, and physiological. A detailed analysis of these processes exceeds the scope of this chapter. However, where radiological techniques have impacted the study of muscle contraction merits discussion because the noninvasive nature of these tools advances the ability of scientists to probe the basic mechanisms of muscle contraction.

In an effort to improve biomechanical modeling of complex musculoskeletal motion, advantage is taken of the flexibility of MRI pulse sequence schemes. In one

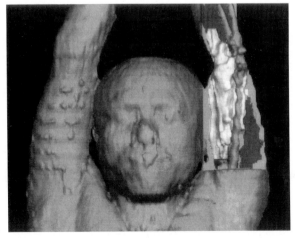
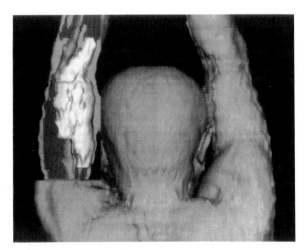

A   B

FIGURE 7.3. Three-dimensional renderings of postinjury axial T_2-weighted images superimposed on high-resolution T_1-weighted images shown in (A) anterior and (B) posterior projections reveal high signal intensity primarily localized to biceps and brachialis muscles.

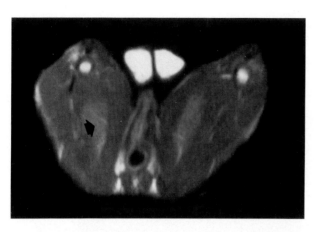

FIGURE 7.4. Physiological variations of muscle on MRI in a rabbit model. Fiber-type heterogeneity can be stuided by MRI of quiescent muscle, as demonstrated in a 2000/60 coronal image of New Zealand White rabbit thighs in which the semi-tendinosus muscle (arrow), composed purely of type 1 fibers, shows much higher signal intensity than nearby muscles composed of more nearly purely type 2 fibers. This is a normal finding in this breed of rabbit.

approach, a grid of radiofrequency-tagged planes is deposited simultaneously and changes in their position following contraction allows assessment of muscle motion.[32] However, rapid fading of the tags due to T_1 decay limits the efficacy of the technique. An alternative technique to monitor muscle displacements involves phase contrast measurement and encoding of velocities of muscle movement during contraction. This was initially established as a means to measure and analyze one-dimensional longitudinal velocity vectors of cyclic human muscle motion.[30] Subsequently, the technique was extended to analyze spatial trajectories in multiple dimensions.[31] Although in an early state of development, biomechanical studies currently suggested by the available technology include assessments of regional deformation, shear strain, tensile strain, strain development rate, and possibly muscle activation patterns. Although clinical studies have yet to be conducted, one reasonable application to neuromuscular disease relates to studies designed to probe mechanisms underlying improvements observed in contractile function in patients with muscular dystrophy after treatment with electrical stimulation or lengthening procedures.

Technical developments in ultrasound imaging have also been applied to biomechanical aspects of muscle contraction. The velocity profiles of isometric muscle contraction, passive muscle motion, and tendon reflex intensity have been studied using a modified Doppler ultrasound technique. In an initial investigation of muscle contraction, Grubb et al.[6] studied time to peak velocity, velocity range, and relaxation times. For reflex contractions, the latency period, area under the velocity curve, and duration of contraction were assessed. Isometric muscle contraction was distinguishable from passive movement by a higher tissue velocity range, by a more rapid initial acceleration slope, and by the velocity differential across the muscle. The convenience of the ultrasound technique is particularly attractive in this application. This study, together with others that indicate the sensitivity of ultrasound in evaluating muscle morphology and fasciculations,[5] argues for a growing potential for ultrasound imaging in evaluating patients with neuromuscular diseases.

Radiology of Muscle Water Shifts During Exercise

One of the first biological applications of proton magnetic resonance was of skeletal muscle stimulation.[37] In that study, an increase in the T_2 relaxation time of frog muscle was observed to occur after a series of stimulated contractions. This change in T_2 was argued to result from liberation of water from that fraction normally bound to macromolecules in the basal state. Years later, similar changes in proton T_2 were shown to occur in stimulated rabbit muscle in which blood flow had ceased due to aortic occlusion, indicating that perfusion was not the cause of the changes.[38] In humans, the same effect on muscle T_2 relaxation times has been the subject of considerable interest. These exercise-induced changes occur as part of a transient, normal phenomenon resulting from a complex combination of physiological and physical processes that merit further consideration.

A number of putative effectors of exercise-induced changes in muscle proton T_2 relaxation times have been put forth since the original description of the effect in 1988.[39] An obvious candidate, postexercise hyperemia, has been intensively studied. Interestingly, blood flow is neither required[36,38,39] nor sufficient[20] for the effect to be observed, although an intact circulation appears to be necessary for the maximal T_2 change to occur[36,39] (Figure 7.5).

The most important effector of postexercise muscle T_2 changes is the increase of muscle water content that occurs transiently as a normal result of exercise. During low-intensity muscular contractions, this increase of muscle water primarily occurs in the extracellular space. During maximal-intensity exercise, an increase also occurs in the intracellular water space.[78,79] These changes in muscle water content/compartmentation occur on a time scale that closely approximates transient increases in muscle T_2 times.[36,39,44,53,60]

An important role for increased extracellular water in mediating transient muscle T_2 changes is supported by the observation that the T_2 time of extracellular water

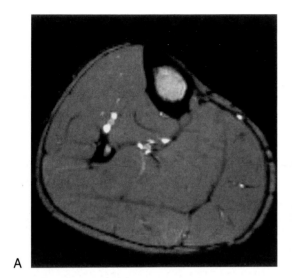

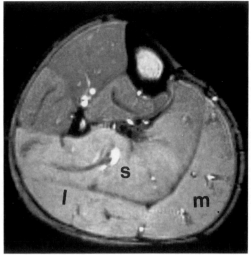

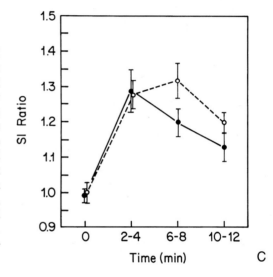

FIGURE 7.5. Acute changes of muscle signal intensity on MRI during exercise. Axial gradient echo (500/30, 30° flip angle) images of the leg before (A) and during the first 4-min period after 2 min of plantarflexion (B). Note increased signal intensity in intensely recruited soleus (s) and medial (m) and lateral (l) gastrocnemius muscles compared to less active muscles. The time course of such changes can be expressed by plotting the ratio of signal intensity of active to inactive muscle (filled circles, C). At rest (time 0), the ratio is 1.0. Following a peak in the first 2 to 4 min, the ratio falls toward the baseline with a half-life of approximately 10 min. When blood flow is occluded, such as by a tourniquet, one can see that the postexercise signal intensity ratio is not altered at 2 to 4 min (empty circles). However, when blood flow is restored, at 6 to 8 min, augmentation in the ratio is observed, prior to a return to baseline.

has a much longer T_2 time than intracellular water.[59,69] Small increases in extracellular water can therefore account for considerable increases in the muscle T_2 relaxation time. In fact, this mechanism was supported by data from studies of rabbit muscle in which shifts of muscle water compartmentation were induced by stimulation and/or diuresis.[59,69] In humans, a significant increase in the image contrast between active and inactive muscles after exercise was observed following application of a preirradiation magnetization transfer contrast (MTC) pulse.[40,41] This was also interpreted to substantiate an important role for extracellular water as a key effector of muscle T_2 variability.[40,41] These studies must be viewed with caution, however, because different investigators arrived at opposing results and conclusions.[42]

Regardless of the precise compartmentation of water changes that occurs after exercise and their relative contributions to the MRI-visible alterations of muscle, there is general agreement that an increase in muscle water is important. This occurs by development of increased muscle osmolarity due to accumulation of lactate and other ions. Increased osmotic strength of muscle causes increased diffusion of water from the vasculature to the extravascular space.[78,79] As argued by Sjøgaard et al.,[80] however, increased hydrostatic pressure is probably also important in mediating the increase in muscle water. This may account for why an intact vasculature appears required to observe the maximal increase in muscle T_2 after exercise.[36,39]

That the mechanism underlying the exercise-induced increases in T_2 relaxation time of muscle relies substantially upon a build-up of osmotic strength in muscle was first suggested by a study comparing normal volunteers to patients with McArdle's disease, in whom glycogenolysis and lactate production are blocked at the level of phosphorylase.[20] The observation that the normal increase in muscle T_2 relaxation times in these patients was also blocked supported the view that intact glycogenolysis is critical in mediating the normal T_2 change brought on by exercise.[20,38] The fact that these patients failed to increase muscle proton relaxation times despite the fact that work was controlled for, in both absolute and relative terms, indicated that a reduced work capacity could not account for those patients' deviation from normal (Figure 7.6). Also, because postexercise hyperemia is normal or even exaggerated following exercise, a role for hyperemia in mediating the normal increase in T_2 was refuted.[38] Findings similar to those in McArdle's disease were demonstrated in patients with other blocks in lactate production due to inherited enzymatic errors in glycogenolysis, including phosphofructokinase deficiency, glycogen debrancher deficiency, and lactate dehydrogenase deficiency (unpublished observations). These data indicate that the block in T_2 signal intensity enhancement is not peculiar to a single enzyme defect (phosphorylase deficiency) but rather is common to those defects in which accumulation of lactate ion is blocked.

Because lactate is quantitatively the most important osmotic effector in the postexercise state, the data together support the idea that a lactate-enhanced osmotic gradient provides a critical means for water to accumulate in the extravascular space and thereby cause an increase in proton T_2 relaxation times. This conclusion is further substantiated by an unimpeded increase in T_2 after exercise in patients with inherited enzyme defects of muscle oxidative metabolism in whom lactic acidemia is marked after exercise (unpublished observations). Additional support for an important role for lactate-mediated water translocation as the critical event in postexercise T_2 changes comes from three studies that found strong correlations between postexercise acidosis with the T_2 change.[43,44,60]

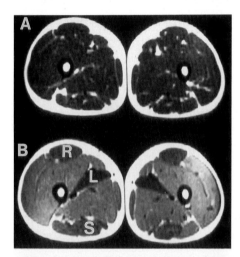

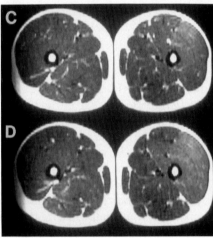

FIGURE 7.6. Absence of exercise-induced T_2 changes in patients with impaired glycogenolysis. Axial 1000/60 thigh image in normal subject before (A) and after (B) cycling at peak oxygen consumption. Most muscles become hyperintense, although the rectus femoris (R), adductor longus (L), and semimembranosus (S) remain relatively unchanged. Similar images from a patient with phosphorylase deficiency show no change in signal intensity from before (C) to after maximal exercise (D).

Practical Applications of Exercise-Induced Proton T_2 Changes of Skeletal Muscle

Although the precise mechanism(s) involved in exercise-induced changes of muscle during exercise remain incompletely understood, the changes in image contrast between metabolically stressed muscle and less active muscle have potentially important practical applications in the science of exercise physiology as well as in the clinical arenas of sports medicine and neuromuscular disease.

Skeletal Muscle Recruitment Patterns

The first practical application of exercise enhancement of muscles on MRI was the demonstration of muscle recruitment patterns that are relevant to MR spectroscopy (MRS) studies of exercise (Figure 7.7),[50] an application that was subsequently repeated and enlarged upon.[54,57] It was shown, for example, that many early MRS studies used surface coils that were larger in diameter than the width of the muscles that they were attempting to study; this meant that admixture of more active and less active muscles were included in the sensitive volume of the coil, underlining the need for reevaluation of results and interpretations of "pioneering" MRS studies.[50] Exercise-enhanced MRI also confirmed the inaccuracy of physical examination in localizing muscles actually stressed during handgrip exercise protocols, emphasizing the need for MRI integration into MRS studies to ensure appropriate placement of surface coils.[50]

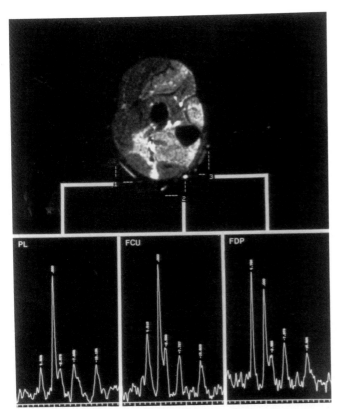

FIGURE 7.7. Effect of coil position on ³¹P-MRI spectra. Post-handgrip STIR (1500/30/100) image shows three coil positions used for forearm spectroscopy relative to muscles in the proximal forearm (top panel). Coil positions were chosen to sample the palmaris longus (PL), flexor carpi ulnaris (FCU), and flexor digitorum profundus (FDP). Although comparable exercise was performed with the coil in each position, ³¹P spectra show markedly different results depending solely on coil position. This difference is most obvious for the variability of inorganic phosphate accumulation and phosphocreatine breakdown. ³¹P peaks represent, from left to right, inorganic phosphate, phosphocreatine, gamma adenosine triphosphate (ATP), alpha ATP, and beta ATP.

MRI also documented a high degree of intersubject variability of muscle recruitment during a "standard" wrist flexion exercise protocol,[50] an application expanded to show a similarly high degree of intrasubject variability, depending upon slightly different changes in forearm position.[54] This variability of muscle recruitment was also shown to exist in handgrip exercise protocols in which finger-specific subvolumes of the flexor digitorum superficialis and profundus were shown to importantly affect MRS data, depending upon the positions of the surface coils in relationship to fingers favored by exercising subjects.[51,57]

The ability of exercise-enhanced MRI to isolate specific muscles involved in a given activity can be exploited commercially in the design and, potentially, marketing of exercise devices. One need only inspect instructions enclosed with most commercially obtained exercise devices to realize the dependence of the industry upon speculative drawings and grandiose, sweeping claims of the muscles supposedly stressed by the exercise advertised to realize a reasonable place for MRI of exercise: Truth in advertising. For example, one device advertised widely on American television shows a scantily clad celebrity describing how to "squeeze . . . your way to beautiful hips and thighs." MRI of exercise using the device shows that only two small groin muscles are stressed by the exercise. Another device by a large American manufacturer makes the reasonable guess that "fly" exercise builds up "the pectorals." MRI revealed that whereas the pectoralis major is recruited, the pectoralis minor is not. Also, the manufacturer does not gain advantage of the truth in that additional muscles other than the pectorlalis muscles are stressed (Figure 7.8). Given the power of MRI to delineate the muscles stressed by exercise equipment, and therefore to validate vendors' claims of muscle recruitment, the dearth of exploitation of MRI for this purpose is perplexing.

Another arena where MRI of muscle recruitment may be important is in the evaluation of physical rehabilitation programs. For example, MRI was used to examine recruitment patterns of lumbar muscles in "Roman chair" trunk extension exercise,[55] a commonly performed rehabilitation activity employed in rehabilitating patients with chronic low back pain. In this investigation, normal subjects, patients with chronic low back pain without surgery, and patients with chronic low back pain with surgery participated. The exercise produced increased signal intensity on MR images in lumbar paraspinal muscles within a few repetitions. The multifidus and

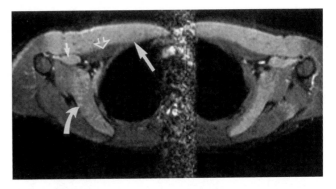

FIGURE 7.8. Truth in advertising: the MRI lie detector. The instructions provided with a well-known exercise device stated that when "fly exercise" is performed with the product, the "pectorals" are the muscles stressed by the activity. However, axial STIR image (1500/30/100) shows that although the pectoralis major is stressed (arrow), the pectoralis minor is not (arrowhead). The coracobrachialis (small arrow) and subscapularis (curved arrow) muscles are, however, strongly recruited.

longissimus/iliocostalis signal intensities were different at peak exercise levels for the different subject groups, and suggested a preferential utilization of the multifidus. MRI also demonstrated between-group differences in lumbar paraspinal musculature in the resting state as well as during exercise, in that patients with chronic low back pain with prior surgery had increased MR signal intensity of the multifidus and longissimus/iliocostalis at rest and an attenuated signal intensity response after exercise compared to normal subjects. The baseline paraspinal muscle changes of the operated patients was attributed to either residual injury or denervation, whereas the attenuated exercise enhancement was speculated to relate to metabolic deconditioning of the muscles.

Exercise-Enhanced MRI of Muscle and Work "Type"

An early study sought to determine if the type of work performed might be important in determining the T_2 response of muscle to exercise. Concentric (shortening) actions were found to be much more potent in eliciting MRI changes than were eccentric (lengthening) actions performing the same amount of work[62] (Figure 7.9). At equivalent workloads, concentric contractions consume much more energy than do eccentric contractions and concentric work is associated with increased oxygen consumption, more activated motor units, and more lactate production for the same power output.[81–84] Taken together, these data indicate that the quantitative dependence of muscle T_2 relaxation times upon work intensity

depends strongly on the relative amount of concentric or eccentric activity performed in the exercise, a point later substantiated by another group.[49]

Exercise-Enhanced MRI of Muscle as an Index of Work "Intensity"

The initial study of muscle proton T_2 changes with hand-grip exercise in humans reported a positive correlation between the signal intensity change and the amount of work performed.[39] However, the correlation was only moderate for one finger flexor and it was poor for the other finger flexor. Although these data provided weak support for a linear correlation between work intensity and muscle T_2 change, subsequent investigators argued that the correlation between muscle T_2 signal intensity changes and work intensity is indeed linear.[46,48,56,63] For example, Fisher et al.[46] reported a strong, linear correlation between force and percent change in T_2 relaxation time. That analysis was criticized and the data reinterpreted to support new data confirming that a limit exists to the magnitude that muscle proton T_2 can change as a function of work[52] (Figure 7.10). The concept of a limit is supported by investigations employing percutaneous muscle stimulation,[49] maximal voluntary contractions,[52] and graded exercise.[44] Concurring that a limit exists to the T_2 increase, Jenner et al.[56] observed that the T_2 response curve was linear over a finite range of submaximal work intensities, supporting the work of Adams et al.,[48] who found a strong linear correlation between electromyographic activity and muscle contrast changes on MRI.

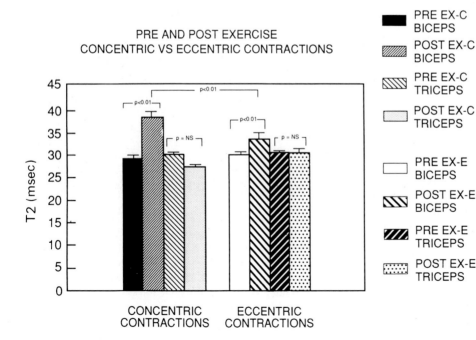

FIGURE 7.9. Quantitative depiction of the relative importance of concentric work in eliciting acute T_2 changes of muscle during work. Graph shows T_2 values of biceps and triceps measured before and after extremities performed concentric and eccentric actions. Values are means + SD. EX-C = concentric actions; EX-E = eccentric actions.

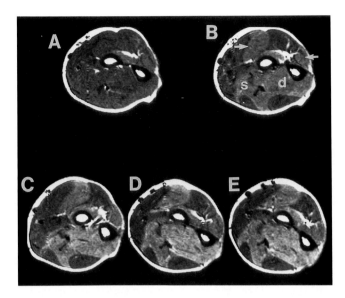

FIGURE 7.10. Nonlinearity of muscle T_2 changes with work duration. Modestly T_2-weighted spin echo images (1000/60) of the forearm at rest (A), and after successive handgrip exercise bouts (B–E). After 10 maximal effort handgrip contractions (B), obvious signal intensity increases are visible within deep (D) and superficial (S) finger flexors, as well as in synergistically recruited wrist extensors (arrows). Note that when twice the number of repetitions is performed, the signal change is more prominent (C). However, additional doublings of the number of MVCs are not associated with proportionate increases in signal of any muscles (D, E).

Subsequently, Cheng et al.[44] studied the T_2 response over a wider range of work intensities than previously studied, including low intensities. This study found that T_2 fails to increase linearly at low work intensities. Taken together, the available data indicate that a sigmoidal curve probably best defines the nature of the dependence of muscle T_2 on work intensity. Hence, the ability to precisely determine the work performed by a muscle on the basis of its T_2 change remains problematic.

It appears quite clear that changes in signal intensity seen on MR images of skeletal muscle provide at least a rough measure of relative muscle use. The relationship between muscle activity and signal intensity changes seen on MRI is apparently a function of the type of exercise performed and physical training level of the subject,[61] among other factors. Therefore, a linear relationship between exercise intensity and T_2 changes should not be assumed for a given protocol unless documented in multiple subjects using MRI criteria.

Dynamic Muscle MRI as a Diagnostic Test in Patients

Changes in proton relaxation times of skeletal muscle during exercise have not only been applied to probe physiological issues in healthy subjects but have also been studied in patient groups. The application in patients with metabolic myopathies has already been commented upon. However, as Jehenson et al.[58] emphasized, detection of subnormal increases in T_2 values in exercised muscle might enable the noninvasive diagnosis of muscle glycogenoses, thereby obviating the need for the less available and more technically challenging test of phosphorus MR spectroscopy. The role of MRI in evaluating pathophysiological mechanisms of muscle disease in patients with defects in muscle energy metabolism is detailed in Chapter 19.

Acute changes of muscle on MRI as a result of exercise have also been touted as a technique to identify patients with chronic compartment syndromes.[85] In these patients, a prolonged increase in the T_1, but not the T_2 time, of muscle was reported to be the abnormal finding. T_1 relaxation time increases are more complicated to measure, however, because T_1 increases are much smaller than those of T_2 and because T_1 times must be measured on scans acquired successively over a time interval that T_2 undergoes large changes. Hence, the role of dynamic MRI to diagnose chronic compartment syndromes deserves further investigation.

Acute changes in skeletal muscle T_2 have also been addressed in patients with congestive heart failure.[64] In patients with mild (New York Heart Association Classes I–II), but not advanced (Classes III–IV), heart failure, the correlation between work and T_2 was found to be linear. However, in all classes, the T_2 change increased linearly with acidosis. These data support conclusions stated above that the linkage between muscle T_2 and work intensity cannot be assumed in any patient population and that acute changes in muscle T_2 fundamentally depend upon lactic acidosis-related phenomena. The data also support an exaggerated dependence of muscle in patients with advanced heart failure upon anaerobic metabolism, possibly as an adaptation to poor oxygen delivery.

Skeletal Muscle Pathophysiology

Pathological conditions of skeletal muscle can readily be studied using standard MRI techniques, as chronicled throughout the chapters of this book. However, some conditions that are suspected to involve the muscles may show no abnormality despite the use of sophisticated radiological techniques. In such instances, such as fibromyalgia, even the negative finding is a clue that whatever the pathology is, it does not cause substantial muscle deterioration.[68] Furthermore, the negative MRI finding in such cases supports other data suggesting that muscle is not primarily affected.

Other painful conditions, although of great interest in the exercise sciences, are not considered to be diseases per se. Examples include DOMS and chronic overuse syndrome.[65] These seemingly benign and self-limited conditions are important clinical entities. The former is important because it is exceedingly common and yet may be the only symptom in patients with specific diseases, such as in enzyme deficiencies associated with defects of muscle energy metabolism. The latter is important because as its name implies, it is only a syndrome that is poorly defined and yet accounts for a large number of patient complaints related to occupational activities and as such accounts for a significant toll to the workplace.[86]

Radiology of skeletal muscle can help evaluate such ill-defined conditions by confirming the presence or absence of parenchymal abnormalities in these disorders. In still other poorly understood clinical occurrences, such as muscle contracture and rhabdomyolysis in myopathies, the distribution of lesions and time course of healing or progression to irreversible fatty atrophy can be documented to help understand basic issues in those diseases (see Chapter 19).

Delayed Onset Muscle Soreness

Delayed onset muscle soreness refers to muscle pain that begins several hours to days after an activity to which one is unaccustomed. This condition contrasts muscle strain in which pain occurs acutely during or immediately following a muscle contraction.[73–75,81–84,86–89] The painful symptoms associated with DOMS typically increase in intensity during the first 24 h after exertion, peak from 24 to 72 h, and then subside. The degree of soreness is related to both the intensity of the muscular contraction and the duration of exercise, with intensity appearing to be the most important factor.

The pathophysiology of DOMS is incompletely understood and remains a subject of great interest in exercise science. Contributing etiologies include a disruption of the connective tissue elements in the muscles and/or their attachments, increased intramuscular fluid pressure, and inflammation. Depending on the severity of DOMS, a variety of clinical findings become apparent, including elevations in plasma enzymes, myoglobinemia, pigmenturia, and abnormal muscle histology and ultrastructure. In severe cases, biopsies may reveal free erythrocytes, leukocytes, and mitochondria within the extracellular spaces, myofibrillar disorganization, and Z-band alterations. In milder cases, sarcomere disruption may be the only finding, occurring at approximately 24 to 48 h with regeneration beginning within 3 days after exertion.

One of the major hindrances to the investigation of DOMS, as is the case in all muscle pathologies, is the inability to precisely localize the involved muscle and to characterize the extent and severity of the lesion. The ability of MR imaging techniques to probe beneath the surface of skin to characterize muscle abnormalities associated with DOMS has yielded considerable insight into its pathophysiology.

The overall MRI appearance of DOMS is quite similar to that of other muscle injuries (Figures 7.11 to 7.14). Muscle proton T_1 and T_2 relaxation times increase, consistent with the presence of edema.[74,75] In both DOMS and strains, perifascial fluid collections are sometimes seen in the early phase of injury (see Chapters 25 and 33).[74] These recede as symptoms abate and creatine kinase and other enzyme levels normalize. The similarity in MRI appearances of strains and DOMS makes it difficult to distinguish between the two syndromes on the basis of MRI change alone.

The first study of the MRI appearance of DOMS employed an unquantitated ankle plantarflexion protocol and reported that whereas both the medial and lateral heads of the gastrocnemius and the soleus were stressed by the exercise (by MRI criteria), this did not accurately predict which muscles subsequently became injured.[74] When pain and rhabdomyolysis developed 24 to 72 h after the activity (i.e., DOMS), MRI showed markedly edematous alteration restricted to the medial head of the gastrocnemius, consistent with necrosis.[19]

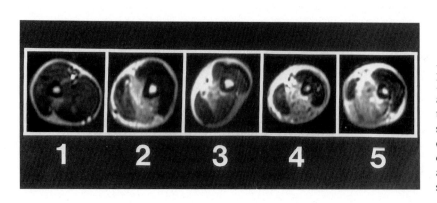

FIGURE 7.11. Variable MRI appearance of DOMS after exercise involving eccentric actions. T_2-weighted (2000/80) images obtained from the middle arms of five different subjects (numbered at bottom) on the fifth day after exercise. Note variability in pattern of signal changes of biceps and brachialis and that the long head of biceps tends to be spared.

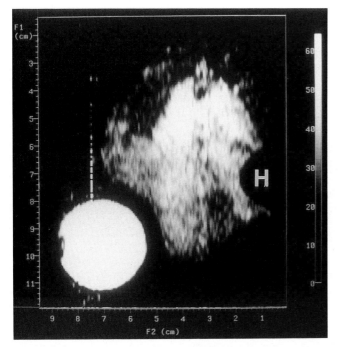

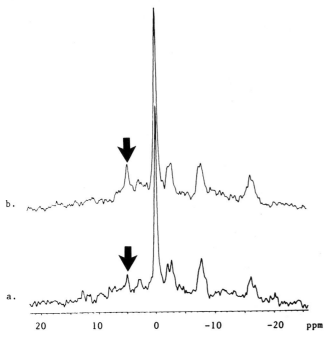

FIGURE 7.12. MRI (top) and ^{31}P-MR spectroscopic data (bottom) from biceps and brachialis following DOMS related to bicep curls performed 2 days earlier. A spherical external marker was placed on top of the painful arm, where a surface coil was placed to acquire ^{31}P-MR spectra. The humerus (H) is visible in the posterior portion of the arm. The stacked plot of ^{31}P spectra shows a typical result in DOMS. The spectrum from the painful muscles is shown in plot b; that from the contralateral normal arm is shown in a. The increased height of the inorganic phosphate peak (arrow) from the painful arm is a nonspecific alteration that occurs in a great variety of muscle disorders. (Case courtesy of Navin Bansal, Ph.D).

A subsequent study supported the long-standing belief that eccentric muscle actions (i.e., those performed while the muscle lengthens) produced DOMS and attendant MRI abnormalities, whereas concentric muscle actions (i.e., those performed while the muscle shortens) produced neither.[75] Recall that this is opposite the case for changes in muscle signal intensity that occur acutely with exercise and that the acute changes were linked to the higher energy consumption that occurs with concentric work.[62] Therefore, the energy production per se would appear to be relatively unimportant in producing DOMS whereas mechanical forces, such as shear or strain, may be more important in eliciting the MRI-visible tissue injury associated with DOMS. This study also demonstrated unexpected findings that forced re-evaluation of traditional approaches to studying this pathophysiology.

First, MRI showed that the spatial extent and distribution of muscle injury varied considerably among individuals (Figure 7.11). For example, although the biceps brachii muscle is the target of many "bicep curls" studies of DOMS, the biceps was quite variably injured by the exercise, and the nearby brachialis muscle was more reliably injured. This emphasized the need to integrate diagnostic imaging into scientific studies to ensure that an injured muscle is actually probed and the results therefore meaningful. Such a directed approach can be employed in magnetic resonance spectroscopy (MRS) (Figure 7.12).

Second, signal intensity within injured muscles may persist for long after cessation of all clinical evidence of injury[73-75] (Figures 7.13, 7.14). This finding suggests that subclinical pathological changes can be documented and monitored noninvasively. The implication that persisting abnormality remains functionally impaired remains to be studied but gains support from the observation of a correlation between strength decrements and peak T_2 relaxation times and signal intensity increases, as well as with volume of abnormal appearing muscle on MRI.[15]

Third, MRI studies on DOMS found a discordance between the onset of severe symptoms and signal abnormalities on MRI, suggesting that clinical findings do not comprehensively describe the severity or extent of muscle injury associated with DOMS.[73-75] This is not unexpected in the setting of very mild DOMS in which only mild ultrastructural changes may result, albeit in association with MRI-visible alterations[73] (Figure 7.15). On the basis of these findings, MRI appears useful to detect subclinical injuries and to monitor the course of DOMS. Awareness of the possibility of detecting subclinical pathological changes resulting from muscle overactivity is particularly interesting clinically when one shifts the focus from injury resulting from exercise to which one is unaccustomed to that encountered in situations where

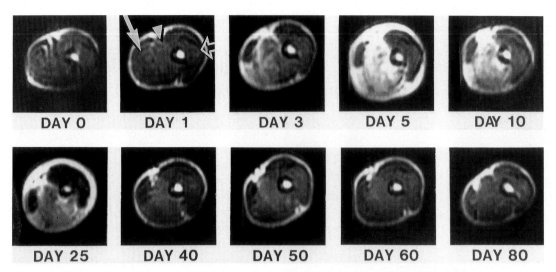

FIGURE 7.13. Long-lived MRI changes associated with DOMS. Axial T_2-weighted (2000/80) images obtained from the middle arm of a healthy volunteer before (day 0) and serially after performance of eccentric muscular actions. Anatomic detail is limited but is best depicted on the day 1 image (biceps, arrow; brachialis, closed arrowhead; triceps, open arrowhead). A subtle increase in signal intensity is seen in the biceps and brachialis muscles on day 1 image after exercise. Day 3 image shows a more diffuse pattern of markedly increased signal intensity in the brachialis and the short head of the biceps. Note sparing of the long head of the biceps, which remains unaffected throughout the experiment. The peak increased signal intensity is seen on day 5. The signal alteration is diminished on days 10 and 25 compared with that on 5 and further diminishes on days 40, 50, and 60. Note also the marked increase in circumference of the affected muscles, which is most apparent on images obtained on days 3, 5, 10, and 25. The image obtained on day 80 shows a return to baseline with regard to signal intensity and muscle size.

the activity is one to which the subject is well accustomed, such as in occupational overuse.

Chronic Overuse Syndrome

Chronic overuse syndrome refers to a broad group of disorders characterized by pain or stiffness that develops in certain occupations (e.g., typists, musicians, etc.) or in recreational activities (running, pitching, etc.).[90-97] This syndrome has also been called chronic injury, chronic strain, chronic myalgia, repetition strain injury, overuse injury, and cumulative trauma disorder. Chronic overuse syndrome is a relatively common condition, occurring in up to 15 to 20% of employees with certain occupations, according to estimates from the National Institute of Occupational Safety and Health.[90]

Chronic overuse syndrome has various presentations. For example, there may be irritation at the musculotendinous junction or tenosynovitis may occur along with an inflammatory reaction caused by adhesions between the tendon and surrounding synovium. If the stress at this site is not eliminated, chronic inflammatory reaction results with further pain, swelling, and edema.

Like other categories of exertional injury, chronic overuse syndrome is poorly understood, in part because of the traditional lack of objective tests to confirm the presence of tissue abnormality. For example, it has been stated that traditional diagnostic radiological tests tend to be normal in such cases.[91] MRI would appear to fill this void in the diagnostic approach, as exemplified in cases of recurrent exertional pain syndromes in which mild edema-like change is evident in muscle–tendon units on MRI (Figures 7.16 to 7.20).

The fact that the MRI appearance of chronic muscle overuse is indistinguishable from that of mild DOMS,

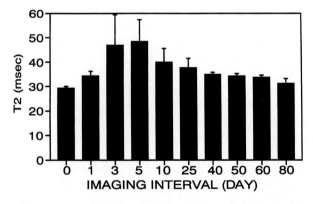

FIGURE 7.14. Quantitative analysis of MRI changes associated with DOMS. Graph shows T_2 relaxation times of the muscles before (day 0) and after (days 1, 3, 5, 10, 25, 40, 50, 60, and 80) the subjects performed exercise involving eccentric actions. A statistically significant ($p < 0.05$) increase in T_2 relaxation times existed for each subsequent postexercise imaging interval compared with T_2 relaxation times before exercise (day 0). Values are means; error bars represent +1 SD.

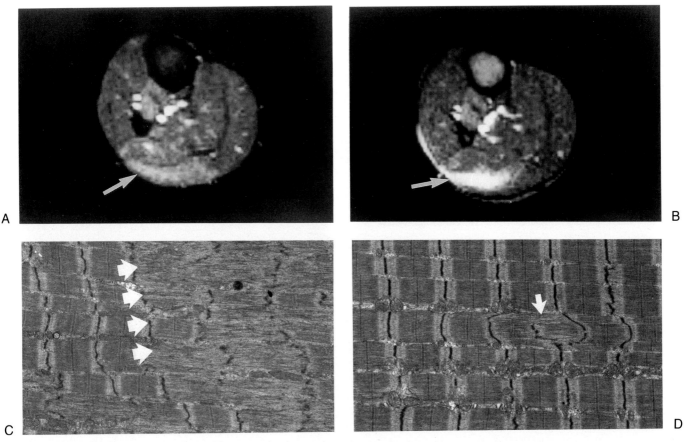

FIGURE 7.15. Ultrastructural changes due to eccentric muscle actions. STIR image (1500/30/100) obtained 48 h after eccentric exercise shows signal intensity increase in lateral head of gastrocnemius (arrow, A). STIR image (1500/30/100) obtained after biopsy of the abnormal muscle confirms site of tissue sampling (arrow, B). Electron micrograph of specimen from biopsy site shows extensive structural disorganization (arrowheads, C). Electron micrograph from another region of same biopsy sample shows structural disorganization involving only two sarcomeres (arrowhead, D).

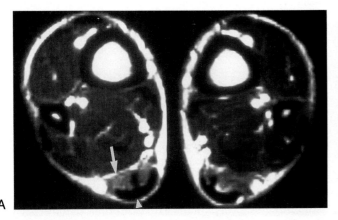
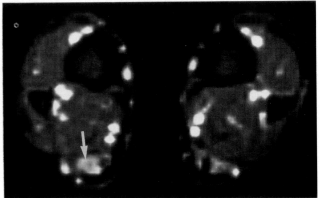

FIGURE 7.16. Recreational overuse syndrome: marathoner's ankle. This runner was training for a marathon but had to cut back his training schedule because of "Achilles' tendinitis." The T_2-weighted image (2000/60) shows abnormal signal intensity in the myotendinous junction of the soleus muscle bilaterally (arrow, A) but no abnormality within the tendons (arrowhead). The lower resolution STIR image (1500/30/100) required less than half the time of the first image and the muscle edema is more conspicuous than in the former (arrow, B).

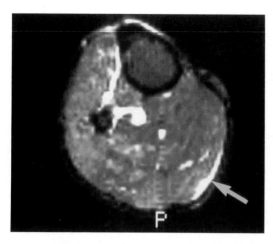

FIGURE 7.17. Recreational overuse syndrome: marathoner's calf. This runner complained of chronic posterior leg pain. Axial STIR image (1500/30/100) shows a peripheral rim of fluid at the painful site (arrow), consistent with the clinical diagnosis of "myofascial strain."

and that similar ultrastructural changes occur in mild forms,[73,92,93] provides a theoretical argument for overlap in the pathophysiology of repetitive strain injury and mild DOMS. It is logical that muscle fibers that have undergone ultrastructural deformation and have reduced

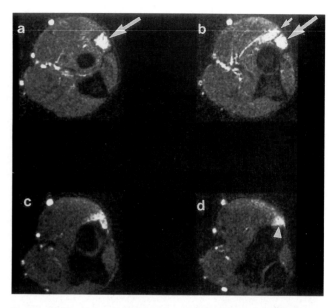

FIGURE 7.19. Recreational overuse syndrome: tennis elbow. Because of progressively increasing exertional pain over the lateral humeral epicondyle, this patient curtailed his frequency of playing tennis. Contiguous 1-cm axial STIR images (1500/30/100), proceeding from distal (a) to proximal (b), show focal signal intensity increase in the extensor digitorum communis (long arrow) and extensor carpi radialis brevis (short arrow) where they originate from the lateral epicondyle (arrowhead).

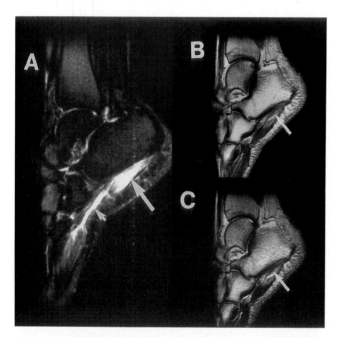

FIGURE 7.18. Recreational overuse syndrome: "plantar fasciitis." Progressive heel pain during aerobics exercise led this patient to stop her workouts. Sagittal STIR (1500/30/100) shows extensive edema in the flexor digitorum brevis (large arrow, A). A prominent vein is also evident (small arrow). On comparable 2000/40 (B) and 2000/80 (C) images, the muscle edema is less conspicuous (arrows).

functional capacity on that basis, when exposed to a constant workload, such as encountered in occupational stresses, would be subjected to a "vicious cycle" wherein sarcomere disruption is propagated. The occurrence of faint edema-like abnormalities on MRI in the legs of marathoners raises the question of whether such findings are best categorized as DOMS, strain, or chronic overuse (Figures 7.16, 7.17).[74] Although this remains a speculative discussion, the cases exemplify that MRI can confirm the presence of tissue abnormality in chronic overuse syndromes and suggest that the degree of muscle abnormality may be understimated in such conditions.

Pathophysiology in Myopathies

The pathophysiology of myalgia and impaired muscular performance in the vast majority of neuromuscular disease remains incompletely defined. Just as MRI has opened the door to a better ability to probe basic issues in the physiology of muscle use and oveüse an healthy individuals, so has it aided the noninvasive study of pathophysiology in patients with neuromuscular diseases. For example, the absence of normal exercise-induced T_2 increases in patients with inherited blocks of glycogenolysis and the attendant implications in diagnosing metabolic myopathies has already been mentioned. However, the same finding provides potential hints to an important

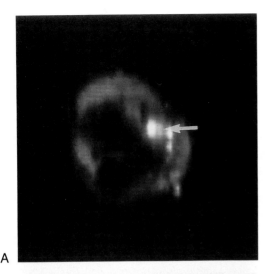

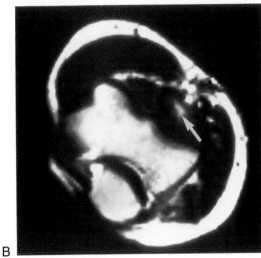

FIGURE 7.20. Occupational overuse syndrome: "waitress elbow." A waitress complained of several days of progressive pain near her elbow, which was exacerbated by holding her cocktail tray, ultimately forcing her to stop work. A 1.1-min, low-resolution STIR (1500/30/100) "scout" sequence provided 16 1-cm slices, one of which showed a small focus of increased signal intensity in the distal brachialis (arrow, A). This led to a higher-resolution (1000/80) sequence, at approximately the same level, which confirmed the focus of edema (arrow, B). The same region was isointense with muscle on the T_1-weighted image (not shown). The entire exam required less than 8 min. Both the MRI abnormality and symptoms resolved during 1 wk off work, and symptoms did not recur.

clinical problem in such patients, muscle contracture and rhabdomyolysis.

In McArdle's disease (muscle phosphorylase deficiency) and other glycogenoses, patients sustain recurrent episodes of exertional muscle pain that precede myoglobinuria. The myalgia is differentiated from a cramp by the characteristic absence of electrical activity on EMG during the painful muscle shortening. Why muscle that is deficient in specific glycogenolytic muscle enzymes and is prone to undergo contracture is unknown. However, observations made on MRI provide some insight.

The well-documented lack of normal, transient exercise-mediated changes in muscle proton MRI in glycogenoses and attenuated increases in muscle CSA together suggest a lack of normal muscle water accumulation during exercise in glycogenoses. Because water constitutes the denominator of solute concentrations, a blunted increase in muscle water necessarily results in exaggerated increases in extracellular solute concentrations, including those of potassium and calcium. Excess muscle concentrations of these and other metabolites that could contribute to cessation of electrical conductance through sarcomeres should therefore be scrutinized as potential contributors to the overall pathophysiology of the disease. These ionic alterations could contribute not only to muscle fatigue, cramps, and necrosis but also to the hyperkinetic cardiovascular response to exercise in glycogenoses.[20]

In addition to providing insight into the mechanism by which muscle contracture develops, MRI has suggested additional functional significance to the occurrence of contracture and rhabdomyolysis in glycogenoses. Employed as a screening test for assessing the incidence of muscle lesions in glycogenoses, MRI revealed an association between the potentially reversible acute injury pattern and irreversible fatty atrophy.[71] Concurrence of muscle edema and fatty infiltration in patients in whom contracture occurs supports the notion that exertion-induced myonecrosis, sustained during activities of daily living, may predispose to progressive muscle deterioration, fatty muscles, and development of "fixed weakness" on that basis. Previous to these observations, no objective evidence existed to support a theory for the cause of fixed weakness in these patients.

The application of imaging, specifically MRI, to probing the mysteries of exercise intolerance in myopathies is clearly in its infancy. However, based on results to date, particularly in glycogenoses, it seems clear that further investigation is indicated.

Conclusions

The role of radiology in the evaluation of muscle physiology remains to be defined. However, the potential exists for MRI of muscle at rest and during and after contraction to unveil new insights and aid in the design of new approaches to problems encountered in exercise science.

References

1. Houghton PL, Turlington LM. Application of ultrasound for feeding and finishing animals: a review. J Anim Sci 1992;70:930–941.

2. Alexander RM, Vernon A. The dimensions of knee and ankle muscles and the forces they exert. J Hum Mov Stud 1975;1:115–123.

3. Ikai M, Fukunaga T. A study on training effect on strength per unit cross-sectional area of muscle by means of ultrasonic measurement. Int Z Angew Physiol Einschl Arbeitsphysiol 1970;28:173–180.

4. Young A, Hughes I, Russell P, Parker MJ, Nichols PJR. Measurement of quadriceps muscle wasting by ultrasonography. Rheumatol Rehabil 1980;19:141–148.

5. Reimers CD, Muller W, Schmidt-Aschert M, Heldwein W, Pongratz DE. Sonographische erfassung von faszikulationen. Ultraschall 1988;9:237–239.

6. Grubb RG, Fleming A, Sutherland GR, Fox KAA. Skeletal muscle contraction in healthy volunteers: assessment with Doppler tissue imaging. Radiology 1995;194:837–842.

7. Reimers CD, Lochmüller H, Goebels N, et al. Der Einfluß von Muskelarbeit auf das Myosonogramm. Ultraschall Med 1995;16:79–83.

8. Sipilä S, Suominen H. Muscle ultrasonography and computed tomography in elderly trained and untrained women. Muscle Nerve 1993;16:294–300.

9. Huang HK, Suarez FR. Evaluation of cross-sectional geometry and mass density distributions of humans and laboratory animals using computerized tomography. J Biomech 1983;16:821–832.

10. Maughan RJ, Watson JS, Weir J. Strength and cross-sectional area of human skeletal muscle. J Physiol 1983;338:37–49.

11. Engstrom CM, Loeb GE, Reid JG, Forrest WJ, Avruch L. Morphometry of the human thigh muscles. A comparison between anatomical sections and computer tomographic and magnetic resonance images. J Anat 1991;176:139–156.

12. McColl RW, Fleckenstein JL, Bowers J, Theriault G, Peshock RM. Three dimensional reconstruction of skeletal muscles from MRI. Comput Med Imaging Graphics 1992; 16:363–371.

13. Fukunaga T, Roy RR, Shellock FG, et al. Physiological cross-sectional area of human leg muscles based on magnetic resonance imaging. J Orthop Res 1992;10:926–934.

14. Roman WJ, Fleckenstein J, Stray-Gundersen J, Alway SE, Peshock R, Gonyea WJ. Adaptations in the elbow flexors of elderly males following resistance training. Spine 1993;18:582–586.

15. Shellock FG, Fukunaga T, Day K, Edgerton V, Mink JH. Serial MRI and Cybex testing evaluations of exertional muscle injury: concentric vs. eccentric actions. Med Sci Sports Exerc 1990;22:S110.

16. Narici MV, Roi GS, Landoni L, Minetti AE, Cerretelli P. Changes in force, cross-sectional area and neural activation during strength training and detraining of the human quadriceps. Eur J Appl Physiol 1989;59:310–319.

17. Kariya Y, Itoh M, Nakamura T, Yagi K, Kurosawa H. Magnetic resonance imaging and spectroscopy of thigh muscles in cruciate ligament insufficiency. Acta Orthop Scand 1989;60:322–325.

18. LeBlanc A, Gogia P, Schneider V, Krebs J, Schonfeld E, Evans H. Calf muscle area and strength changes after five weeks of horizontal bed rest. Am J Sports Med 1988;16:624–629.

19. LeBlanc A, Evans H, Schonfeld E, et al. Changes in nuclear magnetic resonance (T2) relaxation of limb tissue with bed rest. Magn Reson Med 1987;4:487–492.

20. Fleckenstein JL, Haller RG, Lewis SF, Parkey RW, Peshock RM. Absence of exercise-induced MRI enhancement of skeletal muscle in McArdle's disease. J Appl Physiol 1991;71:961–969.

21. Adams GR, Harris RT, Woodard D, Dudley GA. Mapping of electrical muscle stimulation using MRI. J Appl Physiol 1993;74:532–537.

22. Beneke R, Neuerbug J, Bohndorf K. Muscle cross-section measurement by magnetic resonance imaging. Eur J Physiol 1991;63:424–429.

23. Narici MV, Roi GS, Landoni L. Force of knee extensor and flexor muscles and cross-sectional area determined by nuclear magnetic resonance imaging. Eur J Appl Physiol 1988;57:39–44.

24. Narici MV, Landoni L, Minetti AE. Assessment of human knee extensor muscle stress from in vivo physiological cross-sectional area and strength measurements. Eur J Appl Physiol 1992;65:438–444.

25. LeBlanc AD, Schneider VS, Evans H, Pientok C, Rowe R, Spector E. Regional changes in muscle mass following 17 weeks of bed rest. J Appl Physiol 1992;73: 2172–2178.

26. Hather BM, Adams GR, Tesch PA, Dudley GA. Skeletal muscle responses to lower limb suspension in humans. J Appl Physiol 1992;72:1493–1498.

27. Martin PE, Mungiole M, Marzke MW, Longhill JM. The use of magnetic resonance imaging for measuring segment inertial properties. J Biomech 1989;22(4):367–376.

28. Joy M, Scott G, Henkelman M. In vivo detection of applied electric currents by magnetic resonance imaging. Magn Reson Imaging 1989;7:89–94.

29. English AE, Joy MLG, Henkelman RM. Pulsed NMR relaxometry of striated muscle fibers. Magn Reson Med 1991;21:264–281.

30. Drace JE, Pelc NJ. Measurement of skeletal muscle motion in vivo with phase-contrast MR imaging. J Magn Reson Imaging 1994;4:157–163.

31. Drace JE, Pelc NJ. Tracking the motion of skeletal muscle with velocity-encoded MR imaging. J Magn Reson Imaging 1994;4:773–778.

32. Niitsu M, Campeau NG, Holsinger-Bampton AE, Riederer SJ, Ehman RL. Tracking motion with tagged rapid gradient-echo magnetization-prepared MR imaging. J Magn Reson Imaging 1992;2:155–163.

33. Adzamli IK, Jolesz FA, Bleier AR, et al. The effect of gadolinium DTPA on tissue water compartments in slow- and fast-twitch rabbit muscles. Magn Reson Med 1989;11:172–181.

34. Kuno S, Katsuta S, Inouye T, Anno I, Matsumoto K, Akisada M. Relationship between MR relaxation time and muscle fiber composition. Radiology 1988;169:567–568.

35. Kuno S, Katsuta S, Akisada M, Anno I, Matsumoto K. Effect of strength training on the relationship between relaxation time and muscle fiber composition. J Appl Physiol Occup Physiol 1990;61:33–36.

36. Archer B, Fleckenstein JL, Bertocci LA, Haller RG, Barker B, Parkey RW, Peshock RM. Effect of perfusion on exercised muscle: MRI evaluation. J Magn Reson Imaging 1992;2:407–413.

37. Bratton CB, Hopkins AL, Weinberg JW. Nuclear magnetic resonance studies of living muscle. Science 1965;147:147–148.

38. Fleckenstein JL, Haller RG, Bertocci LA, Parkey RW, Peshock RM. Glycogenolysis, not perfusion, is the critical mediator of exercise-induced muscle modifications on MR images. Radiology 1992;183:25–27.

39. Fleckenstein JL, Canby RC, Parkey RW, Peshock RM. Acute effects of exercise on MRI of skeletal muscle in normal volunteers. AJR 1988;151:231–237.

40. Zhu XP, Zhao S, Isherwood I. Magnetization transfer contrast (MTC) imaging of skeletal muscle at 0.26 T—changes in signal intensity following exercise. Br J Radiol 1992;65:39–43.

41. Yoshioka H, Takahashi H, Onaya H, Anno I, Niitsu M, Itai Y. Acute changes of exercised muscle using magnetization transfer contrast MR imaging. Magn Reson Imaging 1994;12:991–997.

42. Mattila KT, Komu ME, Koskinen SK, Niemi PT. Exercise-induced changes in magnetization transfer contrast of muscles. Acta Radiol 1993;34:559–562.

43. Weidman ER, Charles HC, Negro-Vilar R, Sullivan MG, MacFall JR. Muscle activity localization with 31P spectroscopy and calculated T2-weighted 1H images. Invest Radiol 1991;26:309–316.

44. Cheng HA, Robergs RA, Letellier JP, Caprihan A, Icenogle MV, Haseler LJ. Changes in muscle proton relaxation and acidosis during incremental exercise and recovery. J Appl Physiol. In press.

45. Le Rumeur E, Carre F, Bernard AM, Bansard JY, Rochcongar P, De Certaines J. Multiparametric classification of muscle T1 and T2 relaxation times determined by magnetic resonance imaging. The effects of dynamic exercise in trained and untrained subjects. Br J Radiol 1994;67:150–156.

46. Fisher MJ, Meyer RA, Adams GR, Foley JM, Potchen EJ. Direct relationship between proton T2 and exercise intensity in skeletal muscle MR images. Invest Radiol 1990;25:480–485.

47. de Kerviler E, Leroy-Willig A, Jehenson P, Duboc D, Eymard B, Syrota A. Exercise-induced muscle modifications: study of healthy subjects and patients with metabolic myopathies with MR imaging and P-31 spectroscopy. Radiology 1991;181:259–264.

48. Adams GR, Duvoisin MR, Dudley GA. Magnetic resonance imaging in electromyography as indexes of muscle function. J Appl Physiol 1992;73:1578–1583.

49. Adams GR, Harris RT, Woodard D, Dudley GA. Mapping of electrical muscle stimulation using MRI. J Appl Physiol 1993;74:532–537.

50. Fleckenstein JL, Bertocci LA, Nunnally RL, Parkey RW, Peshock RM. Variation in forearm structure and function: importance in MR spectroscopy. AJR 1989;153:693–698.

51. Fleckenstein JL, Watumull D, Bertocci LA, Parkey RW, Peshock RM. Finger-specific flexor recruitment in humans: depiction by exercise-enhanced MRI. J Appl Physiol 1992;72:1974–1977.

52. Fleckenstein JL, Watumull D, McIntire DD, Bertocci LA, Chason DP, Peshock RM. Muscle proton T2 relaxation times and work during repetitive maximal voluntary exercise. J Appl Physiol 1993;74:2855–2859.

53. Fleckenstein JL, Adams GR. Muscle water shifts, volume changes and proton T2 relaxation times after exercise [letter]. J Appl Physiol 1993;74:2047–2048.

54. Fleckenstein JL, Watumull D, Bertocci LA, et al. Muscle recruitment variations during wrist flexion exercise: MRI evaluation. J Comput Assist Tomogr 1994;18:449–453.

55. Flicker PL, Fleckenstein JL, Bond K, et al. Lumbar muscle usage in chronic low back pain: MRI evaluation. Spine 1993;18:582–586.

56. Jenner G, Foley JM, Cooper TG, Potchen EJ. Changes in magnetic resonance images of muscle depend on exercise intensity and duration, not work. J Appl Physiol 1994;76:2119–2124.

57. Jeneson JAL, Taylor JS, Vigneron DB, et al. 1H MR imaging of anatomical compartments within the finger flexor muscles of the human forearm. Magn Reson Med 1990;15:491–496.

58. Jehenson P, Leroy-Willig A, de Kerviler E, Duboc D, Syrota A. MR imaging as a potential diagnostic test for metabolic myopathies: importance of variations in the T2 of muscle with exercise. AJR 1993;161:347–351.

59. Le Rumeur E, De Certaines J, Toulouse P, Rochcongar P. Water phases in rat striated muscles as determined by T2 proton NMR relaxation times. Magn Reson Imaging 1987;5:267–272.

60. Morvan D, Vilgrain V, Arrive L, Nahum H. Correlation of MR changes with Doppler US measurements of blood flow in exercising normal muscle. J Magn Reson Imaging 1992;2:645–652.

61. Ploutz LL, Tesch PA, Biro RL, Dudley GA. Effect of resistance training on muscle use during exercise. J Appl Physiol 1994;76:1675–1681.

62. Shellock FG, Fukunaga TF, Mink JH, Edgerton VR. Acute effects of exercise on MR imaging of skeletal muscle: concentric vs eccentric actions. AJR 1991;156:765–768.

63. Yue G, Alexander AL, Laidlaw DH, Gimitro AF, Unger EC, Enoka RM. Sensitivity of muscle spin-spin relaxation time as an index of muscle activation. J Appl Physiol 1994;77:84–92.

64. Morvan D, Cohen-Solal A, Laperche T, Arrive L. Relationship between anaerobic metabolism involvement and proton T2 in skeletal muscle of patients with heart failure. Proc Soc Magn Reson 1994;1:251.

65. Fleckenstein JL, Weatherall PT, Bertocci LA, et al. Locomotor system assessment by muscle magnetic resonance imaging. Magn Reson Q 1991;7:79–103.

66. LeBlanc A, Evans H, Schonfeld E, et al. Relaxation times of normal and atrophied muscle. Med Phys 1986;13:14–517.

67. Murphy WA, Totty WG, Carroll JE. MRI of normal and pathologic skeletal muscle. AJR 1986;146:565–574.

68. Kravis MM, Munk PL, McCain GA, Vellet Ad, Levin MF. MR imaging of muscle and tender points in fibromyalgia. J Magn Reson Imaging 1993;3:669–670.

69. Polak JF, Jolesz FA, Adams DF. NMR of skeletal muscle differences in relaxation parameters related to extracellular/intracellular fluid spaces. Invest Radiol 1988;23:107–112.

70. Scholz TD, Fleagle SR, Burns TL, Skorton DJ. Tissue determinants of nuclear magnetic resonance relaxation times. Effect of water and collagen content in muscle and tendon. Invest Radiol 1989;24:893–898.

71. Fleckenstein JL, Peshock RM, Lewis SF, Haller RG. Magnetic resonance imaging of muscle injury and atrophy in glycolytic myopathies. Muscle Nerve 1989;12:849–855.

72. Fleckenstein JL, Archer BT, Barker BA, Vaughan JT, Parkey RW, Peshock RM. Fast, short-tau inversion-recovery MR imaging. Radiology 1991;179:499–504.

73. Nurenberg P, Giddings C, Stray-Gundersen J, Fleckenstein JL, Gonyea WJ, Peshock RM. MR imaging-guided muscle biopsy for correlation of increased signal intensity with ultrastructural change and delayed-onset muscle soreness after exercise. Radiology 1992;184:865–869.

74. Fleckenstein JL, Weatherall PT, Parkey RW, Payne JA, Peshock RM. Sports-related muscle injuries: evaluation with MR imaging. Radiology 1989;172:793–798.

75. Shellock FG, Fukunaga T, Mink JH, Edgerton VR. Exertional muscle injury: evaluation of concentric versus eccentric actions with serial MR imaging. Radiology 1991;179:659–664.

76. Mehta RC, Marks MP, Hinks RS, Glover GH, Enzmann DR. MR evaluation of vertebral metastases: T1-weighted, short inversion time inversion recovery, fast spin echo and inversion recovery fast spin echo sequences. AJNR 1995;16:281–288.

77. Houmard JA, Smith R, Jendrasiak GL. Relationship between MRI relaxation times and muscle fibers. J Appl Physiol 1995;78:807–809.

78. Lundvall J, Mellander S, Westling H, White T. Fluid transfer between blood and tissues during exercise. Acta Physiol Scand 1972;85:258–269.

79. Sjøgaard G, Saltin B. Extra- and intracellular water spaces in muscles of man at rest and with dynamic exercise. Am J Physiol 1982;12:R271–R280.

80. Sjøgaard G, Adams RP, Saltin B. Water and ion shifts in skeletal muscle of humans with intense dynamic knee extension. Am J Physiol 1985;17:R110–R196.

81. Armstrong RB. Mechanisms of exercise-induced delayed onset muscular soreness: a brief review. Med Sci Sports Exerc 1984;16:529–538.

82. Abraham WM. Factors in delayed muscle soreness. Med Sci Sports 1977;9:11–20.

83. McCully KK, Faulkner JA. Characteristics of lengthening contractions associated with injury to skeletal muscle fibers. J Appl Physiol 1986;61:293–299.

84. Clarkson PM, Tremblay I. Exercise-induced muscle damage, repair, and adaptation in humans. J Appl Physiol 1988;65:1–6.

85. Amendola A, Rorabeck CH, Vellett D, Vezina W, Rutt B, Nott L. The use of magnetic resonance imaging in exertional compartment syndromes. Am J Sports Med 1990;18:29–34.

86. Evans WJ, Cannon JG. The metabolic effects of exercise-induced muscle damage. In: Holloszy JO, editor. Exercise and sport sciences reviews. Baltimore: Williams & Wilkins, 1991:99–125.

87. Friden J, Sfakianos PN, Hargens AR. Muscle soreness and intramuscular fluid pressure: comparison between eccentric and concentric load. J Appl Physiol 1986;61:2175–2179.

88. Jones DA, Newham DJ, Round JM, Tolfree SEJ. Experimental human muscle damage: morphological changes in relation to other indices of damage. J Physiol 1986;375:435–448.

89. Newham DJ, McPhail G, Mills KR, Edwards RHT. Ultrastructural changes after concentric and eccentric contractions of human muscle. J Neurol Sci 1983;61:109–122.

90. Frymoyer JW, Mooney V. Occupational orthopaedics. J Bone Joint Surg 1986;68:469–474.

91. Ireland DCR. Repetitive strain injury. Aust Fam Physician 1986;15:415–418.

92. Dennett X, Fry HJ. Overuse syndrome: a muscle biopsy study. Lancet 1988;1(8591):905–908.

93. Larsson SE, Bengtsson A, Bodegard L, Henricksson KG, Larsson J. Muscle changes in work-related chronic myalgia. Acta Orthop Scand 1988;59:552–556.

94. Lockwood AH. Medical problems of musicians. N Engl J Med 1989;320:221–227.

95. Stern PJ. Tendinitis, overuse syndromes, and tendon injuries. Hand Clin 1990;6:467–476.

96. Simons D. Muscle pain syndromes, part 1. Am J Phys Med 1975;54:289–311.

97. Simons D. Muscle pain syndromes, part 2. Am J Phys Med 1976;55:15–42.

8
^{1}H-MRS of Muscle Physiology and Pathophysiology

Ponnada A. Narayana, Edward F. Jackson, and Ian J. Butler

Skeletal muscle constitutes nearly 40% of the human body by volume and accounts for major energy consumption. Unlike brain, muscle tissue relies on both aerobic and anaerobic metabolism for its energy needs. The major fuels that support muscular activity are phosphocreatine (PCr), glucose (or glycogen), and lipids. The relative importance of these substrates as fuels depends on the nature of muscular activity. For instance, PCr is utilized to meet the immediate needs for muscle activity. On the other hand, lipids are preferentially utilized during prolonged exercise.

Abnormalities in muscle metabolism are often more pronounced when the muscle is stressed in the form of controlled exercise. Therefore, characterization of muscle tissue for possible metabolic defects involves probing its response during and following exercise. Muscle response to controlled stress is generally evaluated by analyzing blood gases or muscle biopsy samples for more definitive evaluation. Clearly a noninvasive method to accomplish this goal is preferable. This is particularly important with pediatric patients involving serial evaluations. Image-guided in vivo magnetic resonance spectroscopy (MRS) has the potential for noninvasively characterizing muscle tissue.

Concentrations of various substrates and their changes in response to controlled stress provide important information about the state of muscle tissue health. There are a number of nuclei that could be used to monitor the levels of these substrates with MRS. These include ^{1}H, ^{13}C, and ^{31}P. Phosphorus MRS allows the detection of high-energy phosphates such as ATP and PCr. It is also possible to estimate the intracellular pH with ^{31}P-MRS. For these reasons, ^{31}P-MRS has been extensively used to study muscle metabolism.[1] In spite of its low natural abundance, MRS studies of ^{13}C have been successfully performed for monitoring in vivo levels of lipids and glycogen (and glucose) in human muscle.[2–5] However, the relatively low sensitivity of these nuclei (and low natural abundance of ^{13}C) imposes limitations on the achievable spatial and temporal resolution with ^{31}P- and ^{13}C-MRS. Proton MRS (^{1}H-MRS) allows monitoring of lipids and tissue water with a high degree of spatial and temporal resolution.[6,7] In addition, it is also possible to detect in vivo various amino acids, such as carnosine, and other biochemicals, such as creatine, choline, lactate, etc., with ^{1}H-MRS.[8] Recent reports also suggest that it is possible to detect in vivo deoxymyoglobin,[9] glycogen,[10] PCr, and ATP/ADP[11] using ^{1}H-MRS. Furthermore, the positions of carnosine resonances seen on ^{1}H-MRS are sensitive to the intracellular pH.[12] Thus, ^{1}H-MRS has many desirable features for probing muscle physiology and metabolism. The purpose of this chapter is to review the recent progress that has been made with ^{1}H-MRS in understanding muscle metabolism and physiology, and to encourage researchers to enter this exciting and very fertile research area.

The remainder of this chapter is divided into three parts. The first part deals with the basics of in vivo proton MRS. Proton MRS studies of exercised muscle are briefly reviewed in the second part. Finally, the use of water-suppressed ^{1}H-MRS to visualize weak resonances in muscle tissue is briefly described in the third part.

Proton Magnetic Resonance Spectroscopy

Proton as a probe nucleus for MRS studies offers a number of advantages over other nuclei. It has the highest magnetic resonance sensitivity among all stable nuclei. This, combined with high concentration of water and lipids in tissue, allows the acquisition of MRS data with good temporal and spatial resolution. The high temporal resolution is necessary to follow relatively rapid changes in lipid and water during and following exercise.[6,7] The high spatial resolution allows MRS data to be acquired exclusively from muscle tissue that is selectively stressed.

A prerequisite for in vivo MRS studies is the ability to precisely localize the region-of-interest (ROI) based on a standard magnetic resonance image. There are a number of localization schemes for image-guided in vivo MRS studies.[13,14] These schemes can be divided into single voxel and chemical shift or spectroscopic imaging techniques.[15] As the name implies, in a single voxel technique data are acquired from one voxel at a time. On the other hand, in a chemical shift imaging technique spectra are acquired simultaneously from a number of voxels. Advantages of single voxel techniques include shorter acquisition times and superior spectral resolution. The disadvantage of the single voxel technique is that data can be acquired from only a single ROI at a time. The main advantage of multivoxel techniques is the visualization of the spatial distribution of various chemicals. The disadvantage of these techniques is the long acquisition times resulting in poor temporal resolution. In addition, in a multivoxel technique it is often difficult to obtain the degree of magnetic field homogeneity necessary for good spectral resolution. For MRS studies of exercised muscle that require good temporal resolution, single voxel techniques are preferable. Of all single voxel techniques, the stimulated echo localization scheme (Figure 8.1) has attracted the greatest attention.[16-18]

A typical proton spectrum from a 1-cc tissue volume located in the gastrocnemius muscle (Figure 8.2A) of a normal volunteer is shown in Figure 8.2B. This spectrum, which was acquired using the stimulated echo sequence, consists of a strong water peak at 4.76 ppm and a relatively weak peak from lipids around 1.5 ppm. The corresponding water suppressed spectrum for visualizing weak resonances is shown in Figure 8.2C.

MRS of Exercised Muscle

As indicated above, response of muscle to controlled exercise provides valuable information about the tissue state. More often than not this exercise has to be performed inside the magnet bore to allow for acquiring MRS data during and immediately following exercise. In addition, for selectively stressing the muscle group of interest the exercise device used for such studies should also provide quantitative information about the degree of stress to which the muscle is subjected. Thus, the exercise device is an integral part of muscle MRS studies. Therefore, a brief review of these devices used by various investigators is presented.

Exercise Devices

Any exercise device used for quantitating the degree of stress to which the muscle is subjected must not contain ferromagnetic or any other materials that might disturb the magnetic field within the MR scanner. Recently, some suppliers of force transducers have begun to develop nonmagnetic models (such as West Coast Research Corporation, Los Angeles, CA), and others supply models that can be modified to operate in magnetic environments (such as those supplied by Alphatron, Inc., Elburn, IL). Another requirement is that any associated electronics must be able to withstand the static magnetic field effects as well as the applied gradient and radio frequency (RF) pulses, and must not generate noise that may be detected by the sensitive RF detection subsystem of the MR scanner. Also, the exercise apparatus must be accommodated within the confined space of the MR scanner magnet bore. Finally, the exercise protocol and apparatus should ideally stress

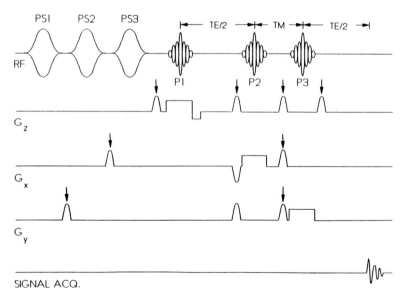

FIGURE 8.1. Stimulated echo localization pulse sequence. The three slice selective RF pulses P1, P2, and P3 in the presence of three orthogonal gradients excite the ROI. Three chemically selective RF pulses PS1, PS2, and PS3 provide water suppression (see text). Arrows indicate the spoiler gradients for dephasing unwanted magnetization from outside the ROI.

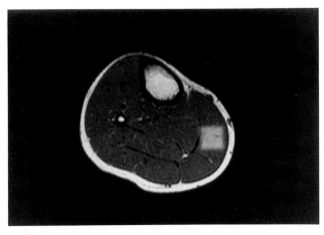

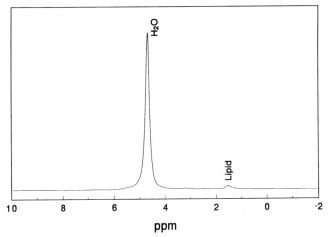

A

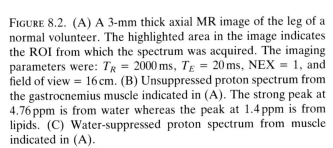

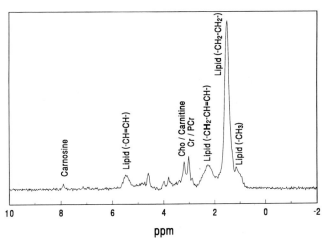

B

C

FIGURE 8.2. (A) A 3-mm thick axial MR image of the leg of a normal volunteer. The highlighted area in the image indicates the ROI from which the spectrum was acquired. The imaging parameters were: $T_R = 2000$ ms, $T_E = 20$ ms, NEX = 1, and field of view = 16 cm. (B) Unsuppressed proton spectrum from the gastrocnemius muscle indicated in (A). The strong peak at 4.76 ppm is from water whereas the peak at 1.4 ppm is from lipids. (C) Water-suppressed proton spectrum from muscle indicated in (A).

only the muscle group of interest without coactivation of other muscle groups. Together, these requirements make the design of a quantitative exercise apparatus technically challenging.

Some of the earliest exercise protocols were designed specifically for stressing the flexor muscles of the forearm. The simplest exercise devices consisted of elastic bands fixed at one end to a stationary object, such as the MR scanner table. Used alone, these devices do not facilitate accurate determination of workload, but can be used in studies in which fatigue is the only aim of the exercise protocol. Such studies have been reported by Fleckenstein et al. in ¹H-MRI of finger-specific flexor recruitment.[19] Somewhat more involved designs for forearm stress consisted of modified dynamometers as originally reported by Chance et al.[20] These devices have been used extensively by the University of Pennsylvania group for ³¹P-MRS studies of human forearm musculature.[20–22] Fleckenstein et al.[23] and Archer et al.[24] have used similar techniques for ¹H-MRI studies of normoxic and ischemic muscle. Exercise protocols consisting of lifting known weights to variable heights and using the weight–distance product to quantitate the workload

have also been utilized for forearm muscle ³¹P-MRS and ¹H-MRI studies.[25–27]

The response to exercise stress by muscles used in flexion of the knee have also been studied with magnetic resonance imaging (MRI) and MRS. Cohen et al.[28] used elastic bands to generate fatigue in order to examine various muscle groups using ¹H-MRI and diffusion imaging. Icenogle and Griffey[29] utilized a weight lift technique for ³¹P-MRS and ¹H-MRI studies. Furthermore, Weidman et al.[30] examined isometric exercise effects using ³¹P-MRS and ¹H-MRI by having subjects perform knee extensions by vertical ankle lifts against a nonmagnetic strain gauge. In this study, the subjects were given feedback of performance via a large LED display, thereby allowing for self-monitoring of performance.

Although some early MR-compatible exercise devices had been designed for nonselective stress of leg muscle in order to aid in evaluation of myocardial function using MRI,[31] devices that selectively stress particular leg muscle groups of interest are preferable for studying metabolism and physiology. Plantar flexion of the foot has been used to selectively stress the posterior compartment of the calf, including gastrocnemius and soleus muscle. Fleckenstein et al.[23] examined the effect of plantar flexion by simply having subjects stand on their toes before [1]H-MRI scans. In a more quantitative approach, Quistorff et al.[32] proposed the use of a pedal-based device for plantar flexion where force was generated against a compressed air cavity. This device provided for calibrated readings of workload, audible feedback to the subject for rhythmic exercise, and external triggering of the RF pulses. Fotedar et al.[6] utilized elastic cables that were previously calibrated with respect to force vs. distance stretched outside the magnet using a force transducer. Subjects generated force against the resistance by plantar flexion, which allowed for examination of the effect of stress on gastrocnemius tissue water using ^{1}H-MRS. For studying muscle glycogen levels using ^{13}C-MRS, Price et al.[4] used a weighted pedal arrangement that, for a given rotation angle, lifted a known weight by a measurable distance, thereby allowing for quantitation of workload. With this technique and proper subject positioning, this group reported that the gastrocnemius muscle was activated almost in isolation with respect to the remaining posterior compartment muscles.

Finally, dorsiflexion of the foot has commonly been used to stress the anterior compartment of the calf. Fisher et al.[33] used elastic bands coupled with a custom-designed boot fitted with microfoil strain gauges to quantitate the workload during exercise-induced stress of the tibialis anterior (TA). Weiner et al.[34] and Boska et al.[35] utilized a nonmagnetic force transducer coupled with visual feedback to the subject to allow for selective stress of the anterior compartment in order to study muscle energetics and intracellular pH using ^{31}P-MRS. Jackson et al.[36] reported water and lipid changes using ^{1}H-MRS and MRI with a similar exercise device. Finally, Morvan et al.[37] examined blood flow, tissue energetics and pH, and water changes using ^{31}P-MRS, [1]H-MRI, and Doppler ultrasound. In this study, anterior compartment muscle stress was generated by having subjects dorsiflex the foot against a half-hemisphere of a rubber ball. The level of exercise was determined by goniometric measurement of the angle of the foot relative to leg.

Regardless of the mechanism utilized for generating exercise-induced stress, for a meaningful interpretation of the data it is essential that the force be reproducible, preferably easily quantitated and recordable, and that the muscle or muscles activated by the protocol be accurately determined. The latter requirement is most easily met by [1]H-MRI. As first noted by Fleckenstein et al.,[23] MR images obtained following exercise at moderate to high intensities demonstrate increased signal intensity within the actively stressed muscle. This hyperintensity is most readily apparent on T_2-weighted or, preferably, fat-suppressed images such as those generated from short tau inversion recovery (STIR) or chem-

ically selective fat saturation sequences.[23,36,38] Finally, the optimum exercise protocol will selectively stress only the muscle group of interest, although this is in general very difficult due to the synergistic behavior of many muscle groups.

Exercised-Induced Water Changes

It is known that exercise alters relative tissue water concentrations in different compartments resulting in alteration of the electrolyte balance.[39,40] This, in turn, has a significant effect on the tissue metabolism.[41] Therefore, ^{1}H-MRS of tissue water in exercised muscle provides important information about tissue state. In addition, the exercise-induced water changes also allow probing of muscle vasculature integrity.[6] It is important to recognize that it is generally not possible to distinguish between intracellular and extracellular water with ^{1}H-MRS. In order to interpret the MRS-observed water changes it is also important to realize that the contribution of metabolically produced water to the total muscle water is negligible.[42] Furthermore, based on the studies by Sjøgaard and Saltin,[39] there appears to be little fluid transfer between the exercising and nonexercising muscle. It is, therefore, reasonable to assume that MRS-observed exercise-induced water changes mainly reflect fluid exchange between muscle and vasculature.

Normal Tissue

The first image-guided volume localized in vivo MRS of exercised muscle to investigate the water changes in human gastrocnemius muscle during and following isometric contraction was reported by Fotedar et al.[6] These investigations utilized a graded and quantifiable isometric exercise protocol to selectively activate the gastrocnemius muscle as verified by the STIR MRI (Figure 8.3). This ability to visualize the activated muscle, combined with the excellent spatial localization provided by the stimulated echo sequence, assured that MRS data was acquired exclusively from the stressed muscle. The temporal variation of the fractional water change

$$\frac{(\text{water peak area}) - (\text{water peak area at rest})}{\text{water peak area at rest}} \times 100$$

observed by these investigators during rest and following exercise performed at 20% MVC (maximum voluntary contraction) is reproduced in Figure 8.4. From this plot the behavior of water during recovery appears to be particularly interesting. Soon after the cessation of exercise an increase in the water level as a result of reactive hyperemia and hypertonicity of the muscle due to accumulation of products of glycogenolysis is observed. (Although both increased blood flow and hypertonicity of

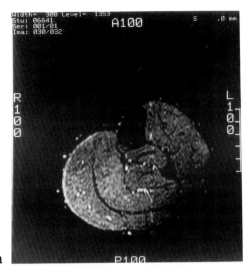
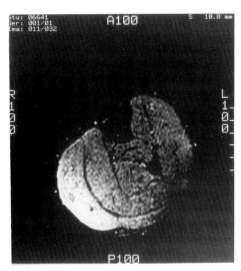

FIGURE 8.3. Axial MR images of leg before (a) and immediately after (b) plantar flexion. Muscle groups that are stressed with this exercise protocol appear brighter in (b). Images were acquired with the STIR sequence. Imaging parameters were T_I = 160 ms, T_E = 30 ms, T_R = 1000 ms, slice thickness = 5 mm, and number of excitations = 1. (Adapted from ref. 6.)

the muscle may contribute, for our discussion we refer to this as simply a hyperemic response.) This hyperemic response, in part, is a result of the release of mechanical compression experienced by vessels of the muscle during isometric contraction.[43,44] The degree of hyperemic response is an indicator of the vessel pliability and provides information about the tissue health. The exponential decay that is observed in these studies following hyperemia is similar to that observed by Dornhorst and Whelan.[45] Although the precise mechanism that is responsible for this decay is not known, it was shown from classical studies that the rate at which the water level decays following hyperemia is an indicator of tissue health. For example, the hyperemic decay was shown to be significantly slower in patients with occlusive vascular disease compared to normals.[46,47]

The behavior of water following ischemic exercise (Figure 8.5a) is observed to be somewhat different from that seen with exercise alone. Immediately upon cessation of exercise an increase in the water due to reactive hyperemia is observed. However, the decay of water to the basal value following hyperemia is observed to be biexponential (Figure 8.5b) with short and long time constants of 1 to 3 min and 7 to 30 min, respectively. Based on the invasive studies by Lundvall et al.[48] and Sejersted et al.,[49] the fast component represents the clearance rate of the pooled blood in the vessels of the exercising muscle whereas the slower component represents the fluid uptake by the capillaries. The slower component, therefore, depends on the density of local capillaries and their capacity to absorb the accumulated fluid.

Jackson et al.[36] have extended these studies to investigate water behavior in the human TA muscle at 40%

MVC employing a sophisticated exercise device with on-line force-time measurements and a visual feedback system. The exercise protocol employed by these authors consists of acquisition of two control spectra to provide baseline data from resting muscle followed by the determination of MVC. The subject performed a 6-s maximum dorsiflexion of the right foot three times with each contraction separated by 1 min. The average of the three measured values was then defined as the MVC force. Immediately following the last maximum contraction, two consecutive spectra were acquired with the subject at rest. The subject then dorsiflexed the foot to generate and sustain a force of 40% MVC for 3 min during which three spectra were acquired. During the 3 min of contraction the transducer output was displayed on a large, custom-built LED readout mounted directly above the subject for visual feedback. The output was also sampled at a 5-Hz rate by a PC-based analog-to-digital converter (LabPC, National Instruments, Austin, TX), converted to force vs. time, and stored for postprocessing. Beginning immediately after cessation of exercise, spectra were acquired every minute for 10 min and subsequently every 2 min until recovery had been monitored for 22 min. Repeatability of the results, which was established by performing the studies on a given subject more than once but on different days, was found to be within 5%. The efficacy of the exercise apparatus and protocol was verified by STIR MR images taken at rest and immediately after the cessation of exercise (Figure 8.6). In the TA muscle at 40% MVC, these authors observed reactive hyperemia immediately upon the cessation of exercise (Figure 8.7). However, the decay of water to the control level was found to be biexponential. The short time constant was estimated to be 0.5 to 3 min whereas the

138 P.A. Narayana, E.F. Jackson, and I.J. Butler

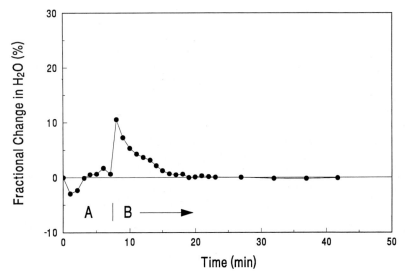

FIGURE 8.4. Temporal variation of the fractional changes in the gastrocnemius muscle water during sustained isometric exercise at 20% MVC (period A) and recovery (period B). (Adapted from ref. 6 with modification.)

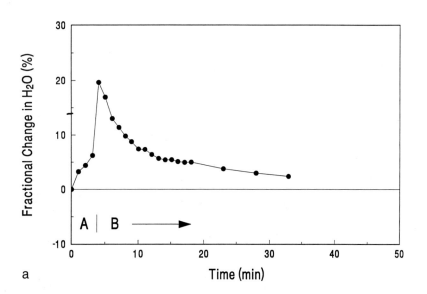

a

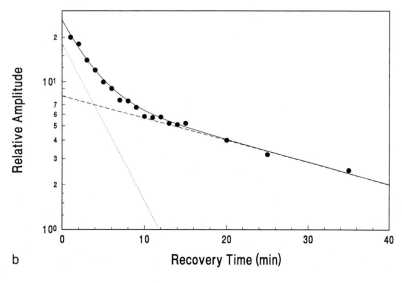

b

FIGURE 8.5. (a) Temporal variation of the fractional changes in the gastrocnemius water during sustained ischemic isometric exercise at 20% MVC (period A) and recovery (period B). (b) Plot showing the decomposition of the bi-exponential clearance of water during recovery (period B). Dashed line, best-fit long component; dotted line: best-fit short component. (Adapted from ref. 6 with modifications.)

FIGURE 8.6. STIR images acquired (a) at rest and (b) immediately after cessation of exercise at 40% MVC. The marked increase in signal intensity in the TA muscle following dorsiflexion of the ankle demonstrates the efficacy of the protocol for stressing this particular muscle group in isolation of other muscles.

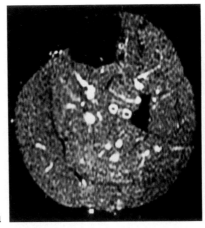
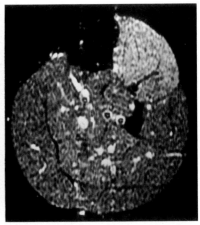

a   b

long time constant was in the range of 5 to 17 min. In the tightly compartmentalized TA muscle, even at submaximal exercise level, substantial intramuscular pressure is expected to yield partial vascular occlusion which may result in pooled blood within the muscle. As in the case of ischemic-exercised gastrocnemius muscle, the fast decay component most probably represents the rate at which the pooled blood disappeared from vessels of previously exercising muscle and the slow component represents the rate at which the accumulated fluid was cleared by the capillaries.

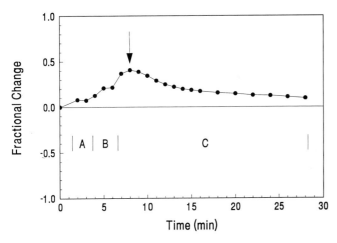

FIGURE 8.7. Temporal variation of water in the TA muscle for one subject. Baseline spectra from resting muscle were acquired before $t = 0$ [i.e., before the determination of maximum voluntary contraction (MVC)]. Periods A, B, and C represent the 2-min rest following the MVC determinations, the 3-min exercise period, and recovery, respectively. The hyperemia reaches its peak (indicated by arrow) within 2 min following the cessation of exercise.

Pathological Tissue

It is clear from the above studies on normal muscle that the MRS-observed exercise-induced water changes have the potential to noninvasively provide valuable information about the vascular integrity of the muscle. Slopis et al.,[50] utilizing the exercise protocol employed by Jackson et al.,[36] studied pathological muscle tissue in a 13-year-old patient with juvenile dermatomyositis. Juvenile dermatomyositis is an inflammatory disorder of muscle, cutaneous, and connective tissue. The pathophysiology of this disease involves an autoimmune complex membrane attack directed against capillaries of the involved tissue, which leads to tissue edema and affects perfusion.[51] The STIR MRI of the leg (Figure 8.8a) of this patient showed hyperintense areas in the various muscle groups indicating inflammation. MRS-observed water changes in the TA muscle during and following exercise are shown in Figure 8.9a. The remarkable lack of hyperemia in this patient, in contrast to that observed in normal muscle, suggests compromised vasculature. This is consistent with electron microscopy of the biopsied tissue, which indicated several necrotic capillaries and undulating tubules in the smooth endothelial reticulum of some endothelial cells.[52] Following 9 months of steroid therapy STIR MRI indicated reduced muscle involvement (Figure 8.8b). The MRS-observed water behavior during the identical exercise protocol used in the pretreatment studies is shown in Figure 8.9b. The reactive hyperemia with subsequent decay of muscle water level to the preexercise level can be appreciated in this figure. In other words, the exercise-induced water change appears to be almost identical to that seen in normal muscle.

MRS data suggest that the functional significance of the autoimmune process in juvenile dermatomyositis extends beyond leaky capillaries and tissue edema. MRS-observed water changes give dramatic evidence of the impact of vasculopathy on tissue perfusion. Impaired

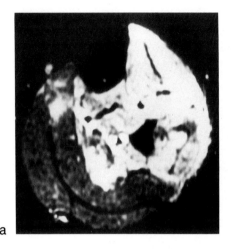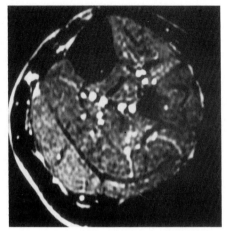

a   b

FIGURE 8.8. Preexercise STIR MR image of the right calf of the patient with juvenile dermatomyositis (a) prior to treatment and (b) following 9 months of steroid therapy. The resolution of inflammation-related edema-like signal intensity changes can be appreciated in (b). (Adapted from ref. 50.)

perfusion results from functionally impaired vasculature, which can be demonstrated on MRS of exercised muscle. Although quantitative studies relating the degree of hyperemia and fluid clearance to the clinical status have not been reported so far, it is clear that the behavior of water following exercise has a great potential in customizing treatment.

Exercise-Induced Lipid Changes

Muscle tissue depends on lipids as an energy substrate during exercise as well as at rest.[53] Any defect in fatty acid metabolism may result in fatigue and other clinical problems. In spite of the crucial role of fatty acid metabolism in day-to-day life, relatively few MRS studies have addressed this problem.

Normal Tissue

The first truly volume localized MRS of exercise-induced lipid changes in normal human TA muscle were reported by Jackson et al.[36] using the same exercise apparatus and protocol that was employed for investigating the water changes. The temporal variation of muscle lipids along with water changes during and following isometric contraction at 40% MVC is shown in Figure 8.10. The most striking observation is the increase in lipids by about 50% during exercise. Soon after the cessation of exercise, the lipid levels fall very rapidly to below the baseline value and recover to basal levels with a relatively long time constant. A similar increase in lipids during exercise was also observed in vivo by Quistorff et al.[54] The reasons for the increased lipids during exercise are not well under-

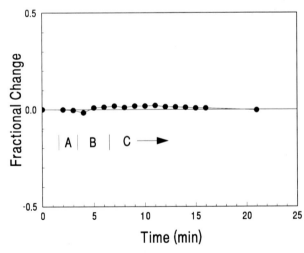

a

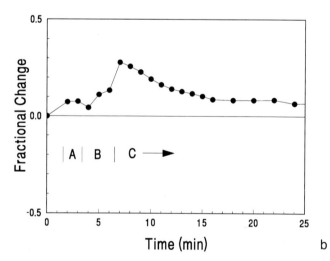

b

FIGURE 8.9. (a) Temporal variation of the TA muscle water peak in the juvenile dermatomyositis patient prior to treatment. Note the absence of reactive hyperemia following the cessation of exercise. (b) Corresponding variation after treatment. Note the marked hyperemia after the cessation of exercise. The periods A, B, and C are same as those defined in Figure 8.7. (Adapted from ref. 50.)

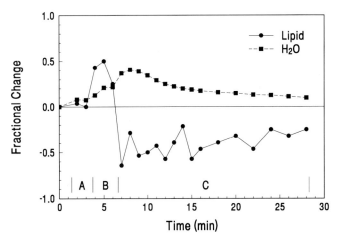

FIGURE 8.10. Temporal variation of lipid along with water changes in the TA muscle in normal volunteers. The exercise protocol is identical to that described in Figure 8.7. (Adapted from ref. 36.)

appears to result from pooled blood, this observation suggests that the increase in the lipids may be a result of blood-borne fatty acids and, possibly, from an early increase in lipid mobilization due to exercise. The sub-baseline values following exercise and relatively long recovery might be explained, however, by the utilization and gradual replenishment of the intramuscular lipid pools. For instance, it was demonstrated by Hopp and Palmer[56] that this pool, even during exercise, is in dynamic equilibrium. Whatever the explanation for this increased MRS-observed lipid levels during exercise might be, the exercise-induced lipid variation can help monitor the effects of therapy and provide an insight into the etiology of the disease, as shown above.

stood. Because the STE sequence used for spatial localization in these studies introduces T_2 weighting, any increased T_2 (spin–spin relaxation) value of lipids during exercise may result in increased lipid signal seen on MRS. Another possible explanation is that the increased mobility of the glycerol core of triglycerides and/or phospholipids as a result of increased intramuscular temperature may make them more MR visible.[55] Such an explanation appears to be unlikely because of the brevity of the contraction period employed by Jackson et al.[36] Furthermore, such a mechanism would not be consistent with the observed rapid recovery of the lipid signal to or below the basal value upon the cessation of exercise. A likely explanation for this behavior is based on the observations summarized in Figure 8.10, which shows simultaneous changes in water and lipid induced by exercise. During exercise the lipid behavior parallels that of water (i.e., an increase in lipid signal is associated with an increase in water). Because the increase in water

Pathologic Tissue

Narayana et al.[7] have demonstrated the utility of monitoring the exercise-induced lipid changes in a patient with unilateral hypertrophy of the TA muscle. The patient was a 32-year-old man with enlargement of the TA muscle for 2 years prior to the initial MR studies. Frequent and complex repetitive discharges were seen on electromyography during exercise. Biopsy of the affected muscle did not show any evidence of inflammatory or malignant cells. A comparison of the water-suppressed proton spectra of the affected and normal TA muscle showed a remarkably depressed lipid level in the hypertrophied muscle (Figure 8.11). Because of low lipid levels seen in this patient, water-suppressed spectra were acquired to gain a better appreciation of the lipid peak (see below). Unfortunately, MRS of exercised muscle to monitor lipid changes could not be performed prior to treatment because of the extremely weak lipid signals seen in the hypertrophied muscle. MRS data acquired at 3 months after treatment with botulinum toxin (Figure 8.12) showed a significant improvement in the lipid levels in the hypertrophied muscle. The changes in the lipid levels during and

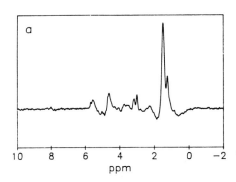

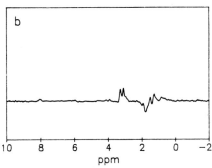

FIGURE 8.11. Proton spectra from TA muscle of the patient with focal hypertrophy prior to treatment. (a) Right leg and (b) left (hypertrophied) leg. Note the depressed lipid levels in the hypertrophied muscle relative to the control. The volume of the ROI was 8 cc. The acquisition parameters were $T_E = 20$ ms, $T_M = 77$ ms, and $T_R = 3000$ ms. (Adapted from ref. 7.)

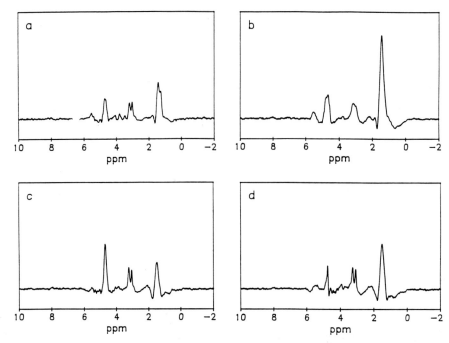

FIGURE 8.12. Proton spectra from TA muscle of the patient with focal hypertrophy. Spectra (a) and (b) are from the control right leg TA before and during exercise. The corresponding spectra from the left affected TA muscle acquired after 3 months of the treatment are shown in (c) and (d), respectively.

The increase in the lipids in the hypertrophied muscle following treatment can be clearly seen. In addition, following treatment the control and hypertrophied muscles exhibit similar exercise-induced lipid changes. (Adapted from ref. 7.)

following exercise at this time indicated a significantly different behavior between the right and left TA muscles (Figure 8.13). For instance, unlike in the normal muscle, a decrease in lipid levels was observed during exercise in the hypertrophied muscle. The lipid levels, however,

showed an increase after the cessation of exercise before approaching the basal value. Three months following treatment, MRS studies indicated that the lipid levels were comparable to that of the contralateral leg. In addition, the exercise-induced lipid changes (Figure

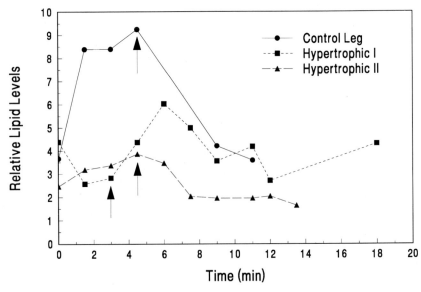

FIGURE 8.13. Temporal variation of lipid peak area during and following exercise in the patient with focal hypertrophy. Right control TA muscle (●), left affected TA muscle 2 weeks after

treatment (■), and left affected TA muscle 3 months after the treatment (▲). The start of exercise is at time = 0 and the arrow indicates the end of the exercise. (Adapted from ref. 7.)

8.13) almost approached that observed in the normal muscle.

These studies also provide some insight into the etiology of the muscle hypertrophy. The spontaneous and action-induced complex repetitive muscle discharges on electromyography seen in this patient indicate that the TA muscle is overstimulated. Chronic stimulation in animals has been shown to produce a transformation of normally fast-twitch TA muscle into a slow-twitch muscle.[57] This is accompanied by an increase in the enzyme activities of fatty acid oxidation (i.e., an increase in aerobic-oxidative capacity). Because lipid is a primary fuel that can sustain prolonged aerobic activity, it appears that in a chronically stimulated muscle lipids are continuously utilized. Narayana et al.[7] have suggested that this may be the reason for low lipid levels observed in the hypertrophied muscle. Botulinum toxin blocks the nerve impulse, thereby removing the stimulus for muscle activity.[58,59] It is known from animal studies that the muscle reverts back to its normal state once the abnormal stimulus has been removed.[60] Thus, following the administration of botulinum toxin a decrease in the utilization of lipids is expected. This could explain the restoration of muscle lipids to almost the control level following treatment.

As mentioned earlier, in normal leg muscle (also in a large number of normal volunteers), an increase in the muscle lipids is observed during isometric contraction whereas the hypertrophied muscle shows a decrease 2 weeks following treatment. Because the muscle at this stage is still hypertrophied, isometric contraction superimposed on abnormal stimulation utilizes more lipids to maintain the muscle activity. However, following 3 months of treatment, at which stage the involuntary contractions have significantly decreased, the trend in the lipid variation is observed to be very similar to that observed in the control leg.

These studies thus demonstrate that carefully executed MRS of exercised muscle provides an improved understanding of the pathophysiology of hypertrophied muscle. More importantly, this technique will allow for noninvasively and objectively following the efficacy of treatment.

Water-Suppressed Proton Magnetic Resonance Spectroscopy

It is possible to suppress the strong water peak using saturation pulses in order to visualize the weak peaks from tissue biochemicals. There are a number of schemes proposed for suppressing the water peak without a concomitant and significant suppression of other peaks. These include use of long echo time, the water eliminated Fourier transform technique (WEFT), and use of saturation pulses. Some of these water-suppression techniques

have recently been reviewed by Hore.[61] For in vivo proton MRS studies, water suppression has to be combined with spatial localization schemes. Use of three RF saturation pulses, followed by appropriate dephasing gradients, combined with the STE localization sequence appears to work well for in vivo proton MRS[62] (Figure 8.1).

The first volume localized in vivo proton MRS of human gastrocnemius muscle was reported by Narayana et al.[63] Subsequently, similar data were reported by a number of other groups.[8,64] A typical water-suppressed proton spectrum from a 1-cc tissue volume located in the gastrocnemius muscle is shown in Figure 8.2C. Besides the relatively strong lipid peaks, well-resolved resonances can be seen from creatine/phosphocreatine (3.0 ppm), choline/carnitine (3.2 ppm), and carnosine (~8.0 ppm) can also be observed. The assignments of these resonances are based on tissue extracts and two-dimensional NMR techniques.[12,65–69] The resonance from histidine protons of carnosine is particularly interesting. Yoshizaki et al.[12] showed that the position of this resonance is sensitive to the intracellular pH and useful in determining tissue pH in vivo.

Despite this spectral richness relatively few proton MRS studies of pathological muscle tissue have been reported. Bongers et al.[70] have shown a relative decrease of choline/carnitine in a patient suffering with Bechet but not in patients with myositis, suggesting the use of proton MRS in differential diagnosis of muscle disease. These authors have also shown complete absence of choline/carnitine resonance in a patient following irradiation of the medial vastus lateralis muscle, suggesting radiation-induced necrosis. These studies indicate a role for proton MRS in noninvasively monitoring radiation damage.

Schick et al.[71] recently performed detailed analysis of lipid signals seen in vivo in human soleus muscle. Based on their analysis, it appears that lipid signals from fat cells embedded within the muscle tissue resonate at a slightly different frequency (0.2 ppm difference) compared to intracellular lipids presumably located in vacuoles within the cytoplasm of muscle cells. This frequency shift appears to be the result of susceptibility differences between interior and exterior of muscle cells. This frequency shift may be useful in determining the source of lipids utilized during exercise. However, such studies have not been reported so far.

The positions, relative intensities, and differences in fat composition of lipids in resting muscle also appear to provide important information about muscle tissue health. For instance, Narayana et al.[72] observed abnormally low levels of lipids in muscle in a family with mitochondrial cytopathy and suggested a defective fatty acid metabolism to explain the weakness and the fatigue these patients experienced in day-to-day life. However, it could not be inferred from ^{1}H-MRS studies if the abnormal mitochondrial ultrastructure seen on electron microscopy represents a primary abnormality or is secondary to defective fatty acid metabolism. Bárány et al.[73] studied a number of patients with neuromuscular diseases. They observed a significant increase in the fat/water ratio (0.5 to 3.5) in patients with cerebral palsy and spina bifida, depending on the progression of the disease, compared to normals (0.05 to 0.07). This increase appears to be more dramatic in patients with Duchenne dystrophy, polio and postpolio muscular atrophy, and myotonic dystrophy (in the range of 1 to 6). Bárány et al.[73] also observed multiple peaks in the aromatic region between 5.5 to 7.0 ppm arising from —CH = CH— protons in polyunsaturated fatty acids in diseased muscle. These resonances are attributed to membrane phospholipid breakdown products that are apparently characteristic of neuromuscular diseases. These authors postulated that these differences in lipid resonances in proton MRS should be useful in distinguishing healthy muscles from those affected by neuromuscular diseases.

Lactate is an important metabolite and plays a central role in exercise physiology. Its concentration in tissue provides fundamental information about ischemia and vascular diseases in muscle. Because lactate has resonances at 4.1 and 1.3 ppm, it is possible to detect tissue lactate levels with proton MRS. Unfortunately, the former resonance is masked by the intense water peak at 4.7 ppm whereas the latter resonance is dominated by strong lipid peaks. Fortunately, it is possible to exploit the spin–spin coupling between the α-CH and β-CH$_3$ protons to selectively detect lactate. The editing techniques for lactate detection include simple homonuclear editing sequences, multiple quantum coherence methods, and two-dimensional techniques.[74–78] However, some of these techniques work well only at high magnetic fields, which may not be appropriate for human studies, whereas others lack the temporal resolution needed for exercise studies.

Perhaps the most convincing studies aimed at following the temporal changes of lactate in an exercised muscle were reported by Hetherington et al.[79] and Pan et al.[80] These studies were performed on healthy human forearm muscle at 4.7 T using a homonuclear editing pulse sequence that incorporated water and lipid suppression. These studies employed a surface coil and, in order to achieve proper localization, depth pulses and surface dephasing gradients were used. Pan et al.[80] monitored the pH using carnosine resonances and lactate using the above sequence in an interleaved fashion and showed substantially different rates of recovery of pH and lactate following exhaustive exercise. In particular, these studies demonstrated the lactate recovery (10.6 min) to be

slower than pH (4.7 min). These measured rates of recovery are in agreement with results obtained by Juel[81] and Medbø and Sejersted.[82] This is the first in vivo study that noninvasively demonstrated the disassociation between pH and lactate in an exercised muscle. In spite of these exquisite studies, routine lactate detection at clinical field strengths in exercised muscles has not, so far, been convincingly demonstrated. Such studies, especially when correlated with blood flow measurements, should provide very fundamental physiologic information.

Potpourri

Direct measurement of tissue oxygenation provides an important physiologic parameter. Hitherto this information has been indirectly obtained by monitoring the arterio-venous oxygen difference. The recent in vivo demonstration by Wang et al.[83] that deoxymyoglobin in tissue can be measured with adequate signal-to-noise (SNR) in a relatively short time opens up an exciting possibility of gaining a better insight into tissue metabolism, especially under ischemic conditions. Myoglobin is an intracellular protein that binds oxygen reversibly to facilitate delivery of oxygen to the tissue. Under physiologic conditions the concentration of myoglobin in tissue is between 0.1 and 0.5 mM, and the resonances from myoglobin are generally overwhelmed by those from other tissue biochemicals. However, deoxymyoglobin is paramagnetic and the proximal histidyl NH protons experience a large chemical shift (~80 ppm) due to hyperfine interaction. Because this region is free of other resonances, it is possible to detect deoxymyoglobin without any interference from other resonances. It is, therefore, possible to monitor tissue oxygenation with this resonance. Jue and Anderson[9] validated the assignment and utility of this peak as a marker of tissue oxygenation using perfused rat heart. Wang et al.[83] demonstrated that the deoxymyoglobin peak seen around 80 ppm has very little contribution from deoxyhemoglobin.

The in vivo detection sensitivity of deoxymyoglobin in skeletal muscle was also investigated by Wang et al.[83] These authors determined that the spin–lattice relaxation time T_1 of proximal histidyl NH protons of deoxymyoglobin is 9.9 ms. This short relaxation time enables rapid signal averaging and allowed these authors to acquire an in vivo spectrum of deoxymyoglobin from cuffed human forearm muscle with an acceptable SNR in 2 s. Such a short acquisition time allows the monitoring of changes in tissue oxygenation with excellent temporal resolution. Wang et al.[84] compared proton MRS of deoxymyoglobin with optical absorption studies in a canine gastrocnemius muscle and validated the quantitative tissue deoxygenation determination with ¹H-MRS. In an elegant study, Noyszewski et al.[85] acquired interleaved ¹H- and ³¹P-MRS from human forearm muscle during exercise and ischemia to determine if the muscle performance is limited by oxygen delivery to mitochondria. By correlating the temporal changes in inorganic phosphate and deoxymyoglobin, they showed that the muscle performance was not limited by the oxygen supply. This is a fundamental observation. Although still preliminary and requiring independent confirmation, these studies nevertheless provide an inkling into the potential of this technique for answering very basic questions about tissue metabolism and physiology.

Due to the relatively low sensitivity, the above studies were performed using a surface coil. Unfortunately, surface coils provide very poor spatial localization. Thus, the observed deoxymyoglobin signal will have contributions both from active and resting muscle, which complicates the interpretation. The utility of this technique would be greatly enhanced if spectra could be acquired exclusively from the active muscle. Because T_2 of histidine protons is on the order of a few milliseconds, localization sequences such as STE, which introduce T_2 weighting, are not suitable.

Glycogen is a very important energy substrate for muscular function. In vivo glycogen levels are generally monitored with ¹³C. However, due to its low natural abundance, ¹³C-NMR studies cannot be performed with good temporal and spatial resolution. Zhao et al.[10] recently reported the detection of glycogen in vivo from a human forearm. Unfortunately, the proton signal is broad and resonates at 3.7 ppm, which is not too far from the strong water peak. Therefore, it is doubtful that glycogen levels can be reliably monitored with ¹H-MRS.

Conclusion

In this chapter, we briefly reviewed ¹H-MRS of normal and pathological muscle. These studies demonstrate the feasibility of ¹H-MRS in providing fundamental information about metabolism and physiology in normal and pathological muscles. In addition, these studies underscore the role of ¹H-MRS in patient management. However, all these observations are based on studies that are preliminary in nature. More controlled and independent studies are needed before the role of ¹H-MRS in studying muscle physiology and metabolism is firmly established.

Acknowledgments. This work is supported by Muscular Dystrophy Association, Shriners Hospital for Crippled Children, and the Dunn Foundation.

References

1. Radda GK. Control, bioenergetics, and adaptation in health and disease: noninvasive biochemistry from nuclear magnetic resonance. FASEB J 1992;6:3032–3038 (and references therein).
2. Beckmann N, Müller S. Natural-abundance ¹³C spectroscopic imaging applied to humans. J Magn Reson 1991;93: 186–194.
3. Avison MJ, Rothman DL, Nadel E, Shulman RG. Detection of human muscle glycogen by natural abundance ¹³C NMR. Proc Natl Acad Sci USA 1988;85:1634–1636.
4. Price TB, Rothman DL, Avison MJ, et al. ¹³C NMR measurements of muscle glycogen during low-intensity exercise. J Appl Physiol 1991;70:1836–1844.
5. Shulman GI, Rothman DL, Jue T, et al. Quantitation of muscle glycogen synthesis in normal subjects and subjects with non-insulin dependent diabetes by ¹³C nuclear magnetic resonance spectroscopy. N Engl J Med 1990;322: 223–228.
6. Fotedar LK, Slopis JM, Narayana PA, et al. Proton magnetic resonance of exercise-induced water changes in gastrocnemius muscle. J Appl Physiol 1990;69:1695–1701.
7. Narayana PA, Slopis JM, Jackson EF, et al. Proton magnetic resonance spectroscopic studies of hypertrophied muscle. Effect of botulinum toxin treatment. Invest Radiol 1991;26:58–64.
8. Bruhn H, Frahm J, Gyngell ML, et al. Localized proton NMR spectroscopy using stimulated echoes: applications to human skeletal muscle in vivo. Magn Reson Med 1991; 17:82–94.
9. Jue T, Anderson S. ¹H NMR observation of tissue myoglobin: an indicator of cellular oxygenation in vivo. Magn Reson Med 1990;13:524–528.
10. Zhao P, Wang Z, Wang D, Leigh JS. In vivo ¹H NMR spectroscopy of glycogen [abstract]. Soc Magn Reson Med 1990;1225.
11. Pan JW, Hetherington HP, Vaughan JT, et al. In vivo ¹H NMR observation of ATP and ADP in human skeletal muscle at 4.1 T [abstract]. Soc Magn Reson Med 1991;113.
12. Yoshizaki K, Seo Y, Nishikawa H. High resolution proton magnetic resonance spectra of muscle. Biochim Biophys Acta 1981;678:283–291.
13. Aue WP. Localization methods for in vivo nuclear magnetic resonance. Rev Magn Reson Med 1986;1:21–72.
14. Narayana PA, Delayre JL. Localization methods in NMR. In: Partain CL, ed. Magnetic resonance imaging, 2nd ed. Philadelphia, PA: W.B. Saunders Co., 1988:1609–1630.
15. Brown TR, Kincaid BM, Ugurbil K. NMR chemical shift imaging in three dimensions. Proc Natl Acad Sci USA 1982;79:3523–3526.
16. Granot J. Selected volume excitation using stimulated echoes (VEST); application to spatially localized spectroscopy and imaging. J Magn Reson 1986;70:488–492.
17. Kimmich R, Hoepfel D. Volume-selective multipulse spin-echo spectroscopy. J Magn Reson 1987;72:379–384.
18. Frahm J, Merboldt K-D, Hänicke W. Localized proton spectroscopy using stimulated echoes. J Magn Reson 1987; 72:502–508.

19. Fleckenstein JL, Watumull D, Bertocci LA, et al. Finger-specific flexor recruitment in humans: depiction by exercise-enhanced MRI. J Appl Physiol 1992;72:1974–1977.

20. Chance B, Eleff S, Leigh JS Jr, et al. Mitochondrial regulation of phosphocreatine/inorganic phosphate ratios in exercising human muscle: a gated ^{31}P-NMR study. Proc Natl Acad Sci USA 1981;78:6714–6718.

21. Argov Z, Bank WJ, Maris J, et al. Bioenergetic heterogeneity of human mitochondrial myopathies: phosphorus magnetic resonance spectroscopy studies. Neurology 1987; 37:257–262.

22. Argov A, Bank WJ, Maris J, et al. Muscle energy metabolism in human phosphofructokinase deficiency as recorded by ^{31}P nuclear magnetic resonance spectroscopy. Ann Neurol 1987;22:46–51.

23. Fleckenstein JL, Canby RC, Parkey RW, Peshock RM. Acute effects of exercise on MR imaging of skeletal muscle in normal volunteers. AJR 1988;151:231–237.

24. Archer BT, Fleckenstein JL, Bertocci LA, et al. Effect of perfusion on exercised muscle: MR imaging evaluation. J Magn Reson Imaging 1992;2:407–413.

25. Katayama K, Naruse S, Tanaka C, et al. Correlation between ^{31}P-MRS and ^{1}H-MRI changes in the quantitative muscle exercise [abstract]. Soc Magn Reson Med 1990;367.

26. Mizuno T, Takanashi Y, Yamamoto H, et al. ^{31}P-MRS change during exercise in polymyositis and dermatomyositis [abstract]. Soc Magn Reson Med 1990;882.

27. Rajagopalan B, Conway MA, Massi B, Radda GK. Alterations of skeletal muscle metabolism in humans studied by phosphorus 31 magnetic resonance spectroscopy in congestive heart failure. Am J Cardiol 1988;62:53E–57E.

28. Cohen MS, Shellock F, Nadeau KA, et al. Acute muscle T2 changes during exercise [abstract]. Soc Magn Reson Med 1991;107.

29. Icenogle MV, Griffey RH. Exercise induced skeletal muscle proton image enhancement correlates with chemical shift imaging of phosphorus metabolism [abstract]. Soc Magn Reson Med 1989;300.

30. Weidman ER, Charles HC, Negro-Vilar R, et al. Muscle activity localization with ^{31}P spectroscopy and calculated T2-weighted ^{1}H images. Invest Radiol 1991;26:309–316.

31. Schaefer S, Peshock RM, Parkey RW, Willerson JT. A new device for exercise MR imaging. AJR 1986;147: 1289–1290.

32. Quistorff B, Nielsen S, Thomsen C, Jensen KE, Henriksen O. A simple calf muscle ergometer for use in a standard whole-body MR scanner. Magn Reson Med 1990;13: 444–449.

33. Fisher MJ, Meyer RA, Adams GR, et al. Direct relationship between proton T_2 and exercise intensity in skeletal muscle MR images. Invest Radiol 1990;25:480–485.

34. Weiner MW, Moussavi RS, Baker AJ, et al. Constant relationships between force, phosphate concentration, and pH in muscles with differential fatigability. Neurology 1990;40:1888–1893.

35. Boska MD, Moussavi RS, Carson PJ, et al. The metabolic basis of recovery after fatiguing exercise of human muscle. Neurology 1990;40:240–244.

36. Jackson EF, Slopis JM, Narayana PA, Butler IJ. Proton magnetic resonance spectroscopy and imaging in isometric

exercise of tibialis anterior muscle [abstract]. Soc Magn Reson Med 1991;544.

37. Morvan D, Vilgrain V, Arrive L, Nahum H. Correlation of MR changes with Doppler US measurements of blood flow in exercising normal muscle. J Magn Reson Imaging 1992; 2:645–652.

38. Fleckenstein JL, Archer BT, Barker BA, et al. Fast short-tau inversion-recovery MR imaging. Radiology 1991;179: 499–504.

39. Sjøgaard G, Saltin B. Extra- and intracellular water space in muscles of man at rest and with dynamic exercise. Am J Physiol 243 (Regul Integr Comp Physiol 12):1982; R273–R280.

40. Miles DS, Sawka MN, Glaser RM, Petrofsky JS. Plasma volume shifts during progressive arm and leg exercise. J Appl Physiol 1983;54:490–495.

41. Sjøgaard G. Water and electrolyte fluxes during exercise and their relation to muscle fatigue. Acta Physiol Scand 1986;128 Suppl 556:129–136.

42. Edwards RH, Wiles CM. Energy exchange in human skeletal muscle during isometric contraction. Circ Res 1981;48 Suppl I:I11–I17.

43. Barcroft H, Millen JLE. The blood flow through muscles during sustained contractions. J Physiol (Lond) 1939;97: 17–31.

44. Järvholm U, Styf J, Suurkula M, Herberts P. Intramuscular pressure and muscle blood flow in supraspinatus. Eur J Appl Physiol Occup Physiol 1988;58:219–224.

45. Dornhorst AC, Whelan RF. The blood flow in muscle following exercise and circulatory arrest: the influence of reduction in effective local blood pressure of arterial hypoxia and of adrenaline. Clin Sci 1953;12:33–40.

46. Shepherd JT. The blood flow through the calf after exercise in subjects with arteriosclerosis and claudication. Clin Sci 1950;9:49–58.

47. Edholm OG, Howarth S, Sharpey-Schafer EP. Resting blood flow and blood pressure in limits with arterial obstruction. Clin Sci 1951;10:361–367.

48. Lundvall J, Mellander EJ, Westling H, White T. Fluid transfer between blood and tissues during exercise. Acta Physiol Scand 1972;85:258–269.

49. Sejersted OM, Vollestad NK, Medbo JI. Muscle fluid and electrolyte balance during and following exercise. Acta Physiol Scand 1986;128 Suppl 556:119–127.

50. Slopis JM, Jackson EF, Narayana PA, et al. Proton magnetic resonance imaging and spectroscopic studies of the pathogenesis and treatment of juvenile dermatomyositis. J Child Neurol 1993;8:242–249.

51. Dalakas MC. Polymyositis, dermatomyositis, and inclusion-body myositis. N Engl J Med 1991;325:1487–1498.

52. Kissel JT, Halterman RK, Rammohan KW, Mendell JR. The relationship of complement-mediated microvasculopathy to the histologic features and clinical duration of disease in dermatomyositis. Arch Neurol 1991;48:26–30.

53. Gollnick PD. Metabolism of substrates: energy substrate metabolism during exercise and as modified by training. Fed Proc 1985;440:353–357.

54. Quistorff B, Wicklund S, Leigh JS, Chance B. Natural abundance 13-C-MRS of the exercising human quadriceps muscle: exercise elicited 2.5-fold increase of a 63 ppm

glycerol-ester resonance [abstract]. Soc Magn Reson Med 1988;312.

55. Doyle DD, Chalovich JM, Bárány M. Natural abundance ¹³C NMR spectra of intact muscle. FEBS Lett 1981;131:147–150.

56. Hopp JF, Palmer WK. Electrical stimulation alters fatty acid metabolism in isolated skeletal muscle. J Appl Physiol 1990;68:2473–2481.

57. Reichmann H, Hoppler H, Mathieu O, et al. Biochemical and ultrastructural changes of skeletal muscle mitochondria after chronic electrical stimulation in rabbits. Pflugers Arch 1985;404:1–9.

58. Kao S, Drachman DB, Price DL. Botulinum toxin: mechanism of presynaptic blockade. Science 1976;193:1256–1258.

59. Simpson LL. Molecular pharmacology of botulinum toxin and tetanus toxin. Annu Rev Pharmacol Toxicol 1986;26:427–453.

60. Eisenberg BR, Brown JM, Salmons S. Restoration of fast muscle characteristics following cessation of chronic stimulation. Cell Tissue Res 1984;238:221–230.

61. Hore PJ. Solvent suppression in nuclear magnetic resonance, part A: spectral techniques and dynamics. In: Oppenheimer NJ, James TL, eds. Methods in enzymology, nuclear magnetic resonance; part A, vol. 176. New York: Academic Press, Inc., 1989:64–77.

62. Moonen CTW, van Zijl PCM. Highly effective water suppression for in vivo proton NMR spectroscopy (DRY-STEAM). J Magn Reson 1990;88:28–41.

63. Narayana PA, Jackson EF, Hazle JD, et al. In vivo localized proton spectroscopic studies of human gastrocnemius muscle. Magn Reson Med 1988;8:151–159.

64. Bárány M, Venkatasubramanian PN. Volume-selective water-suppressed proton spectra of human brain and muscle in vivo. NMR Biomed 1989;2:7–11.

65. Arús C, Bárány M. Application of high-field ¹H-NMR spectroscopy for the study of perfused amphibian and excised mammalian muscles. Biochim Biophys Acta 1986;886:411–424.

66. Arús C, Bárány M. ¹H NMR of intact tissues at 11.1 T. J Magn Reson 1984;57:519–525.

67. Arús C, Bárány M, Westler WM, Markley JL. Proton nuclear magnetic resonance of human muscle extracts. Clin Physiol Biochem 1984;2:49–55.

68. Venkatasubramanian PN, Arús C, Bárány M. Two-dimensional proton magnetic resonance of human muscle extracts. Clin Physiol Biochem 1986;4:285–292.

69. Alonso J, Arús C, Westler WM, Markley JL. Two-dimensional correlated spectroscopy (COSY) of intact frog muscle: spectral pattern characterization and lactate quantitation. Magn Reson Med 1989;11:316–330.

70. Bongers H, Schick F, Skalej M, et al. Localized in vivo ¹H spectroscopy of human skeletal muscle: normal and pathologic findings. Magn Reson Imaging 1992;10:957–964.

71. Schick F, Eismann B, Jung W-I, et al. Comparison of localized proton nmr signals of skeletal muscle and fat tissue in vivo: two lipid compartments in muscle tissue. Magn Reson Med 1993;29:158–167.

72. Narayana PA, Slopis JM, Jackson EF, et al. In vivo muscle magnetic resonance spectroscopy in a family with mitochondrial cytopathy: a defect in fat metabolism. Magn Reson Imaging 1989;7:133–139.

73. Bárány M, Venkatasubramanian PN, Mok E, et al. Quantitative and qualitative fat analysis in human leg muscle of neuromuscular diseases by ¹H MR spectroscopy in vivo. Magn Reson Med 1989;10:210–226.

74. Rothman DL, Arias-Mendoza F, Shulman GI, Shulman RG. A pulse sequence for simplifying hydrogen NMR spectra of biological tissues. J Magn Reson 1984;60:430–436.

75. Williams SR, Gadian DG, Proctor E. A method for lactate detection in vivo by spectral editing without the need for double irradiation. J Magn Reson 1986;66:562–567.

76. Hanstock CC, Bendall MR, Hetherington HP, et al. Localized in vivo proton spectroscopy using depth-pulse spectral editing. J Magn Reson 1987;71:349–354.

77. Sotak CH, Freeman DM, Hurd RE. The unequivocal determination of in vivo lactic acid using two-dimensional double-quantum coherence-transfer spectroscopy. J Magn Reson 1988;78:355–361.

78. Sotak CH, Freeman DM. A method for volume-localized lactate editing using zero-quantum coherence created in a stimulated-echo pulse sequence. J Magn Reson 1988;77:382–388.

79. Hetherington HP, Hamm JR, Pan JW, et al. A fully localized ¹H homonuclear editing sequence to observe lactate in human skeletal muscle after exercise. J Magn Reson 1989;82:86–96.

80. Pan JW, Hamm JR, Hetherington HP, et al. Correlation of lactate and pH in human skeletal muscle after exercise by ¹H NMR. Magn Reson Med 1991;20:57–65.

81. Juel C. Intracellular pH recovery and lactate efflux in mouse soleus muscles stimulated in vitro: the involvement of sodium/proton exchange and a lactate carrier. Acta Physiol Scand 1988;132:363–371.

82. Medbø JI, Sejersted OM. Acid-base and electrolyte balance after exhausting exercise in endurance-trained and sprint-trained subjects. Acta Physiol Scand 1985;125:97–109.

83. Wang Z, Wang D-J, Noyszewski EA, Bogdan AR, et al. Sensitivity of in vivo MRS of the N-δ proton in proximal histidine of deoxymyoglobin. Magn Reson Med 1992;27:362–367.

84. Wang D-J, Wang Z, Noyszewski E, et al. Correlation of optical and ¹HNMR of Hb and Mb deoxygenation in canine gastrocnemius [abstract]. Soc Magn Reson Med 1990;1:175.

85. Noyszewski EA, Wang Z, Leigh JS. Observations of ¹H MRS signals from deoxymyoglobin acquired simultaneously with ³¹P spectra during exercise and ischemia in human [abstract]. Soc Magn Reson Med 1991;1:11.

9
^{31}P-MRS of Muscle Physiology

Loren A. Bertocci

The primary function of skeletal muscle is to convert the chemical energy in food to the kinetic energy of motion. Without a properly functioning skeletal muscle system, we could not perform most of the activities necessary to sustain life. In performing this basic function, skeletal muscle exhibits its most distinctive characteristic: a large metabolic dynamic range. Unlike most tissues in the body, the metabolic rate of resting skeletal muscle is very low. During exercise, however, its metabolic rate increases greatly, and during peak exercise it can be almost two orders of magnitude greater than it is during rest. This differentiates skeletal muscle from all the other tissues of the body and makes it an attractive subject of study by ^{31}P magnetic resonance spectroscopy (^{31}P-MRS). This chapter will focus on two of the most commonly used applications of ^{31}P-MRS: (1) monitoring energy metabolism during the transition from rest to exercise and (2) using these measurements to understand the underlying biochemistry and physiology of skeletal muscle in vivo.

A Simplified View of Muscle Biochemistry

Production of ATP

Muscle activity requires energy in a usable form. The original source of this energy is found in the carbon-carbon bonds of the food we eat. In a multistep biochemical process, muscle cells convert the chemical energy of its available fuels into the kinetic energy of motion. These fuels, more correctly called substrates (Figure 9.1), are supplied by the blood (mostly in the form of glucose, fatty acids, or amino acids) or are found within the muscle cells themselves (mostly in the form of glycogen, triglycerides, and amino acids). Most of the energy in these cells is produced by a process called oxidative phosphorylation, which occurs in the mito-

chondria inside the cells themselves (Figure 9.2). The process of burning, or oxidizing, these substrates is coupled to the synthesis, or phosphorylation, of adenosine diphosphate (ADP), to form adenosine triphosphate (ATP), hence the term oxidative phosphorylation. The complete, or end-terminal, oxidation of these oxidizable substrates releases energy. This energy is used to bind a phosphate group to an ADP molecule via an ester linkage to make an ATP molecule. The net chemical reactions describing the oxidation of a typical carbohydrate unit (such as glucose) and fatty acid unit (such as palmitate) are described in equations (9.1) and (9.2), respectively.

$$C_6H_{12}O_6 + 6O_2 \Leftrightarrow 6CO_2 + 6H_2O + \text{energy} \tag{9.1}$$

$$C_{16}H_{32}O_2 + 23O_2 \Leftrightarrow 16CO_2 + 16H_2O + \text{energy}. \tag{9.2}$$

So far we have only addressed the production of ATP from ADP by oxidative processes. However, ATP can be produced by chemical processes that do not require oxygen. The two such reactions most relevant to the function of skeletal muscle, particulary during exercise, are catalyzed by creatine kinase (CK) and myoadenylate kinase (MK), described in equations (9.3) and (9.4), respectively

$$\text{ATP} + \text{Cr} \overset{\text{CK}}{\rightleftharpoons} \text{ADP} + \text{PCr} + \text{H}^+ \tag{9.3}$$

$$2\text{ADP} \overset{\text{MK}}{\rightleftharpoons} \text{ATP} + \text{AMP}. \tag{9.4}$$

Although these two reactions differ fundamentally from the reactions of mitochondrial oxidative phosphorylation, they are similar in that they both are designed to respond to increases in ADP by creating ATP via a process called substrate-level phosphorylation.

Breakdown of ATP

By what processes is ATP hydrolyzed to ADP? Remember that during rest, the metabolic rate of skeletal

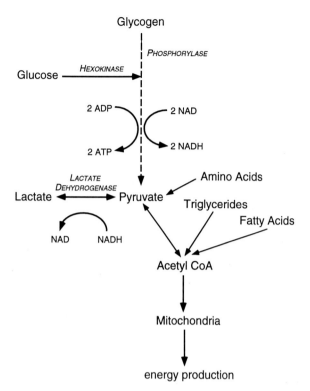

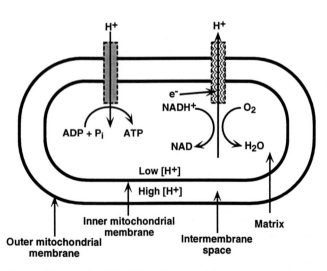

FIGURE 9.1. A simplified description of the major routes of substrate entry into the energy-producing processes of mitochondria. During rest, skeletal muscle produces most of its energy by oxidizing fatty acids. As exercise intensity increases, the relative proportion of energy derived from fat oxidation decreases, and that from carbohydrate oxidation increases. Although skeletal muscle can use several different forms of carbohydrate, and can make usable carbohydrate from several different sources, its preferred carbohydrate fuel is glycogen.

FIGURE 9.2. A simplified description of the important aspects of mitochondrial oxidative phosphorylation. One can see the proton channels, and their linkage to electron transport, end-terminal oxidation, and phosphorylation of ADP to ATP.

muscle is very low. That is because most of the energetic demands of resting skeletal muscle arise from the maintenance of normal transmembrane ionic gradients, mostly the Na^+/K^+ ATPase and the Ca^{2+} pumping of the sarcoplasmic reticulum, and from biosynthetic processes. The sum total demand for ATP from these processes is very low. Things change rapidly during exercise. Muscle contraction, the interaction of actin and myosin protein filaments, only occurs via the activity of actomyosin ATPase. During the transition from rest to maximal exercise, the activity of this enzyme can increase the demand rate for ATP by almost two orders of magnitude. Futhermore, it can occur nearly instantaneously: when making a sudden transition from rest to maximal exercise, the newly increased ATP demand associated with exercise can be reached in less than 1 s.

Balance Between Energy Supply and Demand

Considering the great metabolic needs of skeletal muscle, it may not be surprising that several biochemical mechanisms are at work to regulate the intracellular balance between energy production and energy demand. Because most energy-requiring reactions in the cell are fundamentally thermodynamically dependent processes, that is, they require an excess of ATP compared to ADP, the regulation of the ratio of available ATP to ADP is central to proper cellular function.

Preservation of this ratio can be accomplished by two fundamental strategies: (1) tight coupling of the rate of oxidative ATP production to the rate of ADP production, and (2) linking the normal increases in ADP to phosphoryl transfer reactions whose rates will accelerate via mass action effects. In the first case, studies of the regulation of mitochondrial respiratory control indicate that there is a very tight coupling between an increase in free cytosolic [ADP] and increases in mitochondrial oxygen consumption and thus oxidative phosphorylation.[1] In the second case, there are several different chemical reactions that interact to stabilize the [ATP]/[ADP] ratio. The most prominent of these is the CK reaction [equation (9.3)], where any tendency to cause a depletion of ATP, either from increased utilization (such as during exercise) or decreased production (such as during ischemia), will cause this reaction to shift to the left. Additionally, conditions that induce ATP depletion are often accompanied by intracellular lactic acidosis (Figure 9.3). The resultant accumulation of H^+ also acts to increase ATP by inducing a leftward shift in the steady-state concentrations of the reactants in the CK reaction. Additional stability is provided by the MK reaction [equation (9.4)], where any increase in ADP will increase MK activity, resulting in a general rightward shift in the steady-state concentrations of the reactants, one product of which is ATP.

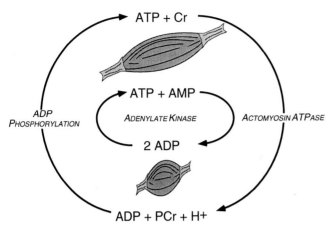

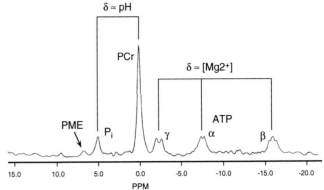

FIGURE 9.3. Interconversion of chemical energy forms required for normal skeletal muscle activity. During muscle contraction, ATP is converted to ADP by the action of actomyosin ATPase. The ADP which is produced is rephosphorylated to ATP by several enzyme-catalyzed chemical reactions. Most of this occurs via oxidative phosphorylation within mitochondria. However, some nonoxidative phosphorylation also occurs, most prominently via the action of creatine kinase, adenylate kinase, or substrate level phosphorylation occurring at several steps of glycogenolysis and the Krebs cycle.

FIGURE 9.4. A ³¹P-MR spectrum collected during rest from the proximal flexor digitorum profundus of a normal, healthy subject. The spectra were collected using a surface coil, a 1.9-T horizontal bore magnet, blocks of 2-min duration, a signal average of 80 RF pulses, and a T_R = 1.5 s. The peaks arising from phosphomonoesters (PME), inorganic phosphate (P_i), phosphocreatine (PCr), and the γ, α, and β phosphates of adenosine triphosphate (ATP) are labeled. The PME region is composed of peaks arising from moieties such as inosine monophosphate (IMP), adenosine monophosphate (AMP), glucose-6-phosphate (G-6-P), fructose-6-phosphate (F-6-P), glyceraldehyde-3-phosphate (G-3-P), and dihydroxyacetone phosphate (DHAP). At this field strength, these individual compounds cannot be deconvoluted. Chemical shift (δ) differences between the P_i and PCr peaks, and between the γ, α and β peaks of ATP are depicted.

What does all this have to do with ³¹P-MRS? All of the major reactants of each of these reactions produce visible peaks in a ³¹P-MR spectrum (Figure 9.3). And by careful analysis of a spectrum collected during a single ³¹P-MRS experiment (Figure 9.4), one can use the relative size of these spectral peaks to determine the free intracellular [ATP], [ADP], phosphocreatine [PCr], inorganic phosphate [P_i], magnesium [Mg^{2+}], and the intracellular pH, and to estimate [AMP], [IMP], [fructose-6-phosphate], and [glucose-6-phosphate]. Thus, one can derive all the measurements necessary for the study of many of the major biochemical processes involving energy production and utilization occurring in skeletal muscle cells. Additionally, because ³¹P-MRS provides the only known method of acquiring these values noninvasively, all of these values represent the truest description of the metabolic events in skeletal muscle occurring in vivo. And perhaps even more importantly, because these measurements are made noninvasively, it is possible to make serial measurements (Figure 9.5) over even very short time periods so that rapidly changing events can be followed.

Application of ³¹P-MRS to the Study of Energy Metabolism

Because one may utilize ³¹P-MRS to determine the relative concentration of many of the most important chemical moieties involved in skeletal muscle energy

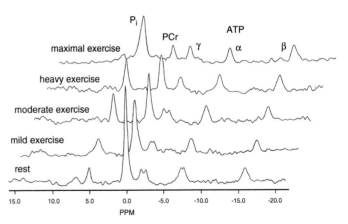

FIGURE 9.5. A stacked plot of ³¹P-MR spectra, collected as described in Figure 9.4 from a normal, healthy subject during rest and during rhythmic isometric handgrip exercise of increasing intensity. The peaks arising from P_i, PCr, and the γ, α, and β phosphates of ATP are labeled. Note the progressive increase in the size of the P_i peak and the decrease in the size of the PCr peak. Not obvious, but occurring, is an upfield shift in the resonance frequency of P_i as the pH of the muscle declines with increasing exercise intensity.

production and utilization, this technology lends itself to study of skeletal muscle. The following includes a description of the means by which ^{31}P-MR spectra can be collected and analyzed in the process of making some of the most scientifically interesting and/or clinically useful measurements. Liberal references to the literature are made for readers interested in a more detailed examination of the topic.

Measurement of Metabolite Concentrations in Skeletal Muscle In Vivo

It is customary to measure the concentration of a compound found in a bodily tissue by obtaining a biopsy sample and assaying it using some commonly accepted biochemical measurement procedure. Generally, such measurements are made in skeletal muscle from homogenates of freshly biopsied or previously frozen samples. The concentration of the metabolites of interest in these homogenates are measured using one or more measurement methods, such as enzyme-linked spectrophotometry or fluorometry, high pressure liquid chromatography (HPLC), histology, or immunocytochemistry. Although the results of these measurements are relatively easy to quantitate, the consequences of tissue collection, preparation, and the assay itself are that the actual measurements are made of the processed tissue sample and may not really represent the concentration of the moiety of interest in the milieu of the intact cells in the tissue.

One of the fundamental advantages inherent to the use of ^{31}P-MRS in vivo is that measurements of the amount of signal from many of the most important phosphorus-containing metabolites in skeletal muscle, those involved in energy production and utilization, can be detected noninvasively. And for biophysical reasons related to relaxation times of the magnetically susceptible nuclei in the liquid vs. the solid state (in a cell, usually membrane, protein, or enzyme bound), the signals actually visible in a ^{31}P-MR spectrum are probably those arising from those moieties that are actually unbound and available for interaction with the physicochemical processes of the cell.

The problem is that it is very difficult to use these MR signals to arrive at a truly quantitative value for a concentration. In reality, all one really knows is that the signal intensities in a ^{31}P-MR spectrum represent the relative amounts of those metabolites that are exposed to similar biophysical environments (for example bound vs. unbound), and one cannot know what fraction of an individual moiety is "NMR invisible" due to various biophysical interactions. Attempts have been made to use strategies based on RF signal detection theory[2] or by comparison with an internal signal arising from a moiety with a known concentration.[3–5] Unfortunately, such

methods provide only estimates (albeit sometimes very good estimates) of real concentration.

For these reasons, one of the earliest uses of ^{31}P-MRS was monitoring the bioenergetics of skeletal muscle and comparing those results with those determined using classical biochemical techniques. Initially, ^{31}P-MRS was used to examine intact, but isolated, skeletal muscles in animals, using vertical bore, high-resolution MR systems.[6–8] The earliest such demonstration used isolated frog and toad muscle, suspended in a 7.5-T vertical bore MR system. The muscles were immersed in circulating oxygenated buffer, and contractions were induced by direct electrical stimulation.[6] As experimental techniques improved, ^{31}P-MRS began to be applied to animal[9–11] and human[12] skeletal muscle. These types of studies indicated that the ratios of the peaks arising from the high-energy phosphate moieties corresponded to the values determined by direct biochemical measurement of tissue samples. They furthermore indicated that ^{31}P-MRS was sensitive to the changes in concentration of the high-energy phosphates that normally accompany muscle contractile activity (Figure 9.5).

Measurement of Intracellular [ADP]

ADP is intimately involved in most cellular processes requiring energy. Thus, in the study of skeletal muscle energetics, one of the fundamental questions to be answered is "what is the intracellular [ADP]?" This is a relevant parameter in the study of the coupling of energy production to demand. During periods when [ADP] increases (as in exercise), it would be important to the cell if the magnitude of the increase in ADP were closely coupled to the oxidative phosphorylation rate of ADP to ATP since this would keep [ADP] from increasing excessively. Hence, excessive [ADP] could signify an uncoupling between ADP and ATP production, a low capacity for ATP production, or excessive production of ADP. Any of these would limit the metabolic work rate of the cell.

Although accurate measurement of intracellular [ADP] is essential for a proper understanding of the regulation of these energy-dependent processes, for several reasons an accurate measurement of [ADP] is very difficult. In most cases, the desired value is that for the free cytosolic form of ADP, which is the form of the compound most thermodynamically or kinetically relevant to the physiologist or biochemist. Difficulties in measuring free cytosolic [ADP] arise because (1) it is usually quite low, on the order of 15 μmol/kg,[13] (2) total (both bound and free) intracellular [ADP] is much higher, on the order of 5 mmol/kg,[14] and (3) ADP is usually released during standard biochemical assays due to ATP hydrolysis.[15] Thus, traditional, direct measurements of intracellular [ADP] can result in values several orders of magnitude higher than the actual free, biochemically available and active [ADP].[14] Prior to the advent of ^{31}P-MRS, free cytosolic [ADP] could only be calculated after measurements of the remaining individual components of one of the energetic or oxidative reactions involving ADP.

Most of the ATP required for muscle cell function is produced by mitochondrial oxidative phosphorylation (Figures 9.1, 9.2). Because of the importance of ATP production to the normal functioning of skeletal muscle cells, the regulation of mitochondrial respiration, which is the process by which most cellular ATP is produced, has been a topic of research for over 40 years.[16] Prior to the advent of MRS, early estimates of the free cytosolic [ADP] in skeletal muscle were estimated to be approximately $20 \mu M$ by using the optical technique of oxygen polarimetry.[16,17] These estimates were in agreement with calculated values based on biochemical reactions of metabolic intermediates which are in rapid exchange and are near steady state.[18] However, use of the direct measurements of muscle cell [ADP] using standard enzyme linked biochemical techniques results in values on the order of 1 to 2 mmol/kg muscle.[19] It was suspected that such direct measurements of ADP were higher because the measurement process caused hydrolysis of ATP, and thus overestimated the real free, cytosolic [ADP] found in the cell. Therefore, it was evident that it was very difficult to know the concentration of the available, and therefore biochemically active, ADP. One solution to this problem is to apply ^{31}P-MRS in vivo,[13,20] where it is possible to make direct measurement of all the moieties involved in the creatine kinase reaction [equation (9.3)].

From a single ^{31}P-MR spectrum (Figure 9.4), one can determine the relative amount of PCr, P_i, and ATP, and the pH. If one knows the absolute concentration of any one of these individual moieties, one can calculate the others by reference to the relative areas of their peaks. Generally, this is done by collecting a muscle biopsy sample and using standard biochemical assays to measure the absolute [ATP], usually expressed in $\mu mol\, g^{-1}$, and total creatine [TCr]. If one then assumes that these moieties are in rapid exchange via the activity of CK [equation (9.3)], it is a simple matter to calculate the free, cytosolic [ADP], generally in $nmol\, g^{-1}$.

What Is/Are the Factor(s) That Regulate Skeletal Muscle Mitochondrial Respiration?

The effective use of ^{31}P-MRS to reexamine the regulation of cellular respiration in vivo was demonstrated initially in preparations of animal muscles where comparisons could be made between muscle fiber types with vastly different metabolic profiles and oxidative capacities.[8,21] These types of studies have been further developed to

investigate the interactions occurring in vivo between energy supply and demand. As an example of this, Meyer proposed a linear model to describe the regulation of mitochondrial respiration based on the time course of changes in PCr concentration in electrically stimulated rat muscle.[22] These data provide in vivo support for the hypothesis that adenine nucleotides exert their respiratory control in a linear, nonequilibrium process at stimulation rates requiring less than the maximal oxidative capacity of the muscle. In another study, Kushmerick et al. used ^{31}P-MRS methods to collect data that suggest that there may be fundamental differences in mechanism of respiratory control in muscles of different oxidative capacities or fiber types.[11]

In view of the potential for noninvasive examination of skeletal muscle bioenergetics, it is not surprising that ^{31}P-MRS methods have been applied to man. Shortly after the first demonstration of the possible utility of ^{31}P-MRS to study mitochondrial respiratory control in situ,[13,23] this technique was applied to human patients with disorders of skeletal muscle energy metabolism. In these types of patients, muscle activity would be expected to result in abnormal changes in [PCr], $[P_i]$, or pH. Among the earliest demonstrations were reports of studies on patients with disorders of glycolysis,[24-26] mitochondrial respiration,[27-29] and other more diverse myopathies.[30-32] As an example of the power of such studies, abnormal high-energy phosphate metabolism was observed in human patients with an inherited deficiency of skeletal muscle phosphofructokinase[33] and the clinical effectiveness of a treatment was demonstrated.[34] In these patients, ^{31}P-MRS was used to diagnose the disorder, was the basis for a suggested course of treatment, and was used to assess the efficacy of the treatment. These results highlighted the advantages of this experimental procedure (see Chapter 10).

Metabolic Regulation via the Creatine Kinase Reaction

^{31}P-MRS in skeletal muscle can be used to measure the functionality of the enzyme that catalyzes the reaction that transfers phosphoryl groups between ATP and PCr [equation (9.3)]. Why is this important? One answer arises from the relationship between intracellular [PCr] and the energy demands of actively contracting muscle. As mentioned earlier, the two forms of so-called "high-energy phosphates" in skeletal muscle are ATP (the direct energy donor)[35,36] and PCr.[37,38] These two compounds are often considered storage forms of chemical energy in the cell, and this is considered to be particularly so for PCr. In typical resting mammalian skeletal muscle, [ATP] is about 5.5 and [PCr] is about $25\ \mu mol\, g^{-1}$.[39] During maximal exercise, the rate of ATP hydrolysis can exceed $3\ \mu mol\, g^{-1} s^{-1}$.[40] After comparison with the

maximal theoretical rates of ATP synthesis from both substrate level and oxidative phosphorylation, it is clear that less than 10 s of maximal exercise would deplete the entire PCr supply. That this does not actually occur indicates that PCr cannot exist solely as an energy buffer as is commonly believed. In fact, it may not have that function at all in normal physiologic states.

If PCr is not a storage form of muscle cell energy, what is it doing in the cell in such large concentration? One of the most promising hypotheses is that PCr is the essential chemical mediator that transfers phosphoryl groups to ADP from ATP, or perhaps to transfer phosphoryl groups (or their equivalents) between the sites where ADP is generated (the myofibrils or the ion pumps) and the sites where ATP is generated (primarily the mitochondria). Such a so-called "creatine-phosphocreatine energy shuttle"[41,42] has been proposed to explain the observed changes in intracellular concentration of high-energy phosphates during exercise and the many regulatory effects of Cr-PCr on mitochondrial respiratory control. If such a phosphate energy shuttle exists, then one would expect that the unidirectional fluxes through CK would increase dramatically during the rest to exercise transition in skeletal muscle where it is known that TCA cycle flux and oxygen consumption can increase by more than two orders of magnitude to a rate as high as $350\,\mu l\ O_2\ g^{-1}\ min^{-1}$.[43] However, such increases in CK flux do not appear to occur in vivo in an uncomplicated manner.

Therefore, the role of CK as a factor in the maintenance of adequate amounts of chemical energy in the cell is of great interest. The enzyme CK catalyzes the near equilibrium reaction [equation (9.3)], which transfers a phosphoryl group from PCr to ADP to make ATP and creatine (Cr).[37] Insofar as this reaction contains all the moieties involved in the energy-requiring processes of the cell (PCr and ATP), as well as the moiety generally regarded as the primary stimulus to mitochondrial respiration (ADP),[16] it is easy to see that ^{31}P-MRS is ideally suited to examine the functionality of CK in vivo.

CK activity is often measured by what is called magnetization transfer.[44,45] This general type of method allows determination of the unidirectional flux of a chemical exchange reaction. As an example of the classical type of this method, it can be used to measure the unidirectional flux through the enzyme CK from ATP to PCr [equation (9.5)]

$$ATP + Cr \xrightarrow{CK} ADP + PCr + H^+. \qquad (9.5)$$

This reaction catalyzes the transfer of the terminal γ phosphate moiety of ATP to free Cr to form PCr. In this method, the magnetization of the peak arising from the γ-phosphate of ATP (Figure 9.6) is saturated. If there were no exchange, the resultant spectrum would have

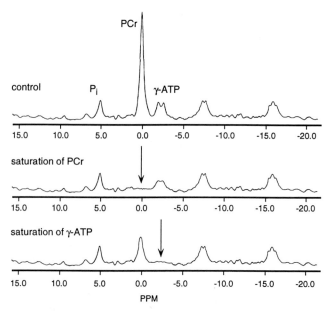

FIGURE 9.6. Noninvasive measurement of the unidirectional flux through creatine kinase in skeletal muscle. A stacked plot of ^{31}P-MR spectra, representing the kinds of data one gets following selective irradiation to saturate the PCr or γ-ATP peaks. The upper spectrum is from normal resting muscle. The center spectrum is the result of saturation of the PCr peak. The lower spectrum is the result of saturation of the γ-ATP peak. Note that the PCr peak is more attenuated when the irradiation is on the γ-ATP than is the γ-ATP peak when PCr is saturated. This is because of the involvement of competing side reactions involving ATP, but PCr is only involved with the CK reaction.

no peak at -2.7 ppm (where the γ-phosphate of ATP resonates) but elsewhere would look like an otherwise normal spectrum. However, if there were chemical exchange between the γ-phosphate of ATP and the phosphate moiety of PCr, as there would be if there were an enzyme-catalyzed transfer of a phosphate from ATP to Cr to produce PCr, then the γ-phosphates of ATP (whose spins are saturated) would be transferred to PCr, causing the net magnetization of PCr to decline, resulting in the PCr peak being smaller than it was originally. After making corrections for T_1 and off-resonance effects, one can calculate the rate of chemical exchange there must have been in order to cause that amount of PCr peak saturation.

Now let us consider the reaction in the reverse direction, the unidirectional flux through the enzyme CK from PCr to ATP [equation (9.6)]

$$ATP + Cr \xleftarrow{CK} ADP + PCr + H^+. \qquad (9.6)$$

Here, CK catalyzes the transfer of the phosphate moiety of PCr to ADP to form ATP. The phosphoryl moiety of PCr thus becomes the γ-phosphate of ATP. In this method, the magnetization of the peak arising from the phosphate of PCr (Figure 9.6) is saturated. As described above, this causes a loss of magnetization of the phosphate of PCr. If there were no exchange, the resultant spectrum would have no peak at 0 ppm (where the PCr resonates) but elsewhere would look like an otherwise normal spectrum. However, if there were chemical exchange between the phosphate moiety of PCr and the γ-phosphate of ATP, then the phosphates of PCr (whose spins are saturated) would be transferred to become the γ-phosphate of ATP causing the net magnetization of the γ ATP peak to decline. This experiment ultimately produces values for each unidirectional CK rate constant.[8] Although early MRS measurements of CK in vivo were in simple preparations, such as aerobic *Escheria coli* cells,[46] this method was soon extended to frog,[47] rat,[10] and ultimately human[48] muscle.

Although the biophysics of this MR technique, as well as the chemical reactions involved, are well described, there is often a difference between the calculated unidirectional fluxes through CK [equations (9.5 and 9.6)]; specifically, flux calculated for the forward direction [equation (9.5)] is usually smaller than flux calculated for the reverse direction [equation (9.6)].[8,49] At first examination of the reactions involved, this would appear to be impossible. The phosphate group must either be on ATP or PCr. However, an explanation has been proposed: that there is some degree of intracellular compartmentation,[49] which prevents immediate and rapid exchange between the production and utilization of ATP. In this theory, the microarchitecture of the cell is arranged into individual compartments between which chemical processes do not freely exchange. As a prominent example of this idea, it is probable that the ADP generated by the contractile proteins does not freely diffuse to the mitochondria to be oxidatively phosphorylated.[42] Although to some this may seem like a novel idea, there are many other examples of such compartmentation, outside the scope of this chapter, to which the reader is referred.[50]

There may also be a methodological explanation for this discrepancy between unidirectional flux rates, due to the exact manner in which the nuclear spin states are saturated. As support for this, there is some evidence that this discrepancy between unidirectional flux rates is less evident when using an inversion recovery as opposed to saturation transfer methods.[51] However, the simplest and most complete explanation for the discrepancy is that there are several competing reactions that require the phosphoryl transfer associated with ATP hydrolysis, and none for phosphoryl transfer associated with PCr hydrolysis.[52]

Another way to examine the role of CK in muscle energy metabolism is to examine PCr-deficient muscle. Such experiments have provided hints that the function of CK in skeletal muscle may not be so simply described. PCr deficiency has been induced by chronic dietary administration of the creatine analog β-guanidino-propionic acid (β-GPA). This simple expedient has been used in electrically stimulated rat hindlimb muscles to examine the role of PCr in achieving normal contractile and metabolic function. Such a study has been used to demonstrate that PCr is not required as a moiety involved in intracellular energy transfer.[53] More recently, genetic overexpression in transgenic mouse muscle of the β subunit of CK has been proposed as a means for determining the role of CK in vivo.[54] It may be that such over- or underexpression of one or more CK isozymes will provide the essential information regarding the actual function of CK in skeletal muscle contractile and metabolic function.

Monitoring Muscle Cell Energy Metabolism During Exercise

As mentioned above, one of the distinctive characteristics of skeletal muscle is its large metabolic dynamic range. The huge increases in both the rates of ATP utilization and ATP production that occur during exercise make this tissue, particularly during exercise, well suited to study using ^{31}P-MRS. Unfortunately, the difficulties inherent in using ^{31}P-MRS to make quantitative measurements of muscle energy metabolites make it important to express the results of a ^{31}P-MRS study in meaningful ways. The most meaningful way to express the results of a ^{31}P-MR spectrum is to use the relative areas under the spectral peaks of interest. Having done this, it is then the task of the investigator or clinician to relate these peak area ratios to other meaningful biochemical or physiologic measurements.

Although Hoult published the first application of ^{31}P-MRS to the study of skeletal muscle energetics,[7] it was Chance and his coworkers who first demonstrated the utility of ^{31}P-MRS to study fundamental muscle bioenergetics.[23] They developed a model that related the changes in the ratio of free cytosolic $[P_i]$ and [PCr] to the free energy of hydrolysis of ATP ($\Delta G°'$) and thus to the phosphorylation potential ($[ATP]/[ADP][P_i]$).[13] Other investigators have used slightly different formulae to bring biochemical meaning to the relative sizes of the relevant spectral peaks in a ^{31}P-MR spectrum. The most common of these other formulae are mole fraction-type expressions, for example, $[PCr]/([PCr] + [P_i])$,[20,55] and [PCr], $[P_i]$, or [ATP] divided by the total visible phosphate signal ($[P_i] + [PCr] + [\beta\text{-ATP}]$).[11,21,56]

Regardless of the method of expressing the results, muscle exercise causes dramatic and well-documented changes to the ^{31}P-MR spectra collected during the exercise. As exercise intensity increases, one sees a gradual increase in the size of the P_i peak, a decrease in the size of the PCr peak, and usually a fall in pH (Figure 9.5). These generalized effects have been used to readdress, in intact tissue, previous questions regarding the (1) metabolic effect of exercise on skeletal muscle, and (2) fundamental regulation of energy utilization and energy production.[13,20,23,57] Although it is outside the scope of this chapter, ^{31}P-MRS has also been used quite extensively to make clinical diagnoses, propose treatments, and to determine the biochemical consequences of these treatments in patients whose symptoms include impairments in skeletal muscle energy metabolism.[55]

Determination of Muscle Fiber Type

Biochemical and Physiological Bases of Muscle Fiber Type

Another purpose for which ^{31}P-MRS may be used is the determination of skeletal muscle fiber type. Although much has been written about the typing of individual skeletal muscle fibers, it may be useful to briefly review the relevant issues.[58,59] A skeletal muscle fiber performs its primary function, contraction, by means of the physical interaction of myosin and actin, its component "contractile proteins." The interaction between these proteins occurs at a rate dictated by the catalytic activity of the actomyosin–ATPase enzyme and requires energy in the form of ATP. In so-called "fast-twitch" muscle fibers, where the maximal rate of this enzyme is high, the speed of muscle contraction is also high; in so-called "slow-twitch" muscle fibers, where the maximal rate of this enzyme is low, the speed of muscle contraction is low. Thus, this general classification of muscle fiber type is by speed of contraction, which is based on the $t_{1/2}$ (half time) to peak tension.

The other half of this actomyosin–ATPase interaction is related to the balance of the rate of ATP utilization (proportional to speed to contraction) and the capacity for ATP production. In muscle fibers with the greatest capacity for ATP production, generally those in which the overall mitochondrial oxidative capacity is greatest, contractile activity may proceed for the longest periods of time, and these fibers demonstrate the greatest resistance to fatigue. Muscle fibers with the greatest fatigue resistance are called "oxidative" fibers; those with the least fatigue resistance are called "nonoxidative" or "glycolytic" fibers. Thus, this general classification of muscle fiber type is by oxidative metabolic capacity, which is related to such things as the capillary to fiber ratio and concentration of mitochondria.

The two principal methods that have been used for the determination of muscle fiber type are (1) histological or immunocytochemical staining of frozen muscle sections, and (2) measurement of substrate concentrations or enzyme activities in muscle sections or in tissue homogenates. These tests can be tailored to assess the expression of myosin corresponding to a particular speed of contraction, the concentration and activity of metabolic enzymes associated with glycolytic or oxidative metabolism, or the density of capillaries per unit fiber or cross-sectional area. The principal drawback of all these tests is that they must be performed on a muscle tissue sample. This requires obtaining a biopsy sample, which is an invasive surgical procedure, associated with sometimes considerable discomfort, and requires the assumption that the characteristics of the sample are representative of the entire muscle. To avoid this (and other) disadvantages, it would be a great advantage if it were possible to determine the fiber type of skeletal muscle noninvasively, as would be the case if the determination were made using ^{31}P-MRS.

It is well known that the metabolic capacity of skeletal muscle depends primarily on the state of exercise training.[59] The skeletal muscles of physically inactive individuals, whether due to some underlying clinical pathology or simply through general disuse, have low exercise capacity, low concentrations of mitochondria and myoglobin, and a low ratio of capillary to fiber area. In contrast, skeletal muscles in exercise-trained individuals have the opposite characteristics. ^{31}P-MR spectra can be used to characterize the bioenergetics of the cell by determining the relative amounts of the moieties involved in the production and utilization of energy (Figure 9.3).

Either during rest or during exercise, ^{31}P-MR spectra can be used to generate ratios representative of the balance between the rate of energy utilization and energy production. Although it is true that the peak rate of ATP breakdown is faster in fast-twitch than in slow-twich fibers, these differences are considerably smaller than the peak rate of ATP production in highly trained and highly oxidative fibers vs. untrained and low-oxidative fibers. Thus, any attempt to describe the fiber type of skeletal muscle based only on metabolic methods evaluates metabolic and not contractile characteristics.

Determination of Metabolic Capacity Alone Based on Changes in Metabolites During Exercise

However, such a selection is not entirely a disadvantage, because much functional information can be derived from such studies. Because ^{31}P-MRS lends itself to the measurement of changes in muscle cell metabolites during exercise, many of the first attempts to determine muscle fiber type used the patterns of changes of these metabolites in the transition from rest to exercise and during exercise of graded intensity. As an example, let us consider a study where one analyzes the pattern of P_i accumulation during exercise. It is expected that exercise would cause an increase in the size of the P_i peak coincident with a chemical shift due to lactic acidosis. In highly oxidative muscle, one would expect that the amount of lactic acidosis would be less than in poorly oxidative muscle, even if the exercise work rate caused the same absolute amount of P_i accumulation and PCr depletion. Careful analysis of the changes in the peaks areas and the resultant pH can provide much information about the metabolic capacity of the muscles.

This principle was exploited in some of the earliest attempts to determine muscle fiber type noninvasively using ^{31}P-MRS. In these studies, the increases in the size and shape of the P_i peak were related to the muscle "fiber type." These studies attempted to identify subregions within the P_i peak with characteristic rates of magnitude increase and acid shift as exercise intensity increased. When peak deconvolution and least-squares curve-fitting methods were applied to the P_i spectral region, "individual peaks" within the general P_i region were identified. These individual spectral components were assigned to metabolic subtypes of skeletal muscle.[60-63] Among the more compelling data that the so-called "splitting" of the P_i resonance into identifiable subcomponents is due to subpopulations of muscle fibers of different metabolic capacities or of recruitment order was by the demonstration that partial curarization of exercising muscle abolished P_i splitting.[61] Such methods suggest a means for making functional metabolic classifications of skeletal muscle using ^{31}P-MRS. However, it remains clear that care must be taken to avoid errors due to anatomical compartmentation of exercising and nonexercising muscle,[64,65] variations in patterns of motor recruitment,[66] misinterpretation of noise for signal, and variability in spectral deconvolution schemes.

Unfortunately, MRS methods have yet to address the more fundamental aspect of muscle fiber typing, that is, the intrinsic speed of contraction. This is a much more intractable problem, inasmuch as the only direct measurements available using ^{31}P-MRS are of a metabolic nature. There have been two basic approaches to this problem. One is based on observable differences between different muscles in the ratios of PCr, P_i, and ATP during rest; the other is based on the likelihood of changes in PCr and P_i accurately reflecting changes in ATP and ADP.

Determination of Actomyosin Type and Metabolic Capacity Based on Distribution of Metabolites During Rest

How can one link the relative amounts of phosphate-containing moieties to the contractile characteristics of

the individual muscle fiber types? To do this, one should first consider that the ratios of PCr, P_i, and ATP may be different in different muscles, an observation that dates back to studies of bioenergetics in cat muscle.[21] Specifically, not only were there metabolic differences in the responses of isolated feline biceps and soleus muscle during electrically stimulated contraction, there were differences in the ratios of PCr, P_i, and ATP during rest. Such an observation prompted a broader study adding rat and mouse muscle to the comparison.[56] In this study, the ratios of PCr, P_i, and ATP during rest were compared to traditional biochemical and functional characterizations of different skeletal muscle types. Based on these results, algorithms were derived to relate the metabolite ratio data to muscle fiber types, based upon the activity of myosin ATPase (the intrinsic speed of contraction). These algorithms were used to accurately predict the distribution of skeletal muscle fiber types in other muscles.

Determination of Actomyosin Type and Metabolic Capacity Based on Changes in Metabolites During Exercise

A more recent study may provide the necessary key to the solution to this problem, and does so by attempting to take advantage of the fundamental relationships between actomyosin–ATPase and the rate of ATP utilization and separating this from the metabolic component related to ATP production. This ^{31}P-MR-based fiber-type method, which yields myosin ATPase-type data, is based on two intriguing notions: (1) that in the absence of oxygen, the initial rate of decline in PCr during a maximal tetanic contraction must equal the maximal ATPase rate, and (2) after hypoxic tetanic contraction has depleted all the PCr, that the initial rate of PCr resynthesis during recovery in the presence of oxygen must equal the maximal functional rate of oxidative capacity.[67] In these studies, prolonged vascular occlusion was used to deplete the skeletal muscles of their O_2 stores. The initial rate of decline in PCr during ischemic maximal tetanic stimulation was then used to characterize the myosin ATPase fiber type. Contraction was halted when the PCr decline and P_i accumulation were maximal. Then the initial rate of PCr resynthesis during recovery with hyperemic reflow was used to characterize the oxidative capacity of the fibers. Thus, in one simple, noninvasive ^{31}P-MRS experiment, a complete characterization of muscle fiber type, analogous to both a myosin ATPase and oxidative capacity measurement, would be achieved. Although more research is indicated, this method holds considerable promise as a noninvasive means of characterizing both the intrinsic rate of the contractile proteins as well as the oxidative capacity of the entire muscle.

Summary

Perhaps the singular hallmark of biological science in the modern era is the application of micromethodology to the study of physiological systems. Although such a reductionist approach provides infomation unavailable by any other means, the challenge of integrating such results into a broader regulatory picture remains. One of the distinguishing features of ^{31}P-MRS as a technology for the study of skeletal muscle physiology is its ability to make bioenergetic measurements of intact muscle in situ. Although this text only described some of its capabilities, the attempt was to put these capabilities into an appropriate context. As the future brings us new applications of MRS, most eagerly awaited will be those where ^{31}P-MRS is combined with molecular studies where the micro results are integrated into an understandable physiological context.

References

1. Jacobus WE, Moreadith RW, Vandegaer KM. Mitochondrial respiratory control. J Biol Chem 1982;257: 2397–2402.
2. Cady EB. Absolute quantitation of phosphorus metabolites in the cerebral cortex of the newborn human infant and in the forearm muscles of young adults using a double-tuned surface coil. J Magn Reson 1990;87:433–446.
3. Shapiro JI, Chan L. In vivo determination of absolute molar concentrations of renal phosphorus metabolites using the proton concentration as an internal standard. J Mag Reson 1987;75:125–128.
4. Wray S, Tofts PS. Direct in vivo measurement of absolute concentrations using ^{31}P nuclear magnetic resonance spectroscopy. Biochim Biophys Acta 1986;886:399–405.
5. Wray S, Wilkie DR. Quantitation of metabolites in NMR spectra from isolated tissues, using ^{15}N spectroscopy and nitrate to determine tissue volume. NMR Biomed 1992;5: 137–141.
6. Dawson MJ, Gadian DG, Wilkie DR. Contraction and recovery of living muscles studied by ^{31}P nuclear magnetic resonance. J Physiol (Lond) 1977;267:703–735.
7. Hoult DI, Busby SJW, Gadian DG, Radda GK, Richards RE, Seeley PJ. Observation of tissue metabolites using ^{31}P nuclear magnetic resonance. Nature 1974;252:285–287.
8. Meyer RA, Kushmerick MJ, Brown TR. Application of ^{31}P-NMR spectroscopy to the study of striated muscle metabolism. Am J Physiol 1982;242:C1–C11.
9. Argov ZJ, Maris J, Damico L, Koruda M, Roth Z, Leigh JS, Chance B. Continuous, graded steady-state work in rats studied by in vivo ^{31}P-NMR. J Appl Physiol 1987;63: 1428–1433.
10. Bittl JA, DeLayre J, Ingwall JS. Rate equation for creatine kinase predicts the in vivo reaction velocity: ^{31}P NMR surface coil studies in brain, heart, and skeletal muscle of the living rat. Biochemistry 1987;26:6083–6090.
11. Kushmerick MJ, Meyer RA, Brown TR. Regulation of oxygen consumption in fast- and slow-twitch muscle. Am J Physiol 1992;263:C598–C606.
12. Bangsbo J, Johansen L, Quistorff B, Saltin B. NMR and analytic biochemical evaluation of CrP nucleotides in the human calf during muscle contraction. J Appl Physiol 1993;74:2034–2039.
13. Chance B, Eleff S, Leigh JS, Sokolow D, Sepega A. Mitochondrial regulation of phosphocreatine/inorganic phosphate ratios in exercising human muscle: a gated ^{31}P NMR study. Proc Natl Acad Sci USA 1981;78:6714–6718.
14. Karlsson J. Lactate and phosphagen concentrations in working muscle of man. Acta Physiol Scand 1971;82:1–72.
15. Pasonneau JV, Lowry OH. Enzymatic analysis: a practical guide. Totowa, NJ: Humana Press, 1993:403.
16. Lardy HA, Wellman H. Oxidative phosphorylations: role of inorganic phosphate and acceptor systems in control of metabolic rates. J Biol Chem 1952;195:215–225.
17. Chance B, Williams GR. Respiratory enzymes in oxidative phosphorylation. J Biol Chem 1955;217:383–393.
18. Veech RL, Lawson JWR, Cornell NW, Krebs HA. Cytosolic phosphorylation potential. J Biol Chem 1979;254: 6538–6547.
19. Karlsson J, Diamant B, Saltin B. Muscle metabolites during submaximal and maximal exercise in man. Scand J Clin Lab Invest 1971;26:358–394.
20. Taylor DJ, Bore PJ, Styles P, Gadian DG, Radda GK. Bioenergetics of intact human muscle: a ^{31}P nuclear magnetic resonance study. Mol Biol Med 1983;1:77–94.
21. Meyer RA, Brown TR, Kushmerick MJ. Phosphorous nuclear magnetic resonance of fast- and slow-twitch muscle. Am J Physiol 1985;248:C279–C287.
22. Meyer RA. A linear model of muscle respiration explains monoexponential phosphocreatine changes. Am J Physiol 1988;254:C548–C553.
23. Chance B, Eleff S, Leigh JS. Noninvasive, nondestructive approaches to cell bioenergetics. Proc Natl Acad Sci USA 1980;77:7430–7434.
24. Lewis SF, Haller RG, Cook JD, Nunnally RL. Muscle fatigue in McArdle's disease studied by ^{31}P-NMR: effect of glucose infusion. J Appl Physiol 1985;59:1991–1994.
25. Ross BD, Radda GK. Application of ^{31}P NMR to inborn errors of muscle metabolism. Biochem Soc Trans 1983;11: 627–630.
26. Ross BD, Radda GK, Gadian DG, Rocker G, Esiri M, Falconer-Smith J. Examination of a case of suspected McArdle's syndrome by ^{31}P nuclear magnetic resonance. N Engl J Med 1981;304:1338–1342.
27. Argov Z, Bank WJ, Maris J, Eleff S, Kennaway NG, Olson RE, Chance B. Treatment of mitochondrial myopathy due to complex III deficiency with vitamins K3 and C: a ^{31}P NMR follow-up study. Ann Neurol 1986;19: 598–602.
28. Arnold DL, Matthews PM, Radda GK. Metabolic recovery after exercise and the assessment of mitochondrial function in vivo in human skeletal muscle by means of ^{31}P NMR. Magn Reson Med 1984;1:307–315.

29. Eleff S, Kennaway NG, Buist NRM, et al. ^{31}P NMR study of improvement in oxidative phosphorylation by vitamins K3 and C in a patient with a defect in electron transport at complex III in skeletal muscle. Proc Natl Acad Sci USA 1984;81:3529–3533.

30. Arnold DL, Bore PJ, Radda GK, Styles P, Taylor DJ. Excessive intracellular acidosis of skeletal muscle on exercise in a patient with a post-viral exhaustion/fatigue syndrome. Lancet J 1984;23:1367–1369.

31. Heerschap A, den Hollander JA, Reynen H, Goris RJA. Metabolic changes in reflex sympathetic dystrophy: a ^{31}P NMR spectroscopy study. Muscle Nerve 1993;16:367–373.

32. Taylor DJ, Rajagopalan B, Radda GK. Cellular energetics in hypothyroid muscle. Eur J Clin Invest 1992;22:358–365.

33. Bertocci LA, Haller RG, Lewis SF, Fleckenstein JL, Nunnally RL. Abnormal high-energy phosphate metabolism in human muscle phosphofructokinase deficiency. J Appl Physiol 1991;70:1201–1207.

34. Bertocci LA, Lewis SF, Haller RG. Lactate infusion in human muscle PFK deficiency. J Appl Physiol 1993;74:1342–1347.

35. Cain DF, Davies RE. Breakdown of adenine triphosphate during a single contraction of working muscle. Biochem Biophys Res Comm 1962;8:361–366.

36. Infante AA, Davies RE. Adenosine triphosphate breakdown during a single isotonic twitch of frog sartorius muscle. Biochem Biophys Res Comm 1962;9:410–415.

37. Lohmann K. Über die enzymatische Aufspalyung ser kreatinphosphorsäure; zugleich ein Beitrag zum Chemismus der Muskelkontraktion. Biochem Z 1934;271:264–277.

38. Lundsgaard E. Über die Energetik der anaeroben Muskelkontraktion. Biochem Z 1931;233:322–343.

39. Sahlin K, Harris RC, Hultman E. Creatine kinase equilibrium and lactate content compared with muscle pH in tissue samples obtained after isometric exercise. Biochem J 1975;152:173–180.

40. Crow MT, Kushmerick MJ. Chemical energetics of slow- and fast-twitch muscles of the mouse. J Gen Physiol 1982;79:147–166.

41. Bessman SP, Geiger PJ. Transport of energy in muscle: the phosphorylcreatine shuttle. Science 1981;211:448–452.

42. Jacobus WE. Respiratory control and the integration of heart high-energy phosphate metabolism by mitochondrial creatine kinase. Annu Rev Physiol 1985;47:707–725.

43. Anderson P, Saltin B. Maximal perfusion of skeletal muscle in man. J Physiol (Lond) 1985;366:233–249.

44. Forsén S, Hoffman RA. Study of moderately rapid chemical exchange reactions by means of nuclear magnetic double resonance. J Chem Phys 1963;39:2892–2901.

45. Morris G, Freeman R. Selective excitation in fourier transform nuclear magnetic resonance. J Magn Reson 1978;29:433–462.

46. Brown TR, Ugurbil K, Shulman RG. ^{31}P nuclear magnetic resonance measurements of ATPase kinetics in aerobic *Escheria coli* cells. Proc Natl Acad Sci USA 1977;74:5551–5553.

47. Gadian DG, Radda GK, Brown TR, Chance EM, Dawson MJ, Wilkie DR. The activity of creatine kinase in frog skeletal muscle studied by saturation transfer nuclear magnetic resonance. Biochem J 1981;194:215–228.

48. Rees D, Smith MB, Harley J, Radda GK. In vivo functioning of creatine phosphokinase in human forearm muscle, studied by ^{31}P NMR saturation transfer. Magn Reson Med 1989;9:39–52.

49. Nunnally RL, Hollis DP. Adenosine triphosphate compartmentation in living hearts: a phosphorus nuclear magnetic resonance saturation transfer study. Biochemistry 1979;18:3642–3646.

50. Sumegi B, Porpaczy Z, McCammon MT, Sherry AD, Malloy CR, Srere PA. Regulatory consequences of organization of citric acid cycle enzymes. In: Stadtman ER, Chock PB, eds. From metabolite to metabolism, to metabolon. San Diego: Academic Press, Inc., 1992:246–260.

51. Hseih PS, Balaban RS. Saturation and inversion transfer studies of creatine kinase kinetics in rabbit skeletal muscle in vivo. Magn Reson Med 1988;7:56–64.

52. Ugurbil K, Petein M, Maidan R, Michurski S, From AHL. Measurement of an individual rate constant in the presence of multiple exchanges: application to myocardial creatine kinase reaction. Biochemistry 1986;25:100–107.

53. Shoubridge EA, Radda GK. A gated ^{31}P NMR study of tetanic contraction in rat muscle depleted of phosphocreatine. Am J Physiol 1987;252:C532–C542.

54. Brosnan MJ, Raman SP, Chen L, Koretsky AP. Altering creatine kinase isoenzymes in transgenic mouse muscle by overexpression of the B subunit. Am J Physiol 1993;264:C151–C160.

55. Radda GK. The use of NMR spectroscopy for the understanding of disease. Science 1986;233:640–645.

56. Kushmerick MJ, Moerland TS, Wiseman RW. Mammalian skeletal muscle fibers distinguished by contents of phosphocreatine, ATP, and P_i. Proc Natl Acad Sci USA 1992;89:7521–7525.

57. Taylor DJ, Styles P, Matthews PM, et al. Energetics of human muscle: exercise-induced ATP depletion. Magn Reson Med 1986;3:44–54.

58. Åstrand P-O, Rodahl K. Textbook of work physiology. New York: McGraw Hill, 1986.

59. Saltin B, Gollnick PD. Skeletal muscle adaptability: significance for metabolism and performance. Bethesda, MD: American Physiological Society, 1983:555–631.

60. Achten E, van Cauteren M, Willem R, et al. ^{31}P-NMR spectroscopy and the metabolic properties of different muscle fibers. J Appl Physiol 1990;68:644–649.

61. Mizuno M, Justesen O, Bedolla J, Friedman DB, Secher NH, Quisorff B. Partial curarization abolishes splitting of the inorganic phosphate peak in ^{31}P-NMR spectroscopy during intense forearm exercise in man. Acta Physiol Scand 1990;139:611–612.

62. Park JH, Brown RL, Park CR, et al. Functional pools of oxidative and glycolytic fibers in human muscle observed by ^{31}P magnetic resonance spectroscopy during exercise. Proc Natl Acad Sci USA 1987;84:8976–8980.

63. Vandenborne K, McCully K, Kakihira H, et al. Metabolic heterogeneity in human calf muscle during maximal exercise. Proc Natl Acad Sci USA 1991;88:5714–5718.

64. Fleckenstein JL, Bertocci LA, Nunnally RL, Peshock RM. Exercise-enhanced MR imaging of variations in forearm muscle anatomy and use: importance in MR spectroscopy. Am J Roentg 1989;153:693–698.

65. Fleckenstein JL, Watumull D, Bertocci LA, Parkey RW, Peshock RM. Finger-specific flexor recruitment in humans: depiction by exercise-enhanced MRI. J Appl Physiol 1992; 72:1974–1977.

66. Henneman E, Mendell LM. Functional organization of motoneuron pool and its inputs. Bethesda, MD: American Physiological Society, 1981:423–507.

67. Blei ML, Conley KE, Kushmerick MJ. Separate measures of ATP utilization and recovery in human skeletal muscle. J Physiol (Lond) 1993;465:203–222.

10
^{31}P-MRS of Muscle Pathophysiology

Kevin McCully, Krista Vandenborne, Glenn Walter, and William Bank

Muscle fatigue and weakness are common clinical complaints, the underlying causes of which are often difficult to determine. The advent of ^{31}P-MRS has provided a powerful tool to identify and study muscle disease.[1] Indeed, some of the first in vivo studies employing ^{31}P-MRS were studies of muscle pathologies.[2,3] This chapter will review some of the muscle pathologies that have been studied using ^{31}P-MRS.

Background

As described in Chapter 9, ^{31}P-NMR permits the continuous and noninvasive measurement of the phosphate compounds involved in muscle metabolism.[4] Concentrations of inorganic phosphate (P_i), phosphocreatine (PCr), adenosine triphosphate (ATP), phosphomonoesters, and phosphodiesters can be measured directly. Free adenosine diphosphate (ADP) concentrations, too low to be directly measured, can be calculated via the creatine kinase equilibrium reaction.[5] ADP concentrations are important as ADP (or ADP*P_i) is thought to be the major metabolic controller of mitochondrial respiration.[6,7] P_i/PCr ratios and rates of PCr resynthesis reflect changes in ADP and are useful measures of mitochondrial function, as long as there are no significant changes in muscle pH. ^{31}P-NMR also offers an alternative method to measure the intracellular pH, based on the pH-dependent chemical shift of P_i. Changes in muscle pH can be used to monitor the onset and extent of glycolysis. In addition, pH changes at the onset and offset of exercise can be used to measure buffering capacity by measuring the actual change in pH compared to the predicted change in H^+ levels from the PCr levels due to the creatine kinase equilibrium.[8]

The relative concentrations of the above-mentioned phosphates, together with the intracellular pH, reflects the metabolic state of a tissue. Dramatic alterations in these parameters are observable in muscle pathologies.

At rest the most important parameter is the P_i/PCr ratio (Figure 10.1).[7] The metabolic response to exercise has been characterized by the relationship between the P_i/PCr ratio and mechanical power output.[2] The P_i/PCr ratio is measured under steady-state conditions at a number of different exercise levels. The initial slope of the P_i/PCr ratio to power output has been shown to be an indicator of the oxidative capacity of the muscle. Subjects with impaired mitochondrial function demonstrate abnormally high P_i/PCr ratios at any given level of power output and have lower initial slopes.[10] Another indicator of oxidative metabolism is the rate of PCr resynthesis following submaximal exercise.[11] Slower rates of PCr resynthesis after exercise can indicate impaired oxidative metabolism. The rate of P_i recovery, on the other hand, has been used to indicate alterations in ion transport.[12] Impairments in the glycolytic pathway are detected by an abnormal degree of acidosis, measured by the intracellular pH, and the amount of PME accumulation, during exercise.[13,14] PME levels are usually low at rest, and when elevated indicate either large increases in sugar phosphate content or breakdown in ATP levels. ATP levels remain relatively constant during low submaximal levels of exercise and only seem to be decreased in a few pathologies.[15]

Recent advances in the development of localization techniques have created a new wave of possibilities. Most clinical NMR studies have been limited to the study of entire muscle groups, such as the wrist flexor muscles and the triceps surae complex. The development of multivolume localization techniques, such as chemical shift imaging (CSI) and Hadamard spectroscopic imaging (HSI), provide an opportunity to monitor the phosphate metabolites in several muscles simultaneously.[16] This will be particularly important in the study of muscle disease that attack specific muscles, such as the proximal muscle weakness of Duchenne and Becker's dystrophies and the lower leg circulatory problems with peripheral vascular disease (PVD). Under these circum-

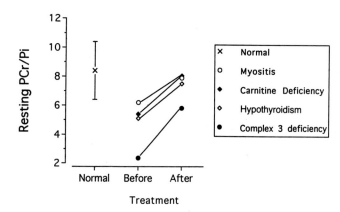

FIGURE 10.1. Resting PCr/P$_i$ in normal subjects with various pathologies. This figure shows that not only are resting PCr/P$_i$ values lower in these groups of patients but that treatment that improves symptoms of the disease improves the ^{31}P-MRS results.

stances, it is important to know the degree of involvement in the muscle that is being tested. Single-volume localization techniques also present an opportunity to actually follow the rate of PCr resynthesis in single muscles.

The first major problem when testing patients with suspected pathologies is to be able to distinguish between a normal and an abnormal response. As with many other physiological measurements, ^{31}P-MRS measurements can show a wide range of results among normal subjects. Significant differences have been found among groups of normal control subjects who have been selected from different population groups.[17] Many of the initial ^{31}P-MRS studies of muscle metabolism used volunteers out of the laboratory as normal controls. These subjects were often quite athletic and not representative of the normal population. Thus, patients from specific subpopulations (older, more sedentary, different muscle fiber compositions) may appear to be abnormal just because they do not fit the tested "normal" population.

Metabolic Myopathies

Disorders in the Glycolytic Pathway

The most important glycolytic disorders include McArdle's disease and phosphofructokinase (PFK) deficiency. McArdle's disease patients lack the enzyme phosphorylase, the first enzyme in the glycolytic pathway, responsible for the breakdown of glycogen into glucose. PFK-deficient patients, on the other hand, lack the enzyme PFK, necessary for the formation of fructose-6-P, a major step in the glycolytic pathway. As a result, both glycolytic disorders lack the ability to produce lactate and hydrogen ions. Spectra collected during strenuous exercise in these patients show marked deple-

tion of PCr, but no change in muscle pH[2,5,10] (Figure 10.2). In contrast, comparable levels of PCr depletion in normal subjects are associated with a significant decline in pH. A short duration (1 to 3 min), high-intensity exercise protocol has been developed that is similar to the forearm ischemic exercise test developed by McArdle to identify these patients.[18] The MRS version of this test has the advantages of knowing the metabolic intensity of the exercise test (based on the ratio of P$_i$/PCr) and thus eliminating questions of how much effort the patient put into the exercise. Exercise can therefore be performed until the appropriate drop in PCr has been achieved, and need not be continued to the point of muscle injury. ^{31}P-MRS measurements have also been useful in detecting partial blocks in glycolytic metabolism,[5,19] indicating that it is a sensitive tool to identify metabolic pathologies. Currently, the ^{31}P-MRS tests that are of the greatest clinical value are those that identify or rule out the presence of glycolytic disorders.

During strenuous exercise patients with PFK deficiency also show elevated PME levels, consistent with the accumulation of sugar phosphate compounds. Large elevations in PME levels are not seen in either normals or McArdle's disease patients. This parameter allows easy discrimination between McArdle's disease patients and PFK-deficient patients. PFK-deficient muscle appears to have reduced levels of ATP (approximately 70% of normal) at rest.[15,20] The significance of this finding is not presently known, but it is not seen in McArdle's patients.

MRS studies have also shown impaired oxidative metabolism (approximately 50% of normal) during

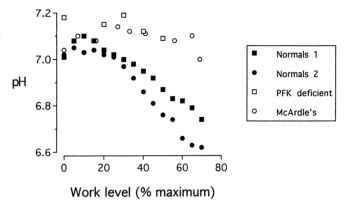

FIGURE 10.2. Muscle pH measurements made in the wrist flexor muscles during repeated isokinetic exercise. Each subject performed 12 contractions a minute of gradually increasing intensity. The force level of each contraction was normalized to each subject's single repetition maximum. Normal subjects (n = 6 in each group, all male) differed in age and race and had a statistically different response. PFK-deficient and McArdle's patients (both male) are single representative cases that are typical of these diseases.[2,5,13,15]

steady-state exercise in both McArdle's and PFK-deficient patients.[5,14] ³¹P-MRS studies have also shown that intravenous glucose infusion in patients with McArdle's disease improves oxidative metabolism, and may indicate the "second wind" phenomenon seen in this condition.[14] These results demonstrate the interaction and importance of glycolytic pathways in the regulation of oxidative metabolism.

Mitochondrial Disorders

Patients with mitochondrial disorders of muscle present with limb weakness and fatigue, "ragged red fibers" in muscle biopsy, and biochemical evidence of impaired mitochondrial function. Mitochondrial disorders include defects of the transport of pyruvate into the mitochondria, lack of the enzyme pyruvate dehydrogenase, and defects in the electron transport chain, all of which reduce oxidative metabolism. Patients with these disorders show a very heterogeneous response to rest and exercise measurements with ³¹P-MRS from near normal to very abnormal. The abnormal responses include elevated P_i/PCr ratios at rest and during exercise, which reflects impairment in the ability to do work.[19,21] The rate of PCr/P_i recovery after exercise in 12 patients with proven mitochondrial diseases varied from normal to 20% of normal, depending on the specific defect and its severity.[19] A ³¹P-NMR follow-up study showed an improvement in oxidative metabolism in a severely affected complex III-deficient patient treated with vitamin K3 and vitamin C for a year.[22]

Systemic Diseases

A number of disease states that do not primarily affect muscle have been shown to affect exercise tolerance, and ³¹P-MRS has been used to show that reduced muscle metabolism is a factor in these diseases (Figure 10.3). Patients with heart failure have increased ratios of P_i/PCr during exercise, suggesting impaired muscle metabolism[23] that may not be related to reduced muscle blood flow.[24] Other studies have demonstrated decreased rates of PCr resynthesis in patients with renal failure.[25] Similarly, patients with complicated migraine have shown both increased P_i/PCr ratios during exercise and slower rates of PCr resynthesis following exercise.[26] The significance of these abnormalities in oxidative metabolism is unclear and may reflect a "detraining" effect due to reduced activity levels caused by the diseases, or specific inhibitions of muscle metabolism. Further studies will be needed to address this question. Some of the lowest rates of PCr recovery observed in calf muscles were measured in peripheral vascular disease patients, with rates three- to fivefold slower than normal healthy volunteers.[27–29]

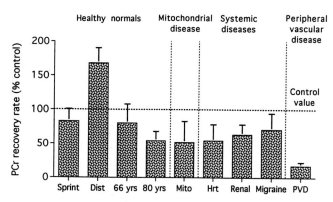

FIGURE 10.3. Relative rate of PCr recovery as a percent of control. For each group the control value was determined from matched controls. Values for Mito (mitochondrial myopathies) and Hrt (heart failure) were determined from data on rate of recovery of PCr/P_i ratios.[10,23] The error bars indicate standard deviations and each group had at least six subjects. All groups are significantly different ($p < 0.05$) from control except the sprint and 66-year-old groups.

The reductions in PCr recovery rates in these patients are consistent with known reductions in leg blood flow.

Muscular Dystrophies

Muscular dystrophies include many hereditary muscle disorders that cause progressive fiber destruction and replacement of muscle cells with fat and connective tissue. Patients with Duchenne muscular dystrophy, a most serious type of muscular dystrophy, demonstrate elevated P_i/PCr ratios at rest.[9] The ratio increases with age and correlates with the progression of the disease[30] (Figure 10.4). Other destructive muscle disorders, such as Becker's dystrophy, myotonic dystrophy, polymyositis, and acute myoglobinuria, also show similar elevations in resting P_i/PCr.[31] Interestingly, similar changes in resting P_i/PCr are seen in normal subjects following transient exercise-induced muscle injury.[31] This suggests that elevated resting P_i/PCr ratios are nonspecific and indicate muscle destruction.

Patients with muscular dystrophy are difficult to exercise due to their young age and severe muscle wasting. However, some exercise studies were performed and no abnormality in muscle metabolism was reported.[32] MRS studies were also used to confirm that treatment with allopurinol has no effect on muscle metabolism in these patients.[31] An interesting finding in Duchenne and Becker's dystrophy patients is a prolonged recovery of P_i following exercise[33] and maybe an indication that H^+ transport in muscle cells is impaired. Thus, measurements of P_i transport may supply clues as to the mechanism of muscle damage in these patients.

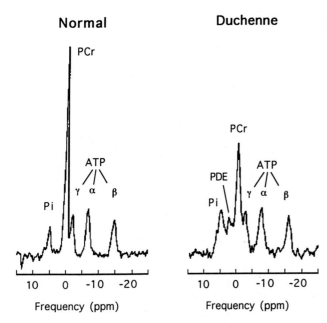

FIGURE 10.4. Resting ^{31}P-MRS spectra from a normal boy and a patient with Duchenne muscular dystrophy. Spectra show typical differences between normals and Duchenne muscle, that is, high P_i and low PCr values, with an increased phosphodiester (PDE) peak.

Miscellaneous Diseases

Other causes of muscle weakness and exercise intolerance have been studied using MRS. One of the most controversial is chronic fatigue syndrome because there is no known mechanism for this condition.[34] There are conflicting results concerning whether peripheral changes occur in these patients. ^{31}P-MRS studies have provided valuable information on this question in the they have shown no evidence to support that metabolic abnormalities exist in the muscles of these patients.[35]

Summary

In this chapter we provided a sampling of the wide range of muscle diseases that have been studied with ^{31}P-MRS. Although ^{31}P-MRS is not a common diagnostic tool, it can be highly useful in identifying and confirming diseases, can provide insight into the severity of the disease, and can follow up on the effectiveness of a treatment. Resting P_i/PCr values can indicate either metabolic abnormalities or the presence of muscle injury. The oxidative capacity can be measured from the P_i/PCr ratios during submaximal exercise or from the rate of PCr resynthesis following exercise. This can be useful in monitoring the peripheral effects of various systemic diseases as well as characterizing the relatively rare mitochondrial disorders. The level of acidosis during strenuous exercise is a simple but powerful parameter to identify glycolytic disorders. In addition, the presence of increased PME levels discriminates between McArdle's disease and PFK deficiencies. Finally, subtle changes, such as a slowed P_i recovery, might provide evidence of abnormal membrane function. Thus, MRS has been used to characterize muscle metabolism in a wide variety of patients, and can be useful in future studies of muscle weakness and exercise intolerance.

References

1. Radda GK, Rajagopalan B, Talyor DJ. Biochemistry in vivo: an appraisal of clinical magnetic resonance spectroscopy. Magn Reson Q 1989;5:122–151.
2. Chance B, Eleff S, Bank W, et al. 31P NMR studies of control of mitochondrial function in phosphofructokinase-deficient human skeletal muscle. Proc Natl Acad Sci USA 1982;79:7714–7718.
3. Gadian DG, Radda RK, Ross BD, et al. 31P NMR examination of a myopathy. Lancet 1981;2:744–775.
4. Chance B, Leigh JS, Kent J, et al. Multiple controls of oxidative metabolism of living tissues as studied by 31-P MRS. Proc Natl Acad Sci USA 1986;83:9458–9462.
5. Bertocci LA, Haller RG, Lewis SF, et al. Abnormal high-energy phosphate metabolism in human muscle phosphofructokinase deficiency. J Appl Physiol 1991;70:1201–1207.
6. Blei ML, Conley KE, Kushmerick MJ. Separate measures of ATP ultilization and recovery in human skeletal muscle. J Physiol (Lond) 1993;456:203–222.
7. Kemp GJ, Radda GK. Quantitative interpretation of bioenergetic data from ^{31}P and ^{1}H magnetic resonance spectroscopic studies of skeletal muscle: an analytical review. Mag Res Quart 1994;10:43–63.
8. Adams GR, Foley JM, Meyer RA. Muscle buffer capacity estimated from pH changes during rest-to-work transitions. J Appl Physiol 1990;69:968–972.
9. Bank W, Argov Z, Leigh JS, Chance B. The value of 31P NMR in the diagnosis and monitoring the course of human myopathies. Ann NY Acad Sci 1986:448–450.
10. Argov Z, Bank WJ, Maris J, et al. Bioenergetic heterogeneity of human mitochondrial myopathies: phosphorus magnetic resonance spectroscopy study. Neurology 1987;37:257–262.
11. McCully K, Vandenborne K, De Meirleir K, et al. Muscle metabolism in track athletes using 31-P magnetic resonance spectroscopy. Can J Physiol Pharmacol 1992;70:1353–1359.
12. Barbiroli B, Funicello R, Iotti S, et al. 31P NMR spectroscopy of skeletal muscle in Becker dystrophy and DMD/BMD carriers: altered rate of phosphate transport. J Neurol Sci 1992;109:188–195.
13. Lewis SF, Haller RC. The pathophysiology of McArdle's disease: clues to regulation in exercise and fatigue. J Appl Physiol 1986;61:391–401.
14. Taylor DJ, Styles P, Matthews PM, et al. Energetics of human muscle; exercise induced ATP depletion. Magn Reson Med 1986;3:44–54.

15. Argov Z, Bank WJ, Maris J, et al. Muscle energy metabolism in human phosphofructokinase deficiency as recorded by 31P nuclear magnetic resonance spectroscopy. Ann Neurol 1987;16:529–538.

16. Goelman G, Walter G, Leigh JS Jr. Hadamard spectroscopic imaging technique as applied to study human calf muscles. Magn Reson Med 1992;25:349–354.

17. McCully KK, Kent JA, Chance B. Muscle injury and exercise stress measured with 31-P magnetic resonance spectroscopy. In: Paul R, Elzinga G, Yamada K, eds. Muscle energetics. Progress in clinical and biological research. vol. 315. 1989:197–207. New York, Alan R Liss, Inc.

18. McArdle B. Myopathies due to a defect in muscle glycogen breakdown. Clin Sci 1951;10:13–35.

19. Argov Z, Bank WJ, Boden B, et al. Phosphorus magnetic resonance spectroscopy of partially blocked muscle glycolysis: an in vivo study of phosphoglycerate mutase deficiency. Arch Neurol 1987;44:614–617.

20. Giger U, Argov Z, Schnall M, et al. Metabolic myopathy in canine muscle-type phosphofructokinase deficiency. Muscle Nerve 1988;11:1260–1265.

21. Eleff S, Kennaway NG, Buist NRM, et al. 31P NMR study of improvement in oxidative phosphorylation by vitamins K₃ and C in a patient with a defect in electron transport at complex III in skeletal muscle. Proc Natl Acad Sci USA 1984;81:3529–3533.

22. Argov Z, Bank WJ, Maris J, et al. Treatment of mitochondrial myopathy due to complex III deficiency with vitamins K₃ and C: a ³¹P-NMR follow-up study. 1986;19:598–602.

23. Wilson JR, Fink L, Maris J, et al. Evaluation of energy metabolism in skeletal muscle of patients with heart failure with gated phosphorus-31 nuclear magnetic resonance. Circulation 1985;71:57–62.

24. Wiener DH, Fink LI, Maris J, et al. Abnormal skeletal muscle bioenergetics during exercise in patients with heart failure: role of reduced muscle blood flow. Circulation 1986;73:1127–1136.

25. McCully KK, Posner JD. Measuring exercise-induced adaptations and injury with magnetic resonance spectroscopy. Int J Sports Med 1992;13(Suppl 1):S147–S149.

26. Barbiroli G, Montagna P, Cortelli P, et al. Complicated migraine studied by phosphorus magnetic resonance spectroscopy. Cephalalgia 1990;10:264–272.

27. Hands L, Bore P, Galloway B, et al. Muscle metabolism in patients with peripheral vascular disease investigated by 31P nuclear magnetic resonance spectroscopy. Clin Sci 1986;71:283–290.

28. Keller U, Oberhansli R, Huber P, et al. Phosphocreatine content and intracellular pH of calf muscle measured by phosphorus NMR spectroscopy in occlusive arterial disease of the legs. Eur J Clin Invest 1985;15:382–388.

29. Zatina M, Berkowitz H, Gross G, et al. 31-P nuclear magnetic resonance spectroscopy: noninvasive biochemical analysis of the ischemic extremity. J Vasc Surg 1986;3:411–420.

30. Younkin DP, Berman P, Sladky J, et al. 31P NMR studies in Duchenne muscular dystrophy: age-related metabolic changes. Neurology 1987;37:165–169.

31. McCully KK, Argov Z, Boden BP, et al. Detection of muscle injury in humans with 31-P magnetic resonance spectroscopy. Muscle Nerve 1988;11:212–216.

32. Griffiths RD, Cady EB, Edwards RH, Wilkie DR. Muscle energy metabolism in Duchenne dystrophy studied by 31P-NMR: controlled trials show no efffect of allopurinol or ribose. Muscle Nerve 1985;8:760–767.

33. Barbiroli B, Funicello R, Iotti S, et al. Muscle energy metabolism in female DMD/BMD carriers: altered rate of phosphate transport. J Neurol Sci 1992;109:188–195.

34. Schluederberg A, Straus SE, Peterson P, et al. Chronic fatigue syndrome research: definition and medical outcome assessment. Ann Intern Med 1992;117:325–331.

35. Kent-Braun JA, Sharma K, Massie B, et al. Absence of metabolic abnormalities in patients with chronic fatigue syndrome. Neurology 1993;43:125–131.

Part IV
Neuromuscular Disease

11
Classification of Neuromuscular Diseases

Carl D. Reimers and Dieter E. Pongratz

Neuromuscular disorders are those diseases that involve the motor nuclei of the cranial nerves and anterior horn cells of the spinal cord, the peripheral nerves, the neuromuscular junction, and/or muscle itself.[1] They can be classified according to many different features. In addition to the site of the lesion, they can be differentiated into hereditary and acquired disorders. Hereditary disorders can be subdivided into those with abnormalities of the nuclear or mitochondrial genome. Their mode of inheritance may be autosomal dominant or autosomal recessive, X-linked dominant (very rare) or X-linked recessive. In the case of acquired diseases the next step of classification usually is to order them according to their etiology (e.g., inflammatory, endocrine, toxic). The World Federation of Neurology[2] proposed a classification that includes all these aspects. Generally, the neurogenic disorders are classified according to the site of the major pathological process, and myopathies according to whether they are hereditary or acquired.[3] Table 11.1 lists a considerably abbreviated classification of the World Federation of Neurology, omitting particularly rare disorders.

The clinician usually assesses a variety of features to categorize neuromuscular diseases. Of interest are the time of onset (congenital, childhood, juvenile, or adulthood), the chronicity (acute or chronic), the course of the disease (progressive, intermittent), the absence or presence and the distribution of muscle weakness [diffuse, proximal (Figure 11.1), distal (Figures 11.2 and 11.3), neck (Figures 11.4 and 11.5), facial (Table 11.2), extraocular (Table 11.3), pharyngeal (Table 11.4), bulbar (i.e., weakness and wasting of facial, mandibular, and tongue muscles, dysphagia and dysarthria); and symmetric or asymmetric (Figure 11.6) (Table 11.5)]. The degree of weakness or wasting, muscle atrophy or hypertrophy (Figures 11.7 and 11.8) (Table 11.6), and the presence or absence of muscle pain and its trigger mechanisms (Table 11.7) are of importance.

Muscle imaging provides a differentiation of muscle atrophy and hypertrophy into simple and complex forms (Table 11.8). Additionally, it is the only noninvasive technique giving information about the muscle tissue. As a general rule, muscle wasting in primary myopathies is more marked in proximal than in distal muscles, whereas in neuropathies the opposite is true. However, there are some important exceptions (e.g., proximal spinal muscular atrophies or distal muscular dystrophies). Abnormal fatiguability (Table 11.9), myotonic phenomena (Table 11.10), and fasciculations (Table 11.11) are characteristic features of several disorders. The involvement of other organs, for example, abnormalities of the brain (Table 11.12), spinal cord (Table 11.13), eye (Table 11.14), ear (Table 11.15), heart (Table 11.16), lung (Table 11.17), skin (Table 11.18; Figure 11.9A), bones (Table 11.19), or endocrine glands, or special features such as muscular calcifications (Table 11.20, Figure 11.9B) and fibrous contractures (Figures 11.10 and 11.11) in early stages of the disease (Table 11.21) may be very valuable hints to the diagnosis. Disorders that typically or occasionally exhibit the features mentioned above are listed in the corresponding tables.

The epidemiologist is interested in the frequency, that is, the general and local incidence and prevalence of the diseases. For the patient, the differentiation into treatable and nontreatable disorders is of greatest importance.

TABLE 11.1. Classification of neuromuscular diseases (World Federation of Neurology,[2] modified and abbreviated).

I. Spinal muscular atrophies
   A. Heritable
      A-1 Autosomal recessive
          1. Infantile spinal muscular atrophy type 1 (Werdnig-Hoffmann)
          2. Intermediate spinal muscular atrophy type 2
          3. Juvenile spinal muscular atrophy type 3 (Kugelberg-Welander)
          4. Proximal spinal muscular atrophy of adults
          5. Scapuloperoneal muscular atrophy
          6. Distal spinal muscular atrophy of childhood
          7. Distal spinal muscular atrophy of adults
          8. Other forms
      A-2 Autosomal recessive
          1. Spinal muscular atrophy with hexosaminidase deficiency
          2. Other forms
      A-3 Autosomal dominant
          1. Proximal type of juvenile spinal muscular atrophy (Kugelberg-Welander)
          2. Neuronal type of Charcot-Marie-Tooth disease
          3. Neuronal scapuloperoneal atrophy with cardiopathy (Emery-Dreifuss)
          4. Scapuloperoneal amyotrophy
          5. Distal spinal muscular atrophy
          6. Facioscapulohumeral type of spinal muscular atrophy
          7. Adult type of proximal spinal muscular atrophy (Finkel)
          8. Other forms
      A-4 X-linked recessive
          1. Spinal and bulbar muscular atrophy (Kennedy)
          2. X-linked facioscapulohumeral spinal muscular atrophy
          3. Other forms
      A-5 X-linked dominant (very rare)
   B. Congenital and developmental abnormalities
      B-1 Möbius syndrome
      B-2 Congenital absence of muscles
      B-3 Other forms
   C. Disorders of motor neurons attributed to physical causes
      C-1 Trauma
      C-2 Amyotrophy due to destruction or compression or compressive ischemia of the anterior horn cells
      C-3 Amyotrophy due to ischemia of the anterior horns
      C-4 Amyotrophy after electrical injury
      C-5 Amyotrophy after radiotherapy
   D. Disorders of motor neurons attributed to toxins, chemicals or heavy metals
      D-1 Toxins (tetanus toxin, strychnine, botulinum toxin)
      D-2 Chemicals (e.g., organophosphates)
      D-3 Heavy metals (lead, mercury)
   E. Disorders of motor neurons attributed to viral infection
      E-1 Acute disorders
          1. Paralytic acute anterior poliomyelitidies due to poliomyelitis or coxsackie viruses
          2. Amyotrophy caused by other viral agents
      E-2 Subacute or chronic disorders
          1. Amyotrophy in Creutzfeldt-Jakob disease
          2. Amyotrophy or amyotrophic lateral sclerosis due to human immunodeficiency virus
          3. Late post-poliomyelitis muscular atrophy
          4. Other forms
   F. Disorders of motor neurons with immunological abnormality
      F-1 Motor neuron disease with monoclonal paraproteinemia, Hodgkin's disease or carcinoma
   G. Disorders of motor neurons of undetermined etiology
      G-1 Motor neuron diseases of adults
      G-2 Sporadic juvenile motor neuron diseases
      G-3 Amyotrophy in Shy-Drager syndrome
      G-4 Other forms
   H. Disorders of motor neurons in endocrine disorders
      H-1 Tetany
      H-2 Other forms

Table 11.1. *Continued*

I. Disorders of motor neurons manifest by hyperactivity
- I-1 Ordinary muscle cramps
- I-2 Benign fasciculation-cramps syndrome
- I-3 Occupational cramps
- I-4 Neuromyotonia (Isaacs)
- I-5 Tetanus
- I-6 Strychnine intoxication
- I-7 Stiff man syndrome (Moersch-Woltman)
- I-8 Other forms

II. Disorders of motor nerve roots

III. Disorders of the peripheral nerve
- A. Heritable, biochemical abnormality unknown
  - A-1 Hereditary motor and sensory neuropathy
    1. HMSN I (hypertrophic type)
    2. HMSN II (neuronal type)
    3. HMSN III (Dejerine-Sottas)
    4. X-linked HMSN
  - A-2 Hereditary sensory and autonomic neuropathies
  - A-3 Hereditary neuropathies associated with specific biochemical abnormalities
    1. Autosomal dominant amyloidosis
    2. Autosomal dominant porphyria
    3. An-alpha-lipoproteinemia (Tangier)
    4. A-beta-lipoproteinemia (Bassen-Kornzweig)
    5. Metachromatic leukodystrophy
    6. Globoid cell leukodystrophy (Krabbe)
    7. Niemann-Pick disease
    8. Adrenoleukodystrophy and adrenomyeloneuropathy
    9. Fabry's disease
    10. Refsum's syndrome
    11. Glycogen storage diseases
    12. Primary hyperoxaluria
  - A-4 Miscellaneous hereditary neuropathies
    1. Hereditary liability to pressure palsies
    2. Other forms
- B. Congenital abnormalities (e.g., associated with meningomyelocele)
- C. Traumatic
  - C-1 Physical
    1. Laceration, contusion, compression or distraction of nerves or plexuses
    2. Birth trauma to brachial plexus
    3. Compression neuropathies
    4. Electric shock
    5. Cold injury
    6. Burns
    7. Vibration injury
    8. Radiation injury
    9. Ischemia neuropathy
        a. Vasculitis
        b. Arteriosclerotic occlusive disease
        c. Thromboangiitis obliterans
        d. Embolic infarction of nerve trunks
        e. Hemorrhage into nerve trunks
        f. Occlusion of large arteries by compression
        g. Volkmann's ischemic contracture
        h. Anterior tibial compartment syndrome
  - C-2 Toxic
    1. Drugs (e.g., vinca alkaloids)
    2. Inorganic substances (e.g., lead)
    3. Organic substances (e.g., alcohol)
    4. Toxins derived from bacteria (botulism, diphtheria, tetanus)
    5. Other forms
  - C-3 Of uncertain etiology (e.g., neuropathy in the Spanish toxic oil syndrome)
- D. Infections (e.g., leprosy, herpes zoster, Lyme disease)
- E. Guillain-Barré syndrome and related disorders
  - E-1 Acute inflammatory neuropathy (Guillain-Barré)
  - E-2 Miller-Fisher syndrome
  - E-3 Chronic inflammatory demyelinating polyradiculoneuropathy

Continued

Table 11.1. *Continued*

  F. Neuropathy associated with connective tissue disorders (e.g., systemic lupus erythematosis)

  G. Metabolic neuropathy

    G-1 Nutritional

    G-2 Neuropathies associated with endocrine disorders (e.g., diabetes mellitus)

    G-3 Neuropathies in blood dyscrasias (e.g., polycythemia vera)

    G-4 Neuropathy in renal failure

    G-5 Neuropathy in acute and chronic liver disease

    G-6 Neuropathy associated with paraproteinemia and dysproteinemia

  H. Neuropathy in malignant disease

  I. Neuropathy associated with other systemic or non-hereditary degenerative disorders (e.g., sarcoidosis, acrodermatitis chronica atrophicans)

  J. Chronic neuropathy with no known cause or association

  K. Tumors of nerves

IV. Disorders of the neuromuscular transmission

  A. Heritable

    A-1 Hereditary (congenital and juvenile) myasthenia gravis

    A-2 Pseudocholinesterase deficiency

  B. Congenital or developmental myasthenia

  C. Toxic (e.g., botulism, tick paralysis, penicillamine-induced myasthenia)

  D. Myasthenia gravis

  E. Lambert-Eaton syndrome

  F. Cholinergic paralysis (e.g., poisoning with anticholinesterase compounds)

V. Disorders of muscle

  A. Heritable myopathies

    A-1 Muscular dystrophies

      1. X-linked types

        a. Severe X-linked dystrophy (Duchenne)

        b. Myopathy in manifesting Duchenne carriers

        c. X-linked Duchenne dystrophy due to chromosomal translocation in females or to Turner's syndrome

        d. Mild X-linked dystrophy (Becker)

        e. X-linked recessive myopathy with McLeod syndrome

        f. X-linked recessive dystrophy with contractures and cardiomyopathy (Emery-Dreifuss)

        g. Other forms

      2. Scapuloperoneal muscular dystrophy

        a. Autosomal dominant

        b. X-linked

        c. With inflammatory changes and cardiopathy

      3. Limb-girdle muscular dystrophy

        a. Autosomal recessive or sporadic

        b. Myopathy limited to quadriceps

        c. Autosomal dominant of late onset

      4. Autosomal recessive dystrophy of childhood

      5. Distal muscular dystrophy

        a. Autosomal dominant variety of late onset (Welander)

        b. Autosomal dominant variety with infantile onset

        c. Autosomal recessive variety with rimmed vacuole formation and lamellar bodies

        d. Hereditary distal myopathy with sarcoplasmic bodies and intermediate filaments

        e. Autosomal recessive distal muscular dystrophy with high creatine kinase

      6. Autosomal dominant dystrophy with humeropelvic distribution and cardiomyopathy

      7. Autosomal dominant Emery-Dreifuss dystrophy

      8. Benign muscular dystrophy with contractures but no cardiomyopathy

      9. Autosomal dominant fibrodysplasia ossificans progressiva

     10. Ocular myopathies

        a. Isolated with or without ragged red fibers

        b. With pigmentary retinal degeneration

        c. Kearns-Sayre syndrome

        d. Oculopharyngeal muscular dystrophy

        e. Other forms

    A-2 Congenital myopathies of unknown etiology

      1. Congenital muscular dystrophy

TABLE 11.1. *Continued*

        2. Congenital muscular dystrophy with severe mental retardation (Fukuyama)

        3. Benign congenital myopathy without specific features (Turner)

        4. Central core disease

        5. Nemaline myopathy

        6. Centronuclear myopathy

        7. Familial myosclerosis

        8. Myopathy in Marfan syndrome

        9. Familial congenital myopathy with cataract, gonadal dysgenesis and oligophrenia (Marinesco-Sjögren)

     10. Myopathies with characteristic histochemical abnormalities (e.g., congenital fiber type disproportion, reducing body myopathy)

     11. Myopathies with cytoplasmic inclusions

     12. Multicore disease

     13. Sarcotubular myopathy

     14. Myopathy with tubular aggregates

     15. Other forms

  A-3 Myotonic disorders

        1. Dystrophia myotonica

          a. Adult form

          b. Infantile form (congenital myotonic dystrophy)

        2. Autosomal dominant myotonia congenita (Thomsen)

        3. Autosomal recessive myotonia congenita (Becker)

        4. Chondrodystrophic myotonia (Schwartz-Jampel)

        5. Paramyotonia congenita (Eulenburg)

        6. Rare forms

B. Trauma to muscle by external agents

  B-1 Physical (e.g., crush syndrome, compartment syndromes)

  B-2 Toxic (e.g., Haff disease)

  B-3 Drugs (e.g., steroids, chloroquine, lovastatine)

C. Inflammatory

  C-1 Infections of muscle

        1. Viral myositis (e.g., influenza A and B, Coxsackie B5)

        2. Bacterial (e.g., gas gangrene, tetanus, staphylococci, Lyme disease)

        3. Fungal myositis (e.g., disseminated candidiasis)

        4. Protozoal myositis (e.g., toxoplasmosis)

        5. Cestode myositis (e.g., cysticercosis)

        6. Nematode myositis (e.g., trichinosis)

  C-2 Other inflammatory disorders of muscle

        1. Dermatomyositis

        2. Polymyositis

        3. Polymyositis with autoimmune disease (e.g., systemic lupus erythematosis)

        4. Polymyositis or dermatomyositis with malignant disease

        5. Eosinophilic polymyositis

        6. Inclusion body myositis

        7. Orbital myositis

        8. Polymyositis in AIDS

        9. Polymyositis or dermatomyositis due to penicillamine

  C-3 Inflammatory disorders of muscle of unknown etiology

        1. Sarcoidosis with myopathy

        2. Granulomatous polymyositis

        3. Polymyalgia rheumatica

        4. Localized myositis ossificans

        5. Fibrositis and nodular fasciitis

        6. Other forms

D. Metabolic myopathies

  D-1 Muscle disorders associated with endocrine disease

        1. Thyrotoxicosis

        2. Myxedema

        3. Hypopituitarism with myopathy

        4. Acromegaly with muscle hypertrophy or myopathy

        5. Exophthalmic ophthalmoplegia

        6. Cushing's disease myopathy

        7. Addison's disease with myopathy

        8. Primary aldosteronism

        9. Hyperparathyroidism with myopathy

     10. Hypoparathyroidism with myopathy

Continued

TABLE 11.1. *Continued*

11. Myopathy in other forms of metabolic bone disease
12. Very rare forms

D-2 Heritable myopathies, biochemical abnormality known
    1. Glycogen storage disease involving muscle
        a. Glycogenosis type II (Pompe) due to amylo-1,4-glucosidase deficiency
        b. Glycogenosis type III (Cori-Forbes) due to lack of debrancher enzyme
        c. Glycogenosis type IV (Andersen) due to lack of brancher enzyme
        d. Glycogenosis type V (McArdle) due to phosphorylase deficiency
        e. Glycogenosis type VII (Tarui)
        f. Phosphoglycerate kinase deficiency
        g. Phosphoglycerate mutase deficiency
        h. Lactate dehydrogenase deficiency
        i. Lysosomal glycogen storage disease with acid maltase deficiency
        j. Very rare forms
    2. Other inherited disorders of carbohydrate metabolism
    3. Myoadenylate deaminase deficiency
    4. Familial periodic paralysis and related syndromes
        a. Hypokalemic periodic paralysis
        b. Hyperkalemic periodic paralysis
        c. Normokalemic periodic paralysis
        d. Myotonic periodic paralysis
        e. Thyrotoxic periodic paralysis
    5. Mitochondrial and lipid storage myopathies
        a. Lipid storage myopathies of uncertain origin
        b. Deficiencies involving the carnitine acyl-carnitine carrier system
            i) Muscle carnitine deficiency
            ii) Systemic carnitine deficiency
            iii) Partial muscle carnitine deficiencies
            iv) Carnitine palmitoyl transferase (CPT) deficiency
            v) Combined carnitine and CPT deficiencies
        c. Defects of mitochondrial substrate utilization (e.g., pyruvate decarboxylase deficiency)
        d. Defects of the respiratory chain (e.g., cytochrome c oxidase deficiency)
        e. Defects of energy conservation and transduction (e.g., Luft disease, mitochondrial ATPase deficiency)
        f. Malignant hyperpyrexia myopathy with tubular aggregates
        g. Cytoplasmic body myopathy
        h. Very rare forms

D-3 Other metabolic myopathies
    1. Alcoholic myopathy
    2. Nutritional myopathy
    3. Myoglobinuria (other than that due to glycogen storage disease, mitochondrial or lipid storage disease and CPT deficiency)
        a. Exertion
        b. Crush or ischemic injury
        c. Metabolic depression or distortion (e.g., hypokalemia)
        d. Due to drugs or toxins
        e. Abnormalities of body temperature
        f. Infections
        g. Autoimmune muscle disease
        h. Idiopathic recurrent myoglobinuria
    4. Chronic myopathy due to drugs (e.g., chloroquine, steroids)
    5. Very rare forms

E. Myopathy associated with malignant disease
    E-1 Carcinomatous myopathy (other than polymyositis)
    E-2 Lambert-Eaton syndrome
    E-3 Other forms

F. Myopathy associated with myasthenia gravis

G. Myopathy in thalassemia

H. Other disorders of muscle of unknown or uncertain etiology
    H-1 Acute muscle necrosis
    H-2 Amyloid myopathy
    H-3 Disuse atrophy
    H-4 Muscle cachexia
    H-5 Other forms

I. Tumors of muscle

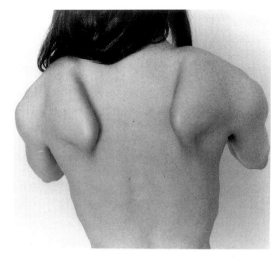

FIGURE 11.1. Facioscapulohumeral muscular dystrophy. Typical symmetric winging of the scapulae results from weakness and wasting of the anterior serratus muscles.

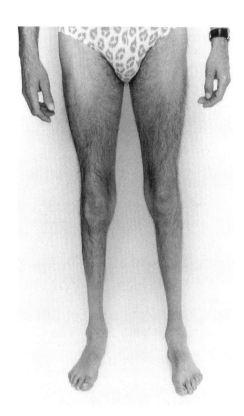

FIGURE 11.2. Distal spinal muscular dystrophy. Although the distal quadriceps are mildly atrophic, extreme wasting of leg and foot muscles is evident.

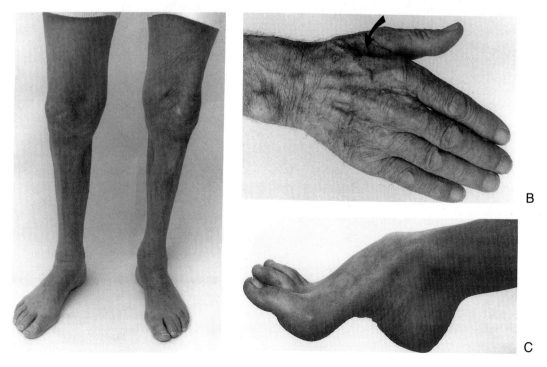

FIGURE 11.3. Hereditary motor and sensory neuropathy. (A) Minimal quadriceps atrophy contrasts with marked wasting of leg and foot muscles. (B) Wasting of the intrinsic hand muscles, particularly the first dorsal interosseus (arrow). (C) Typical pes cavus results from weakness and wasting of intrinsic foot muscles.

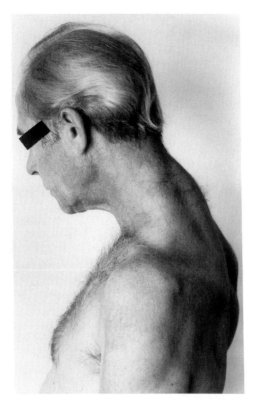

FIGURE 11.4. Chronic polymyositis. The patient is unable to fully extend his head due to wasting of neck extensors, a clinical feature highly suggestive of inflammatory myopathies.

TABLE 11.2. Neuromuscular diseases associated with clear facial involvement.

Neuropathies
  Facioscapulohumeral spinal muscular atrophy
  X-linked bulbospinal muscular atrophy
  Progressive juvenile bulbar palsy (Fazio-Londe disease)
  Progressive bulbar palsy of adults
Disorders of the neuromuscular transmission
  Congenital myasthenia
  Myasthenia gravis
Myopathies
  Facioscapulohumeral muscular dystrophy
  Oculopharyngeal muscular dystrophy
  Congenital myopathies:
    Central core-disease
    Nemaline myopathy
    Centronuclear myopathy
    Minicore disease
    Multicore disease
    Sarcotubular myopathy
    Reducing body myopathy
    Cap disease
    Congenital fiber type disproportion
  Myotonic dystrophy
  Alcoholic myopathy (rarely)

TABLE 11.3. Neuromuscular diseases with external ophthalmoplegia.

Neuropathies
  Progressive juvenile bulbar palsy (Fazio-Londe disease)
  Progressive bulbar palsy with deafness (Brown-Vialetto-van Laere syndrome)
  Spinal muscular atrophy with ophthalmoplegia
  Spinal muscular atrophy with Joseph disease
  Miller-Fisher syndrome
Disorders of the neuromuscular junction
  Myasthenia gravis
  Congenital myasthenia
  Botulism
Myopathies
  Ocular myopathies (e.g., Kearns-Sayre syndrome, oculopharyngeal muscular dystrophy)
  Congenital myopathies
    Multicore disease
    Nemaline myopathy
    Centronuclear myopathy
    Reducing body myopathy
    Myopathy with lysis of myofibrils
    Myopathy with focal loss of cross-striations
  Myotonic dystrophy
  Ocular myositis
  Metabolic myopathies
    Hyperthyroid myopathy
    Mitochondrial encephalomyopathies
    Carnitine deficiency
    Chronic vitamin E deficiency
    Acute alcoholic myopathy

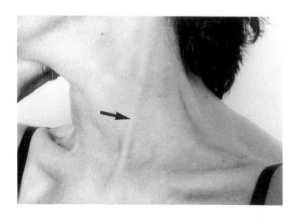

FIGURE 11.5. Adult-onset myotonic dystrophy. A very typical and early feature in this disease is exhibited by the highly atrophic sternocleidomastoid muscles (arrow).

TABLE 11.4. Neuromuscular diseases with involvement of pharyngeal muscles.

Neuropathies
    Bulbar spinal muscular atrophy
    Progressive bulbar paralysis
    Progressive bulbar palsy of childhood (Fazio-Londe disease)
    Progressive bulbar palsy with deafness (Brown-Vialetto-van Laere syndrome)
    Spinal and bulbar muscular atrophy (Kennedy disease)
    Late post-poliomyelitis muscular atrophy
Disorders of the neuromuscular junction
    Congenital myasthenia
    Myasthenia gravis
Myopathies
    Oculopharyngeal muscular dystrophy
    Myotonic dystrophy
    Inflammatory myopathies:
        Poly-/dermatomyositis
        Inclusion body myositis
        Granulomatous myositis
    Hyperkalemic periodic paralysis
    Hyperthyroid bulbar myopathy

TABLE 11.5. Generalized neuromuscular diseases occasionally exhibiting clearly asymmetric muscle involvement.

Neuropathies
    Progressive bulbar palsy of childhood (Fazio-Londe disease)
    Chronic asymmetric spinal atrophy
    Amyotrophic lateral sclerosis
    Monomelic motor neuron disease
    Poliomyelitis
Myopathies
    (Facio-)scapulohumeral muscular dystrophy
    Beginning limb girdle muscular dystrophy
    Polymyositis
    Inclusion body myositis
    Periodic paralysis

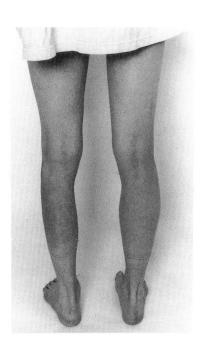

FIGURE 11.6. Facioscapulohumeral muscular dystrophy. Note asymmetric wasting of the left calf muscles. Asymmetry of muscle deterioration is a classic feature of facioscapulohumeral muscular dystrophy, but is uncommon in most other generalized neuromuscular diseases.

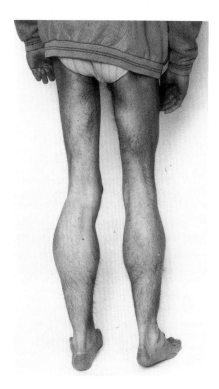

FIGURE 11.7. Progressive muscular dystrophy of Becker type. Note atrophy of thighs in contrast to apparent hypertrophy of calves.

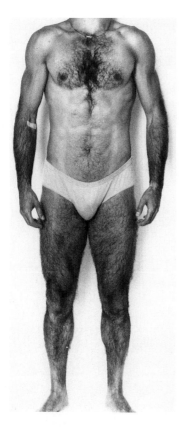

FIGURE 11.8. Congenital myotonia. Note generalized muscle hypertrophy in a sedentary patient.

TABLE 11.7. Neuromuscular disease associated with exercise-induced myalgias.

Myopathy with tubular aggregates
Metabolic myopathies
   Glycogen storage diseases
      Glycogenosis type V
      Glycogenosis type VII
      Phosphoglycerate kinase deficiency
      Phosphoglycerate mutase deficiency
      Lactate dehydrogenase deficiency
   Myoadenylate deaminase deficiency
   Mitochondrial and lipid storage myopathies
      Defects of the respiratory chain
      Defects of energy conservation and transduction
      Primary muscular carnitine deficiency
      Carnitine palmitoyl transferase deficiency

TABLE 11.8. Classification of muscle atrophy and hypertrophy according to imaging findings.

	Gross muscle volume*		
	Normal	Diminished	Augmented
Absence of fat**	normal	simple atrophy	true hypertrophy
Presence of fat**	fat replacement	complex atrophy	pseudohypertrophy

* Cross-sectional area within the muscle fascia, ** proven by histopathology or muscle imaging modalities.

TABLE 11.6. Neuromuscular diseases presenting with generalized muscle hypertrophy.

(Strength training)
Hypertrophia musculorum vera
Congenital myopathies
   Centronuclear myopathy
   Congenital lipoatrophic diabetes
Myotonic disorders
   Myotonia congenita
   Paramyotonia congenita Eulenburg
   Chondrodystrophic myotonia Schwartz-Jampel
Metabolic disorders
   Hypothyroid myopathy
   Acromegaly
   Glycogenosis type III and V
Myositides
   Sarcoid myositis
   Cysticercosis
Muscle amyloidosis
Cornelia de Lange syndrome

TABLE 11.9. Neuromuscular disease associated with abnormal fatigability.

Neuropathies
   Motor neuron diseases
Disorders of the neuromuscular transmission
   Myasthenia gravis
   Lambert-Eaton syndrome
Myopathies
   Glycogenoses type III, V and VII
   Mitochondrial myopathies
   Endocrine myopathies
      hypothyroid myopathy
      hyperthyroid myopathy
      myopathy in Cushing's syndrome
      myopathy in Addison's disease
      myopathy in Conn's syndrome
      hypocalcemia

TABLE 11.10. Myotonic disease.

Congenital myotonia (Thomsen)
Autosomal recessive myotonia (Becker)
Paramyotonia congenita (Eulenburg)
Chondrodystrophic myotonia Schwartz-Jampel
Myotonic dystrophy
Drug-induced myotonia (e.g., 20,25-diazocholestrol, clofibrate)
Myopathy with cylindric spirals
Myxedema

TABLE 11.11. Disorders often exhibiting widespread fasciculations.

Spinal muscular atrophies
Hereditary motor and sensory neuropathies
Post-poliomyelitis muscular atrophy
Neuromyotonia
Morvan syndrome
Benign fasciculation-cramp syndrome
Hyperthyroid myopathy

TABLE 11.12. Neuromuscular diseases with cerebral/cerebellar abnormalities.

Neuropathies
  Heritable spinal muscular atrophies
    Friedreich's ataxia
    Sjögren-Larsson syndrome
    Spinal muscular atrophy with hexosaminidase deficiency
    Amyotrophic lateral sclerosis—parkinsonism—dementia complex
      of Guam
    Amyotrophic lateral sclerosis with dementia
    Spinal muscular atrophy with Joseph disease
    Amyotrophic lateral sclerosis with Pick disease
  Amyotrophy in Creutzfeldt-Jakob disease
  Disorders involving peripheral nerves
    Hereditary motor and sensory neuropathy type II with ataxia
      and tremor
    Hereditary neuropathies associated with specific biochemical
      abnormalities:
    An-alpha-lipoproteinemia (Bassen-Kornzweig disease)
    a-beta-lipoproteinemia (Tangier disease)
    Metachromatic leukodystrophy
    Globoid cell leukodystrophy (Krabbe disease)
    Niemann-Pick disease
    Adrenoleukodystrophy
    Fabry's disease
    Refsum's syndrome
Myopathies
  X-linked recessive muscular dystrophy of Duchenne type
  Congenital muscular dystrophy with severe mental retardation
    (Fukuyama)
  Fingerprint myopathy
  Myotonic dystrophy
  Chondrodystrophic myotonia Schwartz-Jampel
  Kearns-Sayre syndrome
  Familial congenital myopathy with cataract, gonadal dysgenesis and
    oligophrenia (Marinesco-Sjögren syndrome)
  Mitochondrial encephalomyopathies

TABLE 11.13. Neuromuscular diseses with abnormalities of the spinal cord.

Spinal muscular atrophy with retinitis pigmentosa and hereditary
   spastic paraplegia
Troyer syndrome
Friedreich's ataxia
Sjögren-Larsson syndrome
Amyotrophic dystonic paraplegia
Amyotrophic lateral sclerosis
Hereditary motor and sensory neuropathy type V
Adrenomyeloneuropathy

TABLE 11.14. Neuromuscular disease with abnormalities of the eye.

Neuropathies
  Rare syndromes with heritable spinal muscular atrophies
  Disorders involving peripheral nerves
    Hereditary motor and sensory neuropathy types III and VII
    Hereditary neuropathies associated with specific biochemical
     abnormalities
     An-alpha-lipoproteinemia (Tangier disease)
     A-beta-lipoproteinemia (Bassen-Kornzweig syndrome)
     Metachromatic leukodystrophy
     Globoid cell leukodystrophy (Krabbe disease)
     Niemann-Pick disease
     Fabry's disease
     Refsum's syndrome
Myopathies
  Kearns-Sayre syndrome
  Ocular myopathy with pigmentary retinal degeneration
  X-linked recessive ophthalmoplegia and myopia
  Myotonic dystrophy

TABLE 11.15. Neuromuscular disease with abnormalities of the ear.

Neuropathies
  Progressive bulbar palsy with deafness (Brown-Vialetto-van Laere
   syndrome)
  Friedreich's ataxia
  Hereditary motor and sensory neuropathy type VII
  Refsum's syndrome
Myopathies
  Facioscapulohumeral muscular dystrophy
  Ophthalmoplegia plus

TABLE 11.16. Neuromuscular diseases with cardiac involvement.

Neuropathies
  Neuronal scapuloperoneal atrophy with cardiopathy
   (Emery-Dreifuss)
  Friedreich's ataxia
  Amyloid neuropathies
  An-alpha-lipoproteinemia (Tangier disease)
  Fabry's disease
  Refsum's syndrome
  Acute inflammatory neuropathy
Myopathies
  Muscular dystrophies
    X-linked recessive muscular dystrophies of Duchenne and
     Becker type
    X-linked recessive dystrophy with contractures and
     cardiomyopathy (Emery-Dreifuss)
    Autosomal dominant Emery-Dreifuss dystrophy
    Facioscapulohumeral muscular dystrophy
    Limb girdle muscular dystrophy
    Kearns-Sayre syndrome
  Nemaline myopathy with cardiomyopathy
  Rigid spine-syndrome
  Myotonic dystrophy
  Hyperkaliemic periodic paralysis
  Poly-/dermatomyositis
  Eosinophilic myositis
  Glycogenosis type II
  Carnitine deficiency
  Hypothyroid myopathy
  Hyperthyroid myopathy
  Myopathy in acromegaly
  Alcoholic myopathy
  Carcinoid myopathy

TABLE 11.17. Neuromuscular diseaes associated with early respiratory problems.

Neuropathies
  Amyotrophy with asthma
  Acute inflammatory neuropathy (Guillain-Barré)
Disorders of the neuromuscular transmission
  Myasthenia gravis
  Botulism
Myopathies
  Congenital myopathies
    Nemaline myopathy
    X-linked centronuclear myopathy
    Multicore disease
  Congenital dystrophia myotonica
  Glycogenosis type II (Pompe)
  Dermato-/polymyositis

TABLE 11.18. Neuromuscular diseases with skin abnormalities.

Neuropathies
  Sjögren-Larsson syndrome
  Infantile spinal muscular atrophy in incontinentia pigmenti
    (Bloch-Sulzberger)
  Fabry's disease
  Refsum's syndrome
Myopathies
  Dermatomyositis
  Eosinophilic myositis

TABLE 11.19. Neuromuscular diseases with skeletal abnormalities.

Neuropathies
  Spinal muscular atrophy type II
  Distal spinal muscular atrophy
  Spinal muscular atrophy with mental retardation, seizures, and
    orofacial dysplasia
  Spinal muscular atrophy with Joseph disease
  Hereditary motor and sensory neuropathy type I and III
  Friedreich ataxia
  An-alpha-lipoproteinemia (Tangier)
  Refsum's syndrome
Myopathies
  Kearns-Sayre syndrome
  Congenital myopathies:
    Central-core disease
    Multicore disease
    Nemaline myopathy
    Centronuclear myopathy
    Fingerprint myopathy
    Cytoplasmic body myopathy
    Congenital fibre type disproportion
  Congenital myotonic dystrophy
  Chondrodystrophic myotonia Schwartz-Jampel
  Arthrogryposis multiplex congenita
  Malignant hyperthermia

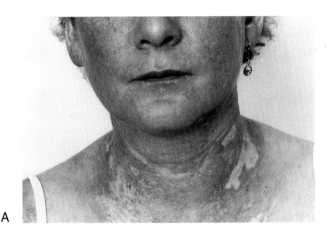

A

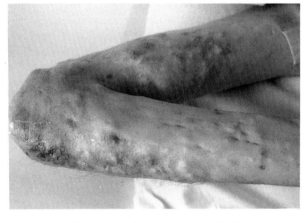

B

FIGURE 11.9. Chronic dermatomyositis. (A) Patchy macular foci of skin de- and hyperpigmentation (poikilodermia). (B) Multiple calcifications of the skin and muscles on the right arm are demonstrated. Such sequelae of childhood-onset dermatomyositis occurs in approximately one-third of patients.

TABLE 11.20. Neuromuscular disease with intramuscular calcifications.

Myodysplasia ossificans progressiva
Dermatomyositis, particularly in childhood
Localized myositis ossificans
Localized nodular myositis
Trichinosis
Cysticercosis

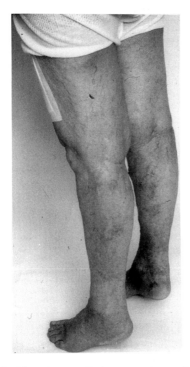

FIGURE 11.10. Chronic granulomatous polymyositis. Although thigh muscle weakness is only moderate, lipomatosis and fibrosis of the foot extensors is marked, resulting in associated contractures of the ankle joints. The patient is attempting to stand on the heels.

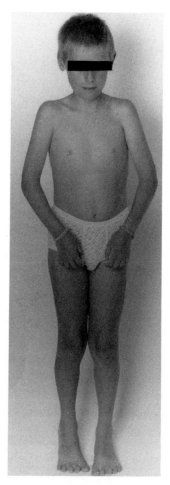

FIGURE 11.11. Emery-Dreifuss muscular dystrophy. A scapuloperoneal distribution of muscle wasting is evident with contractures of the elbows and ankle joints occurring in association with fibrosis of the elbow flexors and foot extensors.

TABLE 11.21. Neuromuscular diseases with early contractures.

Muscular dystrophies
    X-linked recessive dystrophy with contractures and cardiomyopathy
      (Emery-Dreifuss)
    Autosomal dominant Emery-Dreifuss dystrophy
    Benign muscular dystrophy with contractures but no cardiopathy
Congenital myopathies
    Congenital muscular dystrophy with severe mental retardation
      (Fukuyama)
    Central core-disease
    Multicore disease
    Congenital fibre type disproportion
    Congenital myotonic dystrophy
Arthrogryposis multiplex congenita
Familial myosclerosis
Multiple contracture syndrome
Fibrodysplasia ossificans progressiva
Rigid spine syndrome
Granulomatous myositis

References

1. Walton J. A simple classification of neuromuscular diseases. Neuro Muscular diseases News Bulletin. March, 1991:9–10.
2. World Federation of Neurology Research Committee. Research group on neuromuscular diseases. J Neurol Sci 1988;86:333–360.
3. Swash M, Schwartz MS. Neuromuscular diseases. A practical approach to diagnosis and management. 2nd ed. London: Springer, 1988.

12
Histopathological Basis of Muscle Imaging

Carl D. Reimers, Petra Fischer, and Dieter E. Pongratz

Histology of Healthy Skeletal Muscles

The skeletal musculature, consisting of 434 single muscles, comprises approximately 25% to 35% of the total body weight in women and 40% to 50% in men,[1] thus being the largest organ of the body. Every muscle has at least one belly. A few muscles, for example, the rectus abdominis, consist of more than one belly, separated by tendinous intersections. The muscle merges at either end with a tendon, aponeurosis, or the periosteum of the bone.

Muscles consist of polynuclear syncytial cells, called the muscle fibers, with a length of 1 mm to more than 30 cm and a diameter of approximately 10 to 100 μm. Lengths and diameters depend on sex, age, and physical activity. In normal muscle, fiber diameters follow a Gaussian distribution. Neighboring muscle fibers are separated from each other by a thin network of connective tissue, the endomysium, which contains the capillaries supporting the muscle fibers and small nerve endings. Muscle fibers are arranged together in fascicles, surrounded by a thin layer of connective tissue, the perimysium. Every muscle is surrounded by an epimysium composed of collagen fibers. A group of single muscles is surrounded by a fascia.

In cross section, muscle fibers have a polygonal configuration (Figure 12.1). They consist primarily of contractile myofibrils and mitochondria with small lipoid droplets lying between the fibers. The space between the myofibrils and enclosed by the cell membrane, or sarcolemma, is filled with cytoplasm, called the sarcoplasm. The nuclei are situated in the periphery of the fiber, beneath the sarcolemma. In normal muscles, the nuclear number does not exceed six per cross section per fiber.

Enzyme histochemical staining can distinguish two types of muscle fibers, type 1 and type 2 (Figure 12.1). Type 2 fibers can be further subclassified into types 2a, 2b, and 2c (Table 12.1). According to their physiological characteristics, type 1 fibers may be called slow-twitch fibers and type 2 fibers fast-twitch fibers. The different muscle fiber types have differing contents of glycogen, lipids, myoglobin, and mitochondria, and have variable physical properties. The number of surrounding capillaries is also variable, being greater in type 1 than in type 2b fibers. Type 1 fibers are predominantly oxidative, type 2b are glycolytic. In muscles that contract predominantly slowly and for relatively long durations (tonic), such as the erector spinae, there is a predominance of type 1 fibers. In rapidly contracting phasic muscles, such as the vasti, type 2b fibers are relatively numerous. However, intersubject variations in muscle fiber-type proportions are considerable. Properties of type 2a muscle fibers are intermediate between type 1 and 2b fibers. Type 2c fibers are characteristic of fetal muscles and do not normally occur in mature human muscle. A variable number of muscle fibers are innervated by a single anterior horn cell, ranging from about 10 in extraocular muscles to 2000 in leg muscles.[2]

Histopathology of Diseased Skeletal Muscles

Most neuromuscular diseases result in muscle atrophy and/or mesenchymal abnormalities. There are some exceptions, however. In early stages of myasthenia gravis, for example, pronounced muscle weakness may be unrelated with atrophy and mesenchymal abnormality. Disuse typically causes selective atrophy of type 2 fibers. Type 1 fiber atrophy is less common, being found in myotonic dystrophy and several congenital myopathies.

Histopathology distinguishes neurogenic and myogenic patterns of abnormalities. In neuropathies, atrophy may occur focally or diffusely, depending upon the size and distribution of the motor unit(s) involved. The atrophic fibers occur singly or in small groups corresponding to the arrangement of muscle fibers within the territory of the motor unit. The atrophic fibers are separated by

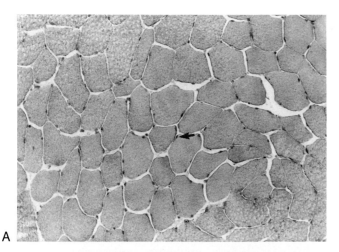

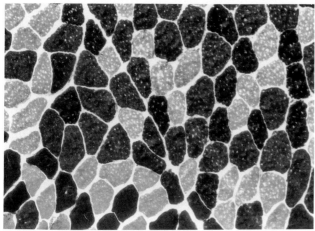

FIGURE 12.1. Light microscopy of normal skeletal muscle. (A) Note polygonal shape of muscle fibers in cross section and eccentric nuclei (arrow) on hematoxylin and eosin-stained specimen (magnification ×400). (B) Fiber types are differentiated by use of ATPase stain at pH 9.4. Note normal checkerboard pattern of type 1 (bright) and type 2 (dark) muscle fibers (magnification ×400).

fibers of normal size belonging to intact motor units whose territories overlap with that of the denervated motor unit. Reinnervation occurs by collateral sprouts from nearby normal nerve fibers. As a result, there is an increase in the number of muscle fibers of the same histological type appearing immediately adjacent to each other (type grouping). "Target"-shaped muscle fibers occur in areas of denervation in which reinnervation has recently occurred.

A multitude of microscopic changes are visible in myopathies. These changes are frequently nonspecific, but in some cases are of sufficiently high specificity to allow a single diagnosis. In other cases, histopathologic features are nonspecific but characteristic of certain diseases. Examples of characteristic features include,

degenerative (Figures 12.2, 12.3), congenital (Figure 12.4), metabolic (Figure 12.5), and inflammatory myopathies (Figure 12.6). For example, inflammatory infiltrates containing lymphocytes and histiocytes are found in the different types of inflammatory myopathies (Figure 12.6). Overabundances of glycogen and lipid in muscle fibers are the main features of the so-called glycogen and lipid storage diseases (Figure 12.5). However, in these cases, the final diagnosis is based on the biochemically or histopathologically proven enzyme deficiency.

Mitochondrial myopathies are characterized by "ragged red fibers" on light microscopy and on electron microscopy by numerically increased, enlarged, or abnormally shaped mitochondria. In many so-called benign congenital myopathies, the recognition of relatively specific histological abnormalities permits the definite diagnosis. For example, the combination of multiple internal nuclei, ring fibers, and sarcoplasmic masses are characteristic of myotonic dystrophy (Figure 12.2). Less specific but valuable clues for differentiating from other myopathies are degenerative changes in muscular dystrophies. Degenerative changes include an increased variability in the size of the muscle fibers, necrosis, splitting, regeneration of fibers, and changes of the nuclei and in the architecture of the intermyofibrillar network (Figure 12.3). Vacuoles with varying features are found in some of the inflammatory, degenerative, and metabolic myopathies (Figure 12.5).

There is yet to be proof that the above-described parenchymal abnormalities can be detected by diagnostic imaging techniques. However, in many diseases, the specific structural abnormalities are associated with more

TABLE 12.1. Properties of the different fibers types.

Property	Type 1	Type 2a	Type 2b
routine ATPase at pH 9.3		pale	dark dark
ATPase at pH 4.6	dark	pale	dark
ATPase at pH 4.3	dark	pale	pale
NADH-TR	dark	intermediate to high	pale
size	small	medium	big
color	intermediate	red	white
myoglobin	plentiful	plentiful	sparse
glycogen	sparse	plentiful	intermediate
neutral lipids	plentiful	sparse	sparse
mitochondria	many	many	few
capillaries	many	many	few
contraction	slow	intermediate	fast
energy supply	oxidative	oxidative/ glycolytic	glycolytic
fatigability	low	low	rapid

ATPase = reactivity to adenosine triphosphatase; NADH-TR = reactivity to nicotinamide adenine dinucleotide hydrogenase-tetrazolium reductase.

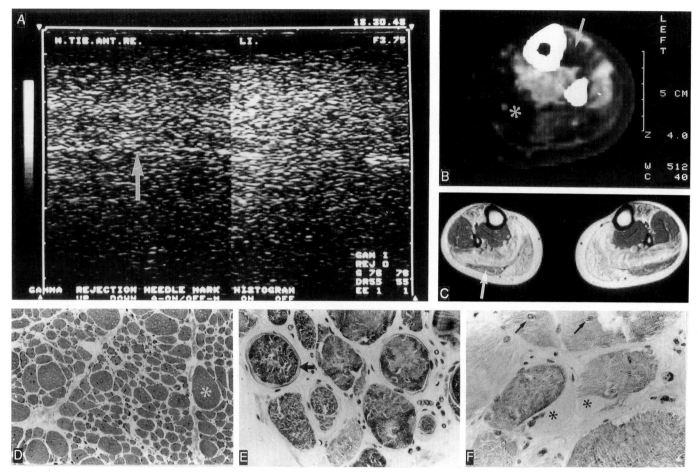

FIGURE 12.2. Radiology/histopathology in myotonic dystrophy. Longitudinal ultrasound scans (3.75 MHz) of the tibialis anterior muscles (patient's right side is on left and patient's left side is on right) show highly increased muscular echointensities that obscure interosseous membrane (arrow) (A). (B) Computed tomography of the left leg shows marked atrophy and hypodensity indicating fatty replacement of the tibialis anterior (arrow) and the soleus (asterisk). (C) The same fatty changes are manifested on "spin density"-weighted MRI (TR 1600 ms, TE 30 ms) by highly increased signal intensities of the tibialis anterior, soleus, and medial head of the gastrocnemius. Note less intense abnormality in the lateral head of the gastrocnemius muscles (arrow). (D) Photomicrograph (hematoxylin and eosin staining, magnification ×100) of the left tibialis anterior muscle shows increased space between fibers (enlargement of the interstitial space) due to fibrosis and lipomatosis. Note highly increased variation of muscle fiber diameters with many atrophic and few hypertrophic fibers (asterisk), abnormally round fibers, and centrally located nuclei. (E, F) Photomicrographs (trichrome staining, magnification ×400) of same specimen shows abnormally rounded muscle fibers, internal nuclei (white arrow), and ring "binds" consisting of displaced myofibrils (black arrow). (F) Note sarcoplasmic masses (asterisks) and central nuclei (arrows). The combination of numerous central nuclei, ring "binds," and sarcoplasmic masses are typical histopathological features of myotonic dystrophy. (CT and MRI courtesy of Professor Dr. T.J. Vogl, Dept. of Radiology, H.A. v. Humboldt University, Berlin, Germany.)

general changes of the muscle that are variably detectable by ultrasound, computed tomography, and/or magnetic resonance imaging (Figures 12.2 to 12.5). The most easily detected mesenchymal abnormality is increased muscle fat content. This is prominent even in early stages of some muscular dystrophies and congenital myopathies (e.g., centronuclear myopathy) (Figure 12.4). It is often accompanied by fibrosis, which predominates or is especially severe in congenital muscular dystrophy, X-linked muscular dystrophy of Duchenne type, rigid spine syndrome, and in muscular dystrophy with early contractures of the Emery-Dreifuss type.

Muscle edema is another nonspecific finding, but is less frequently reported in imaging studies than fatty change and is difficult to demonstrate histopathologically. It may be severe in acute myositis, rhabdomyolysis, and muscle trauma. Muscle calcification/ossification is a rare finding in neuromuscular disease but is easily detected by imaging modalities. Diseases in which this finding might be expected include childhood dermatomyositis,

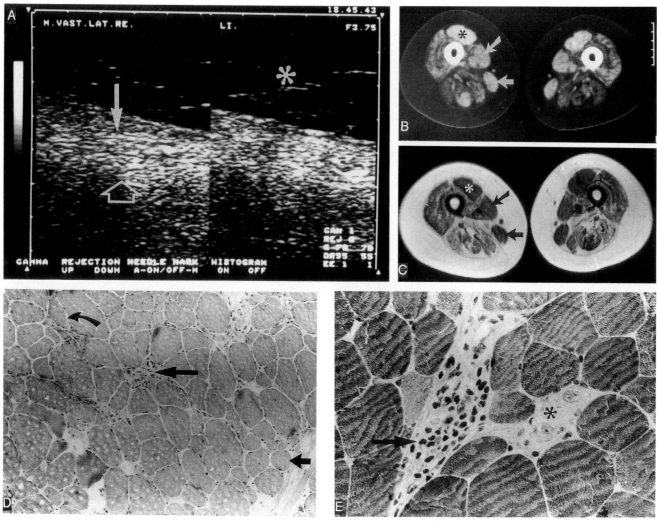

FIGURE 12.3. Radiology/histopathology in autosomal recessive limb girdle muscular dystrophy. (A) Longitudinal ultrasound scans (3.75 MHz) of the vastus lateralis muscles (patient's right side is on left and patient's left side is on right) show increased thickness of subcutaneous fat (asterisk) and atrophic and abnormally echogenic muscles (arrow) indicating fatty infiltration. Note lack of clarity of femur echo (open arrow). (B) Computed tomography of the thighs shows hypertrophy of rectus femoris (asterisk), sartorius (oblique arrow), and gracilis (arrow). Note atrophy and hypodensity of remaining muscles due to fat deposition. (C) "Spin density"-weighted MRI (TR 1600 ms, TE 30 ms) of the thighs shows similar changes as the CT scan.

(D) Light microscopy (hematoxylin and eosin staining, magnification ×100) of the right vastus lateralis muscle shows a nonspecific myopathic pattern with an abnormal mixture of fiber sizes, including some slightly hypertrophic and some atrophic. Some fibers are rounded (short arrow) whereas others are necrotic (long arrow) or split (curved arrow). (E) Photomicrograph of the same specimen (trichrome staining, magnification ×400) shows fiber necroses (asterisk) and accumulation of histiocytes and monocytes removing the cell detritus (arrow). (CT and MRI courtesy of Professor Dr. T.J. Vogl, Dept. of Radiology, H.A. v. Humboldt University, Berlin, Germany.)

myodysplasia fibrosa ossificans, myopathia ossificans localisata, and parasitic myositis.

Correlation of Histopathological and Imaging Findings

Although limited data exist to support definitive correlations between imaging and histopathological findings in neuromuscular diseases, Table 12.2 provides a brief summary of the infuence of intramuscular fat, connective tissue, edema, and calcifications on ultrasound (US), computed tomography (CT), and magnetic resonance (MR) imaging of muscles.

Ultrasound

Several studies established a close relationship between the severity of mesenchymal abnormalities in the muscle

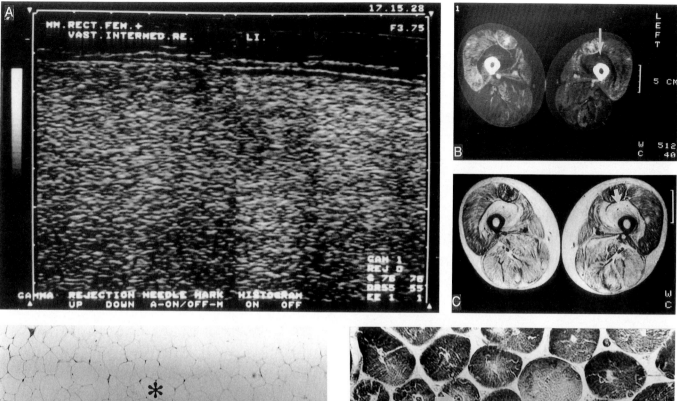

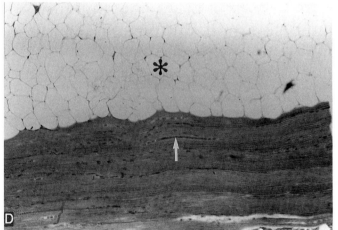

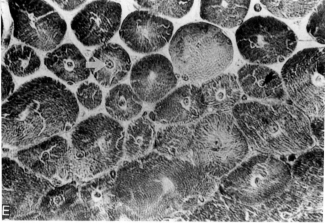

FIGURE 12.4. Radiology/histopathology in adult-onset centronuclear myopathy. (A) Longitudinal ultrasound scans (3.75 MHz) of the rectus femoris and vastus intermedius muscles (patient's right side is on left and patient's left side is on right) show highly increased muscular echointensities indicating lipomatosis. Note that the femur echo is not visible. (B) Computed tomography of the thighs shows homogeneously diminished density, indicating fatty replacement, of many muscles, including the vastus intermedius (arrow). (C) "Spin density"-weighted MRI of the thighs (TR 1600 ms, TE 30 ms) shows similar distribution of fatty change as the CT scan. (D) Light microscopy (hematoxylin and eosin staining, longitudinal section, magnification ×100) of the rectus femoris muscle shows large, confluent area of lipocytes (asterisk) and muscle fibers with long rows of internal nuclei (arrow). (E) Photomicrograph of same specimen (trichrome staining, transverse section, magnification ×400) shows abnormally rounded, partly atrophic muscle fibers with exclusively internal nuclei (arrow). (CT and MRI courtesy of Professor Dr. T.J. Vogl, Dept. of Radiology, H.A. v. Humboldt University, Berlin, Germany.)

biopsy and the echogenicity.[3–5] However, in the case of extreme lipomatosis, echogenicity may be less marked than in moderate lipomatosis.[4,6] Quantitative correlation of muscle lipomatosis and fibrosis with the corresponding echointensities argued that high echogenicity is caused by muscle lipomatosis (Figure 12.4), whereas muscle fibrosis does not substantially influence echogenicity.[4,5] Unfortunately, very thick subcutaneous fat layers can result in an apparent increase of muscle echointensity, probably due to increased through-transmission in the overlying echo-lucent fat layer (Figure 12.3). Muscle edema, either from physiological effects, such as exercise, or from pathological changes, such as necrosis or inflammation, can cause low echointensity and muscle swelling.[5,7] However, in most cases, decreased echointensity due to muscle edema is too small to be readily identified

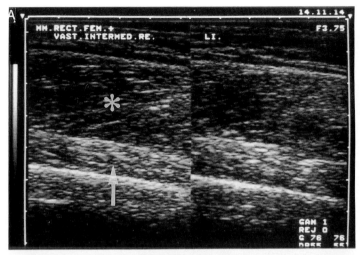

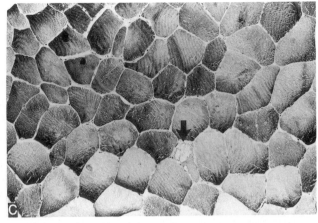

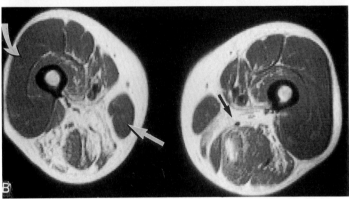

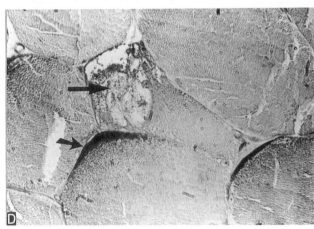

FIGURE 12.5. Radiology/histopathology in adult acid maltase deficiency. (A) Longitudinal ultrasound scans (3.75 MHz) of the rectus femoris and vastus intermedius muscles (patient's right side is on left and patient's left side is on right) show hypertrophy of the rectus femoris (asterisk) and atrophy and moderately increased echointensity of the vastus intermedius (arrow). (B) "Spin density"-weighted MRI (TR 1600 ms, TE 30 ms) shows hypertrophy of gracilis (white arrow) and parts of the quadriceps, including the vastus lateralis (curved arrow). Note associated atrophy and fatty replacement of other muscles, including the adductor magnus (black arrow). (C) Light microscopy (PAS stain, magnification ×100) of the right rectus femoris muscle shows abnormally intense uptake of the stain, indicating increased glycogen content, and vacuoles occurring within a fiber (arrow). (D) Photomicrograph (PAS stain, magnification ×400) of same specimen shows a vacuole containing glycogen (arrow) and subsarcolemmal concentration of glycogen (oblique arrow). (MRI courtesy of Professor Dr. T.J. Vogl, Dept. of Radiology, H.A. v. Humboldt University, Berlin, Germany.)

on ultrasound.[5] As a result, normal ultrasound findings do not exclude neuromuscular disorders.[5,8]

Computed Tomography

The attenuation coefficient for pure muscle tissue is approximately 54 Hounsfield units (H.U.), for fat −106 H.U., and for fibrous tissue +74 H.U.[9] The decrease of attenuation value on CT is related to the degree of muscular degeneration and replacement of fat determined by histopathology (Figure 12.5).[10–12] Because both fat and edema diminish muscle density, they cannot be distinguished by computed tomography. An exception is the case in which the fat content is sufficient in magnitude such that the average pixel H.U. is substantially below that of water. As in ultrasound, not every histopathological lesion is detectable using CT.[12] Artifacts and radiation dosages are significant problems (see Chapter 1). A particularly severe artifact, described as "beam hardening," results in spuriously low muscle density measurements.

Magnetic Resonance Imaging

Fat is characterized by high signal intensity on T_1-, proton-, and T_2-weighted spin echo images[13] because of its short T_1 and long T_2 relaxation times (Figures 12.2 to 12.5). The collagen content of the tissue is inversely

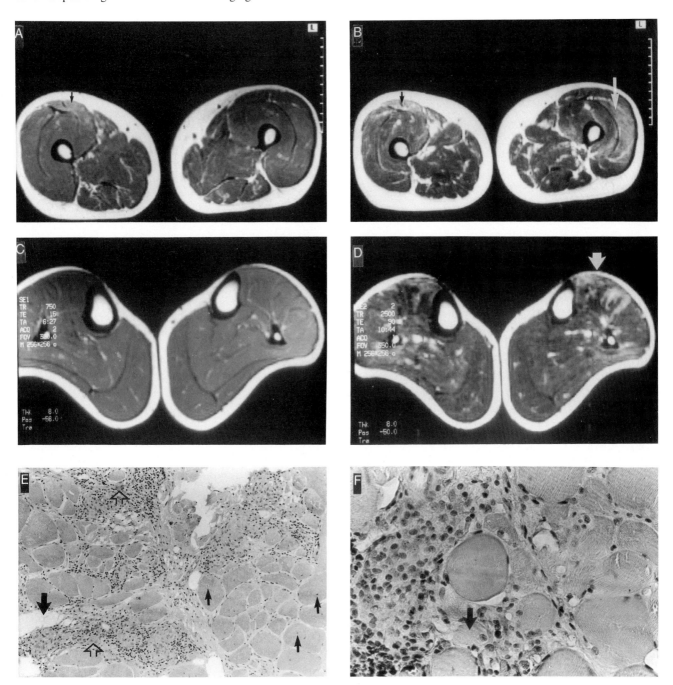

FIGURE 12.6. Radiology/histopathology in inflammatory myopathy. (A) T_1-weighted MRI (TR 750 ms, TE 15 ms) shows slightly increased signal intensity in a relatively few muscles, including the right rectus femoris (arrow). (B) T_2-weighted MRI (TR 1600 ms, TE 90 ms) shows large volumes of diffusely increased signal intensity in a variety of muscles, including the right rectus femoris (black arrow) and the left vastus lateralis (white arrow). The changes in the right rectus femoris indicate the presence of significant amounts of fat (short T_1 and long T_2 relaxation times), while the changes in the left vastus lateralis reflect those typical of muscle edema, i.e., modest T_1 time changes relative to marked increases in T_2 times. (C) T_1-weighted MRI (TR 750 ms, TE 15 ms) of the legs shows no definite abnormality. (D) T_2-weighted MRI (TR 1600 ms, TE 90 ms) shows irregularly marginated zones of hyperintensity, particularly in the tibialis anterior (arrow). These changes, like those in the vastus, reflect muscle edema. In contrast to MRI, specific changes ascribable to edema are not seen histopathologically. (E) Photomicrograph (hematoxylin-eosin staining, magnification ×100) of the left tibialis anterior shows abnormal variability of fiber size and diffuse infiltration of mononuclear cells, a few lipocytes (thick arrow), many atrophic fibers, rounded and necrotic fibers (open arrows) and numerous central nuclei (small arrows). (F) Photomicrograph (hematoxylin-eosin staining, magnification ×400) of the left tibialis anterior shows with better detail the mononuclear cell infiltration and abnormal variability of fiber size. Note abnormally round and variably sized fibers. (MRI courtesy of Professor Dr. T.J. Vogl, Department of Radiology, H.A. v. Humboldt University, Berlin, Germany.)

TABLE 12.2. Correlation of histopathological and imaging findings.

Histopathological abnormality	Ultrasound	Computed tomography	Magnetic resonance imaging*
lipomatosis	hyperechoic	hypodense	high SI on T1 and T2
connective tissue	no significant influence	hyperdense	low SI on T1 and on T2
increased total water content ("edema") or relative increase of extracellular space	hyper- or hypoechoic	hypodense	low SI on T1, high SI on T2 and STIR
calcification	highly echogenic with acoustic shadow	highly hyperdense	very low SI on T1 and T2 (seldom increased SI on T1)

*SI = signal intensity; T1 = T1-weighted image; T2 = T2-weighted image; STIR = short tau inversion recovery.

correlated to the T_1 and T_2 relaxation times.[14] Thus, a high collagen content, such as occurs in fibrosis, can theoretically alter signal intensities on T_1- and T_2-weighted images. An increase in muscle collagen content to greater than 60 mg/g of tissue is needed before changes become visible on MR images.[14] In addition, muscle fibrosis usually occurs in association with lipomatosis, so that the effects of one may obscure those in the other.

The appearance of muscle water is considerably more complicated than that of muscle fat or fibrosis, and a detailed analysis exceeds the scope of this chapter (see Chapter 3). The study of muscle edema in neuromuscular disease is further complicated by the fact that pathological correlation is methodologically difficult because the amount of muscle water is not visible under the microscope, whereas the associated causes, such as inflammation, are relatively conspicuous. However, in simple terms, it can be assumed that the magnitude of muscle water content above the basal state correlates positively with the estimated proton density and measured T_1 and T_2 relaxation times. These changes in relaxation times account for observed signal intensity decreases on heavily T_1-weighted spin echo images and increases on other sequences proportional to their degree of T_2 weighting.

A complicating factor in MRI detection of mild or moderate muscle edema is encountered in cases in which muscle fat content is increased, because the changes in muscle signal intensity may be dominated by the potent effects of intramuscular fat on relaxation times. The search for muscle edema in these cases is greatly simplified by the inclusion of fat suppression imaging schemes. These techniques include the increasingly popular short tau (inversion time) inversion recovery (STIR) sequence and selective fat saturation pulse sequences. In polymyositis, the STIR sequence was documented to provide more sensitive depiction of muscle edema than spin echo sequences that lack additional

inverting pulses.[15,16] This also has been demonstrated in muscle necrosis[17] and muscle injuries.[18]

An appearance similar to muscle edema is also seen in the nonedematous condition of subacute denervation and again the appearance is most conspicuous using the STIR sequence.[19] The "edema-like" appearance of denervated muscle appears to result from the fact that when the muscle fiber atrophies, the fraction of muscle water that is intracellular decreases and, consequently, that of the extracellular space increases. Because extracellular water has a T_2 relaxation time that is far in excess of intracellular water, small increases in the extracellular water fraction account for large increases in the T_2 time[20] and hence increased signal intensity of denervated muscle in neuropathic muscle disease using the STIR and other edema-sensitive sequences.[19]

An additional theoretical determinant of signal intensity of muscle on MRI is the fiber type proportion. This controversial issue is discussed in Chapter 7.

Results to date are inconclusive, with opposing conclusions resulting from animal[20] and human experiments.[21]

References

1. Hollmann W, Hettinger T. Sportmedizin. Arbeits- und Trainingsgrundlagen. 3rd ed. Stuttgart: Schattauer, 1990:30.
2. Sissons HA. Anatomy of the motor unit. In: Walton JN, ed. Disorders of the voluntary muscle. Edinburgh: Churchill Livingston, 1974:1–19.
3. Lamminen A, Jääskeläinen J, Rapola J, Suramo I. High-frequency ultrasonography of skeletal muscle in children with neuromuscular disease. J Ultrasound Med 1988;7: 505–509.
4. Reimers K, Reimers CD, Wagner St, et al. Skeletal muscle sonography: a correlative study between echointensities and morphology. J Ultrasound Med 1993;12:73–77.

5. Reimers CD, Fleckenstein JL, Witt TN, et al. Muscular ultrasound in idiopathic inflammatory myopathies of adults. J Neurol Sci 1993;116:82–92.

6. Nishimura M, Nishimura S, Yamada S. Ultrasound imaging of the muscle in muscular dystrophy. No To Hattatsu 1989;21:234–238.

7. Reimers CD, Lochmüller H, Goebels N, et al. Der Einfluß von Muskelarbeit auf das Myosonogramm. Ultraschall Med 1995;16:79–83.

8. Schedel H, Reimers CD, Naegele M, et al. Imaging techniques in myotonic dystrophy. A comparative study of ultrasound, computed tomography and magnetic resonance imaging of skeletal muscles. Eur J Radiol 1992;15:230–238.

9. Grindrod S, Tofts P, Edwards R. Investigation of human skeletal muscle structure and composition by X-ray computerised tomography. Eur J Clin Invest 1983;13:465–468.

10. Herson D, Larde D, Ferry M, et al. Apport diagnostique du scanner X en pathologie musculaire. Rev Neurol (Paris) 1985;141:482–489.

11. Ohiwa N, Kato T, Ando T, et al. CT findings of skeletal muscles in children with progressive muscular dystrophy. Brain Dev 1981;13:156–159.

12. van der Vliet AM, Thijssen HOM, Joosten E, Merx JL. CT in neuromuscular disorders: a comparison of CT and histology. Neuroradiology 1988;30:421–425.

13. Fleckenstein JL, Weatherall PT, Bertocci LA, et al. Locomotor system assessment by muscle magnetic resonance imaging. Magn Reson Q 1991;7:79–103.

14. Scholz TD, Fleagle SR, Burns TL, Skorton DJ. Tissue determinants of nuclear magnetic resonance relaxation times. Effect of water and collagen content in muscle and tendon. Invest Radiol 1989;24:893–898.

15. Fraser DD, Frank JA, Dalakas MC. Inflammatory myopathies: MR imaging and spectroscopy. Radiology 1991;179:341–342.

16. Hernandez RJ, Keim DR, Chenevert TL, et al. Fat-suppressive MR imaging in myositis. Radiology 1992;182:217–219.

17. Fleckenstein JL, Haller RG, Lewis SF, Parkey RW, Peshock RM. Focal muscle injury and atrophy in glycolytic myopathies. Muscle Nerve 1989;12(10):849–855.

18. Fleckenstein JL, Parkey RW, Peshock RM. Sports-related muscle injuries: evaluation with MR imaging. Radiology 1989;172(3):793–798.

19. Fleckenstein JL, Watumull D, Conner K, et al. Denervated human skeletal muscle: MRI evaluation. Radiology 1993;187:213–218.

20. Polak JF, Jolesz FA, Adams DF. NMR of skeletal muscle differences in relaxation parameters related to extracellular/intracellular fluid spaces. Invest Radiol 1988;23:107–112.

21. Kuno S-y, Katsuta S, Inouye T, et al. Relationship between MR relaxation time and muscle fiber composition. Radiology 1988;169:567–568.

13
Spinal Muscular Atrophy

Asma Q. Fischer and Elwood Longenecker

The spinal muscular strophies (SMA) of childhood are inherited neurodegenerative disorders in which there is progressive weakness and wasting of skeletal muscle secondary to degeneration of the anterior horn cells in the spinal cord and brain stem nuclei.[1] SMA is the second most common serious neuromuscular disease of childhood, affecting one in 10,000 children.[2] SMA of childhood is clinically and genetically a heterogeneous group. Their etiologies are currently unknown, and no specific treatment is available.[3]

Clinical Classification

Although various systems have been used to classify the subtypes of the disease, the current accepted method is division into three main types: type I, or Werdnig-Hoffmann disease; type II, or chronic infantile spinal muscular atrophy; and type III, chronic proximal spinal muscular atrophy, or Kugelberg-Welander disease.[4]

Clinical Features

The onset of type I or Werdnig-Hoffmann disease is no later than the first few months of life with a rapidly progressive course. The patient presents as a floppy infant with symptoms of progressive muscle weakness, including sucking difficulties, postural abnormalities, and respiratory distress.[5-9] Most infants with this disease die in the first year of life due to pneumonia and respiratory failure.[3,4]

The differential diagnosis of a floppy infant is quite extensive, ranging from neuromuscular problems to upper motor neuron lesions and cerebral palsy. Clinical observation of fasciculations, especially in the tongue, would exclude the differential diagnosis of primary muscle disorders.[3] Muscle imaging can be helpful in differentiating between upper motor neuron and most lower motor neuron etiologies in a floppy baby. The findings on muscle imaging of most upper motor neuron lesions are quite unremarkable compared to those of primary muscle diseases.

The existence of type II SMA as a separate disease is in debate. It rarely presents before 6 months of age, but most patients are afflicted by their first year of life. Clinical progression is also very variable, with periods of slow or arrested development in addition to the possibility of rapid deterioration. Untreated children develop scoliosis with further respiratory compromise and increased risk of pneumonia. Prognosis is variable, with many patients surviving into adulthood with marked disability.[4]

Type III or Kugelberg-Welander disease is characterized by a longer course, later onset, and more variable symptoms than the type I disease. It most often begins at age two and survival occurs into the third decade.[3] Clinically, it may resemble a muscular dystrophy with the exception of observable fasciculations.[4] Progression of the weakness may be slow to the point that developmental increases in strength may overtake the disease process. There is great risk of skeletal deformities, such as scoliosis and kyphosis in an ambulatory child and equinovarus deformities in a nonambulatory child.[3]

Diagnosis

The standard tests for establishing a definitive diagnosis of SMA include: (1) a detailed clinical neuromuscular examination, (2) electromyography, (3) nerve conduction studies, and (4) muscle biopsy. Although muscle enzyme levels may occasionally be elevated, they are usually normal. Muscle biopsy is the most specific of these tests. Diagnosis is established by recognizing the typical clinical presentation, with characteristic muscle biopsy findings.

Biopsy Findings

The microscopic findings of grouped atrophic fibers are seen in 85% of the patients with SMA, regardless of the age of onset of the disease. Interstitial fat is seen in 39% of patients. Sixty-eight percent of patients have neuropathic changes, 19% have neuropathic and myopathic changes, 5% of patients have myopathic changes only, and 8% of patients have nonspecific changes or are normal.[10]

Characteristic features would show denervation atrophy.[3] Large groups of atrophic fibers can be seen next to bunches of hypertrophic fibers, suggesting a neuropathy.[1,3,4] These hypertrophic fibers are predominantly type 1 histochemically.[1] However, type 1 and 2 fibers cluster together, reflecting reinnervation.[3] In some biopsies, only sheets of atrophic fibers can be seen, making interpretation more difficult.[1] In type I (Werdnig-Hoffmann) disease, muscle biopsy reveals fascicles containing clusters of hypertrophic type 1 muscle fibers among numerous tiny atrophic fibers of both fiber types.[5-8,11-14] Ultrastructural examination is most remarkable for reduction and disruption of contractile elements attributed to denervation during muscle development.[15-21] Biopsy changes in the chronic forms of SMA are more variable[1] (Table 13.1).

SMA can be distinguished from a peripheral neuropathy by biopsy primarily becuse a peripheral neuropathy is characterized by small-group atrophy, whereas SMA is characterized by large-group atrophy. The changes seen in a peripheral neuropathy are generally not as severe as those seen in SMA.[22]

TABLE 13.1 Microscopic diagnosis and histologic findings in skeletal muscle biopsies of 180 patients with chronic spinal muscular atrophy.[10]

	Percent
Microscopic diagnosis	
Neuropathy	68.2 (60–75)
Neuropathy and myopathy	18.9 (19–26)
Myopathy	4.5 (2–8)
Nonspecific	4.5 (2–8)
Normal	3.9 (2–8)
Histologic findings in 110 patients	
Atrophic muscle fibers	100.0 (97–100)
Grouped atrophic fibers	85.5 (78–92)
Muscle fiber degeneration	22.7 (15–32)
Phagocytosis	7.3 (3–13)
Basophilic muscle fibers	5.5 (2–12)
Increased sarcolemmal nuclei	20.0 (13–28)
Internal nuclei	20.9 (13–30)
Cell infiltration	2.7 (1–8)
Interstitial fat tissue	39.0 (30–48)
Increased connective tissue	33.5 (25–43)

Electrophysiologic Findings

Nerve conduction studies are usually normal or show minimal reductions in conduction velocities.[1] EMG findings include increased insertional activity, abnormal spontaneous activity, impaired recruitment of motor units, and increased amplitude and duration of voluntary motor unit potentials.[1]

Ultrasound in Spinal Muscular Atrophy

Methods

Recent technological improvements have contributed to the increased usage of ultrasound in evaluating neuromuscular diseases (see Chapter 2). In brief, several methods have been described for performance of muscle ultrasound using static and real-time equipment.[23,24] We find it best to perform muscle sonography using a standardized procedure, so that inter-test and inter-patient variability is minimized. This method of muscle ultrasound has been well established:[24] Several non-diseased subjects in the age groups of newborn to 12 months, 12 months to 5 years, and 5 years to adult are sonogrammed to standardize age-matched norms for the individual ultrasound laboratory. The optimized combinations for each age group are then stored in the equipment memory to be used for sonogramming the neuromuscular patients.

Sonographic images in the transverse and longitudinal planes of all four limbs are documented at approximately the midsection of the imaged limb. Using standard high-resolution real-time ultrasound equipment, the depth gain compensation (DGC), overall gain, pre- and post-processing, and persistence are optimized for age and thickness of muscle being examined. Minor instrumental adjustments may be needed while scanning the SMA patients but major departures from the age standardized methods can obscure subtle findings.

Interpretation

Interpretation of the sonograms using a standardized method provides interinterpreter reliability. In any one neuromuscular sonogram, five major findings are described. Subcutaneous fat and muscle thickness measurements are made.[24] In normal muscle, fascial planes and bone edges appear hyperechoic, the bone edge casting a crisp shadow.[25] Normal muscle parenchyma gives a somewhat less intense signal, termed "euechoic." The exact signal intensity corresponding to the term euechoic differs slightly between age groups.[24]

The initial findings of SMA described on static scanning were a generalized increase in echogenicity of the muscle parenchyma.[23] It was not until the advent of the high-resolution real-time computerized ultrasound imaging that the actual pattern within the muscle parenchyma was described.[25] The classical finding in early but established disease in floppy babies with SMA has been described as a pattern of heterogeneous hyperechogenicity is within the muscle parenchyma of each muscle, giving it a "motheaten" appearance[25] (see Figures 13.1 to 13.3). These sonographic findings are usually evident in the midthighs or midarms. The changes in the muscle parenchyma are usually coupled with decreases in the clarity of the bone edge and indistinguishable myofascial interfaces. The bone shadow is preserved until late in the disease process. The earliest diagnostic changes detected by ultrasound are the moth-eaten appearance of the muscle parenchyma.

Two groups found muscle atrophy and increased subcutaneous tissue depth associated with the increased muscle echogenicity of SMA.[26,27] However, though all of their patients with mild or intermediate forms of SMA showed sonographic abnormalities, only 7 of 15 of their patients with severe SMA had abnormal sonograms.[26] Atrophy of the quadriceps and increased subcutaneous tissue thickness has been reported in one study to be of greater significance than the hyperechogenicity of muscle parenchyma.[28]

The ultrasound pattern of peripheral nerve denervation may mimic the SMA ultrasound pattern. However, the abnormal sonographic findings are localized to the muscle supplied by the affected peripheral nerve in peripheral nerve denervation processes, whereas in SMA these findings are usually found diffusely, affecting almost all muscle groups (see Figures 13.4 to 13.7).

Disease Progression

Muscle ultrasound findings change significantly with progression and chronicity of disease. These durational changes can sometimes cause confusion for the interpreter who may be expecting a specific unchanging pattern associated with the disease. Progressive changes in the bone edge, myofascial planes, and the increase in intensity of the echogenicity of the muscle parenchyma become manifest with progression and duration of disease. One cause of increased echogenicity has been attributed to fat replacement.[29] In chronic SMA, it has been noted on CT that as the muscle shrinks, fat replacement occurs.[30] In chronic SMA, the long duration of the disease is reflected in the marked increase in muscle parenchymal echogenicity (see Figures 13.8 to 13.11). The increased echogenicity by itself is a nonspecific finding of disease progression, as this may also be seen in chronic advanced inflammatory myopathic disease[31] and Duchenne muscular dystrophy.[25]

The progression of SMA as indicated by ultrasound has not been well studied in relationship to clinical progression. In the patients we studied over time, progression is noted by increased muscle echogenicity, and loss of muscle mass and muscle anatomical landmarks. Both Duchenne muscular dystrophy and SMAs share this picture at the advanced stages of the diseases. The major differentiation of SMA from Duchenne muscular dystrophy in the advanced state is that in SMA, both the muscle and subcutaneous tissue is lost, whereas in Duchenne the subcutaneous fat may be retained in the face of an extremely dystrophic muscle.[32]

Muscle biopsy findings are important in SMA because they help establish the diagnosis, but they do not help predict the severity of the disease among infants with Werdnig-Hoffmann disease.[33]

It is helpful for the muscle ultrasonographer to become familiar with the normal muscle anatomy,[34] as well as the sonographic patterns in disease. With experience the changes attributed to disease progression can be monitored sonographically with reliability.

Illustrative Case Reports

Three patients are presented, illustrating the variability of the sonographic findings of SMAs according to age of onset and stage of chronicity of the disease.

Case One

This 17-month-old male presented for a neurological evaluation for severe floppiness. Significant clinical features included marked generalized hypotonia, head lag, diffuse generalized muscle weakness, and areflexia. Electromyography revealed a diffuse neuropathic process and biopsy findings were consistent with progressive SMA. A neuromuscular sonogram done at that time revealed the typical moth-eaten picture (Figures 13.1 to 13.3).

Case Two

This patient was diagnosed with SMA type II at age 14 months based on a clinical history, neuromuscular examination, and muscle biopsy. At age 7 years the patient presented for a follow-up examination and a sonogram was performed. At the time, the patient was nonambulatory, scoliotic, with moderate weakness in all four extremities, and had barely detectable deep tendon reflexes. He was having no respiratory difficulties at this time. Sensory examination was reported as normal. His sonogram showed marked increase in heterogeneous echogenicity, with a loss of the classical moth-eaten lesions seen in recently diagnosed SMA patients (Figures 13.4 to 13.7.)

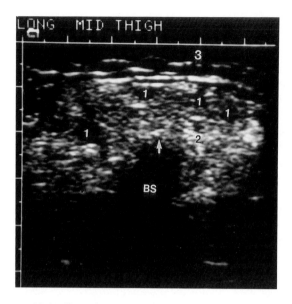

FIGURE 13.1. Case one: transverse sonogram, midthigh, of a 17 month old with severe hypotonia and areflexia. 1 = "moth-eaten" hypoechoic areas within each of the thigh muscles, 2 = background increase in heterogeneous echogenicity, 3 = subcutaneous fat, arrow = marked reduction in clarity and crispness of bone edge, BS = preservation of bone shadow.

Case Three

This patient was diagnosed as having chronic progressive SMA at age 18 months. At age 5 years she demonstrated moderately severe proximal muscle weakness but was ambulatory. A sonogram done at this time revealed an

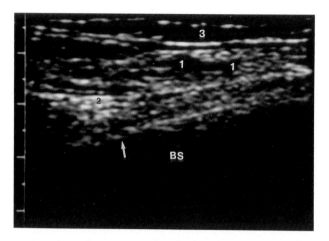

FIGURE 13.3. Case one: longitudinal sonogram, midthigh, of the same patient in Figure 13.1. 1 = "moth-eaten" hypoechoic areas within thigh muscles, 2 = background increase in heterogeneous echogenicity, 3 = subcutaneous fat, BS = preservation of bone shadow, arrow = bone edge.

abnormal increase in heterogeneous echogenicity with the moth-eaten appearance (Figures 13.8, 13.10). She returned at age 8 years after a bout of pneumonia and at that time was moderately weak with some restriction in range of motion and had developed significant scoliosis. A sonogram at this time revealed a progressive increase in muscle parenchymal echogenicity and loss of most of the anatomical landmarks in the muscle (Figures 13.9 to 13.11).

Computed Tomography in Spinal Muscular Atrophy

Computed tomography findings in SMA type I include atrophy of the thigh muscles.[35] In SMA type II, patches of low-density tissue can be demonstrated in the muscles whose motor neurons have been affected. These patches are very small, sharp, and very diffusely distributed throughout the muscles. As the disease progresses these patches become larger and the muscles acquire a ragged outline, and progressively submerge into the panniculus adiposus,[30] Another group described the appearance of SMA type III as having a typical, nonhomogeneous, patchy atrophy.[36]

One group of authors studied 100 patients with a very heterogeneous group of patients with SMA.[37] The patients were divided into four groups based on the severity of their CT scans, grade 1 having slightly abnormal scans and grade 4 having late or end-stage CT appearances. Scans were graded for attenuation values,

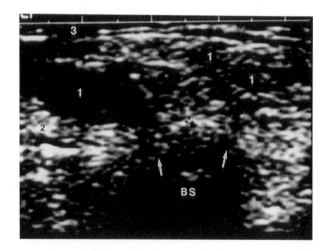

FIGURE 13.2. Case one: high-resolution sonogram, transverse plane, of the same patient in Figure 13.1. 1 = "moth-eaten" hypoechoic areas within muscle parenchyma, 2 = background increase in heterogeneous echogenicity of the muscle parenchyma, 3 = subcutaneous fat, arrows = indistinct bone edge, BS = preservation of bone shadow.

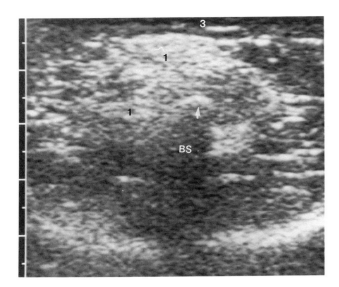

FIGURE 13.4. Case two: transverse sonogram, midarm, in a wheel chair-bound 7 year old diagnosed at age 14 months with SMA (type II) with a moderate decrease in muscle strength and scoliosis. 1 = marked increase in heterogeneous echogenicity and loss of myofascial planes, 3 = subcutaneous fat, arrow = indistinct bone edge, BS = relative preservation of bone shadow despite marked increase in muscle echogenicity.

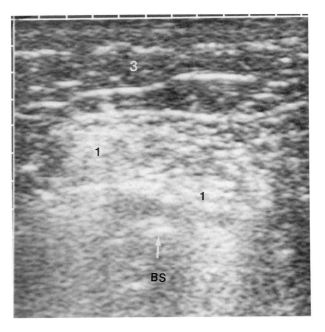

FIGURE 13.6. Case two: sonogram transverse midthigh in same patient as Figure 13.4. 1 = marked increase in heterogeneous echogenicity and loss of myofascial planes, 3 = subcutaneous fat, arrow = indistinct bone edge, BS = bone shadow.

muscle hypertrophy, evidence of asymmetrical involvement, and maintenance of fascial planes within individual muscles. Grade 1 patients had areas of low attenuation in leg muscles, the tibialis anterior usually being spared.

Muscles of the neck, shoulders, abdomen, spine, pelvis, and thigh were normal. In grade 2 patients, the gluteal and leg muscles showed larger areas of low attenuation. In addition, most other muscle groups, with the exception

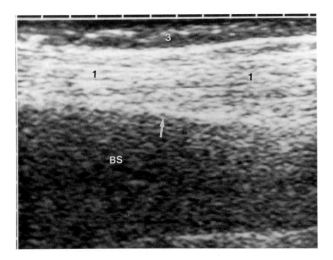

FIGURE 13.5. Case two: sonogram longitudinal plane midarm in the same patient as in Figure 13.4. 1 = marked increase in heterogeneous echogenicity and loss of myofascial planes, 3 = subcutaneous fat, arrow = indistinct bone edge merging with muscle echogenicity, BS = relative preservation of bone shadow despite marked increase in muscle echogenicity.

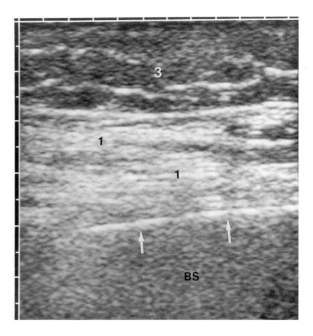

FIGURE 13.7. Case two: sonogram longitudinal midthigh in same patient as Figure 13.4. 1 = marked increase in heterogeneous echogenicity and loss of myofascial planes, 3 = subcutaneous fat, arrows = bone edge, BS = bone shadow.

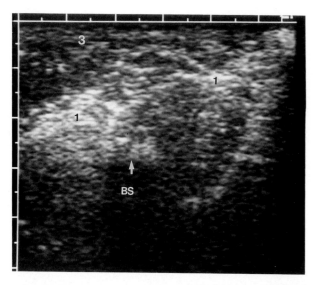

FIGURE 13.8. Case three: transverse sonogram, midarm, of a 5-year-old patient with marked proximal weakness first diagnosed with SMA at age 18 months. 1 = marked increase in heterogenous echogenicity and loss of myofascial planes, 3 = subcutaneous fat, arrow = indistinct bone edge, BS = partial preservation of bone shadow.

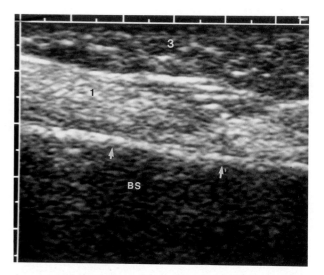

FIGURE 13.10. Case three: longitudinal sonogram, midarm, in the same patient as Figure 13.8 at age 5 years. 1 = marked increase in heterogeneous echogenicity and loss of myofascial planes, 3 = subcutaneous fat, arrows = bone edge, BS = preservation of bone shadow.

of the sternocleidomastoid and shoulder girdle, were affected. In grade 3 patients, the shoulder girdle was also affected, although sternocleidomastoid was usually spared. This group showed the most diagnostic pattern of CT abnormality. Both large and small areas of low attenuation could be seen in most muscles. Thigh abnormalities were often more severe in the hamstrings than in the quadriceps. In grade 4 cases, areas of low

attenuation could be seen in all muscles, including the usually unaffected sternocleidomastoid and psoas. Fascial planes were preserved in the majority of grade 1 and 2 patients, whereas this was the case in about half of the grades 3 and 4 patients. Asymmetry increased with increasing grade, 14% of those in grade 1 having had asymmetrical involvement compared to 47% of those in grade 4.[37]

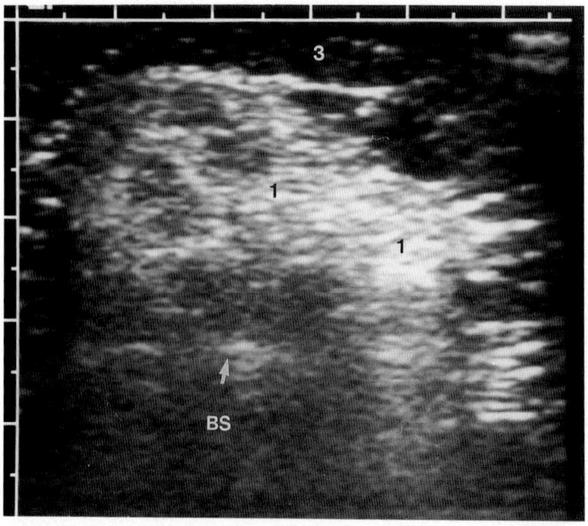

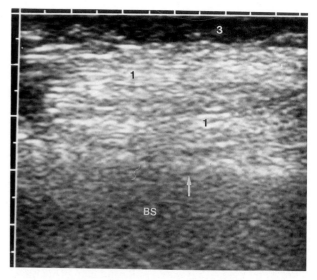

FIGURE 13.9. Case three: transverse sonogram, midarm, in the same patient as Figure 13.8 at age 8 years with moderate progression in muscle weakness and respiratory difficulties. 1 = marked increase in heterogeneous echogenicity and loss of myofascial planes, 3 = subcutaneous fat, arrow = indistinct bone edge, BS = bone shadow.

FIGURE 13.11. Case three: longitudinal sonogram, midarm, in the same patient as Figure 13.8 at age 8 years. 1 = marked increase in heterogeneous echogenicity and loss of myofascial planes, 3 = subcutaneous fat, arrow = indistinct bone edge, BS = indistinct bone shadow.

Two studies compared SMA with muscular dystrophy.[38,39] In one study, it was noted that in Becker-type muscular dystrophy, low-density tissue eventually replaced all normal muscle. In contrast, in SMA, low-density areas were scattered through the muscle.[38] According to one author, types I and II SMA show somewhat more diffuse fatty changes than muscular dystrophy.[39] There was not much preferential muscle involvement in the muscles of SMA patients, which was in contrast to muscular dystrophy.[38]

Spinal muscular atrophy has been reported to resemble Charcot-Marie-Tooth disease with peroneal muscle atrophy upon CT examination.[35,40] A difference that was noted was that there were earlier changes of decreased density in the muscles of the thigh in SMA.[35] Increased thigh muscle definition was noted in the milder cases of SMA, due to atrophy and therefore increased separation.[35] Proximal muscles were seen to be more affected in severe cases.[35] Extreme involvement of some muscles along with sparing of others was generally not seen.[40]

One group of authors examined the CT pattern in patients with bulbar spinal muscular atrophy. They found a varying degree of fatty infiltration in the muscles of the lower extremities and trunk. More infiltration was seen in the flexor compartments of the leg than the extensor compartments. A significant correlation was found between fatty infiltrations in flexors of the lower extremities and duration of the disease. CT evaluation assisted in assessing the muscle distribution and perhaps the duration of disease by the presence and severity of fatty infiltration in the muscles of patients with SMA in this study group.[41]

MRI in Spinal Muscular Atrophy

The use of MRI in evaluation of SMA has been somewhat more limited (Figure 13.12). One recent report described the MRI appearance of denervated muscle, which presumably would have an appearance similar to that of SMA. Subacutely denervated muscles (between 1 month and 1 year) were described as having prolonged T_1 and T_2 and hyperintensity on STIR images. Chronically denervated muscle was described as being markedly atrophic, with fatty infiltration seen on T_1 images and variable changes on STIR images. MRI was less successful in depicting acute denervation of less than 1 month.[42]

Another study compared the MRI appearances of muscles afflicted by Duchenne muscular dystrophy (DMD) and Kugelberg-Welander SMA to each other and to controls. Perhaps these disorders were selected because of their similar clinical picture. Both DMD and Kugelberg-Welander patients had significantly more subcutaneous fat than normals. However, differences in

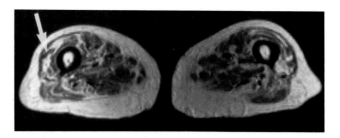

FIGURE 13.12. MRI of spinal muscular atrophy. Axial spin density-weighted image (2000 TR/30 TE) shows relatively preserved fascial boundaries in muscles having undergone extensive deterioration. Note increased signal intensity (fat) in the vastus lateralis where only a small irregularly shaped inner portion of muscle tissue remains present (arrow.) The CT appearance of SMA is very similar.

musculature appearance were noted between the two diseases. The muscles of SMA patients were described as being more completely involved, and it was difficult to distinguish muscles from each other. However, within each muscle, affliction was more heterogeneous than in DMD. Areas of normal signal intensity could be seen in the same muscles as areas of hypo- and hyperintensity. Another distinguishing feature between the disorders was that SMA patients' muscles were affected to the same extent, whereas muscles having more fasttwitch fibers were most affected in DMD.[43]

Role of Imaging in Patient Care

The role of imaging in SMA is that of an adjunct method of confirming a clinical assessment and assisting the clinician in choosing further testing. The most uncomplicated, noninvasive method of imaging is ultrasound because most SMA patients are children with type II onset (47%) and babies with Werdnig-Hoffmann disease (27%).[44] Muscle ultrasound provides ease of performance and interpretation without removing a sick baby from its environment. In experienced and knowledgeable hands, with persistence and patience diseased muscles can be found. With the current sophistication offered in real-time imaging tools the muscles can be exquisitely imaged, and the ideal muscle for biopsy can be chosen during the examination.

Floppy infants are a challenge to the clinician. The question arises, "Are they floppy because of an upper motor neuron lesion a lower motor neuron lesion or myopathy?" In most cases there are clinical suspicions of lower motor neuron disease that can be corroborated by abnormal findings on the sonogram. This can facilitate the decision to obtain a muscle biopsy promptly. A clinical dilemma occurs if the sonogram is normal and the patient does not have hard signs of lower motor neuron disease. Usually in these cases, in our experience, either the disease was so subtle, or was a non-SMA type of congenital muscular dystrophy.

Muscle imaging of SMA in childhood is possible with all three current modalities (i.e., ultrasound, CT, and MRI). The most clinically useful tool currently remains ultrasound by virtue of its noninvasiveness, ease of performance, and relatively lower expense. However, like most ultrasound applications, it demands a basic knowledge of muscle anatomy and pathology of the disease being studied by the sonographer. An uninformed sonographer can miss the characteristic findings.

Neuromuscular ultrasound is used as an adjunct to clinical evaluation and can assist the clinician in choosing further diagnostic studies or can be helpful in the follow-up of patients. Because clinical and ultrasound correlative studies have not yet been performed in chronic SMA patients, the exact severity of the disease cannot be assessed on ultrasound alone; however, this may change in the face of current ongoing investigations in many neuromuscular centers.

Acknowledgments. We would like to thank Sharon Stephens for her assistance in performing the muscle sonograms.

References

1. Wessel HB. Spinal muscular atrophy. Pediatr Ann 1989; 18:421–427.
2. Anonymous. Spinal muscular atrophies. Lancet 1990; 336:280–281.
3. Gordon N. The spinal muscular atrophies. Dev Med Child Neurol 1991;33:934–938.
4. Campbell MJ. Motor neurone diseases In: Disorders of voluntary muscle. Avon: The Bath Press, 1988:754–792.
5. Byers RK, Banker BQ. Infantile spinal muscular atrophy. Arch Neurol 1961;5:140–164.
6. Dubowitz V. Muscle biopsy: a practical approach 2nd ed. London: Baillière Tindall, 1985.
7. Dubowitz V. Muscle disorders in childhood. Philadelphia: W.B. Saunders, 1978.
8. Dubowitz V. Color atlas of muscle disorders in childhood. Chicago: Year Book Medical, 1989.
9. Hausmanowa-Petruseqicz I, Fidzianska-Dolot A. Clinical features of infantile and juvenile spinal muscular atrophy. In: Gamstorp I, Sarnat HB, eds. Progressive spinal muscular atrophies. New York: Raven Press, 1984:31–42.
10. Namba T, Aberfield DC, Grob D. Chronic proximal spinal muscular atrophy. J Neurol Sci 1970;11:401–423.
11. Buchthal F, Olsen PZ. Electromyography and muscle biopsy in infantile spinal muscular atrophy. Brain 1970; 93:15–30.
12. Fenichel GM, Engel WK. Histochemistry of muscle in infantile spinal muscular atrophy. Neurology 1963;13: 1059–1066.
13. Fidzianska-Dolot A, Hansmanowa-Petrusewicz I. Morphology of the lower motor neuron and muscle. In: Gamstorp I, Sarnat HB, eds. Progressive spinal muscular atrophies. New York: Raven Press, 1984:55–89.
14. Sarnat HB. Pathology of spinal muscular atrophy. In: Gamstorp I, Sarnat HB, eds. Progressive spinal muscular atrophies. New York: Raven Press, 1984:91–110.
15. Hausmanowa-Petrusewicz W, Askanas B, Badurska B, et al. Infantile and juvenile spinal muscular atrophy. J Neurol Sci 1968;6:269–287.
16. Shafiq SA, Milhorat AT, Gorycki MA. Fine structure of human muscle in neurogenic atrophy. Neurology 1967;17: 934–948.
17. Fidzianska A. Ultrastructural changes in muscle in spinal muscular atrophy Werdnig-Hoffmann's. Acta Neuropathol 1974;27:247–256.
18. Fidzianska A. Morphological differences between the atrophied small muscle fibers in amyotrophic lateral sclerosis and Werdnig-Hoffmann's disease. Acta Neuropathol (Berl) 1976;34:321–327.
19. Highes JT, Brownell B. Ultrastructure of muscle in Werdnig-Hoffmann's disease. J Neurol Sci 1969;8: 363–379.
20. VanHaelst U. An electron microscopic study of muscle in Werdnig-Hoffmann's disease. Virchows Arch [A] 1970; 351:291–305.
21. Nonaka I, Miike T, Ueno T, et al. An electron microscopic study of biopsied muscle in Werdnig-Hoffmann disease. Brain Dev 1974;6:10–18.
22. Dubowitz V, Brooke MH. Muscle biopsy: a modern approach. Lavenham: The Lavenham Press, 1973.
23. Heckmatt JZ, Dubowitz V. Diagnosis of spinal muscular atrophy with pulse echo ultrasound imaging. In: Gamstorp I, Sarnat HB, eds. Progressive spinal muscular atrophies. New York: Raven Press, 1984:141–152.
24. Fischer AQ, Stephens S. Computerized real-time neuromuscular sonography: a new application, techniques, and methods. J Child Neurol 1988;3:9–74.
25. Fischer AQ, Carpenter DW, Hartlage PL, et al. Muscle imaging in neuromuscular disease using computerized real-time sonography. Muscle Nerve 1988;March:270–275.
26. Heckmatt JZ, Dubowitz V. Real-time ultrasound imaging of muscles. Muscle Nerve 1988;11:56–65.
27. Lamminen A, Jaaskelainen J, Rapola J, Suramo I. High-frequency ultrasonography of skeletal muscle in children with neuromuscular disease. J Ultrasound Med 1988; 7:505–509.
28. Schmidt R, Voit T. Ultrasound measurement of quadriceps muscle in the first year of life. Normal values and appliction to spinal muscular atrophy. Neuropediatrics 1993;24:36–42.
29. Reimers K, Reimers CD, Wagner S, et al. Skeletal muscle sonography: a correlative study of echogenicity and morphology. J Ultrasound Med 1993;2:73–77.

30. Bulcke JAL, Baert AL. Spinal muscular atrophies. In: Clinical and radiological aspects of myopathies. Berlin: Springer-Verlag, 1982:114–122.

31. Fischer AQ, Hartlage PL, et al. Inflammatory myopathies of childhood: diagnosis and follow-up by computerized real-time sonography. Ann Neurology 1987:22(3).

32. Fischer AQ. Pediatric applications of clinical ultrasound. In: Bodensteiner J, ed. Neurologic clinics of North America. Philadelphia: Saunders, 1990;8:759–774.

33. Zalneraitis EL, Halperin JJ, Grunnet ML, et al. Muscle biopsy and the clinical course of infantile spinal muscular atrophy. J Child Neurol 1991;6:324–328.

34. Fornage BD. Ultrasonography of muscles and tendons: examination technique and atlas of normal anatomy of the extremities. New York: Springer-Verlag, 1989.

35. Hawley RJ Jr, Schellinger D, O'Doherty DS. Computed tomographic patterns of muscles in neuromuscular diseases. Arch Neurol 1984;41:383–387.

36. Termote JL, Baert A, et al. Computed tomography of the normal and pathologic muscular system. Radiology 1980; 137:439–444.

37. Sambrook P, Rickards D, Cumming WJK. CT muscle scanning in the evaluation of patients with spinal muscular atrophy (SMA.) Neuroradiology 1988;30: 487–496.

38. de Visser M, Verbeeten B. Computed tomography of the skeletal musculature in Becker-type muscular dystrophy and benign infantile spinal muscular atrophy. Muscle Nerve 1985;8:435–444.

39. Torch WC. Computed tomography (CT) of skeletal muscle in muscular dystrophy (MD) and spinal muscular atrophy (SMA): a method for clinical diagnosis. Muscle Nerve (Suppl) 1986;9:244.

40. Nordal HJ, Dietrichson PE, et al. Fat infiltration, atrophy and hypertrophy of skeletal muscles demonstrated by X-ray computed tomography in neurological patients. Acta Neurol Scand 1988;77:115–122.

41. Koga H, Yamamoto H, Sahashi K, Ibi T, Mori K. Computed tomographic analyses on skeletal muscles in bulbar spinal muscular atrophy. Rinsho Shinkeigaku (Clin Neurol) 1990;30(8):828–834.

42. Fleckenstein JL, Watumull D, et al. Denervated human skeletal muscle: MR imaging evaluation. Radiology 1993; 187:213–218.

43. Suput D, Zupan A, Sepe A, Demsar F. Discrimination between neuropathy and myopathy by use of magnetic resonance imaging. Acta Neurol Scand 1993;87:118–123.

44. Pearn J. Genetics of the spinal muscular atrophies. In: Gamstorp I, Sarnat HB, eds. Progressive spinal muscular atrophies. New York: Raven Press, 1984:19–30.

14
Neuropathies and Motor Neuron Diseases

Berthold C.G. Schalke, Erich Hofmann, Karlheinz Reiners, and Werner Kaiser

Neuropathies are a group of diseases affecting the peripheral nervous system as a whole or only in part. Neuropathies can be classified variously, by course, cause, distribution of affected nerves or functional systems (motor, sensory, autonomic), or by the underlying pathological processes.[1-3]

Pathological Mechanisms

The integrity of the peripheral nerve can be disturbed by various mechanisms, all of which ultimately manifest with nonspecific clinical evidence of neuropathy. Trauma or chronic entrapment can cause Wallerian degeneration of the nerve and thereby lead to denervation of the muscles in the affected nerve territory. Toxic neuropathies are the prototype of acute, subacute, or chronic axonal degeneration. The inflammatory neuropathies, Guillain-Barré-Strohl syndrome (GBS) and chronic inflammatory demyelinating polyneuropathy (CIDP), represent acute and chronic demyelinating neuropathies, respectively. The chronic type of demyelination is also found in hereditary motor and sensory neuropathies (HMSN, formerly called peroneal muscular atrophy, Charcot-Marie-Tooth disease and/or dominantly inherited hypertrophic neuropathy), chronic diabetes mellitus, and dysproteinemias.[2] Degeneration of the nerve cell body (perikaryon), or of the entire neuron, is found in poliomyelitis, spinal muscular atrophy (see Chapter 13), and amyotrophic lateral sclerosis (ALS).[4,5]

Clinical Evaluation and Diagnostic Procedures

Clinical assessment should always include the family history, potential acute or chronic toxic exposures, drugs, recent infections, and metabolic illnesses. It is important to establish the initial clinical presentation, the distribution of abnormalities, and the progression of neuropathic symptoms. The great majority of neuropathies develop insidiously; only patients with an acute type of the disease (e.g., GBS) can precisely date the onset of symptoms. Initial symptoms are primarily sensory, such as paraesthesias, numbness, and pain in a glove- or stocking-like distribution. Physical examination should include detection of trophic abnormalities, detailed sensory testing, and testing of strength, reflex status, limb girth at defined sites, and autonomic function.

The clinical hallmark of motor neuropathy is weakness, either symmetric or asymmetric. Muscle atrophy is a sign of more chronic disease,[4,6] and when it occurs, may arise from either disuse (e.g., following conduction block) or muscle denervation following Wallerian degeneration (axonal damage) of the innervating nerve fibers. Deformities of the spine and/or feet suggest a chronic disease, reflecting imbalance of agonistic and antagonistic muscle groups. Deformities such as pes cavus and hammer toes are especially frequent in hereditary neuropathies.

In general, symptoms are more pronounced distally, with legs being more affected than arms, and extensor and abducting muscles weaker than flexors and adductors. In patients with hereditary neuropathies, symptoms are slowly progressive. Tendon reflexes are diminished or absent. Autonomic symptoms become clinically relevant only late in the course of disease.

Electrophysiology

A detailed review of electrophysiology of muscle and nerve exceeds the scope of this chapter. Suffice to say that electrodiagnostic studies record spontaneous, evoked, or voluntarily generated potentials from nerve or muscle by electrodes placed on the skin or via needle into the muscles themselves. These allow identification of distinctive features that allow determination of the site and type of changes that result from many neuropathies and myopathies. Synchronized discharges can be obtained by electrical stimulation of a nerve to elicit compound nerve action potentials (CNAPs) or compound muscle action potentials (CMAPs). The shapes and velocities of these are of considerable clinical interest. Synchronous activation of groups of muscle fibers can also be obtained by voluntary activation of motor unit potentials (MUPs). Repetitive stimulation tests assess the neuromuscular junction. Electromyography (EMG) records spontaneous and voluntary potentials with a needle electrode in muscle.

Using electrophysiological techniques, it is possible to distinguish between axonal degeneration (reduced CMAPs) or demyelination (slowed nerve conduction velocity), and between a focal or generalized, proximal or distal, nerve root or perikaryal process, thick or thin fiber involvement, pure motor, sensory, autonomic, or mixed neuropathy.[7] EMG of clearly affected muscles is helpful to estimate the chronicity of axonal loss and to establish ongoing Wallerian degeneration of nerve fibers. It also serves to differentiate neurogenic muscle atrophy and paresis from similar symptoms in primary muscle diseases (myopathies). Examination of muscles that are not clinically involved allows identification of subclinical neuropathy and provides a comprehensive understanding of the distribution of neuropathology.

Nerve and Muscle Biopsy

Nerve biopsy, usually taken from the sural nerve, is helpful if history, clinical, electrophysiological, and laboratory examinations do not allow a definite classification of the underlying pathological process. Microscopic examination can provide evidence of inflammation, cellular infiltration, acute and chronic demyelination and remyelination, nerve hypertrophy, axonal degeneration, and may also show the distribution of fiber type involvement. Although microscopy examination is very sensitive for pathological changes, most findings are nonspecific. A specific pathological diagnosis is possible only in a few diseases (e.g., in sarcoidosis, leprosy, amyloidosis, neurofibromatosis, necrotizing angiopathy, and lipid storage diseases). In general, there is no indication for muscle biopsy in peripheral neuropathies because histological findings in the muscle are particularly nonspecific (e.g., fiber type grouping and target formations). Only in inflammatory neuropathies (e.g., vasculitis or sarcoidosis) is a combined nerve/muscle biopsy helpful.[6] Hence, only by analysis of the combined genetic, clinical, electrophysiological, and morphological data can a final classification of the subtype of polyneuropathy be established.

Typical Radiological Findings

Because some electrodiagnostic techniques are painful and somewhat operator dependent, radiological techniques have been explored as potential noninvasive alternatives to electrodiagnostic tests. To date, no diagnostic imaging technique has been reported to be sensitive in detecting very early muscle changes after acute denervation in humans. However, at approximately the same time as EMG becomes abnormal after nerve transection (at more than 1 week), MRI becomes quite sensitive to morphological changes in the muscle. The precise nature of these changes remains unclear. The prolongation of muscle proton relaxation times suggests the presence of edema during this phase. However, because edema would be expected to cause muscle swelling and the prolonged relaxation times are commonly observed while the muscle atrophies, edema per se appears to be an unlikely explanation for the signal intensity changes visible during the first several months of denervation. A more tenable explanation is that as the muscle fibers atrophy, the fraction of water that is intracellular consequently decreases, requiring that the extracellular water fraction increases. Because extracellular water has a much longer T_2 time than intracellular water, such small fractional changes of water likely contribute to the "edema-like" appearance of denervated muscle on MRI.[8–11] Whatever the cause of the edema-like MRI appearance of subacute denervation, the changes in relaxation times result in a conspicuous appearance when edema-sensitive sequences are used (Figure 14.1). It is important to remember that this MRI appearance of denervation is highly nonspecific, having an appearance similar to a wide variety of other neurologic and orthopedic conditions described elsewhere in this book.

Ultrasound is a viable method to evaluate patients with neuropathy because it allows assessment not only of muscle size, and therefore atrophy,[12] but also of fine intramuscular structural alterations in early denervation, with fascial echoes appearing less intense than normal and denervated muscle echoes more intense than normal. In some cases with long-standing denervation, the muscle has an opaque ultrasound appearance.[13] Another advantage of this method is that, like EMG, it can detect one type of spontaneous involuntary muscle activity (i.e., fasciculations) in chronic neuropathies; the ability to evaluate deep muscle layers is an obvious ultrasound advantage over EMG, especially in obese persons.[14] In children, ultrasound is most attractive because it is a screening method that provides additional information and can be used without movement artifacts, sedation of the child, or radiation[15] (see Chapter 13).

CT has yet to be used to systematically evaluate acute denervation. As denervation ensues, however, mesenchymal alteration with progressive deposition of fat and connective tissue can be seen along the fascia and smaller muscle septae, causing the muscle to have a nonspecific "moth-eaten" appearance,[16] easily visible on MRI or CT (see below). The earliest visible CT changes (i.e., the reduction of the muscle cross-sectional area caused by inactivation atrophy, cannot be expected before 3 to 5 weeks after denervation. In fact, the volume of the muscle within fascial boundaries is preserved for long periods of time in many cases.[17] Over successive years of denervation, the density of the muscle further decreases until finally the muscle becomes completely replaced by fat and connective tissue.[18-21]

Degeneration starts distally in polyneuropathies, and later also involves proximal muscle groups. A distal-proximal gradient of degeneration may even be seen in a single muscle.[16] If the denervation is not complete, intermediate stages can be expected. With reinnervation, the muscles may gradually appear normal again.[11] In focal neuropathies, either by transection, compression, or in case of mononeuritis multiplex, pathological changes are restricted to muscles innervated by the individual nerves or spinal roots. Muscle imaging may thus help to detect anatomical variations in nerve supply.[11] In general, however, the clinical information provided by MRI, CT, and ultrasound does not allow for a specific diagnosis in patients with chronic neuropathic disorders.

Indications for Radiological Evaluation of Peripheral Neuropathy

Except in the case of pediatric patients, diagnostic imaging studies are not currently considered first-line tests in evaluating neuropathic patients. However, a variety of settings occur in which radiology can be used to provide supplementary information. These include detection of fasciculation (ultrasound only) or edema-like change as early signs of denervation; estimation of extent of muscle atrophy and fatty change; distribution of affected muscles to aid in determining cause of denervation (focal, multifocal, generalized, asymmetric, or symmetric involvement); detection of specific or focal patterns of neuropathic alterations in generalized neuropathies (e.g., nerve compression syndromes, nerve hypertrophy); noninvasive monitoring of degeneration and regeneration of muscle after transection or compression of the nerve and subsequent reinnervation; selection of muscles for biopsy; and selection of specific procedures for rehabilitation (e.g., arthrodesis, homologous muscle transplantation).[22]

Hereditary Motor and Sensory Neuropathies

HMSN are a group of diverse hereditary disorders having different genetic bases, and variable histopathological, electrophysiological, and clinical findings.[1] In HMSN, the extent and distribution of degeneration in CT or MRI and replacement of the muscle by fat and connective tissue is variable and does not strictly correlate with the duration of disease nor clinically apparent muscle atrophy. A variety of morphological alterations have been reported using imaging techniques. These include selective and generalized involvement of muscle groups with diffuse atrophy, a speckled pattern of fat infiltration, and complete fatty replacement and even true hypertrophy of distal muscle groups.[16-20,22-24] The gross structural changes of muscle in HMSN are, however, nonspecific and imaging studies do not, in general, further refine the diagnostic classification (Figures 14.1, 14.2). In some cases, however, imaging provides very important information when other treatable conditions may be present (Figures 14.3, 14.4).

Other Neuropathies

Transection of a nerve leads to denervation of the supplied muscles followed by complete degeneration and replacement of muscle tissue by fat and connective tissue.[25] This process takes months or even years (Figures 14.5, 14.6).

In contrast to the relatively uncommon occurrence of complete nerve transections, compression of nerves is a very common problem in patient groups. Etiologies include compression of the nerves as they traverse various bony and/or retinacular canals, such as in tarsal or carpal tunnel syndromes (Figure 14.4). Nerve entrapment may also develop when orthopedic trauma to adjacent tissues results in exuberant scar formation and retraction (Figure 14.7). Mass lesions, such as ganglion cysts, may cause nerve compression (see Chapter 25) and primary nerve neoplasms can clinically mimic nerve compression (Figure 14.8).

Compression of spinal nerves by ruptured intervertebral disks is a frequent indication for spinal MRI, and foraminal narrowing due to osteophytic changes of nearby bones similarly may present with nerve root lesions. Surgery itself may cause root damage neuropathy, such as in lumbar diskectomies when posterior rami are sectioned in the approach to the disk. Paraspinal muscle atrophy results in such cases and is arguably a contributor to the failed back syndrome (Figure 14.9).[26]

Metabolic etiologies for peripheral neuropathies are common, with diabetes mellitus probably the most

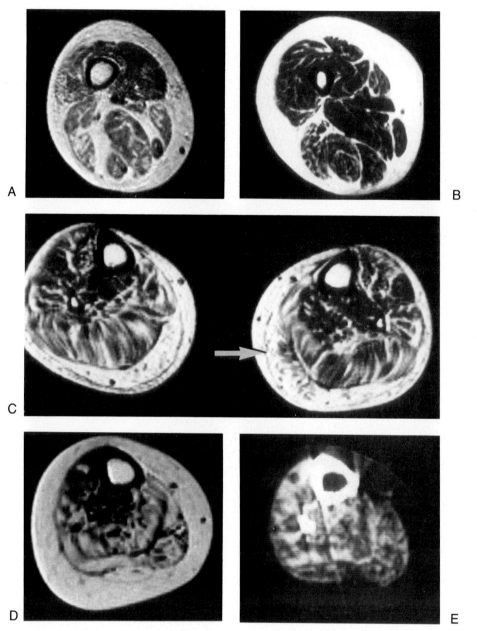

FIGURE 14.1. MRI of lower extremities in HMSN, type I. This 37-year-old woman with only mild neuropathic symptoms has marked edema-like change as a sign of subacute, active denervation. (A,B) This is manifested as abnormally increased signal intensity of multiple thigh muscles to a much greater degree on proton density-weighted image (A) than on T_1-weighted image (B). High signal intensity streaks of muscles in (B) result from the short T_1 time of deposited fat, indicating a chronic component of the denervation. More extensive degeneration with typical fatty infiltration and distribution is seen on T_1-weighted image of the legs. (C) Note particularly severe fatty replacement of the gastrocnemius muscles (arrow). Nerve conduction study of the legs revealed that no compound muscle action potential could be elicited. Histology of the sural nerve revealed severe combined demyelinating neuropathy with axonal degeneration. The patient's son, who had walking problems since age 4, developed an equinus foot deformity. Conduction velocity of the son's right tibial nerve was reduced, as was the compound muscle action potential amplitude. (D,E) The distribution and degree of muscle degeneration in his legs, as determined by T_1-weighted MRI (D) and CT (E), is comparable to his mother, despite the much shorter duration of disease.

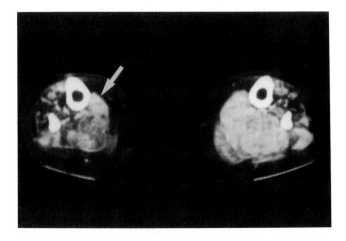

FIGURE 14.2. CT of inactivity as a synergistic cause of muscle atrophy in a patient with chronic neuropathy from infancy. Note that although the left anterior compartment appears severely degenerated, other muscles are relatively preserved. Muscles of the right leg are nearly completely degenerated with the exception of the flexor digitorum longus muscle which appears normal (arrow). Although the patient had arthrodesis of her right ankle years ago (because of foot-drop) this muscle was still functionally intact because the toes were not held rigid by the procedure. Degeneration of the other right-sided muscles, although doubtlessly caused by neuropathy, was apparently augmented by inactivation following fixation.

frequent cause of metabolic neuropathy. In chronic diabetes, muscle atrophy is usually symmetric on MRI.[19,21] Distal muscle groups are more severely involved (Figure 14.10).

In patients with chronic radiculopathy or spinal muscular atrophy, lesions are not always associated with muscle atrophy. Rarely, hypertrophy occurs in the affected muscles, most frequently of the calf. Most of the patients with this unusual clinical finding had an operation for disk prolapse in the past. Muscle hypertrophy with enlargement of the calf muscles is followed by degeneration with replacement by fat and connective tissue during the chronic denervation. Thus, hypertrophic, pseudohypertrophic, and atrophic muscles can appear in parallel, so imaging is helpful for further differentiation.[27–31] Serial imaging supplements the clinical follow-up and can be used to distinguish the relative distribution of muscle hypertrophy, pseudohypertrophy, and atrophy over the years (Figure 14.11).

GBS and CIDP are typical inflammatory demyelinating neuropathies. Although the pathogenesis appears to be different, the primary characteristic in both disorders is demyelination of the spinal roots, and peripheral and cranial nerves. GBS and CIDP are disorders with a potentially severe clinical course. Rodiek described complete replacement by fat and connective tissue of lower leg muscles in an 84-year-old GBS patient.[21]

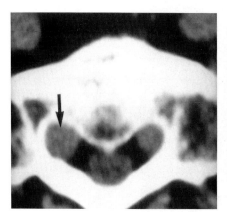

A

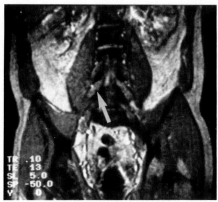

B

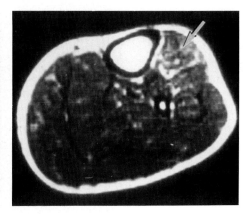

C

FIGURE 14.3. HMSN, type I: CT and MRI findings. Clinical findings included pes cavus, atrophic extremities, thickened nerves, mild sensory disturbance in a sock-like distribution, diminished tendon reflexes, severely reduced motor nerve conduction, and unobtainable sensory nerve action potentials. The family history was positive for similar findings in a sister, nephew, and son. (A) CT of the lumbar spine, performed because of low back pain, shows prominent nerve roots (arrow) but no disk protrusion. (B) Coronal T_1-weighted gradient echo image confirms the presence of hypertrophic nerve roots (arrow). (C) T_1-weighted MRI of the lower leg shows only mild diffuse fatty infiltration in the tibialis anterior muscle (arrow). Whether this change is due to the primary neuropathy or to a superimposed L5 radiculopathy by imbalance of the sizes of hypertrophic nerve root and foramen is unknown. Sural nerve biopsy showed thickened nerve fibers and onion bulb formation with signs of chronic de- and remyelination, thus supporting the clinical diagnosis of HMSN, type I.

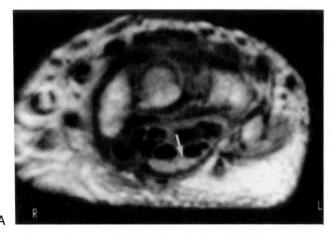
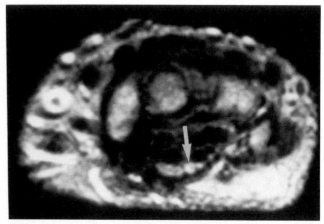

FIGURE 14.4. Role of imaging in clinical problem solving: distinguishing between possible diagnoses. If a patient is suffering from a known neuropathy and, in addition, has typical clinical signs of another condition, such as a nerve entrapment, electrophysiology alone may give equivocal findings because focal reduction of the nerve conduction velocity may be caused either by the hereditary neuropathy or nerve entrapment. This patient presented with HMSN 1 and signs suggesting carpal tunnel syndrome. First (A) and second (B) echoes of a long TR sequence reveal focal edema and swelling of the median nerve (arrow) in the carpal tunnel. This proved to be due to physical entrapment in the carpal tunnel syndrome as an additional and treatable cause for clinical symptoms in the neuropathic patient.

However, the more usual course of GBS is that of acute demyelination, followed soon thereafter by remyelination. Therefore, structural changes with irreversible replacement of muscle tissue usually do not occur. Visible atrophy may be caused by inactivity alone. In the acute phase, MRI examination may be contraindicated in patients with severe GBS because of the necessity of a temporary pacemaker (Figure 14.12).

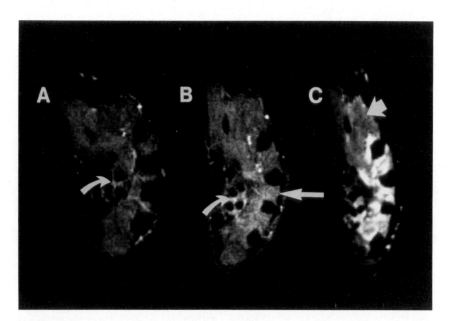

FIGURE 14.5. Denervation following high ulnar nerve transection. (A) Twenty-four days after the injury, STIR image shows edema-like increase of signal intensity in the ulnar-innervated lumbricales (curved arrow). (B) Fourteen days later, signal intensity is further increased within ulnar lumbricales (curved arrow) and progressive changes of interosseous muscles are noted (arrow). (C) Signal intensity changes are much more prominent after an additional 37 days when atrophy of muscles is also prominent. The case is typical of ulnar nerve transections in that muscles are differentially affected. Note apparent sparing of the first dorsal interosseous (arrowhead), which was denervated by EMG criteria.

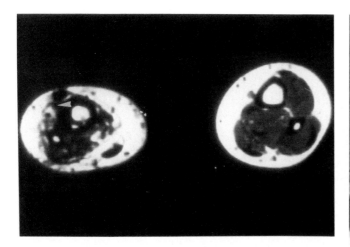

FIGURE 14.6. MRI of remote nerve transection: reinnervation. Complete denervation of the right lower leg muscles resulted from trauma 4 years before imaging was performed. At the time of MRI, reinnervation was found on EMG in the posterior muscles and the tibialis anterior muscle was electrically inactive. T_1-weighted MRI reveals the denervated tibialis anterior muscle to be completely degenerated (arrowhead). The reinnervated posterior muscles are atrophic but were normal in signal intensity on all sequences, indicating at least partial regeneration.

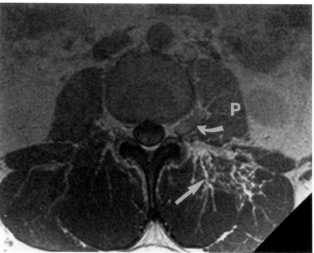

FIGURE 14.8. Paraspinal muscle atrophy as a clue to neoplastic neuropathy. Axial postgadolinium T_1-weighted lumbar spine MRI shows left-sided atrophy and streaky fatty change of iliocostalis (arrow) in a patient with back pain as the reason for the scan. Minimal streaky changes are also present in the left psoas (P). A fusiform, focal mass lesion is noted exiting the neural foramen (curved arrow), which subsequently was proved to be a neurofibroma.

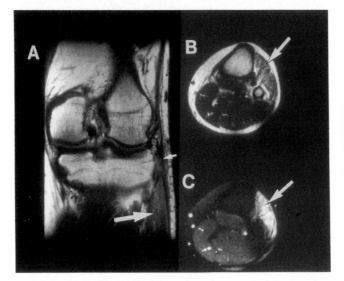

FIGURE 14.7. Edema-like change of muscle denervated due to nerve compression. Following a skiing injury and tearing of the lateral collateral ligament, this patient developed foot-drop. (A) Coronal T_1-weighted MRI of knee shows fibrous thickening of lateral collateral ligament (i.e., scar) in location of peroneal nerve (short arrow). Peroneal muscles are normal in signal (long arrow), indicating lack of fatty change. (B) Axial T_2-weighted image shows increased signal intensity, indicating edema-like change (arrow). (C) Axial fat-suppressed STIR sequence shows the edema-like change much more conspicuously (arrow).

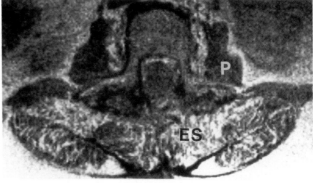

FIGURE 14.9. Iatrogenic peripheral neuropathy. Postoperative paraspinal muscle atrophy is usually unilateral at, and inferior to, the level of disk operated on due to transection of branches of posterior spinal rami. Axial T_1-weighted lumbar spine MRI shows bilateral atrophy of erector spinae (ES) in a patient who had undergone multilevel bilateral laminectomies. Streaky fatty infiltration is visible as high signal intensity material infiltrating the erector spinae. Note that the psoas muscles (P) are unremarkable. Although associated with the "failed back syndrome," a causal role of such atrophy has not been proved.[26]

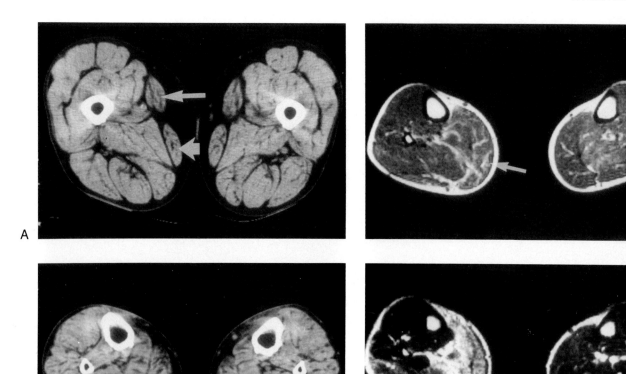

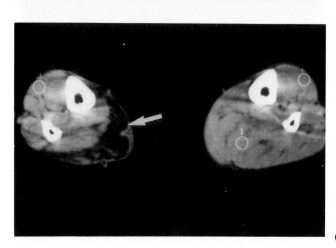

FIGURE 14.10. Polyneuropathy as a complication of long-lasting diabetes mellitus. In the late course of disease, muscles may have a "marbled" appearance as fatty tissue replaces muscle. (A) Transverse image of thighs shows slightly greater involvement of sartorius (arrow) and gracilis (arrowhead). (B) Streaks of fat that parallel the muscular septae are particularly visible in the lower legs, especially the lateral head of the gastrocnemius (arrow).

CIDP patients carry the risk of a long-lasting disease with muscle weakness and sensory disturbances. The structural muscle changes as shown by imaging are comparable to other long-lasting chronic neuropathies (Figure 14.13).

Motor Neuron Disease: Postpoliomyelitis Syndrome

Acute poliomyelitis induces destruction of anterior horn cells leading to perikaryal degeneration and subsequent neuronal loss. Nerve conduction velocity can be normal for long periods of time whereas the CMAP is significantly reduced. This reflects the clinical finding of muscle atrophy with widespread denervation on the

FIGURE 14.11. Increased limb size after lumbar disk rupture. The patient was operated in 1974 and 1983 for herniated lumbar disk, but was never free of symptoms (pain, muscle cramps, sensory disturbance). (A) T_1-weighted MRI, performed in 1987, shows pseudohypertrophy, characterized by increased girth on the right and diffuse, mild fatty infiltration posteromedially (arrow). (B) Marked coexistent edema-like change is visible on the proton density weighted image in the medial portions of the gastrocnemius and soleus muscles (arrow). (C) Progressive atrophy and fatty replacement developed, as demonstrated on CT scan (arrow).

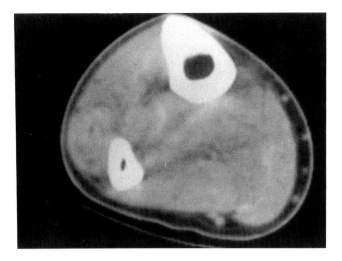

FIGURE 14.12. CT of Guillain-Barré-Strohl syndrome. This patient experienced acute, quadriplegia and required 10 weeks of mechanical ventilation. At the time of CT examination, clinical symptoms were already remitting. Only subtle effacement of muscle septae can be seen, with no replacement or infiltration by fat, edema, or connective tissue.

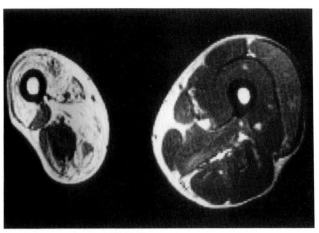

FIGURE 14.14. MRI of postpoliomyelitis syndrome. A typical attack of poliomyelitis occurred at the age of 2 years with subsequent atrophy of the right leg. At age 40, the patient recognized increasing weakness in the left leg, which was ascribed to postpoliomyelitis syndrome. T_1-weighted MRI shows a typical appearance of muscles in polio survivors, characterized by highly asymmetrical fatty infiltration, atrophy, and hypertrophy, reflecting the apparent randomness of attack of anterior horn cells by the polio virus.

electromyogram and no sensory deficits. After a clinically quiescent period of 15 to 30 years, some patients develop a secondary progressive amyotrophy, called postpoliomyelitis syndrome. The reason for this may be the failure of motor neurons to maintain their enlarged territory; a late autoimmune reaction may also contribute.[32–37]

Typical radiological findings of muscle are asymmetric focal muscle atrophy, partial or complete fatty degeneration of single muscles, and hypertrophy of apparently uninvolved muscles (Figure 14.14).[22,25] MRI may sometimes also show edema-like changes, which could be

interpreted either as a sign of recent denervation correlating with the postpoliomyelitis syndrome or due to edema from muscle damage related to overexertion.[10]

Conclusions

Radiological tests of muscle in neuropathies and motor neuron disease are helpful for characterizing pathological

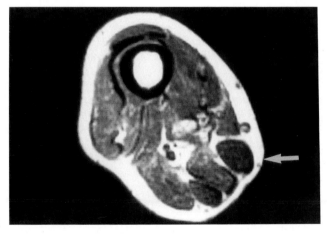

A

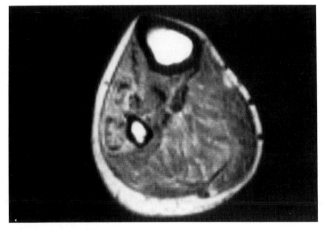

B

FIGURE 14.13. MRI of chronic inflammatory demyelinating polyneuropathy (CIDP). The patient suffered for nearly 3 years from CIDP uninfluenced by an intensive therapeutic regimen. (A) T_1-weighted thigh MRI shows mild muscle atrophy and speckled fatty infiltration, a sign typical of chronic disease. Note peculiar sparing of the gracilis (arrow). Calf muscles were more severely involved, diffusely although heterogeneously (B).

changes, defining distributions of abnormalities, and monitoring progression of disease. Imaging is sensitive, but findings are generally nonspecific and frequently do not allow specific diagnoses. Therefore, it is generally not possible to subclassify neuropathies by MRI, CT, or ultrasound imaging. In summary, radiological tests of muscle in neuropathic patients are complementary to detailed clinical evaluation.

References

1. Dyck PJ, Thomas PK, Griffin JW, eds. Peripheral neuropathy, 3rd ed. Philadelphia: W.B. Saunders Company, 1993.
2. Ashbury AK, Bird SJ. Disorders of peripheral nerve. In: Asbury AK, McKhann GM, McDonald WI, eds. Diseases of the nervous system. Clinical neurobiology. vol. 1. Philadelphia: W.B. Saunders Company, 1992:252–269.
3. Griffin W, Cornblath DR. Diseases of the peripheral nervous system. In: Rosenberg RN, ed. Comprehensive neurology. New York: Raven Press, 1991:421–450.
4. Said G, Thomas PK. Pathophysiology of nerve and root disorders. In: Asbury AK, McKhann GM, McDonald WI, eds. Diseases of the nervous system. Clinical neurobiology. vol. 1. Philadelphia: W.B. Saunders, 1992:241–251.
5. Cha CH, Patten BM. Amyotrophic lateral sclerosis: abnormalities of the tongue on magnetic resonance imaging. Ann Neurol 1989;25:468–472.
6. Banker BQ, Engel AG. Basic reaction of muscle. In: Engel AG, Banker BQ, eds. Myology. vol. 1. New York: McGraw Hill, 1986:845–907.
7. Donofrio PD, Albers JW, AAEM Minimonograph # 34: Polyneuropathy: classification by nerve conduction studies and electromyography. Muscle Nerve 1990;13:889–903.
8. Shabas D, Gerard G, Rossi D. Magnetic resonance imaging examination of denervated muscle. Comput Radiol 1987;11:9–13.
9. Polak JF, Jolesz FA, Adams DF. Magnetic resonance imaging of skeletal muscle, prolongation of T_1 and T_2 subsequent to denervation. Invest Radiol 1988;23:365–369.
10. Fleckenstein JL, Weatherall PT, Bertocci LA, et al. Locomotor system assessment by muscle magnetic resonance imaging. Magn Reson Q 1991;7:79–103.
11. Fleckenstein JL, Watumull D, Connor KE, et al. Denervated human skeletal muscle: MR imaging evaluation. Radiology 1993;187:213–218.
12. Boonstra AM, van Weerden TW, te Strake L, Hillen B. Ultrasonography of the peroneal nerve muscle group in normal subjects and patients with peroneal paresis. J Clin Ultrasound 1988;16:17–24.
13. Gunreben G, Bogdahn U. Real-time sonography of acute and chronic muscle denervation. Muscle Nerve 1991;14:654–664.
14. Reimers CD, Naegele M, Fenzl G, et al. Comparative study of ultrasound, MRI, CT, and myopathological findings in generalized neuromuscular diseases. In: Nadjmi M, ed. Imaging of brain metabolism, spine and cord, interventional neuroradiology. Berlin: Springer, 1989:627–630.
15. Heckmatt JZ, Dubowitz V. Real time ultrasound imaging of muscles. Muscle Nerve 1988;11:56–65.
16. Hawley RJ, Schellinger D, O'Doherty DS. Computed tomographic patterns of muscles in neuromuscular diseases. Arch Neurol 1984;41:383–387.
17. Nordal HJ, Dieterichson P, Eldevik P, Gronseth K. Fat infiltration, atrophy and hypertrophy of skeletal muscles demonstrated by X-ray computed tomography in neurological patients. Acta Neurol Scand 1985;77:115–122.
18. Kaiser W, Schalke BCG. Kernspintomographie bei generalisierten Skelettmuskelerkrankungen. Röntgenpraxis 1989;42:338–345.
19. Bulcke JAL, Baert AL. Clinical and radiological aspects of myopathies. Berlin: Springer, 1982.
20. Kaiser W, Schalke BCG, Rohkamm R. Kernspintomographie in der Diagnostik von Muskelerkrankungen. Fortschr Röntgenstr 1986;145:199–209.
21. Rodiek SO. CT, MR-Tomographie und MR-Spektroskopie bei neuromuskulären Erkrankunge. Stuttgart: F. Enke, 1987.
22. Kaiser WA, Schalke BCG. Kernspintomographie bei generalisierten Skelettmuskelerkrankungen. Untersuchungsmodalitäten und Indikationsempfehlungen. Röntgenpraxis 1989;42:338–345.
23. Pongratz DE, Reimers CD, Hahn D, Nägele M, Müller-Felber W. Atlas der Muskelkrankheiten. München: Urban-Schwarzenberg, 1990:163–172.
24. Visser de M, Hoogendijk JE, Ongerboor de Visser BW, Verbeeten BJ. Calf enlargement in hereditary motor and sensory neuropathy. Muscle Nerve 1990;13:40–46.
25. Rodiek, SO. Kernspintomographie der Skelettmuskulatur bei neuromuskulären Erkrankungen. Fortschr Röntgenstr 1985;143:418–425.
26. Laasonen EM. Atrophy of sacrospinal muscle groups in patients with chronic, diffusely radiating lumbar back pain. Neuroradiology 1984;26:9–13.
27. Mielke U, Ricker K, Emser W, Boxler K. Unilateral calf enlargement following S1 radiculopathy. Muscle Nerve 1982;5:434–438.
28. Visser de M, Verbeeten B, Lyppens KCH. Pseudohypertrophy of the calf following S1 radiculopathy. Neuroradiology 1986;28:279–280.
29. Ricker K, Rohkamm R, Moxley RT. Hypertrophy of the calf with S1 radiculopathy. Arch Neurol 1988;45:660–664.
30. Bernat JL, Ochoa JL. Muscle hypertrophy after partial denervation: a human case. J Neurol Neurosurg Psychiatr 1978;41:719–725.
31. Pareyson D, Morandi L, Scaioli V, Marazzi R, Boiardi A, Sghirlanzoni A. Neurogenic muscle hypertrophy. J Neurol 1989;236:292–295.
32. Mulder DW. Motor neuron disease in adults. In: Engel AG, Banker BQ, eds. Myology. vol. 2. New York: McGraw Hill, 1986:2013–2030.
33. Wiechers DO, Hubbel SL. Late changes in the motor unit after acute poliomyelitis. Muscle Nerve 1981;4:524–528.
34. Dalakas MC. New neuromuscular symptoms in patients with old poliomyelitis: a three year follow-up study. Eur Neurol 1986;25:381–387.

35. Sharief MK, Hentges R, Ciardi M. Intrathecal immune response in patients with post-polio syndrome. N Engl J Med 1991;325:749–755.

36. Bertorini TE, Igarashi M. Post poliomyelitis muscle pseudohypertrophy. Muscle Nerve 1985;8:644–649.

37. Pongratz DE, Reimers CD, Hahn D, Nägele M, Müller-Felber W. Atlas der Muskelkrankheiten. München: Urban-Schwarzenberg, 1990:180–184.

15
Disorders of the Neuromuscular Junction

Berthold C.G. Schalke, Erich Hofmann, and Werner Kaiser

Myasthenia gravis, Lambert-Eaton myasthenic syndrome, and congenital myasthenic syndromes are diseases of the neuromuscular junction. They are characterized by fatiguability on exertion, fluctuating weakness of voluntary muscles, and spontaneous improvement at rest.

Myasthenia Gravis

In acquired myasthenia gravis (MG), autoimmune antibodies directed against the postsynaptic nicotinic acetylcholine receptor (AChR) cause damage to the AChR by complement fixation, activation of the lytic phase, and modulation of AChR turnover by cross-linking or direct blocking of the receptor.[1] The diagnosis is firmly established by a typical history (weakness upon exertion and spontaneous improvement at rest), a positive reaction to anticholinesterase drugs [e.g., edrophonium (Tensilon) or pyridostigmine (Mestinon)], a decremental EMG response on repetitive nerve stimulation, and a positive test for AChR-specific autoantibodies in the patient's serum.

The pathogenesis of MG is incompletely understood but the thymus plays a key role. Approximately 15% of MG cases are a paraneoplastic syndrome, associated with thymomas; in 60% to 70% of patients under the age of 40 thymic lymphoid follicular hyperplasia is the predominant histological finding in the thymus.[2] The treatment of MG may be surgical (i.e., thymectomy or thymomectomy) or medical (e.g., removal of autoantibodies by plasmapheresis or immunadsorption) and/or immunosuppressive drugs such as azathioprine, corticosteroids, cyclosporin A, cyclophosphamide, and immunoglobulins; symptomatic relief employs cholinesterase inhibitors like pyridostigmine.[3]

In only 5% to 10% of chronic MG patients is muscle atrophy present.[4,5] Usually this atrophy is focal but can be found in any voluntary muscle. The extent of atrophy does not correlate with duration or severity of myasthenic symptoms. Muscle atrophy is usually associated with long-standing disease and ineffective immunosuppressive therapy. The electromyogram often is normal. Only in severe cases are typical myopathic or neuropathic changes found. Muscle biopsy is not usually performed but when done in these cases may identify additional diseases known to cause muscle atrophy, and with which MG may overlap, including connective tissue diseases and polymyositis.[1] In the absence of associated diseases, nonspecific neurogenic changes may be seen, such as fiber type grouping and type II fiber atrophy.

Diagnostic imaging studies of MG are few. Bulcke and Baert described a nonspecific "marble-like" linear pattern of fatty change of CT imaging, a pattern they also observed in some cases of polymyositis.[6] In our studies of MG, changes of muscle are minimal on imaging studies, regardless of the technique. When changes are seen, however, we too have found diffuse "marble-like" fatty changes (Figure 15.1). Although no rigorous study has been done, there is no definite difference in findings between MRI and CT imaging, in our experience. On occasion, however, markedly abnormal fatty changes may be seen (Figure 15.2).

Lambert-Eaton Myasthenic Syndrome

Lambert-Eaton myasthenic syndrome (LEMS) refers to a myasthenic syndrome that classically accompanies carcinoma, although other autoimmune diseases may be associated with LEMS including polyneuritis, cerebellar degeneration, and polymyositis. About 60% to 70% of LEMS cases are associated with small-cell lung cancer. LEMS can precede the tumor by years. Clinical signs include weakness of the neck flexors, limbs, and extraocular muscles. Tendon reflexes may be absent initially but are typically present on repeated testing or after a short contraction of the muscle. Weakness also transi-

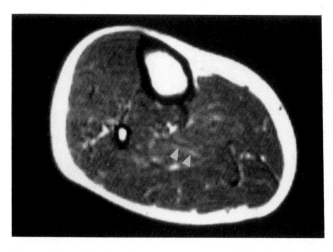

FIGURE 15.1. Myasthenia gravis: typical findings. T_1-weighted MRI of leg muscles of a myasthenia gravis patient with chronic, untreated disease. The nearly normal appearance of the muscles contrasts the marked clinical findings. Only minimal, questionable "marbling" is seen (arrows).

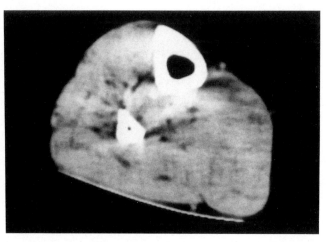

FIGURE 15.3. Lambert-Eaton myasthenic syndrome: Typical CT findings. CT image of the leg muscles shows minimal, questionable hypodensities.

ently improves after maximal muscle contraction. Autonomic symptoms such as dry mouth, obstipation, and sexual impotence are frequently pesent.

The diagnosis is established by an incremental response on repetitive nerve stimulation at high frequencies, and an increase of the initial compound muscle action potential in the EMG after maximal voluntary muscle activation.[7] In LEMS, autoantibodies are

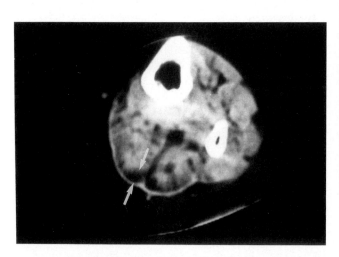

FIGURE 15.2. Myasthenia gravis: uncommon findings. CT shows atrophy and fatty infiltration in left leg muscles of patient with long-standing myasthenia gravis and ineffective therapy. Note relatively severe soleus deterioration that is worst along the fascia (between arrows).

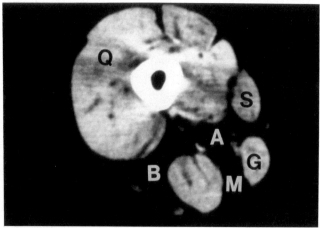

FIGURE 15.4. Lambert-Eaton myasthenic syndrome: unusual findings. CT image of the thigh in a patient with a chronic, untreated, LEMS, not associated with neoplasm. The quadriceps (Q), semitendinosus, sartorius (S), and gracilis (G) are relatively normal. The adductor magnus (A), semimembranosus (M) and biceps femoris muscle (long head) (B) are completely replaced by fat.

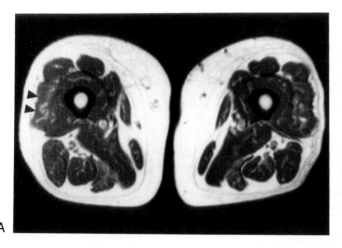

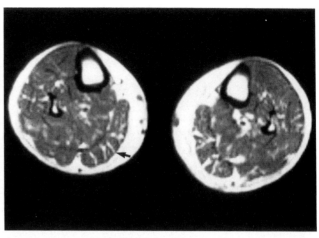

A   B

FIGURE 15.5. Lambert-Eaton myasthenic syndrome: MR findings. T_1-weighted MRI of LEMS in a patient with small-cell lung cancer. Note mild atrophy in thigh, particularly of the vastus lateralis (arrows, A). Diffuse marble-like fatty infiltration is visible, especially in the gastrocnemii of the legs (e.g., arrow, B). The pattern of abnormality is indistinguishable from that in chronic neuropathy.

directed against presynaptic structures, mainly the voltage-gated calcium channel (VGCC), which can be detected by radioimmunoassay.[8]

Symptomatic treatment of muscle weakness is possible with 3,4-diaminopyridine (3,4-DAP), which increases calcium release, and pyridostigmine.[9] Plasma exchange and immunosuppressive corticosteroids, and in non-tumor cases with azathioprine, improves the clinical condition, although often less effectively than in MG. In tumor cases, long-term prognosis is limited by the low survival rate in lung cancer patients.[10]

Muscle morphology in LEMS, as in MG, is frequently only mildly abnormal. Muscle biopsy reportedly shows nonspecific type II fiber atrophy.[11] We had the chance to examine three patients with CT or MRI. On CT, muscle parenchyma appeared minimally "motheaten" with diffuse hypodensities (Figure 15.3), comparable to patients with MG or chronic polyneuropathy. In one chronic case without an associated neoplasm, the adductor magnus, biceps femoris, and semimembranosus were partly replaced by fat whereas the volume of the replaced muscle was normal (Figure 15.4). MRI features of LEMS patients are indistinguishable from patients with chronic neuropathy (Figure 15.5, see Chapter 14).

Congenital Myasthenic Syndromes

Congenital Myasthenic syndromes (CMS) are a group of different hereditary disorders, affecting the neuromuscular junction. Interestingly, up to 12 different subtypes of this rare condition, including both pre- and postsynaptic defects, have been described.[11] All types are negative for autoantibodies against the AChR or VGCC. Unlike MG or LEMS, the various CMS disorders have been associated with diverse findings on muscle histopathology.[11] Some patients respond to treatment with pyridostigmine, 3,4-DAP, or even corticosteroids. Exact subclassification requires special laboratories.

Atrophy in the affected muscles is a frequent finding. CT images of the leg muscles of a patient with CMS do not differ from patients with acquired MG; eye muscles are usually atrophic (Figure 15.6).

Conclusions

MG, LEMS, and CMS are disorders of the neuromuscular junction, usually without structural defects in the affected muscles. In 5% to 10% of MG patients, and in an unknown percentage of LEMS and CMS patients with long duration of symptoms, muscle atrophy may develop. In these cases, it may be helpful to use CT or MRI to distinguish between a partly reversible atrophy, in which an edema-like appearance of muscle is noted, and an irreversible replacement of muscle tissue by fat and connective tissue, which will not respond favorably to therapy. However, imaging findings are nonspecific and do not allow a distinction from other muscle disorders, particularly polyneuropathies.

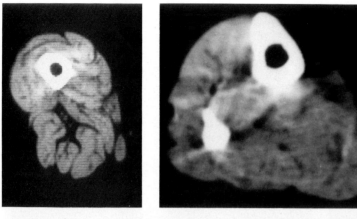

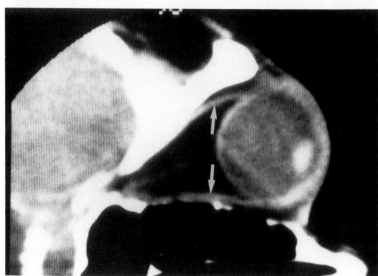

FIGURE 15.6. Congenital myasthenic syndrome: CT findings. CT of the thigh (A) and leg (B) show diffuse atrophy and hypodensity involving all muscles, although posterior involvement is more severe in the leg. Note atrophic extraocular muscles on sagittal orbital CT scan (arrow, C).

References

1. Engel AG. Acquired autoimmune myasthenia gravis. In: Engel AG, Franzini-Armstrong C, eds. Myology. New York: McGraw-Hill Inc., 1994:1769–1797.

2. Kirchner TS, Tzartos S, Hoppe F, Schalke B, Wekerle H, Müller-Hermelink HK. Myasthenia gravis: acetylcholine receptor related antigenic determinants in tumor free thymuses and thymic epithelial tumors. Am J Pathol 1988;130:268.

3. Toyka KV. Myasthenia gravis. In: Johnson RT, ed. Current therapy in neurologic diseases. Philadelphia: Decker, 1990:385.

4. Oosterhuis HJGH. Clinical aspects. In: Baets, de MH, Oosterhuis HJGH, eds. Myasthenia gravis. Boca Raton: CRC Press, 1993:13–42.

5. Schimrigk K, Samland O. Neurogene Muskelatrophien bei Myasthenie. In: Hertel G, Mertens HG, Ricker K, Schimrigk K, eds. Myasthenia gravis und andere störungen der neuromuskulären synapse. Stuttgart: G. Thieme Verlag, 1977.

6. Bulcke JAL, Baert AL. Clinical and radiological aspects of myopathies. Berlin: Springer-Verlag, 1982.

7. O'Neill JH, Murray NM, Newson-Davis J. The Lambert-Eaton myasthenic syndrome: a review of 50 cases. Brain 1988;111:577.

8. Lennon VA, Lambert EH. Antibodies bind solubilized calcium channel-omega conotoxin complexes from small cell lung carcinoma: a diagnostic aid for Lambert-Eaton myasthenic syndrome. Mayo Clin Proc 1989;64:1498.

9. McEvoy KM, Windebank AJ, Daube JR, Low PA. 3,4 Diaminopyridine in the treatment of Lambert-Eaton myasthenic syndrome. N Engl J Med 1989;321:1567.

10. Newsom-Davis J, Murray NMF. Plasma exchange and immunosuppressive drug treatment in Lambert-Eaton myasthenic syndrome. Neurology 1984;34:480.

11. Engel AG. Myasthenic syndrome. In: Engel AG, Franzini-Armstrong C, eds. Myology. New York: McGraw-Hill Inc., 1994:1798–1835.

16
Muscular Dystrophies

Marianne de Visser, Berthold C.G. Schalke, and Carl D. Reimers

Muscular dystrophies are a group of inherited disorders characterized by progressive muscle wasting and weakness, in which muscle histopathology shows certain distinctive features (muscle fiber necrosis, phagocytosis, etc.) and where there is no clinical or laboratory evidence of spinal cord or peripheral nervous system involvement or myotonia.[1] This broad definition includes disorders that are heterogeneous with regard to clinical appearance and mode of inheritance (Table 16.1).

Duchenne Muscular Dystrophy

Duchenne muscular dystrophy (DMD) is an X-linked recessive disorder that results from an "out-of-frame" mutation of a gene located in Xp21.[2] The protein product of this gene, dystrophin, which is localized in the cytoplasmic face of the plasma membrane of muscle fibers, is virtually absent or nonfunctional in DMD.[3]

The proximal muscles of the lower limbs are among the first to be affected. Weakness of the hip and knee extensors results in the so-called Gowers' maneuver. The onset of weakness usually dates to the time of beginning to walk, which is often delayed. Subsequently, proximal muscles of the upper limbs and distal muscles become involved. Calf hypertrophy is often present (Figure 16.1). Around the age of 12 or 13, most boys lose the ability to walk. They usually become respirator-dependent before age 20. Respiratory insufficiency or cardiac failure are the main causes of death.[4]

Muscle pathology includes increased variability of fiber size, foci of necrosis and regeneration, hyaline fibers, and increased endomysial connective and fatty tissue.[5] Diagnosis is based on the clinical picture, a more than 10-fold increase in serum creatine kinase (CK) activity, the above-described alterations in muscle, paucity, or absence of dystrophin, and a frameshift deletion within the dystrophin gene.[6]

Ultrasonography

Ultrasound usually does not detect abnormalities in preclinical[7,8] or even early clinical stages. However, increased echointensities are seen in limb muscles as the disease progresses.[7–12] Echointensities subsequently decrease again when the muscle is completely replaced by fat.[10] In advanced cases, fascia and bone echoes become obscured as the muscle atrophies.[9–11]

Involvement of muscles is frequently not uniform in DMD, a finding supported by ultrasound studies. For example, echointensities are usually higher in gastrocnemius muscles compared to soleus muscles, and hypertrophy of the sartorius muscle can easily be demonstrated[12,13] (Figure 16.2).

Computed Tomography

Computed tomography (CT) has been used to monitor the progression of muscle damage in DMD.[14,15] This method, which quantifies the degree of muscle fiber loss and fat tissue replacement, disclosed a characteristic pattern of involvement. In the early stages, the gluteus maximus and medius, tensor fasciae latae, biceps femoris, adductors, quadriceps femoris, peroneals, and gastrocnemius muscles become infiltrated with fat, manifested on CT by areas of decreased attenuation[15] (Figure 16.3). This fat deposition may increase the girth of the legs prominently (pseudohypertrophy).[16,17] Subsequently, the iliopsoas, quadratus lumborum, paravertebral, semitendinosus, semimembranosus, and tibialis anterior muscles become affected.[15] Degeneration of the lateral portion of the paraspinal muscles is more prominent than the medial portion.[18–21] Loss of muscle and replacement by fat is greater on the concave side of the spinal curvature and at the middle lumbar level.[18,19] The rectus abdominis, internal and external obliques, sartorius, gracilis, and tibialis posterior muscles are relatively preserved until the patients become wheel-

TABLE 16.1. Muscular dystrophies.

Dystrophinopathies
   Duchenne muscular dystrophy
   Becker muscular dystrophy
   Carriers of abnormal dystrophin genes
Limb girdle muscular dystrophy
Emery-Dreifuss muscular dystrophy
Congenital muscular dystrophy
Facioscapulohumeral muscular dystrophy
Distal muscular dystrophy
Oculopharyngeal muscular dystrophy

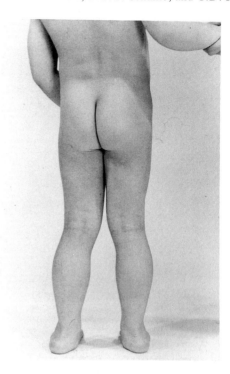

FIGURE 16.1. Enlarged calves of a 3-year-old boy with Duchenne muscular dystrophy.

chair-bound.[15] Preserved synergistic muscles such as the gracilis, sartorius, and semitendinosus may become hypertrophic as if to compensate for the weakened muscles[9,14,22–24] (Figure 16.3). It should be noted, however, that the cause for the selectivity has not been proved. All of these findings are more or less in keeping with studies performed by others.[14,20,22–26] In two studies a significant correlation between CT markers of muscle damage and muscle strength was found.[14,15]

Magnetic Resonance Imaging

In early stages, skeletal muscle degeneration and regeneration result in long T_1 times in the thighs[27] and slightly decreased T_1 times in the calf muscles.[28] With disease progression, T_1 values rapidly decrease due to replacement of muscle by fat.[27–29] In advanced lipomatosis, increased signal intensity is visible on both T_1- and T_2-weighted images in a distribution similar to that reported on CT scans[9,30–33] (Figure 16.4). Asymmetric involvement of the thigh muscles is not unusual.[30,32] As on CT, selective preservation of the gracilis, sartorius,

semitendinosus, and semimembranosus, and true hypertrophy of the gracilis is seen.[30]

MR images of DMD patients also showed that muscles have a longitudinally streaky appearance in a direction parallel to the myofibers, which is more prominent near the myotendinous junction compared to the muscle bellies.[28,34] Other segmental involvement of muscle is also clearly demonstrated by longitudinal MR imaging.[30]

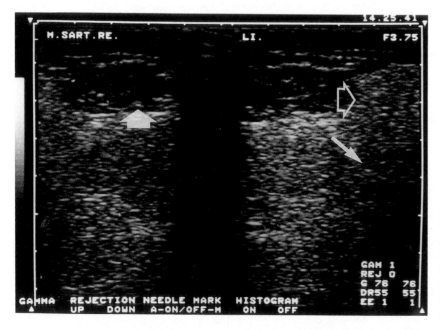

FIGURE 16.2. Duchenne muscular dystrophy: ultrasound findings. Transverse scans of the thighs reveal hypertrophy of the sartorius (arrowhead points to right sartorius). Note that hyperechoic changes of the vastus medialis (open arrowhead) cause poor definition of femur echoes (arrow).

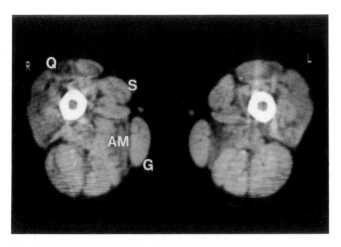

FIGURE 16.3. Duchenne muscular dystrophy: CT findings. Note decreased attenuation, indicating fatty change of the quadriceps femoris (Q) and adductor magnus (AM) muscles. The sartorius (S) and gracilis (G) muscles are hypertrophic.

Although a significant correlation was found between MR data and patients' functional status, age, and disease duration, one study revealed that in half of patients, MRI showed progressive subclinical muscle degeneration.[30] Skeletal muscle degeneration progresses rapidly between 7 and 10 years of age, and then reaches a plateau.[34]

Becker Muscular Dystrophy

Becker muscular dystrophy (BMD) and DMD are both allelic. BMD results from in-frame mutations at Xp21, resulting in an abnormal, partially functional dystro-

phin.[2,35] The clinical picture is quite variable, even within families. At one end of the spectrum there is a distribution of weakness similar to that seen in DMD, although not as rapidly progressive. At the other end of the spectrum, there are patients in whom muscle cramps, calf hypertrophy (Figure 16.5), or congestive cardiomyopathy are the only manifestations of the disease.[36,37]

Histopathological examination of muscle reveals an abnormal variation in diameter of the muscle fibers (single or small groups of atrophic fibers and hypertrophic fibers are scattered throughout the muscle biopsy specimen), foci of regenerating fibers, the occasional necrotic fiber, and an increase in endomysial and fatty tissue.[5] Diagnosis is made on the basis of the clinical and pathological findings in combination with a more than fivefold increase of serum CK activity, rearrangements within the dystrophin gene (usually in-frame deletions), or dystrophin of abnormal size and/or reduced abundance.[6]

Ultrasonography

The findings are similar to those found in DMD (Figure 16.6), although less severe.[13] In the early stages, true hypertrophy of the calf muscles can be confirmed, whereas later pseudohypertrophy occurs.[13]

Computed Tomography

The results of CT studies in BMD resemble those in DMD.[23,26,38–41] Selective involvement of muscles with relative preservation and even hypertrophy of the sartorius, gracilis, adductor longus, semitendinosus, or semimembranosus occurs in BMD[23,26,33,38–41] (Figure

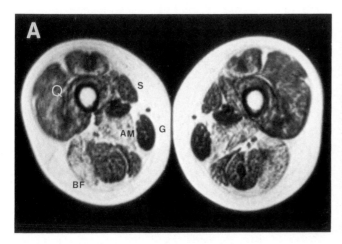

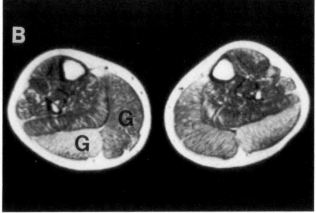

FIGURE 16.4. Duchenne muscular dystrophy: typical degeneration of thigh muscle tissue on MRI. (A) T_1-weighted appearance (T_R 500 ms/T_E 17 ms) of the thighs shows marked fatty deterioration of the adductor magnus (AM) and long head of the biceps femoris (BF), whereas the quadriceps (Q) is less

degenerated. The sartorius (S) and gracilis (G) muscles are preserved, and the latter even has a hypertrophic appearance. (B) T_1-weighted image (T_R 500 ms/T_E 17 ms) of the lower legs shows streaky fatty infiltration of the muscles, particularly the right lateral gastrocnemius (G).

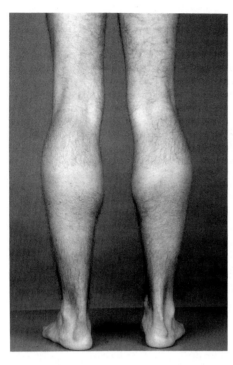

FIGURE 16.5. Enlarged calves of a 17-year-old boy with Becker muscular dystrophy.

16.7). Ultimately, these hypertrophic muscles are infiltrated by fat, initially without wasting (pseudohypertrophy). Clinico-radiological studies showed concordance in two-thirds of the muscles investigated.[38] One explanation for the discordance is partial morphological involvement of a compound muscle, which may progress without weakness.

Magnetic Resonance Imaging

As with the CT examination, the selective pattern of involvement is apparent on MRI.[13,32]

Carriers of the Dystrophin Gene

Due to random inactivation of the X chromosome, so-called manifesting carriers are found to show clinical features of the disease. Between 3% and 10% of DMD carriers have muscle weakness to a certain extent.[1] Manifesting BMD carriers are rare.[42] Muscle weakness has a limb girdle distribution, but is often asymmetrical. Cardiomyopathy may be the sole manifestation.[43] Abnormalities in muscle pathology in carriers are common, varying from minimal myopathic changes to florid dystrophic alterations.[1]

Carrier detection has greatly benefitted from the identification of the dystrophin gene. If a mutation is found in families where DNA samples from affected cases are available, then carrier detection is possible. However, in a proportion of DMD patients (35%), no deletion or duplication is present.[44] In those cases, the probability of a woman being a carrier is determined by indirect DNA methods (e.g., restriction fragment length polymorphisms) combined with estimation of serum CK activity, which is elevated in 60–70% of the carriers.

Ultrasonography

An increased echo within thigh muscles and a poorly defined demarcation of gastrocnemius and soleus muscles are found in DMD carriers.[45] According to some authors, the diagnostic value of ultrasound scanning in DMD/BMD carriers is high,[46] but this is refuted by others.[47–49]

Computed Tomography

In manifesting DMD carriers, areas of decreased attenuation are found in weak muscles but may also be seen in nonparetic muscles.[50,51] Calf pseudohypertrophy is observed in some carriers.[40,50,52] As with the clinical features, CT scan abnormalities are often asymmetric[50–52] (Figure 16.8). Although Stern et al.[53] advocated that CT

FIGURE 16.6. Becker muscular dystrophy: ultrasound findings. (A) Transverse thigh images show highly similar pattern as in Duchenne's dystrophy. Note increased echointensities of the vastus medialis (open arrowhead) and, to a lesser degree, in the sartorius (filled arrowhead). Note also obscure femur echoes (arrow). (B) Longitudinal ultrasound scans of the right (left side of figure) and left (right side of figure) lower legs reveal marked hypertrophy of the gastrocnemius (curved arrow) and soleus (arrowhead) muscles (thickness of both muscles 50% greater than normal, i.e., 6 cm). Slightly increased echointensities of the right gastrocnemius suggests early mesenchymal alteration. (C) In a patient with clinically prominent calves, the large size of the legs was due not to hypertrophy, but rather to increased adiposity of the calf muscles (i.e., pseudohypertrophy). This is indicated by such markedly increased echointensity of the gastrocnemius muscles that the soleus muscles are not visible due to attenuation of the ultrasound waves in the gastrocnemius muscles.

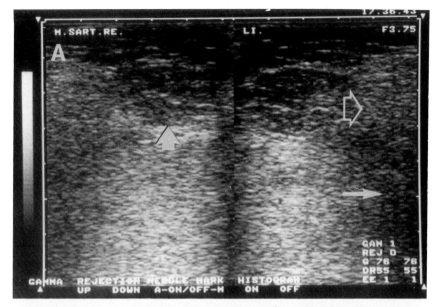

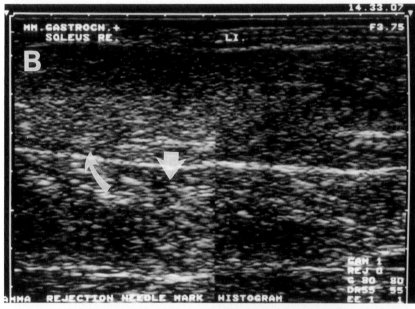

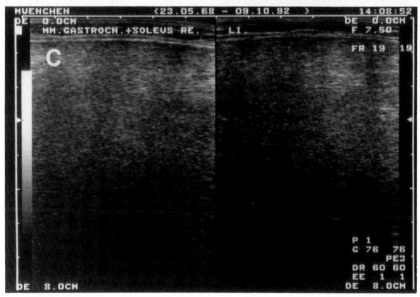

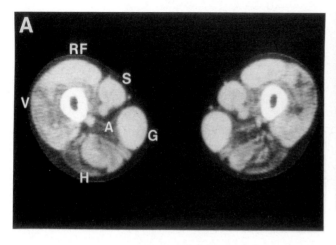
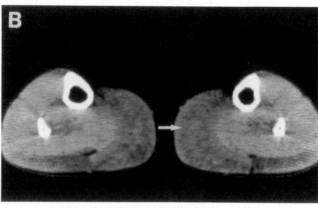

FIGURE 16.7. Becker muscular dystrophy: CT findings. (A) Transverse scan of thighs shows fatty changes of the vasti (V) muscles, adductors (A), and hamstrings (H). Note also hypertrophic appearance of the rectus femoris (RF), sartorius (S), and gracilis (G) muscles. (B) Transverse scan of legs shows fatty change and enlargement (pseudohypertrophy) of the medial gastrocnemius muscles (arrow).

would improve the accuracy of genetic counseling, this is disputed by the fact that one group was unable to detect abnormalities[54] and another detected pathological changes only in carriers above the age of 40.[55]

Magnetic Resonance Imaging

Significantly higher T_1 values caused by degenerative muscular changes accompanied by interstitial edema are found in the proximal muscles of DMD carriers com-

pared to normal females.[56] These data may reflect the edema accompanying muscle fiber degeneration.[56] Manifesting carriers may show asymmetric involvement of proximal muscles of the lower limbs.

Limb Girdle Muscular Dystrophy

Limb girdle muscular dystrophy (LGMD) encompasses a large group of phenotypically and genotypically distinct disorders. One particular form of autosomal recessive LGMD, closely resembling that of DMD or BMD, and therefore called severe childhood autosomal recessive Duchenne-like muscular dystrophy (SCARMD),[57] is considered a well-delineated clinical entity. In contrast to DMD and BMD, cardiomyopathy is not present in the majority of LGMD patients.

Estimation of serum CK activity and histopathological examination of muscle tissue are not very helpful to distinguish between DMD/BMD and autosomal recessive LGMD. Dystrophin analysis and DNA screening of the Xp21 region is required for a distinction between the dystrophinopathies and LGMD and gives an accurate diagnosis in 90% of the cases.[58] In a proportion of SCARMD patients, deficiency or absence of a dystrophin-associated glycoprotein (50 DAG), adhalin, was found.[59] Linkage studies have added to the widely held belief that there is heterogeneity within the group of limb girdle muscular dystrophies, because to date at least four loci on chromosomes 15q, 13q, 2p, and 17q, respectively, are recognized.[60-63]

Autosomal dominant LGMD, which usually has a relatively mild course, gives rise to even more confusion.

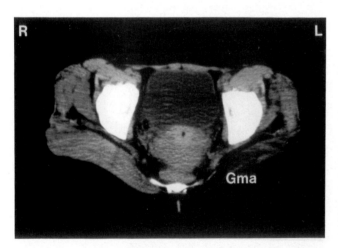

FIGURE 16.8. Radiological investigation of manifesting carrier of the dystrophin gene (mother of a son with Duchenne muscular dystrophy): CT findings. Transverse scan of the pelvic girdle shows wasting and fatty replacement of the left gluteus maximus (GMa) muscle.

A great variety of additional clinical features, such as early contractures, calf hypertrophy, and cardiopathy, may be present but are not consistently seen. Similarly, a spectrum of alterations is found in muscle biopsy, including undetermined myopathic changes and nonspecific structural abnormalities such as rimmed vacuoles or moth-eaten fibers. So far, linkage studies have yielded one locus on chromosome 5q in a single North American family suffering from autosomal dominant LGMD.[64]

Ultrasonography

In autosomal recessive LGMD, atrophy is most prominent in the vastus lateralis and tibialis anterior muscles.[13] Markedly elevated echointensities are found in the biceps brachii, vasti, hamstrings, soleus, and paraspinal muscles[13] (Figure 16.9). Ultrasonography was performed in a large consanguineous Finnish family with two clinically separate phenotypes of muscular dystrophy (i.e., one predominantly proximal and one with a distal

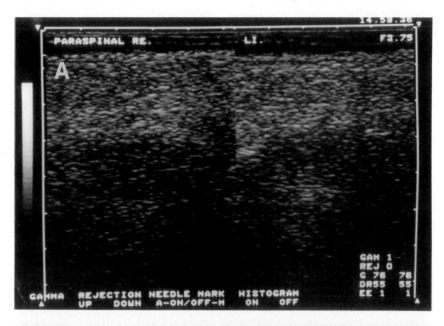

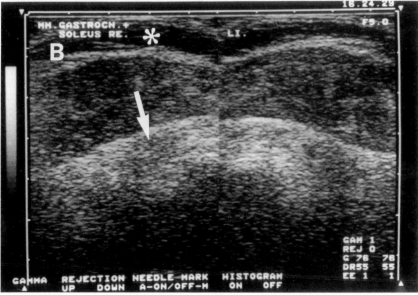

FIGURE 16.9. Autosomal recessive limb girdle muscular dystrophy: ultrasound findings. (A) Longitudinal images of the lumbar erector spinae muscles show markedly increased echointensities. (B) Transverse scans of the gastrocnemius and soleus (arrow) muscles show markedly increased echointensities of the soleus muscles. Asterisk indicates subcutaneous fat.

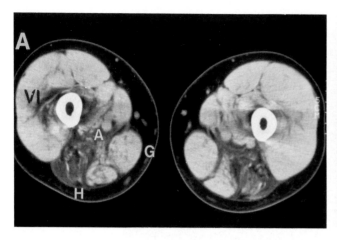

FIGURE 16.10. Autosomal recessive limb girdle muscular dystrophy: CT findings. (A) Transverse scan of the thighs shows preferential involvement of the vastus intermedius (VI) muscles, right more than left. The hamstrings (H) and adductors (A) are severely infiltrated by fat. The gracilis (G) muscles are clearly hypertrophic. (B) Scan of the legs shows decreased attenuation, indicating fatty change, of the soleus (S), and to a greater extent, of the medial head of the left gastrocnemius (GCmh).

distribution of weakness). In family members with limb girdle weakness, increased echogenicity, disintegration of muscular structure, and markedly reduced or completely lost bone echo was found in all limb girdle and lower leg muscles.[65]

Computed Tomography

In autosomal recessive LGMD, CT findings resemble those found in DMD and BMD with selective involvement of the paraspinal, gluteal, and quadriceps femoris muscles, the adductors, hamstrings, and the medial head of the gastrocnemius muscle.[23,66] However, the vastus intermedius and the soleus are more often and earlier affected than in DMD and BMD (Figure 16.10).[13,23,65,67] The sartorius and gracilis muscles are preserved or even show an hypertrophic appearance.[23,66]

In the aforementioned family with autosomal recessive LGMD, in which considerable intrafamilial variation of clinical expression was present, severe atrophy and fatty involvement of all muscles with relative preservation of the distal and paravertebral muscles was observed in affected family members with limb-girdle weakness.[65]

A CT study in one patient with autosomal dominant LGMD showed progressive changes in all thigh muscles, initially with relative preservation of the vastus lateralis, rectus femoris, sartorius, and gracilis muscles.[68] Subsequent, progressive involvement of distal leg muscles occurred with preferential involvement of the calf muscles, particularly the soleus muscle.

In Bethlem myopathy, CT showed more diffuse involvement than expected based on clinical findings. The quadriceps and hamstrings were among the first muscles to be affected. Subclinical, but morphologically severe, involvement of lumbar paravertebral muscles, abdominal muscles, the deltoids, and the lower leg muscles was noted.[69]

Magnetic Resonance Imaging

In autosomal recessive LGMD, abnormalities on MRI are similar to those found on CT[31] (Figure 16.11). MRI was performed in two patients with severe limb-girdle

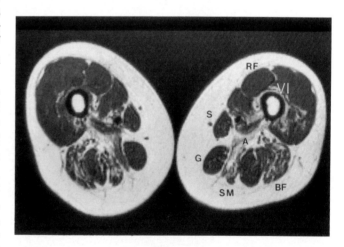

FIGURE 16.11. Autosomal recessive limb girdle muscular dystrophy: MRI findings. T_1-weighted image (T_R 500 ms/T_E 17 ms) of the thighs shows fatty change in the long head of the biceps femoris (BF), semimembranosus (SM), adductors (A), and vastus intermedius (VI) muscles. The rectus femoris (RF), sartorius (S), and gracilis (G) muscles are hypertrophic.

weakness from the aforementioned family with LGMD reported by Udd et al.[65] Abnormal signal intensity in all and distal myopathy muscles was seen, with less extensive changes in the rectus femoris and distal leg muscles.

Images of the thighs obtained from three patients from a large kindred suffering from Bethlem myopathy revealed general atrophy and fatty infiltration of all muscles with a predilection for the quadriceps muscles, and relative sparing of the hamstrings, adductors, gracilis, and sartorius muscles.[70]

Emery-Dreifuss Muscular Dystrophy

Emery-Dreifuss muscular dystrophy (EMD) is a rare, usually X-linked recessive myopathy, but autosomal dominant forms do exist. Genetic linkage studies mapped X-linked EMD to Xq28.[71] EMD is characterized by early contractures of the Achilles tendons, elbows, and spine, slowly progressive muscle wasting and weakness with a predominantly humeroperoneal distribution in the early stages, and cardiac involvement with conduction defects. The latter may cause sudden death preventable by timely insertion of a pacemaker.

Muscle biopsy shows nonspecific myopathic changes. Diagnosis is established by the characteristic clinical picture and the nonspecific histopathology.[72]

Ultrasonography

Heckmatt et al.[8] described selective involvement of the vastus intermedius and sparing of the rectus femoris.

Computed Tomography

In three patients with EMD, areas of lower attenuation were found in the soleus and paravertebral muscles, and in one of these cases the medial head of the gastrocnemius and the hamstrings were affected as well.[23]

Magnetic Resonance Imaging

MRI studies have not been reported in EMD.

Congenital Muscular Dystrophy

The classical form of congenital muscular dystrophy (CMD) is characterized by onset at birth or in the first year of life, hypotonia, generalized muscle weakness and multiple joint contractures, a nonprogressive or slowly progressive course, and the absence of severe impairment of intellectual development.[73] Other forms, including Fukuyama CMD, are associated with severely impaired

intellectual function and/or major malformation of the central nervous system, evident on CT or MRI.

Diagnosis is based on clinical features and muscle histology. Muscle biopsy findings include a marked variability of fibers and severe replacement by fat and connective tissue. Fiber necrosis and regenerative activity are not prominent and when present necessitate the need for analysis of dystrophin, which should be normal.[73] Recently, Fukuyama CMD has been localized to chromosome 9q.[74] Evidence supports that classical CMD results from deficiency of merosin, a subunit of laminin, a major component of the extracellular matrix; subsequently, a form of merosin-negative CMD was localized to chromosome 6q.[75]

Ultrasonography

Markedly elevated echointensities and decreased bone echoes were found in patients with CMD[8,13] (Figure 16.12).

Computed Tomography

A decrease in attenuation values both in proximal and distal muscles of the lower limbs was found.[76] In Fukuyama CMD pseudohypertrophy of the calf muscles was reported.[16]

Magnetic Resonance Imaging

MRI studies have not been reported in CMD, to our knowledge.

Facioscapulohumeral Muscular Dystrophy

Facioscapulohumeral muscular dystrophy (FSHD) is an autosomal dominant myopathy with a variable age of onset and a wide range of clinical expression even within families. Weakness of facial and/or shoulder girdle muscles, often asymmetrical (Figure 16.13), is usually the presenting symptom in the second decade, but early-onset cases occur in about 5% of the cases.[77] The disease runs mostly a progressive course with subsequent involvement of the abdominal, foot-extensor, upper arm, and pelvic girdle muscles. Early-onset FSHD should be regarded as a severe expression of the disease and is usually associated with hearing loss and vascular retinopathy, although the latter symptoms are also found to a lesser extent in mild cases.[77]

Recently, the causative gene defect has been localized to the distal portion of the long arm of chromosome 4. De novo rearrangements in a region on chromosome

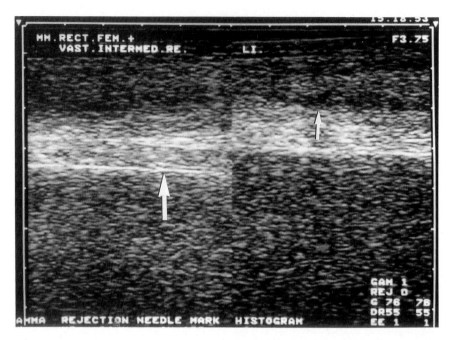

FIGURE 16.12. Congenital muscular dystrophy: ultrasound findings. Longitudinal thigh scans show atrophy and increased echointensity of the vastus intermedius muscles (deep surface marked by large arrow). Note asymmetrical atrophy of the rectus femoris, with the left (deep surface marked by short arrow) smaller than the right.

4q containing homeobox sequences were found in sporadic cases.[78] Although most of the families studied so far showed linkage with chromosome 4 markers, there appears to be heterogeneity.[79]

Muscle pathology is usually nonspecific, showing an increased variation in the size of the fibers. A few scattered small angulated fibers strongly reactive with oxidative enzyme reactions and moth-eaten fibers are also frequently seen. Muscle fiber necrosis and regenera-

tion are not prominent. Sometimes, an extensive mononuclear cell infiltrate is present.[5]

Diagnosis is based on the clinical picture and family history. If there are no affected individuals in the family, a muscle biopsy should be performed in order to rule out other neuromuscular disorders with a scapuloperoneal distribution of weakness.[80] Molecular genetic studies are very helpful in these sporadic cases or in patients with minor signs of muscle weakness.

Ultrasonography

Elevated echointensities were found in atrophic upper arm and tibialis anterior muscles, and also in the brachioradialis and rectus femoris muscles (Figure 16.14). There is often asymmetrical involvement.[13]

Computed Tomography

CT shows the same asymmetric pattern of involvement.[26,66,81,82] The most evident abnormalities occur in the biceps and triceps brachii and in the parascapular muscles[23,66,81] (Figure 16.15). Compound muscles with normal strength on clinical examination, such as the hamstrings, hip adductors, quadriceps femoris, and the gastrocnemius muscles, may also show areas of decreased attenuation in one or more constituent parts.[23,24,66,81] The soleus and lateral head of the gastrocnemius muscle are relatively spared compared to the tibialis anterior

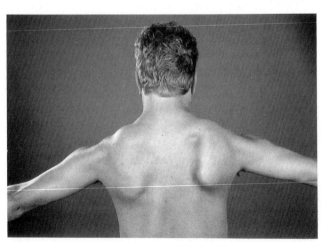

FIGURE 16.13. A 22-year-old man with asymmetric involvement of the periscapular muscles due to facioscapulohumeral muscular dystrophy.

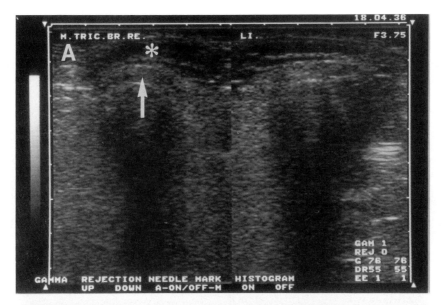

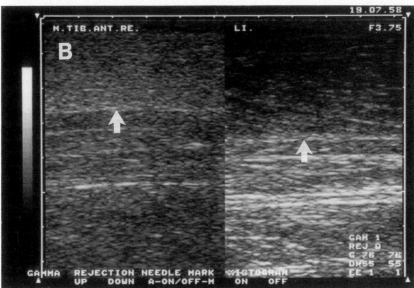

FIGURE 16.14. Facioscapulohumeral muscular dystrophy: ultrasound findings. (A) Transverse scans of the triceps brachii muscles (arrow) show marked atrophy (thickness 6 mm). Asterisk indicates subcutaneous fat. (B) Longitudinal scans of the tibialis anterior muscles reveal atrophy and increased echointensities of the right-sided muscle (left side of figure). Arrows indicate interosseous membrane.

muscle.[82] In the trunk, the abdominal muscles are involved first with subsequent involvement of the gluteal and paraspinal muscles, with the psoas muscles remaining preserved,[23,81,82] sometimes even appearing hypertrophic.[23]

Magnetic Resonance Imaging

MRI findings resemble those on CT[13,32] (Figure 16.16). The distribution of fatty replacement is asymmetric, comparable to the aforementioned imaging methods. In one patient selective involvement of the soleus muscles was observed, whereas the other calf muscles were spared.[31]

Distal Muscular Dystrophy

Muscular dystrophies with predominantly distal involvement constitute a heterogeneous group of disorders. In 1991, Barohn et al.[83] proposed the following classification: late adult-onset autosomal dominant Welander myopathy with onset in the extensors of the fingers, late adult-onset

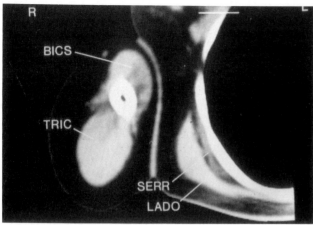

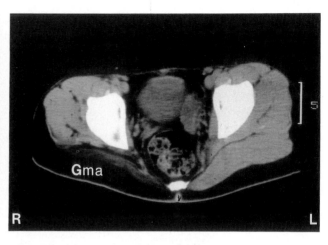

FIGURE 16.15. Facioscapulohumeral muscular dystrophy: CT findings. (A) Transverse scan of the right upper arm and periscapular muscles shows decreased attenuation of the right-sided serratus anterior (SERR) muscle, with relatively normal latissimus dorsi (LADO), triceps (TRIC), and biceps (BICS). (B) Transverse scan of the pelvis shows wasting and replacement by fat of the right-sided gluteus maximus (GMa).

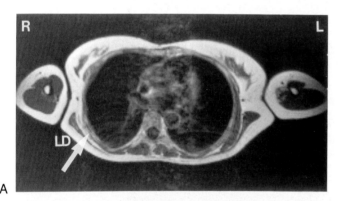

autosomal dominant distal myopathy with onset in the anterior compartment of the legs, early adult-onset autosomal recessive or sporadic distal myopathy with onset in the anterior compartment of the legs, and early adult-onset autosomal recessive or sporadic Miyoshi distal muscular dystrophy with onset in the posterior compartment of the legs (Figure 16.17).

Muscle fiber pathology of Welander myopathy (which is mainly seen in Swedish patients) is characterized by an

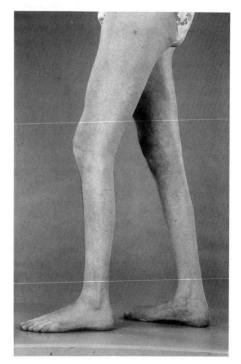

FIGURE 16.16. Facioscapulohumeral muscular dystrophy: MRI findings. (A) T_1-weighted image (T_R 500 ms/T_E 17 ms) of the upper arms and the periscapular muscles shows atrophy and hyperintensity (fatty change) of the right serratus anterior muscle (at tip of arrow) and atrophy of the nearby latissimus dorsi (LD) muscle. (B) T_1-weighted image (T_R 500 ms/T_E 17 ms) of the legs shows complete fatty replacement of the right tibialis anterior (arrow).

FIGURE 16.17. Miyoshi distal muscular dystrophy manifesting as atrophy of the legs in a 32-year-old man.

increased variation in fiber size with angulated and rounded atrophic fibers, as well as rimmed vacuoles. At the ultrastructural level, filamentous inclusions similar to those found in inclusion body myositis are found in connection with these vacuoles.[84] A neurogenic component is suggested by electrophysiological studies and sural nerve abnormalities.[84]

The other late-onset distal muscular dystrophy occurs in non-Scandinavian patients. Muscle biopsy reveals a vacuolar myopathy.[85] Recently, a large Finnish family was described showing an essentially similar clinical picture. However, the muscle biopsy did not reveal vacuoles.[65]

In Miyoshi distal muscular dystrophy, serum CK activity is markedly elevated and the muscle biopsy shows dystrophic changes without vacuoles. The other early adult-onset autosomal recessive type of distal muscular dystrophy has less elevated CK and the muscle biopsy reveals severe rimmed vacuolar myopathy.[86]

Ultrasonography

Both in Welander myopathy and in other forms of distal muscular dystrophy elevated echointensities are found, not only in the clinically affected distal musculature (Figure 16.18) but also in muscles that have

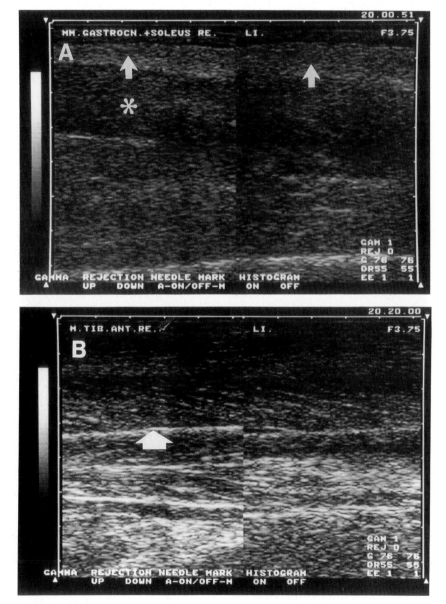

FIGURE 16.18. Miyoshi distal muscular dystrophy: ultrasound findings. (A) Longitudinal scans of the gastrocnemius and soleus muscles show considerable atrophy and slightly increased echointensities of the gastrocnemius (arrows) muscles, whereas the soleus (asterisk) muscles are unremarkable. (B) Longitudinal scans of the anterior legs of the same patient show only normal findings. Arrow indicates interosseous membrane.

normal strength on examination, such as in the thigh and biceps brachii.[13,87]

Udd et al.[65] found increased echogenicity and disintegration of muscle structure in the weak tibialis anterior muscles of eight patients with late-onset autosomal dominant distal muscular dystrophy from the aforementioned family with variable clinical expression. Similar changes can also be observed in the clinically unaffected quadriceps femoris, gastrocnemius, and soleus muscles.

Computed Tomography

CT studies have been carried out in only a limited number of patients with Welander myopathy, revealing pathological changes in the tibialis anterior, soleus, and medial head of the gastrocnemius muscles.[88] In early adult-onset rimmed vacuolar distal muscular dystrophy, extensors and flexors of the lower legs are affected, whereas the latter are not always clinically apparent. In some patients, the flexors are less affected than the extensors. In the thighs, the quadriceps femoris is relatively preserved, but the adductors, hamstrings, and gracilis muscles are severely affected. In the hip girdle, the gluteus minimus and medius muscles are affected earlier than the gluteus maximus. In the lumbar region, the psoas muscles are spared, whereas other paraspinal muscles, quadratus lumborum, and rectus abdominis are severely involved. CT of the upper extremities shows more extensive changes of wrist and finger flexors and more or less equal involvement of the flexors and extensors of the upper arms. Hypertrophy is not found in this early onset distal muscular dystrophy with rimmed vacuoles.[88]

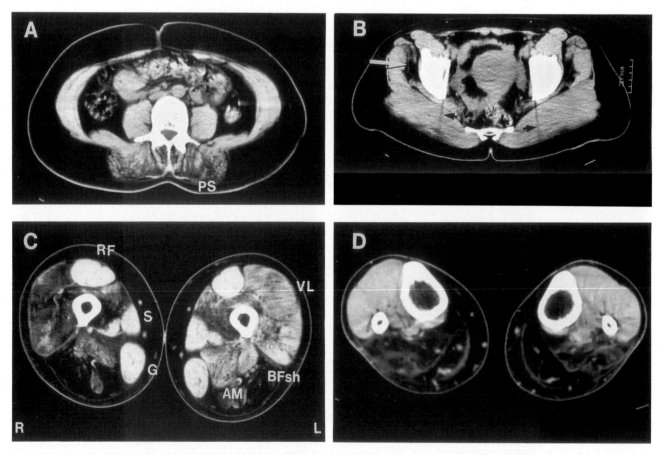

FIGURE 16.19. Miyoshi distal muscular dystrophy: CT findings at four levels in the same patient. (A) Transverse scan at the level of the fourth lumbar vertebra shows diffuse deterioration of paraspinal (PS) muscles. (B) Transverse scan of the pelvis shows nearly complete replacement by fat of both gluteus minimus (arrow) muscles. Note also linear "beam-hardening" artifacts (small arrows). (C) Transverse scan of the thighs shows preservation of the rectus femoris (RF), sartorius (S), and gracilis (G) muscles, whereas all other right-sided muscles have been replaced by fat. On the left, the short head of the biceps femoris (BFsh) is relatively preserved, and the vastus lateralis (VL) and adductor magnus (AM) muscles show areas of partial fatty replacement. (D) Transverse scan of the legs shows calf muscles to be completely replaced by fat.

In Miyoshi distal muscular dystrophy the posterior muscles of the lower legs are preferentially affected, consistent with the clinical findings (Figure 16.19). In all patients, the gluteus minimus muscles show replacement by fat. In addition, considerable changes may be found in the paravertebral and thigh muscles, sometimes accompanied by hypertrophy of the sartorius, semitendinosus, and gracilis muscles.[89]

Udd et al.[65] reported symmetrically reduced attenuation in the anterior tibial muscles of all patients investigated. In addition, asymmetrically distributed areas of lower density were seen in the clinically unaffected posterior muscles of the lower legs, in the thigh muscles (the flexors showing more extensive changes than the extensors and the adductors), and in the gluteal and paraspinal muscles.

Magnetic Resonance Imaging

The distribution of findings on MRI in patients described by Udd et al.[65] was similar to those on CT. In Welander myopathy, abnormalities were seen in the same muscles in which CT had demonstrated low-density changes. Except for a slight increase in T_1 values in the vastus lateralis muscles, proximal muscles were unaffected.[88]

T_1- and T_2-weighted MRI showed high signals, suggesting fatty change, in the adductors of the thigh, the hamstrings, and the lower leg muscles of one patient with distal myopathy with rimmed vacuoles who presented with clinical findings in the lower legs.[90] Similar to CT findings, in two patients with Miyoshi-type distal muscular dystrophy, MRI suggested fatty change in the distal legs with preferential involvement of the flexors, and in the thigh muscles with sparing of the gracilis, sartorius, and short head of the biceps femoris muscle.[91]

Oculopharyngeal Muscular Dystrophy

Oculopharyngeal muscular dystrophy (OPMD) is a late-onset, autosomal dominantly inherited disorder usually presenting with bilateral ptosis, and rarely with dysphagia. Subsequently, progressive extraocular muscle paresis and involvement of limb muscles is observed. Muscle pathology is characterized by rimmed vacuoles and an otherwise unremarkable myopathy.[92]

Computed Tomography

Medici et al.[93] described the presence of areas of lower attenuation in the paraspinal muscles, hamstrings, and soleus muscles of 17 out of 35 patients. In half of

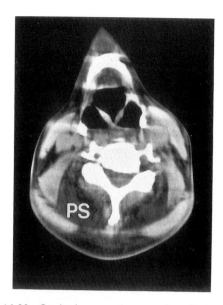

FIGURE 16.20. Oculopharyngeal muscular dystrophy: CT findings. Transverse scan at the level of the spinous process of the sixth cervical vertebra shows complete replacement of multiple paraspinal muscles (PS) by fat.

the clinically normal patients, CT involvement of the paraspinal muscles (Figure 16.20) was detected. Ultrasonography and MRI studies have not been reported in oculopharyngeal muscular dystrophy.

Present and Future Implications on Evaluation of Patients with Muscular Dystrophies

It is of paramount importance to know in fine detail the natural course of progressive neuromuscular diseases in order to provide appropriate rehabilitative care to patients. This can be accomplished by a combination of manual muscle testing, dynamometry, and assessment of the functional status of the patient in a follow-up study. However, muscle imaging investigations are more accurate, because they enable the evaluation of individual constituents of compound muscles and deep-seated muscles. The new quantitative CT method introduced by Liu et al.,[15] which quantifies the degree of muscle fiber loss and fat tissue replacement, is very promising in the assessment of both the rate of progression and the efficacy of therapeutic interventions. Ultrasound and MRI are particularly suitable for studies of children because they avoid the radiation exposure incurred with CT examinations.[94,95] Additionally, MRI is superior to ultrasound and CT in terms of tissue characterization (i.e., fat, fibrosis, and edema).

References

1. Emery AEH. Duchenne muscular dystrophy. Oxford: Oxford University Press, 1993.

2. Kunkel LM. Analysis of deletions in DNA from patients with Becker and Duchenne muscular dystrophy. Nature 1986;322:73–77.

3. Hoffman EP, Fischbeck KH, Brown RH, et al. Dystrophin characterization in muscle biopsies from Duchenne and BMD patients. N Engl J Med 1988;318:1363–1368.

4. Brooke MH, Fenichel GM, Griggs RC, et al. Duchenne muscular dystrophy: patterns of clinical progression and effects of supportive therapy. Neurology 1989;39:475–481.

5. Dubowitz V. Muscle biopsy—a practical approach. 2nd ed. London: Ballière Tindall, 1985.

6. Jennekens FGI, Kate LP ten, Visser M de, Wintzen AR. Diagnostic criteria for Duchenne and Becker muscular dystrophy and myotonic dystrophy (workshop report). Neuromuscul Disord 1991;1:389–391.

7. Forst R, Casser H-R. 7-MHz-real-time-Sonographie der Skelettmuskulatur bei Duchenne-Muskeldystrophie. Ultraschall 1985;6:336–340.

8. Heckmatt JZ, Pier N, Dubowitz V. Real-time ultrasound imaging of muscles. Muscle Nerve 1988;11:56–65.

9. Alanen A, Kantola I, Komu M. New imaging methods in hereditary neuromuscular diseases. Acta Cardiomiol 1989;1:32–45.

10. Nishimura M, Nishimura S, Yamada S. Ultrasound imaging of the muscle in muscular dystrophy. No To Hattatsu 1989;21:234–238.

11. Fischer AQ, Carpenter DW, Hartlage PL, et al. Muscle imaging in neuromuscular disease using computerized real-time sonography. Muscle Nerve 1988;11:270–275.

12. Aizawa H, Kozima S, Takagi A. Ultrasound imaging of muscles in Duchenne muscular dystrophy. Clin Neurol 1989;29:49–53.

13. Pongratz DE, Reimers CD, Hahn D, et al. Atlas der Muskelkrankheiten. Munich: Urban & Schwarzenberg, 1990.

14. Kawai M, Kunimoto M, Motoyoshi Y, et al. Computed tomography in Duchenne muscular dystrophy—morphological stages based on the computed tomographic findings. Clin Neurol 1985;25:578–590.

15. Liu M, Chino, N, Ishihara T. Muscle damage progression in Duchenne muscular dystrophy evaluated by a new quantitative computed tomographic method. Arch Phys Med Rehabil 1993;73:507–514.

16. Kawai M. A computed tomographic study of calf pseudo-hypertrophy in the three types of progressive muscular dystrophy (Duchenne, Becker, and Fukuyama). Brain Dev 1985;17:241.

17. Jones DA, Round JM, Edwards RHT. Size and composition of the calf and quadriceps muscles in Duchenne muscular dystrophy. J Neurol Sci 1983;60:307–322.

18. Stern LM, Clark BE. Investigation of scoliosis in Duchenne dystrophy using computerized tomography. Muscle Nerve 1988;11:775–783.

19. Ando N, Takayanagi T, Fujimoto Y, et al. Mechanism to induce scoliosis in Duchenne muscular dystrophy—a study of paraspinal muscle by X-ray computed tomography. Clin Neurol 1992;32:956–961.

20. Gellerich I, Koch RD. Computertomographische Befunde bei maligner progressiver Muskeldystrophie Duchenne (DMD). Psychiatr Neurol Med Psychol 1990;42:282–290.

21. Lissoni A, Molteni F, Sechi L, Cellotto N. Erector spinae degeneration and scoliosis development in Duchenne muscular dystrophy. Acta Cardiomiol 1991;3:425–429.

22. O'Doherty DS, Schellinger DD, Raptopoulos V. Computed tomographic patterns of pseudohypertrophic muscular dystrophy: Preliminary results. J Comput Assist Tomogr 1977;1:482–486.

23. Serratrice G, Salamon G, Jiddane M, et al. Résultats du scanner X musculaire dans 145 cas de maladies neuro-musculaires. Rev Neurol 1985;141:404–412.

24. Hawley RJ, Schellinger D, O'Doherty DS. Computed tomographic patterns of muscles in neuromuscular diseases. Arch Neurol 1984;41:383–387.

25. Stern LM, Caudrey DJ, Perrett LV, Boldt DW. Progression of muscular dystrophy assessed by computed tomography. Dev Med Child Neurol 1984;26:569–573.

26. Herson D, Larde D, Ferry M, et al. Apport diagnostique du scanner X en pathologie musculaire. Rev Neurol 1985;141:482–489.

27. Matsumura K, Nakano I, Fukuda N, et al. Proton spin-lattice relaxation time of Duchenne dystrophy skeletal muscle by magnetic resonance imaging. Muscle Nerve 1988;11:97–102.

28. Nagao H, Morimoto T, Sano N, et al. Magnetic resonance imaging of skeletal muscle in patients with Duchenne muscular dystrophy—serial axial and sagittal section studies. No To Hattatsu 1991;23:39–43.

29. Lamminen AE, Tanttu JI, Sepponen RE, et al. Magnetic resonance of diseased skeletal muscle: combined T_1 measurement and chemical shift imaging. Br J Radiol 1990;63:591–596.

30. Liu G-C, Jong Y-J, Chiang C-H, Jaw T-S. Duchenne muscular dystrophy: MR grading system with functional correlation. Radiology 1993;186:475–480.

31. Murphy WA, Totty WG, Carroll JE. MRI of normal and pathologic skeletal muscle. AJR 1986;146:565–574.

32. Lamminen AE. Magnetic resonance imaging of primary skeletal muscle diseases: patterns of distribution and severity of involvement. Br J Radiol 1990;63:946–950.

33. Kuryama M, Hayakawa K, Konishi Y, et al. MR imaging of myopathy. Comp Med Imaging Graph 1989;13:329–333.

34. Hasegawa T, Matsumura K, Hashimoto T, et al. Intra-muscular degeneration process in Duchenne muscular dystrophy—Investigation by longitudinal MR imaging of the skeletal muscle. Clin Neurol 1992;32:333–335.

35. Monaco AP, Bertolson CJ, Liechti-Gallati S, et al. An explanation for the phenotypic difference between patients bearing partial deletions of the DMD locus. Genomics 1988;2:90–95.

36. Gospe SM, Lazaro RP, Lava NS, et al. Familial X-linked myalgia and cramps: a non-progressive myopathy associated with a deletion in the dystrophin gene. Neurology 1989;39:1277–1280.

37. Yoshida K, Ikeda S-I, Nakamura A, et al. Molecular analysis of the Duchenne muscular dystrophy gene in patients with Becker muscular dystrophy presenting with dilated cardiomyopathy. Muscle Nerve 1993;16:1161–1166.

38. Visser M de, Verbeeten B Jr. Computed tomography of the skeletal musculature in Becker-type muscular dystrophy and benign infantile spinal muscular atrophy. Muscle Nerve 1985;8:435–444.

39. Bulcke JA, Crolla D, Termote J-L, et al. Computed tomography of muscle. Muscle Nerve 1981;4:67–72.

40. Bulcke JAL, Baert AL. Clinical radiological aspects of myopathies: CT scanning, EMG, radioisotopes. New York: Springer-Verlag, 1982.

41. Termote J-L, Baert A, Crolla D, et al. Computed tomography of the normal and pathologic muscular system. Radiology 1980;137:439–444.

42. Glass IA, Nicholson LVB, Watkiss E, et al. Investigation of a female manifesting carrier. J Med Genet 1992;29:578–582.

43. Mirabella M, Servidei S, Manfredi G, et al. Cardiomyopathy may be the only clinical manifestation in female carriers of Duchenne muscular dystrophy. Neurology 1993;43:2342–2345.

44. Dunnen JT den, Grootscholten PM, Bakker E, et al. Topography of the DMD gene: FIGE- and cDNA analysis of 194 cases reveals 115 deletions and 13 duplications. Am J Hum Genet 1989;45:835–847.

45. Rott H-D, Santellani M, Breimesser FH. Duchenne muscular dystrophy: carrier detection by ultrasound and computerised tomography. Lancet 1984;1:111.

46. Steinbicker V, Rohden L von, Gellerich I, Szibor R. Duchenne carrier diagnosis by use of ultrasonography and computed tomography. Clin Genet 1985;28:468.

47. Uppal G, Dewbury KC, Dennis NR. Carrier detection in DMD. Clin Genet 1987;31:62–63.

48. Schapira G, Laugier P, Rochette J, et al. Detection of Duchenne muscular dystrophy carriers: quantitative echography and creatine kinasemia. Hum Genet 1987;75:19–23.

49. Spiegler AWJ, Schindler S, Herrmann FH. Becker muscular dystrophy: carrier detection by real-time ultrasound. J Neurol 1985;232:307–309.

50. Visser M de, Verbeeten B Jr. Computed tomographic findings in manifesting carriers of Duchenne muscular dystrophy. Clin Genet 1985;27:269–275.

51. Kawai M, Kunimoto M, Kamakura K, et al. Asymmetrical patchy muscle involvement in manifesting carriers of Duchenne muscular dystrophy—computed tomographical and histological study. Clin Neurol 1988;29:23–29.

52. Kikumoto O, Yoshinaga J, Sasaki T, et al. A manifesting carrier of Duchenne muscular dystrophy presenting mosaic distribution of dystrophin negative and positive muscles fibers. Clin Neurol 1990;37:107–109.

53. Stern LM, Caudrey DJ, Clark MS, et al. Carrier detection in Duchenne muscular dystrophy using computed tomography. Clin Genet 1985;27:392–397.

54. Gasto-Gago M, Alonso A, Novo I, Fuster M. Carrier detection of Duchenne muscular dystrophy by computerised tomography. Lancet 1986;i:1039.

55. Rott H-D, Santellani M, Rödl W, Nebel G. Duchenne muscular dystrophy: carrier detection by ultrasound and computerised tomography. Lancet 1983;2:1199–2000.

56. Matsumura K, Nakano I, Fukuda N, et al. Duchenne muscular dystrophy carriers. Proton spin-lattice relaxation times of skeletal muscles on magnetic resonance imaging. Neuroradiology 1989;31:373–376.

57. Ben Hamida M, Fardeau M, Attia N. Severe childhood muscular dystrophy affecting both sexes and frequent in Tunisia. Muscle Nerve 1983;6:469–483.

58. Ginjaar HB, Bakker E, Busch HFM, et al. Toepassing van gecombineerde DNA en dystrofine eiwit-analyse in de diagnostiek van Duchenne en Becker spierdystrofie bij 102 Nederlandse patiënten. Ned Tijdschr Geneesk 1993;137:68–75.

59. Matsumura K, Tomé FMS, Collin H, et al. Deficiency of the 50K dystrophin-associated glycoprotein in severe childhood autosomal recessive muscular dystrophy. Nature 1992;359:320–322.

60. Beckmann JS, Richard I, Hillaire D, et al. A gene for limb-girdle muscular dystrophy maps to chromosome 15 by linkage. CR Acad Sci Paris 1991;312:141–148.

61. Ben Othmane K, Ben Hamida M, Pericak-Vance MA, et al. Linkage of Tunesian autosomal recessive Duchenne-like muscular dystrophy to the pericentromeric region of chromosome 13q. Nature Genet 1992;2:315–317.

62. Bashir R, Strachan T, Keers, et al. A gene for autosomal recessive limb-girdle muscular dystrophy maps to chromosome 2p. Hum Mol Genet 1994;3:455–457.

63. Roberds SL, Leturcq F, Allamand V, et al. Missense mutations in the adhalin gene linked to autosomal recessive muscular dystrophy. Cell 1994;78:625–633.

64. Speer MC, Yamaoka LH, Gilchrist JH, et al. Confirmation of genetic heterogeneity in limb-girdle muscular dystrophy: linkage of an autosomal dominant form to chromosome 5q. Am J Hum Genet 1992;50:1211–1217.

65. Udd B, Lamminen A, Somer H. Imaging methods reveal unexpected patchy lesions in late onset distal myopathy. Neuromuscul Disord 1991;1:279–285.

66. Jiddane M, Gastaut JL, Pellissier JF, et al. CT of primary muscle disease. AJNR 1983;4:773–776.

67. Schwartz MS, Swash M, Ingram DA, et al. Patterns of selective involvement in neuromuscular disease. Muscle Nerve 1988;11:1240–1245.

68. Marconi G, Pizzi A, Arimondi CG, et al. Limb girdle muscular dystrophy with autosomal dominant inheritance. Acta Neurol Scand 1991;83:234–238.

69. Merlini L, Morandi L, Granata C, Ballestrazzi A. Bethlem myopathy: early-onset benign autosomal dominant myopathy with contractures. Description of two new families. Neuromuscul Disord 1994;4:503–511.

70. Nielsen JF, Jakobsen J. A Danish family with limb-girdle muscular dystrophy with autosomal dominant inheritance. Neuromuscul Disord 1994;4:139–142.

71. Hodgson SV, Boswinkel E, Cole C, et al. A linkage study of Emery-Dreifuss muscular dystrophy. Hum Genet 1986;74:409–416.

72. Yates JRW. European workshop on Emery-Dreifuss muscular dystrophy (workshop report). Neuromuscul Disord 1991;1:393–396.

73. Dubowitz V. ENMC sponsored workshop on congenital muscular dystrophy (workshop report). Neuromuscul Disord 1994;4:75–81.

74. Toda T, Segawa M, Nomura Y, et al. Localization of a gene for Fukuyama type congenital muscular dystrophy to chromosome 9q31–33. Nature Genet 1993;5:283–286.

75. Hillaire D, Leclerc A, Fauré S, et al. Localization of merosin-negative congenital muscular dystrophy to chromosome 6q2 by homozygosity mapping. Hum Mol Genet 1994;3:1657–1661.

76. Ohiwa N, Kato T, Ando T, et al. CT findings of skeletal muscles in children with progressive muscular dystrophy. Brain Dev 1981;13:156–159.

77. Brouwer OF, Wijmenga C, Frants RR, Padberg GW. Facioscapulohumeral muscular dystrophy: the impact of genetic research. Clin Neurol Neurosurg 1993;95:9–21.

78. Wijmenga C, Hewitt JE, Sandkuijl LA, et al. Chromosome 4q DNA rearrangements associated with facioscapulohumeral muscular dystrophy. Nature Genet 1992;2:26–30.

79. Gilbert JR, Stajich JM, Wall S, et al. Evidence for heterogeneity in facioscapulohumeral muscular dystrophy (FSHD). Am J Hum Genet 1993;53:401–408.

80. Padberg GWAM, Lunt PW, Koch M, Fardeau M. Diagnostic criteria for facioscapulohumeral muscular dystrophy (workshop report). Neuromuscul Disord 1991;4:231–234.

81. Patijn J. De ziekte van Landouzy-Dejerine; een computertomografische studie van de skeletmusculatuur [thesis]. Amsterdam: Rodopi, 1983.

82. Horikawa H, Takahashi K, Nishio H, et al. X-rays computed tomographic scans of lower limb and trunk muscles in facioscapulohumeral muscular dystrophy. Clin Neurol 1992;32:1061–1066.

83. Barohn RJ, Miller RG, Griggs RC. Autosomal recessive distal dystrophy. Neurology 1991;41:1365–1370.

84. Borg K, Borg L, Lindblom U. Sensory involvement in distal myopathy (Welander). J Neurol Sci 1987;80:323–332.

85. Markesbery WR, Griggs RC, Leach RP, et al. Late onset hereditary distal myopathy. Neurology 1974;23:127–134.

86. Misuzawa H, Kurisaki H, Takatsu M, et al. Rimmed vacuolar distal myopathy: a clinical, electrophysiological, histopathological and computed tomographic study of seven cases. J Neurol 1987;234:129–136.

87. Rohden L von. Ultraschalluntersuchungen an der quergestreiften Muskulatur bei neuromuskulären Erkrankungen. Magdeburg: Habilitationsschrift, 1989.

88. Åhlberg G, Jakobsson F, Fransson A, et al. Distribution of muscle degeneration in Welander distal myopathy—a magnetic resonance imaging and muscle biopsy study. Neuromuscul Disord 1994;4:55–62.

89. Visser M de. Computed tomographic findings of the skeletal musculature in sporadic distal myopathy with early adult onset. J Neurol Sci 1983;59:331–339.

90. Mizuno T, Motonaga T, Yanagida K, et al. MRI findings in studies of distal myopathy with rimmed vacuoles. Clin Neurol 1989;29:1290–1293.

91. Ohsuga H, Oshuga M, Yamamoto Y, Shinohara Y. Skeletal muscle MRI findings in autosomal recessive distal muscular dystrophy (Miyoshi). Clin Neurol 1988;28:1304–1311.

92. Tomé FMS, Fardeau M. Oculopharyngeal muscular dystrophy. In: Engel AG, Franzini-Armstrong C, eds. Myology. 2nd ed. New York: McGraw-Hill, 1994: 1233–1245.

93. Medici M, Tenyi A de, Vincent O, et al. Muscle computed axial tomography features in oculopharyngeal dystrophy. Muscle Nerve 1986;9(Suppl):244.

94. Griggs RC. Quantitation of muscle mass and muscle protein synthesis rate: documenting a response to myoblast transfer. In: Griggs R, Karpati G, eds. Myoblast transfer. New York: Plenum Press, 1990:235–240.

95. Karpati G, Ajdukovic D, Arnold D, et al. Myoblast transfer in Duchenne muscular dystrophy. Ann Neurol 1993;34:8–17.

17
Myotonic Disorders

Carl D. Reimers and Thomas J. Vogl

Myotonic dystrophy was recognized to represent a specific disease by the German internist Hans Steinert[1] and the British neurologists Fred Eustace Batten and H.P. Gibb[2] in 1909. However, the characteristic combination of myotonia and distal muscle weakness was first described by the American physician C.L. Dana in 1888.[3]

Myotonic dystrophy is the most frequent degenerative myopathy in adulthood with a prevalence estimated at 1:7500 inhabitants.[4] It has an autosomal dominant mode of inheritance with a very high penetrance. The DNA defect is localized on the long arm of chromosome 19 (19q13.2–q13.3).[5] Clinical features often worsen from generation to generation[6] due to expansion of an unstable DNA region with an increased number of cytosine-thymidine-guanidine (CTG) trinucleotides.[4] The pathogenesis of the disorder is still unclear.

Clinically, three types of myotonic dystrophy can be distinguished: congenital, childhood, and juvenile or adult-onset types. The congenital type is characterized by severe hypotonia at birth, facial weakness, respiratory insufficiency, and swallowing and sucking difficulties. Skeletal abnormalities and marked delay in motor and intellectual milestones are usually associated. Myotonia (i.e., difficulty in relaxing muscles after contraction) usually occurs after the third year of life. Signs often improve if the patient survives the first year. Children manifesting myotonic dystrophy often present with skeletal abnormalities such as a slender face, thin ribs, or talipes equinovarus. Otherwise this type shows the same features as the juvenile and adult-onset form. In addition to the combination of myotonia and faciocervicodistal muscle wasting, cardiac (conduction defects, arrhythmias), endocrine (gonadal atrophy, insulin-resistant diabetes mellitus), cerebral (intellectual deficits, dementia), and ophthalmologic (cataract, increased intraocular pressure) abnormalities may be present. Often smooth muscles of the pharynx, esophagus, and the gastrointestinal tract are involved. Premature balding is usual in men. The life expectancy is reduced.

The diagnosis of myotonic dystrophy is grounded upon the clinical feature or electromyographical proof of myotonia, that is, high-frequency repetitive discharges with a waxing and waning of amplitude and frequency, combined with muscle wasting. Serum creatine kinase activity is slightly or moderately increased in the majority of patients. The diagnosis can be substantiated by the histopathological finding in muscle of a characteristic triad of numerous internal nuclei, ring fibers, and sarcoplasmic masses. However, these features are usually present only in advanced stages of the disease when the diagnosis is easy due to the typical phenotype. Today the diagnosis can be established by DNA analysis.

Muscle Imaging in Myotonic Dystrophy

Ultrasound

Congenital Type

Von Rohden[7] described coarse, focal hyperechoic structures in the muscles due to increased fat content.

Childhood Type

Lamminen et al.[8] found increased muscle echogenicity resulting in slightly indistinct fascial echoes and a distinct bone echo in two children whose age of onset was not reported.

Juvenile/Adult-Onset Type

A relatively large quantitative study of many muscles offers a comprehensive summary of muscle changes.[9] Common findings include atrophy of the tibialis anterior, triceps brachii, rectus femoris, vastus intermedius muscles, and sternocleidomastoid muscle (Figure 17.1). The study also confirmed that the thickness of subcutaneous fat layers is increased and that a decrease in muscle thickness correlates with weakness.

Muscle echogenicity is increased in the majority of muscles. The tibialis anterior (Figure 17.1), brachioradialis, biceps brachii, peroneus longus, rectus abdominis, and triceps brachii muscles have the highest echointensities. Echointensity correlates well with muscle weakness.[9] The femur echo may be obscure.[10] The abnormalities are usually symmetric, but occasionally may be asymmetric.[9]

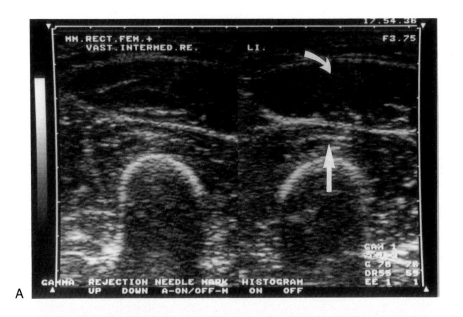

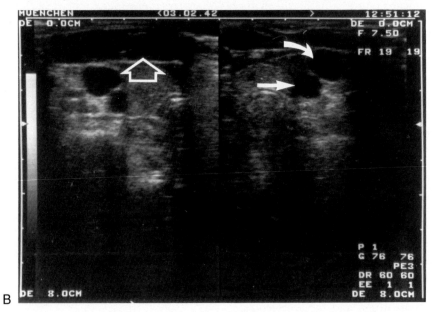

FIGURE 17.1. Adult-onset myotonic dystrophy: ultrasound findings. (A) Transverse scans of the thighs (3.75 MHz; right side of the image = left thigh and vice versa) show normal appearing rectus femoris (curved arrow) and atrophic vastus intermedius (arrow). (B) Transverse ultrasound scans of the lateral neck (7.5 MHz; right side of the image = left neck and vice versa) demonstrate normal thickness and echo texture of sternocleidomastoid muscles (open arrow). (C) Transverse ultrasound scans of the lateral neck (7.5 MHz; right side of the image = left neck and vice versa) demonstrate atrophy of the sternocleidomastoid muscles (open arrow). Curved arrows indicate common carotid arteries, arrows indicate jugular veins. Transverse ultrasound scans of the anterior legs (7.5 MHz; right side of the image = left leg and vice versa) show increased echointensity of the anterior tibialis muscles due to fat infiltration. The interosseous membrane (arrowhead) is nearly invisible. The aponeuroses are not detectable and tibial echoes are blurred (oblique arrow) (D).

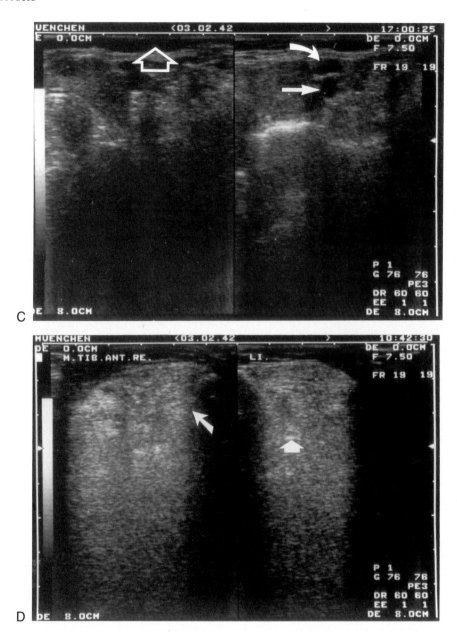

FIGURE 17.1. *Continued*

Computed Tomography

Congenital and Childhood Types

There are no reports available.

Juvenile/Adult-Onset Type

Using a standardized CT approach, the sternocleido-mastoid was determined to be the first muscle involved with atrophy and replacement of muscle fibers by fat[11] (Figure 17.2). In early stages, true hypertrophy can be observed in the rectus abdominis,[11] spinal,[11] rectus femoris,[12–14] adductor magnus and longus,[9] gracilis[12] and biceps femoris muscles[9] and in the lateral head of the gastrocnemius muscle.[9] With progressing disease, atrophy becomes obvious in the extensor muscles of the spine, at first in the thoracolumbar region, and in the tibialis anterior muscle and the medial head of the gastrocnemius muscle. The lateral head of the gastrocnemius muscle[9,11] and the soleus[11] become involved later and to a lesser extent.

Regarding the severity of the abnormalities, Gellerich et al.[15] reported that deep neck muscles show hypodensities in about two-thirds of the patients. Decrease of muscle volume and irregular hypodensities can be seen preferentially in the legs,[16,17] but also in

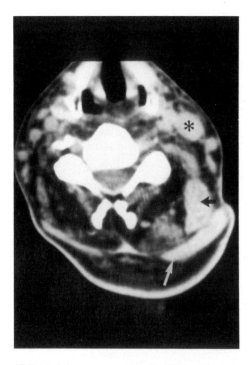

MUENCHEN

FIGURE 17.2. Adult-onset myotonic dystrophy: computed tomography findings in the neck. Axial image of the neck shows asymmetric atrophy and fatty change of the sterno-cleidomastoid (*) and deep neck extensor muscles. Note that sternocleidomastoid, levator scapulae (black arrow) and trapezius (white arrow) are relatively normal on the left and are extremely atrophic on the right.

abdominal and paraspinal muscles and the thighs.[12,16] In the thighs, fatty replacement of muscles is more pronounced in the extensors than in the adductors and flexors.[12,17] Even in early stages, the sartorius and gracilis muscles often show only slight abnormalities[9] (Figure 17.3). Involvement of the extensors often is evidenced by a semilunar region of low density ("halo"), indicating fat around the femoral diaphysis[9,17,18] (Figure 17.3). The fatty change of the tibialis anterior is of the same severity as in the medial head of the gastrocnemius[9,15] (Figure 17.4), or milder.[12,17,19] In the forearm, CT may show hypodensities in deep-seated muscles (Figure 17.5).[9] The abnormalities are usually symmetric,[9,17] but clearly asymmetric in about every third or fourth patient.[9] The levator scapulae, trapezius, psoas major, iliopsoas, gluteus, and tibialis posterior muscles usually show only normal density.[12]

Magnetic Resonance Imaging

Congenital and Childhood Types

There are no reports available.

Juvenile/Adult-Onset Type

The dystrophic process is associated with fatty degeneration of the muscles.[9] Occasionally, visual assessments reveal relative increase of signal intensities in T_2- as opposed to T_1-weighted images, indicating muscle

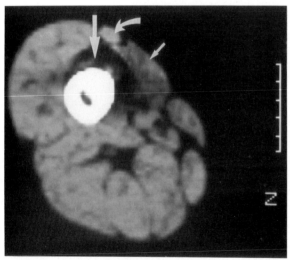

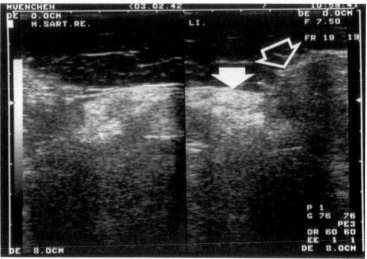

FIGURE 17.3. Adult-onset myotonic dystrophy: thigh variations. (A) Axial CT image of the right thigh shows the vastus intermedius (arrow) to be markedly atrophic and hypodense due to fat infiltration. The vastus medialis (small arrow) shows less severe fatty change. A few small low-density areas are visible in the sartorius and adductor longus. The rectus femoris (curved arrow) is also atrophic. (B) In another patient, transverse ultrasound scans of the thighs (7.5 MHz; right side of the image = left thigh and vice versa) show markedly increased echointensities of the sartorius (arrow) and less marked increases in the vastus medialis (open arrow). The femur echoes are obscured.

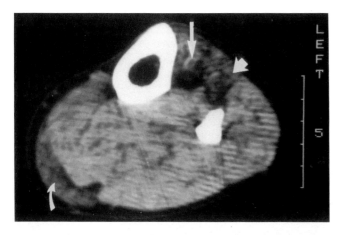

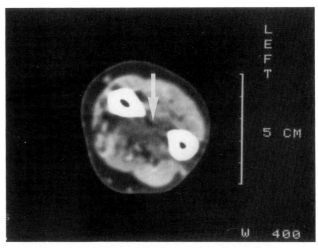

FIGURE 17.4. Adult-onset myotonic dystrophy: computed tomography of the left leg. Confluent low-density areas due to fat can be seen in the tibialis anterior (arrow), extensor digitorum longus (broad arrow), and in the medial head of the gastrocnemius muscle (curved arrow). Small hypodensities are scattered throughout other muscles.

FIGURE 17.5. Adult-onset myotonic dystrophy: computed tomography of the left forearm. Confluent hypodensities due to fatty involution are depicted in the deep finger flexors (arrow).

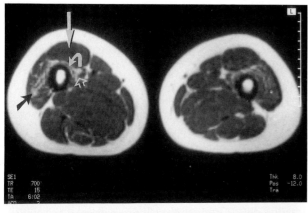

A

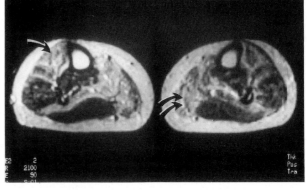

C

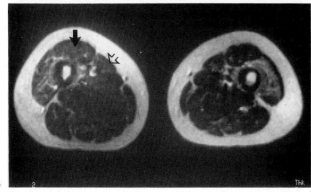

B

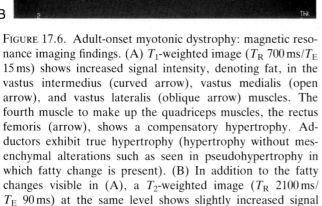

D

FIGURE 17.6. Adult-onset myotonic dystrophy: magnetic resonance imaging findings. (A) T_1-weighted image (T_R 700 ms/T_E 15 ms) shows increased signal intensity, denoting fat, in the vastus intermedius (curved arrow), vastus medialis (open arrow), and vastus lateralis (oblique arrow) muscles. The fourth muscle to make up the quadriceps muscles, the rectus femoris (arrow), shows a compensatory hypertrophy. Adductors exhibit true hypertrophy (hypertrophy without mesenchymal alterations such as seen in pseudohypertrophy in which fatty change is present). (B) In addition to the fatty changes visible in (A), a T_2-weighted image (T_R 2100 ms/T_E 90 ms) at the same level shows slightly increased signal intensities, indicating edema-like change in the right-sided rectus femoris (arrow) and sartorius (open arrow). (C) In the same patient's legs, primarily fatty changes are noted in a slightly asymmetric distribution. Note on the T_1-weighted image (T_R 600 ms/T_E 15 ms), high signal intensity bilaterally in the anterior tibialis (curved arrow) and soleus (arrowhead). Fat is also prominent in the medial head of the gastrocnemius (small arrow) but not in the lateral head (arrow). (D) A T_2-weighted image (T_R 2100 ms/T_E 90 ms) shows signal intensities of the right tibialis anterior (curved arrow) and of the medial head of the left gastrocnemius (double curved arrow) to be relatively higher when compared to those on the T_1-weighted image, indicating edema-like change superimposed on the fatty infiltration. The remaining muscles show the same features as on the T_1-weighted images, indicating muscle lipomatosis only.

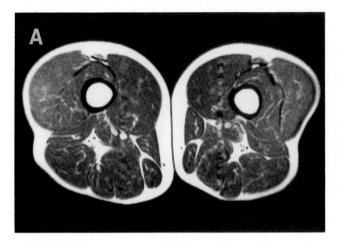 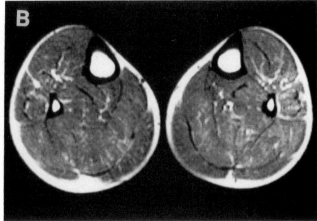

FIGURE 17.7. Myotonia congenita: typical findings. (A,B) T_1-weighted images of thighs (A) and legs (B) show apparently hypertrophic and otherwise normal muscles. (Cases courtesy of Dr. B.C.G. Schalke, Würzburg, Germany.)

edema.[9,20] As is apparent clinically, distal muscles are more severely damaged than proximal ones.[21] However, proximal changes can be noted. For example, in the thighs, the vasti show the highest signal intensities on T_1-and T_2-weighted images, indicating fat, whereas the rectus femoris muscle is generally spared[21] (Figure 17.6). In the legs, the medial head of the gastrocnemius muscle becomes involved earliest.[21] In the majority of patients, the medial head of the gastrocnemius muscle, the tibialis anterior, and the soleus muscles are bilaterally involved[9] (Figure 17.6). The posterior tibialis is relatively spared, even in advanced stages.[21] Occasionally, true muscle hypertrophy occurs[9] (Figure 17.6).

Other Myotonic Disorders

Thomsen's congenital myotonia, an autosomal dominant, Becker's congenital myotonia, an autosomal recessive, and the autosomal dominant Eulenburg's congenital paramyotonia are rare disorders. Like myotonic dystrophy, these disorders are characterized by "uncontrolled temporary stiffness of muscle due to a transient hyperexcitability of the muscle fiber membrane."[22] Of these, congenital myotonia is the more common; these patients frequently look athletic because muscles are hypertrophic. In congenital myotonia, routine muscle histology with conventional stains is usually normal. MRI and sonography confirm muscle hypertrophy without any significant structural changes[23,24] (Figure 17.7).

Impact of Radiology on the Diagnosis and Treatment of Myotonic Dystrophy

Practical indications for radiological tests are currently rather limited in evaluating myotonic disorders, although occasions arise in which the morphological features visible by ultrasound, CT, or MRI may be helpful. For example, in the early stages of myotonic dystrophy, the definite diagnosis may be difficult to establish because myotonia and/or muscle weakness may be very slight. If muscle wasting is only mild, congenital myotonia might be suspected. In this case, visualization of mesenchymal muscle changes by diagnostic imaging can be a valuable hint because muscle wasting is rare in congenital myotonia. In advanced stages of myotonic dystrophy, the diagnosis is usually easy. In this case, imaging can help to assess the degree and distribution of muscle wasting and progression of the disease. Of considerable scientific interest and potential clinical importance will remain the question of the mechanism(s) underlying the peculiar selectivity of muscle deterioration in myotonic dystrophy.

References

1. Steinert H. Myopathologische Beiträge. Über das klinische und anatomische Bild des Muskelschwundes der Myotoniker. Dtsch Z Nervenheilk 1909;37:58–104.
2. Batten FE, Gibb HP. Two cases of myotonia atrophica, showing a peculiar distribution of muscular atrophy. Proc Roy Soc Med, Neurol Section 1909;2:32–33.
3. Dana CL. An atypical case of Thomsen's disease (myotonia congenita). Med Rec 1888;33:433–435.
4. Harley HG, Brook JD, Rundle SA, et al. Expansion of an unstable DNA region and phenotypic variation in myotonic dystrophy. Nature 1992;355:545–546.
5. Brook JD, Shaw DJ, Meredith AL, et al. Localizing the gene for myotonic dystrophy on chromosome 19. J Med Genet 1985;22:396.
6. Höweler CJ, Busch HFM, Geraedts JPM, et al. Anticipation in myotonic dystrophy: fact or fiction? Brain 1989;112:779–797.

7. von Rohden L. Ultraschalluntersuchungen an der querge-streiften Muskulatur bei neuromuskulären Erkrankungen Postdoctoral thesis. Magdeburg: Germany, 1989:16–17.

8. Lamminen A, Jääskelainen J, Rapola J, et al. High-frequency ultrasonography of skeletal muscle in children with neuromuscular disease. J Ultrasound Med 1988;7:505–509.

9. Schedel H, Reimers CD, Nägele M, et al. Imaging techniques in myotonic dystrophy. A comparative study of ultrasound, computed tomography and magnetic resonance imaging of skeletal muscles. Eur J Radiol 1992;15:230–238.

10. Kaschka WP, Druschky K-F, Rott H-D. Myotonic muscular dystrophy: structural changes visualized by ultrasound (letter). J Neurol 1987;234:122–123.

11. Bulcke JAL, Baert AL. Clinical and radiological aspects of myopathies. CR scanning, EMG, radioisotopes. Berlin: Springer, 1982;126–135.

12. Miyashita I, Yamamoto H, Koga H, et al. Computed tomography of skeletal muscles in myotonic muscular dystrophy. Clin Neurol 1990;30:24–28.

13. Nordal HJ, Dietrichson P, Eldevik P, et al. Fat infiltration, atrophy and hypertrophy of skeletal muscles demonstrated by X-ray computed tomography in neurological patients. Acta Neurol Scand 1988;7:115–122.

14. Rodiek S-O. CT, MR-Tomographie und MR-Spektroskopie bei neuromuskulären Erkrankungen. Stuttgart: Enke, 1987:29–30.

15. Gellerich I, Müller D, Koch RD. Computertomographische Untersuchungen bei myotonen Dystrophien. Psychiatr Neurol Med Psychol 1986;38:378–383.

16. Jiddane M, Gastaut JL, Pellissier J, et al. CT of primary muscle diseases. Am J Neuroradiol 1983;4:773–776.

17. Rickards D, Isherwood I, Hutchinson R, et al. Computed tomography in dystrophia myotonica. Neuroradiology 1982;24:27–31.

18. Serratrice G, Salamon G, Jiddane M, et al. Résultats du scanner X musculaire dans 145 cas de maladies neuro-musculaires. Rev Neurol 1985;141:404–412.

19. Wussow W, Mielke U. Computertomographie der Unterschenkel bei Dystrophia myotonica. Verh der Deutschen Gesellschaft für Neurologie 1985;3:833–836.

20. Schedel H, Reimers CD, Vogl T, et al. Kernspintomographische Darstellung des Muskeloedema bei neuromuskulären Erkrankungen. Radiol Diagn 1992;33:29–32.

21. Damian MS, Bachmann G, Herrmann D, et al. Magnetic resonance imaging of the muscle and brain in myotonic dystrophy. J Neurol 1993;240:8–12.

22. Rüdel R, Lehmann-Horn F, Ricker K. The nondystrophic myotonias. In: Engel AG, Franzini-Armstrong C, eds. Myology. New York: McGraw-Hill Inc., 1994;1291.

23. Pongratz DE, Reimers CD, Hahn D, Nägele M, Müller-Felber W, eds. Atlas der Muskelkrankheiten. Wien: Urban und Schwarzenberg, 1990.

24. Fisher AQ, Carpenter DW, Hartlage PL, Caroll JE, Stephens S. Muscle imaging in neuromuscular disease using computerized real time sonography. Muscle Nerve 1988;11:270.

18
Congenital Myopathies

Antti Lamminen and Helena Pihko

Congenital myopathies constitute a rare group of disorders characterized by hypotonia and generalized muscle weakness from birth and structural alterations of muscle fibers. The clinical presentation of congenital myopathies is very similar regardless of the pathological changes in the muscle. The severity of muscle weakness varies, but most often it is mild with a stable or slowly progressive clinical course. Congenital dislocation of hip can be present, and scoliosis, chest and foot deformities can develop. Facial weakness with a high arched palate is common. In severe cases, weakness of respiratory muscles can cause death in infancy or childhood. Exceptional cases have an adult onset and a progressive course. Cardiomyopathy has been described in isolated cases. Serum creatine kinase is normal or slightly elevated, and, like electromyography (EMG), is of very little help in establishing the diagnosis of congenital myopathies. Nerve conduction velocity is normal and EMG may show myopathic changes. Muscle biopsy with histochemical staining of cryostat sections and electronmicroscopic study is essential for the diagnosis of a congenital myopathy. Dystrophic or neurogenic changes are absent and accumulation of fat or increased amount of connective tissues is less typical than in the muscular dystrophies. The classification of congenital myopathies is based on structural changes—presence of cores, rods or myotubes—in the muscle. The majority of the pathological changes are not specific. More than one type of pathological change can be present in one biopsy and similar changes can be seen to a small extent in other conditions.[1-3]

Although sporadic cases exist, there is a strong genetic component in congenital myopathies with dominant, recessive, or X-linked inheritance.

As imaging studies of the congenital myopathies have been scarce and include many case reports, the following presentation first briefly concentrates on the clinical and pathological characteristics of these diseases, fol-lowed by a review of the imaging findings with different modalities.

Disease Descriptions

Central Core Disease

Clinical

Central core disease is named after round, "core"-like areas in the center of individual muscle fibers. The clinical presentation is that of hypotonia and nonprogressive muscle weakness, mainly proximal, which begins at birth and is associated with slightly delayed motor milestones. There is usually no focal muscle atrophy.[3-5] Congenital hip dislocation, scoliosis, and foot deformities are frequent, and slight facial muscle involvement can occur. Adult patients may show mild proximal weakness, resembling limb girdle muscular dystrophy. The condition is usually stable and even improvement of muscle power can occur. Tendon reflexes are usually normal. EMG is normal or myopathic. The disease is sporadic or dominantly inherited. Patients with central core disease have a high susceptibility to malignant hyperthermia. Central core disease has recently been shown[6] to map to the long arm of chromosome 19, very close to the ryanodine receptor locus, which is a candidate gene for malignant hyperthermia syndrome.[7]

Pathology

The disease is characterized by the well-defined circular core area, extending through the whole length of the normal-looking muscle fiber. There can be more than one core in a muscle fiber. The cores, which can be overlooked in paraffin sections, show a striking lack of reaction with oxidative stains in cryostat section. Fiber size variation with predominance of type 1 fibers is

245

common, but necrosis, fibrosis, and fat accumulation are uncommon. Cores are usually present in type 1 fibers only. On electron microscopy the cores are packed with myofilaments and show absence of mitochondria with disruption of sarcomeric organization. Cores are not present in all fibers and there is no correlation between the number of cores and the clinical severity of the disease.[2]

Myotubular (Centronuclear) Myopathy

Clinical

Myotubular myopathies are clinically heterogeneous disorders characterized by large, centrally located nuclei in muscle fibers. The fibers resemble fetal myotubes, but many authors believe that the resemblance may be more apparent than real and prefer the term "centronuclear" myopathy. The centronuclear myopathies can be divided into several clinical groups:[8–10] a severe X-linked recessive, a congenital autosomal recessive, an autosomal dominant, and a late-onset sporadic form. The X-linked neonatal form has an intrauterine onset with diminished fetal movements and polyhydramnios. Severe hypotonia, sucking difficulties, and respiratory weakness requiring artificial ventilation are common. The disease is usually fatal in infancy. A linkage to Xq28 has recently been shown.[11–13]

The autosomal recessive, dominant and sporadic forms vary in clinical severity. The disease can manifest in infancy as severe muscle weakness with delayed motor milestones. The muscle weakness is diffuse; there is a waddling gait, and the flexors of the feet are affected. Ptosis, ophthalmoplegia, and facial weakness are common. The symptoms can be slowly progressive and lead to wheelchair by adolescence. Another variety of the disease can manifest in adults and show a relatively mild limb girdle-type proximal muscle weakness with facial involvement.

Pathology

The pathological change in the muscle—large, centrally placed nuclei surrounded by a halo—are readily visible. The central localization of the nuclei is well demonstrated in longitudinal sections of the muscle fibers. There is usually a type 1 fiber predominance with normal size type 2 fibers. The pathological process of the muscle, at least in the infantile form, is suspected to be arrested fetal development of the fibers at the myotubular stage.[14] In adult cases, where differentiation into fiber types has occurred, regression of adult myofibers to a fetal stage has been suggested.[15] Ultrastructural changes consist of absence of myofibrils and accumulations of mitochondria and glycogen in the perinuclear central zone.[16]

Nemaline Myopathy

Clinical

Nemaline myopathy is characterized by weakness and hypotonia from birth and by the presence of thread-like particles (Greek nema = thread) in muscle biopsy. Muscle weakness is most severe in the limb girdle muscles and distally in the limbs, whereas the proximal limb muscles are better preserved. Facial myopathy is common and the respiratory muscles are often affected. Arthrogryposis is not a feature of nemaline myopathy, but later in life there is a tendency to develop contractures and skeletal deformities such as high arched palate, chest deformities, and scoliosis.

Banker[9] recognized four forms of nemaline myopathy: a severe infantile form, a congenital nonprogressive form, an asymptomatic form recognized on biopsy only, and an adult form. Dominant inheritance with variable penetrance has been reported. Wallgren-Pettersson,[17] in her study of 13 patients and their parents, found one slowly progressive clinical entity with variable severity. The disease was recessively inherited. The gene of the dominant form of nemaline myopathy has been assigned to chromosome 1 in one kindred.[18]

Pathology

The morphological changes consist of accumulations of small rod-like particles, the nemaline bodies, in the subsarcolemmal region of muscle fibers. The rods are easily recognized with the Gomori-trichrome stain, which stains the nemaline bodies red. The rods are at least partly composed of alpha-actin and with electron microscopy they are shown to originate from the Z discs. There is also a type 1 fiber predominance and deficient differentiation of type 2 fibers. The presence of rods is a nonspecific finding, because similar structures are seen in small quantities in other unrelated conditions.

Neurophysiological studies have shown neurogenic and myogenic changes in nemaline myopathy. In her study of 13 patients, Wallgren-Pettersson[19] found the EMG in proximal muscles myopathic and explained the neuropathic unit potentials seen in distal muscles by the degenerating–regenerating activity secondary to the myopathic process.

Multicore (Minicore) Disease

Clinical

The characteristic finding of this congenital myopathy is the presence of multifocal degeneration of the muscle fibers associated with a prevalence of type 1 fibers. The clinical presentation is that of delayed motor milestones and proximal muscle weakness from early childhood. Mild distal weakness occurs, occasionally more pronounced in the upper extremities. Facial muscle involvement, including ptosis, has been observed. The development of scoliosis and contractures has been reported and a few exceptional cases have died of respiratory insufficiency in infancy. Serum creatine kinase values and EMG are often normal. The mode of inheritance is recessive or sporadic.

Pathology

The typical finding is type 1 fiber predominance and hypotrophy. Occasional large type 2 fibers are seen. Small focal areas of degeneration, which do not extend the whole length of the muscle fiber, are seen. Ultrastructurally these lesions are devoid of mitochondria and consequently are best identified by focal lack of staining with oxidative enzyme methods. The myofibrils and cross striations are abnormal in the cores. The histochemical abnormalities tend to increase with age without concurrent progression in the clinical symptoms.[9,20]

Congenital Fiber Type Disproportion

Clinical

The predominance and hypotrophy of type 1 fibers with hypertrophic type 2 fibers associated with a clinical entity was first described by Brooke.[3,21] Symptoms consist of weakness and hypotonia apparent in infancy and delayed motor development with a nonprogressive course. Respiratory problems can occur and a few cases with a rapidly fatal course in infancy have been described. Because predominance of type 1 fibers is a common finding in other congenital myopathies as well as in various neurological disorders of central origin,[22–24] the existence of congenital fiber type disproportion as an independent disorder has been questioned.

Pathology

The characteristic feature is the disparity of size between type 1 and type 2 fibers with predominance of type 1 fibers. The type 1 fibers are in the low-normal and type 2 fibers are in the high-normal range in diameter. There is no grouping of fiber types and ultrastructural changes have not been reported.

Imaging Findings in Congenital Myopathies

Ultrasonography

Application of ultrasound (US) to the study of congenital myopathies is beset with the same problems as the use of ultrasonography in general: the ultrasonic characteristics are dependent upon technical and positional factors and on the state of muscular relaxation, the identification of individual muscles may present difficulties, and the visual interpretation is quite operator dependent. Although detailed in Chapter 2, brief review of muscle ultrasound follows.

Heckmatt et al.[25,26] were the first to report US findings for skeletal muscle in various neuromuscular diseases, including congenital myopathies. Static B-mode US equipment was used with a 5-MHz transducer, which was placed in direct contact with the skin. Normal muscle was echo-poor, and the echo reflected from the underlying bone was clearly seen. Muscular dystrophies were associated with increased echoes from muscle and with reduced or absent bone echo. Changes of similar type were found in four out of five patients with congenital myopathies, namely central core disease and multicore (minicore) disease. Differentiation between the dystrophies and congenital myopathies was not possible.

Heckmatt et al.[27] later confirmed their earlier static B-scan results in a report of real-time US imaging of muscles. In that paper, they demonstrated the usefulness of follow-up studies; in a 4-year-old child with congenital nemaline myopathy, inital US studies were normal, but a year later, abnormal echogenicity was seen in the vastus intermedius. In a larger study of 12 patients with nemaline myopathy, Wallgren-Pettersson et al.[28] demonstrated abnormal echogenicity especially in the dorsiflexors and plantarflexors of the feet. Most of their patients also had abnormal but less severe US findings in the rectus femoris and vastus intermedius muscles. The distribution of muscle involvement in nemaline myopathy appears to differ from that observed in central core disease: in the latter form of congenital myopathy, the rectus femoris muscles and the dorsiflexors of the feet seem to be selectively spared, whereas the sartorius, gracilis, and soleus muscles tend to be more severely affected.[29,30]

In an effort to minimize US image variation from study to study, and thereby reduce operator dependence, computer-assisted real-time ultrasonography has been utilized in muscle diseases,[31] and the results appear favorable. Dock et al.[32] presented a method based on an analysis of the number of what they regarded as perimysial septa in the US image; however, this method produced no differences between patients with mitochondrial myopathy and normal controls.

In a comparative study between muscle US and muscle biopsy findings in 8 children with progressive muscle dystrophies and 11 children with congenital myopathies[39] (five fiber type disproportion diseases, two multicore diseases, four unclassified congenital myopathies), the US image was clearly abnormal in all the patients with progressive dystrophy, and in the majority of those with congenital myopathies; the principal changes were increased muscle echogenicity with a reduced bone surface echo, and disturbance of muscle architecture. When the semiquantitatively graded US findings were compared with those of similarly graded muscle biopsy specimens, a clear correlation was found between the severity of the microscopic changes and the degree of abnormality of the US image. Also, some differentiation between the two conditions was possible; the dystrophies had a higher score of both US and microscopic findings, whereas the congenital myopathies had a lower score (Figure 18.1).

Computed Tomography

O'Doherty et al.[34] were among the first to apply computed tomography (CT) to the evaluation of muscle diseases. They reported a basic finding of replacement of normal muscle by tissue of low density, equivalent to the range of fatty tissue. They also described two different intramuscular patterns, characterized as diffuse or patchy replacement. The CT images were marred by beam-hardening artifacts from dense cortical bone. A later report by the same group,[35] based on a larger series of patients with various neuromuscular diseases, described characteristic differences between the CT findings of muscles in myopathic and neurogenic diseases. Neurogenic diseases were first apparent as muscle atrophy, and a decrease in the density of the muscles appeared later in the course of the disease. In primary muscle diseases, decreased density of the muscle was an early sign, with atrophy occurring later. Their patient material included one case with congenital, nonprogressive myopathy, but no specific features were described. Termote et al.[36] emphasized the selective muscle sparing seen also in congenital myopathies; in a 15-year-old boy with congenital fiber type disproportion, the most severe changes were seen in the tibialis anterior, tibialis posterior, and

soleus muscles, whereas the caput mediale of the gastrocnemius was spared. This is in direct contrast with the findings in muscular dystrophies, where the tibialis posterior often remains relatively unaffected even in end-stage cases, and the caput mediale of the gastrocnemius is involved quite early in the disease process.[37,38]

In central core disease, the distribution patterns are also in contrast with those seen in muscular dystrophies; the sartorius and gracilis, which are often spared in dystrophies,[38] are prone to atrophy and fatty degeneration in central core disease,[29,30] a feature shared with mitochondrial myopathies (see Chapter 19).

In nemaline myopathy, a substantial number of cases imaged by CT have been reported.[28,39–41] Wallgren-Pettersson et al.[28] presented a relatively large series of 12 patients with congenital nemaline myopathy. Eight patients were ambulatory and four were wheelchair bound. The pattern of selective muscular involvement and sparing changed during progression of the disease: in the ambulatory patients, all components of the quadriceps femoris and soleus were spared (Figure 18.2), but in the wheelchair stage, the rectus femoris and vastus intermedius components of the quadriceps and the soleus had become affected. The dorsiflexors of the feet and the gastrocnemius were selectively affected early in the disease, whereas the tibialis posterior and gracilis were spared even in the advanced stage. In general, the distal muscles appeared to be more severely affected than the proximal ones.

Magnetic Resonance Imaging

The application of nuclear magnetic resonance in skeletal muscle diseases began with the evaluation of normal and abnormal relaxation times; early investigations concentrated on the muscular dystrophies or the inflammatory myopathies. To date, very few magnetic resonance (MR) studies have been published on the congenital myopathies. Borghi et al.,[42] in their in vitro study of relaxation times of normal and pathological human skeletal muscle, included samples from nine patients with congenital myopathies: four cases of fiber type disproportion, two cases each of central core disease and centronuclear myopathy, and one case of nemaline myopathy. They found abnormally shortened T_1 relaxation time values in all patients with congenital myopathy, as well as in other patient groups including muscular dystrophies and spinal muscular atrophies. However, these samples represented cases with severe morphologic changes in muscle, and the effect of accompanying secondary changes like fatty and fibrous infiltration must be considered.

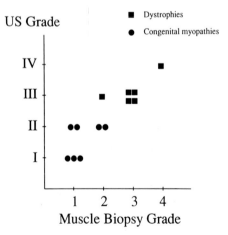

FIGURE 18.1. Relationship between ultrasound and muscle biopsy findings in muscular dystrophies and in congenital myopathies, graded in order of increasing severity.[33]

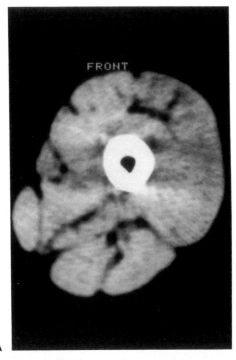

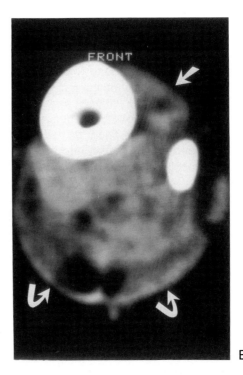

FIGURE 18.2. CT of left thigh (A) and leg (B) of a 15-year-old girl with nemaline myopathy in the ambulatory stage. Atrophy and fatty degeneration of the tibialis anterior and extensor digitorum longus muscles (arrow) and the gastrocnemius muscle (curved arrows) are evident, whereas the quadriceps femoris and soleus muscles are affected to a lesser degree. The gracilis and tibialis posterior muscles appear normal.

In clinical studies, intramuscular fatty degeneration which can be seen also in the congenital myopathies,[28] has been shown to decrease the T_1 and increase the T_2 values of muscle.[43–45] In a study of Duchenne muscular dystrophy, abnormally high T_1 values of skeletal muscle were measured at a field strength of 0.1 T in the preclinical stage of the disease; with progression of the dystrophy, the T_1 values rapidly decreased below the control values.[46] The latter phenomenon was assumed to be due to progressive fatty infiltration of muscles.

This effect of fatty infiltration was also confirmed in the congenital myopathies; in a study of tissue characterization by MR relaxometry and chemical shift imaging in our institution,[47] differential T_1 relaxation time measurements were performed with a low-field imager in 19 patients with muscle disease and in eight healthy controls. Nine patients had congenital myopathies, including four nemaline myopathies, two multicore myopathies, and three unclassified myopathies. Images were obtained with a gradient echo chemical shift technique based on the 3-Hz frequency difference between fat and water. A magnitude image and a phase image were reconstructed from the raw data, and from these, the final composite images and separate water and fat images were produced (Figure 18.3). T_1 values for muscle tissue were measured from the primary composite images, and differential T_1 values were calculated separately from the water and fat

images. These calculations were made from measurements of images based on inversion recovery pulse sequences. The longitudinal relaxation times of skeletal muscle were significantly increased both in dystrophies (mean, 145.9 ms) and in the congenital myopathies (mean, 141.1 ms); the mean T_1 of muscle in the controls was 126.0 ms. In addition, comparison of the differential T_1 measurements indicated that secondary fatty infiltration of muscles attenuates the increases in T_1 values associated with muscle disease. In the congenital myopathy group, the mean muscle T_1 value further increased to

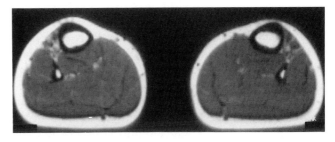

FIGURE 18.3. T_1-weighted (T_R/T_E, 500/15 ms) 1.0 T MR image of legs of an 11-year-old boy with nemaline myopathy. Note selective atrophy and fatty degeneration of tibialis anterior and extensor digitorum longus muscles, more advanced in the right leg.

149.0 ms, when the measurement was performed from the water images with no fat signal. In the muscular dystrophies with more advanced fatty infiltration, the corresponding mean T_1 value increased to 167.2 ms after exclusion of the fat signal. This phenomenon may affect measurement results when tissue characterization of skeletal muscle diseases is based on conventional measurements of T_1 relaxation times. Thus, the effect of secondary fatty infiltration must be taken into account, and separate measurements of the fat and water components should be made.

Clinical MR imaging studies of patients with different neuromuscular diseases show varying patterns of changes in the size and signal intensity of muscles.[28,38,43,45,48] The overwhelming majority of the MR investigations and case reports deal with disorders other than the congenital myopathies. Wallgren-Patterson et al.[28] reported MR findings in four patients with congenital nemaline myopathy; chemical shift imaging was also used to confirm fatty degeneration in the muscles. They suggested that the presence of intramuscular fatty infiltration supported the histologic findings of disease activity[49] and the electromyographic abnormalities,[19] indicating that in nemaline myopathy, contrary to what had been believed, there is active degeneration and regeneration of muscle fibers. In patients with nemaline myopathy, the distal limb muscles appear to be more severely affected than the proximal ones. The most advanced imaging findings are often seen in the tibialis anterior and extensor digitorum longus muscles (Figure 18.3), whereas the tibialis posterior, soleus and quadriceps femoris (excepting the rectus femoris) muscles are generally well preserved. This type of selective muscle involvement differs from that observed in the muscular dystrophies or in central core disease; in those, the rectus femoris and the dorsiflexors of the feet are often selectively spared, and the soleus is often affected early in the disease process.[29,30,38,50]

Lamminen[38] performed a comparative MR imaging study of the lower extremity musculature in a total of 51 patients, representing three different categories of muscle disease: 32 cases of muscular dystrophies, 11 cases of congenital myopathies, and 8 cases of polymyositis. In the congenital myopathy group, there were three cases of fiber type disproportion disease, two multicore myopathies, and 6 cases of unclassified congenital myopathy. The distribution patterns were slightly different between congenital myopathies and dystrophies: the overall involvement was significantly less severe in the congenital myopathies, but the dorsiflexors of the feet (tibialis anterior and extensor digitorum longus) were more involved than the other muscles (Figures 18.4, 18.5).

In conclusion, MR imaging, with its excellent soft tissue contrast resolution, seems very suitable for muscle

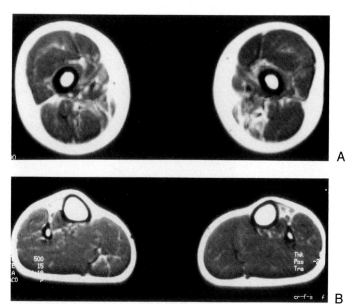

FIGURE 18.4. T_1-weighted (T_R/T_E, 500/15 ms) 1.0 T MR images of a 12-year-old girl with multicore myopathy. In the thighs (A), the adductor muscles are affected. In the legs (B), very selective atrophy and fatty degeneration of the dorsiflexors of the feet is seen.

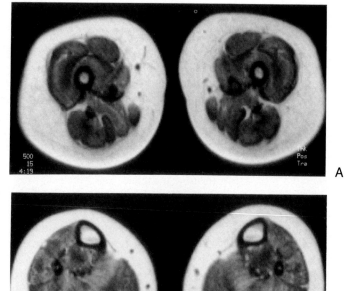

FIGURE 18.5. T_1-weighted (T_R/T_E, 500/15 ms) 1.0 T MR images of a 4-year-old boy with congenital fiber type disproportion. Diffuse fatty infiltration is seen in nearly all thigh muscles (A), with relative sparing of both semitendinosus muscles. In the legs (B), the diffuse intramuscular fatty infiltration spares the gastrocnemius muscles.

evaluation in the congenital myopathies. As the inter-pretation of US studies is very dependent on the experi-ence of the individual operator, and CT may be degraded by beam-hardening artifacts, MR emerges as the optimal imaging modality in primary skeletal muscle diseases.

References

1. Fitzsimons RB, McLeod JG. Myopathy with pathological features of both centronuclear myopathy and multicore disease. J Neurol Sci 1982;57:395–405.
2. Fardeau M. Congenital myopathies. In: Mastaglia FL, Walton Sir John, eds. Skeletal muscle pathology. London: Churchill and Livingstone, 1983:161–203.
3. Brooke MH. Congenital (more or less) muscle disease. In: Brooke MH, ed. A clinician's view on neuromuscular disorders, 2nd ed. Baltimore: Williams & Wilkins, 1986: 340–380.
4. Byrne E, Blumberg PC, Hallpike JF. Central core disease. Study of a family with five affected generations. J Neurol Sci 1982;53:77–83.
5. Shuaib A, Passuke RT, Brownell KW. Central core disease. Clinical features in 13 patients. Medicine (Baltimore) 1987; 66:389–396.
6. Hann EA, Freemantle CJ, McCure JA, et al. Assignment of the gene for central core disease to chromosome 19. Hum Gent 1990;86:187–190.
7. Mulley JC, Kozman HM, Phillips A, et al. Refined genet-ic localization for central core disease. Am J Hum Genet 1993;52:398–405.
8. Heckmatt JZ, Sewry CA, Hodes D, Dubowitz V. Congen-ital centronuclear (myotubular) myopathy. A clinical, pathological and genetic study in eight children. Brain 1985;108:941–964.
9. Banker B. The congenital myopathies. In: Engel A, Banker B, eds. Myology. New York: McGraw-Hill, 1986: 1527–1581.
10. Oldfors A, Kyllerman M, Wahlstrom J, et al. X-linked myotubular myopathy: clinical and pathological findings in a family. Clin Genet 1989;36:5–14.
11. Darnfors C, Larsson HE, Oldfors A, et al. X-linked myotubular myopathy: a linkage study. Clin Genet 1990; 37:335–340.
12. Lehesjoki AE, Sankila EM, Miao J, et al. X-linked neonatal myotubular myopathy: one recombination detected with four polymorphic DNA markers from Xq28. J Med Genet 1990;27:288–291.
13. Thomas NS, Williams H, Cole G, et al. X-linked neonatal centronuclear/myotubular myopathy: evidence for linkage to Xq28 DNA marker loci. J Med Genet 1990;27:284–287.
14. Sarnat HB. Myotubular myopathy: arrest of morphogenesis of myofibres associated with persistence of fetal vimentin and desmin. Four cases compared with fetal and neonatal muscle. Can J Neurol Sci 1990;17:109–123.
15. Misra AK, Menon NK, Mishra SK. Abnormal distribution of desmin and vimentin in myofibers in adult onset myotub-ular myopathy. Muscle Nerve 1992;15:1246–1252.
16. Dubowitz V. Congenital myopathies. In: Dubowitz V, ed. Muscle biopsy: a practical approach, 2nd ed. London: Baillière Tindall, 1985:405–464.
17. Wallgren-Pettersson C. Congenital nemaline myopathy. A clinical follow-up study of twelve patients. J Neurol Sci 1989;89:1–14.
18. Laing NG, Majda BT, Akkari PA, et al. Assignment of a gene (NEMI) for autosomal dominant nemaline myo-pathy to chromosome 1. Am J Hum Genet 1992;50:576–583.
19. Wallgren-Pettersson C, Sainio K, Salmi T. Electromyo-graphy in congenital nemaline myopathy. Muscle Nerve 1989;12:587–593.
20. Martin JJ, Bruyland M, Busch HF, et al. Pleocore disease. Multi-minicore disease and focal loss of cross striations. Acta Neuropathol (Berl) 1986;72:142–149.
21. Brooke MH. Congenital fiber type disproportion. In: Kakulas BA, ed. Clinical studies in myology. Amsterdam: Excerpta Medica, 1971:147–159.
22. Clancy RR, Kelts KA, Oehlert JW. Clinical variability in congenital fiber type disproportion. J Neurol Sci 1980; 46:257–266.
23. Torres CF, Moxley RT. Early predictors of poor outcome in congenital fiber-type disproportion myopathy. Arch Neurol 1992;49:855–856.
24. Kyriakides T, Sillberstein J, Jongpiputvanich S, et al. The clinical significance of type 1 fiber predominance. Muscle Nerve 1993;16:418–423.
25. Heckmatt JZ, Dubowitz V, Leeman S. Detection of patho-logical change in dystrophic muscle with B-scan ultrasound imaging. Lancet 1980;i:1389–1390.
26. Heckmatt JZ, Leeman S, Dubowitz V. Ultrasound imaging in the diagnosis of muscle disease. J Paediatr 1982;101: 656–660.
27. Heckmatt JZ, Pier N, Dubowitz V. Real-time ultrasound imaging of muscles. Muscle Nerve 1988;11:56–65.
28. Wallgren-Pettersson C, Kivi L, Jääskeläinen J, et al. Ultrasonography, CT, and MRI of muscles in congenital nemaline myopathy. Pediatr Neurol 1990;6:20–28.
29. Bulcke JAL. Ultrasound and CT scanning in the diagnosis of neuromuscular disease. In: Gamstorp I, Sarnat HB, eds. Progressive spinal muscular atrophies. New York: Raven Press, 1984:153–161.
30. Arai Y, Sumida S, Osawa M, et al. Skeletal muscle CT scan and ultrasound imaging in two siblings with central core disease. No To Hattatsu 1990;22:55–60.
31. Reimers CD, Müller W, Schmidt-Achert M, et al. Quanti-tative skeletal muscle sonography: a useful tool in differen-tial diagnosis of generalized neuromuscular diseases? In: Bondestam S, Alanen A, Jouppila P, eds. Euroson '87 Proceedings. Helsinki: Finnish Society for Ultrasound in Medicine and Biology, 1987:241.
32. Dock WD, Happak W, Grabenwöger F, et al. Neuromus-cular diseases: evaluation with high-frequency sonography. Radiology 1990;177:825–828.
33. Lamminen A, Jääskeläinen J, Rapola J, Suramo I. High-frequency ultrasonography of skeletal muscle in children with neuromuscular disease. J Ultrasound Med 1988;7: 505–509.

34. O'Doherty DS, Schellinger D, Raptopoulos V. Computed tomographic patterns of pseudohypertrophic muscular dystrophy: preliminary results. J Comput Assist Tomogr 1977;1:482–486.

35. Hawley RJ, Schellinger D, O'Doherty DS. Computed tomographic patterns of muscles in neuromuscular diseases. Arch Neurol 1984;41:383–387.

36. Termote J-L, Baert A, Crolla D, et al. Computed tomography of the normal and pathologic muscular system. Radiology 1980;137:439–444.

37. Bulcke JAL, Baert AL. Clinical and radiological aspects of myopathies. Berlin: Springer, 1982.

38. Lamminen AE. Magnetic resonance imaging of primary skeletal muscle disease: patterns of distribution and severity of involvement. Br J Radiol 1990;63:946–950.

39. Maruyama T, Hanyu N, Maruyama K, et al. Clinical and pathological studies on two patients with adult-onset nemaline myopathy. Rinsho Shinkeigaku 1990;30:738–744.

40. Noda Y, Sakai K, Tojo M, et al. Nemaline myopathy of severe infantile type: a case report of a 9-year-old girl. No To Hattatsu 1990;22:82–85.

41. Shimizu J, Matsumura K, Noguchi H. A case of severe infantile form of congenital nemaline myopathy with extensive fatty replacement of the skeletal muscles. Rinsho Shinkeigaku 1990;30:1123–1127.

42. Borghi L, Savoldi F, Scelsi R, Villa M. Nuclear magnetic resonance of protons in normal and pathological human muscles. Exp Neurol 1983;81:89–96.

43. Rodiek SO. Kernspintomographie der Skelettmuskulatur bei neuromuskulären Erkrankungen. RÖFO 1985;143:418–425.

44. Fisher MR, Dooms CG, Hricak H, et al. Magnetic resonance imaging of the normal and pathologic muscular system. Magn Reson Imaging 1986;4:491–496.

45. Kaiser WA, Schalke BCG, Rohkamm R. Kernspintomographie in der Diagnostik von Muskelerkrankungen. RÖFO 1986;145:195–205.

46. Matsumura K, Nakano I, Fukuda N, et al. Proton spin-lattice relaxation times of Duchenne dystrophy skeletal muscle by magnetic resonance imaging. Muscle Nerve 1988;11:97–102.

47. Lamminen AE, Tanttu JI, Sepponen RE, et al. Magnetic resonance of diseased skeletal muscle: combined T1 measurement and chemical shift imaging. Br J Radiol 1990;63:591–596.

48. Murphy WA, Totty WG, Carroll JE. MRI of normal and pathologic skeletal muscle. Am J Roentgenol 1986;146:565–574.

49. Wallgren-Pettersson C, Rapola J, Donner M. Pathology of congenital nemaline myopathy. A follow-up study. J Neurol Sci 1988;83:243–257.

50. Udd B, Lamminen A, Somer H. Imaging findings reveal unexpected patchy lesions in late onset distal myopathy. Neuromuscul Disord 1991;1:279–285.

19
Inherited Defects of Muscle Energy Metabolism: Radiologic Evaluation

James L. Fleckenstein, Carl D. Reimers, and Ronald G. Haller

Disorders of muscle energy metabolism constitute an extremely diverse group of inherited defects that are generally associated with impaired aerobic and/or anaerobic muscle cell metabolism. These disorders can be categorized as defects of lysosomal glycogen handling, classic glycolysis, lipid metabolism, or mitochondrial structure and/or function.[1–4]

An imbalance between energy supply and demand during muscular exercise ultimately accounts for the majority of signs and symptoms in these myriad diseases. Symptomatology stems directly from failure in energy-dependent processes necessary for powering muscle contraction (exertional fatigue, weakness), for mediating muscular relaxation (muscle tightness, cramping), and/or for maintaining ion gradients necessary for normal membrane excitability (fatigue, weakness) and muscle cell integrity (muscle pain, injury, myoglobinuria). In contrast to the prominence of symptoms during exercise, symptoms and signs are often absent or inapparent at rest, when energy demands are low. The exercise intolerance of these patients is therefore frequently attributed to "being out of shape" and the true nature of the genetic defect goes undiagnosed until detailed exercise testing is performed.[1]

Abnormal biochemistry is clearly a critical mediator of fatigue and weakness in patients with defects of muscle energy metabolism. On the other hand, loss of muscle contractile mass (i.e., muscle atrophy), a common contributor to clinical deficits in many myopathies, is clinically recognized in only a few disorders of muscle energy metabolism (e.g., lysosomal glycogen storage disease, acid maltase deficiency).[2] In classic glycolytic defects, such as myophosphorylase and phosphofructokinase deficiencies, the cause of a form of weakness that is unrelated to fatigue ("fixed weakness") has therefore been difficult to elucidate.[3] The ability of radiological tools, and in particular magnetic resonance imaging (MRI), to noninvasively identify focal regions of clinically inapparent muscle atrophy is but one example of the capability of these noninvasive techniques to aid our understanding of mechanisms underlying functional deficits in myopathies. This chapter reviews clinically important structural and functional deficits in this diverse group of diseases, and reviews the impact of modern radiological techniques in their elucidation.

Genetic Defects of Muscle Glycogen Metabolism

Type I Glycogenosis

Chemically, glycogen is a branched homopolymer of glucose, an extremely large starch molecule resembling a tree with many secondary and tertiary branches.[4] For glycogen synthesis to occur, glucosyl units must be available, the primary source of which is glycogen breakdown in, and glucose release from, the liver. Hepatic glucose production is dependent upon the presence of normal activity of the enzyme glucose-6-phosphatase. When this enzyme is absent or defective, as in type I glycogen storage disease (Von Gierke's disease), glycogen accumulation occurs in the liver and kidneys, resulting in organomegaly and related alteration.[2] Although this was the first-named glycogenosis, Von Gierke's disease merits no further discussion here because the enzyme involved is normally absent from muscle and myopathy is not a feature of the disease.

Upon entry to the muscle cell, glucose is phosphorylated to glucose-6-phosphate, which can then be converted to glycogen to store energy, or can be metabolized to release energy via glycolysis.[3] Defects in these metabolic pathways result in the majority of recognized glycogenoses, which have been assigned Roman numerals in approximate agreement with their order of discovery (Figure 19.1). The most common glycogenosis, type II, however, does not involve either of the major catabolic or anabolic pathways, but rather involves a rather enig-

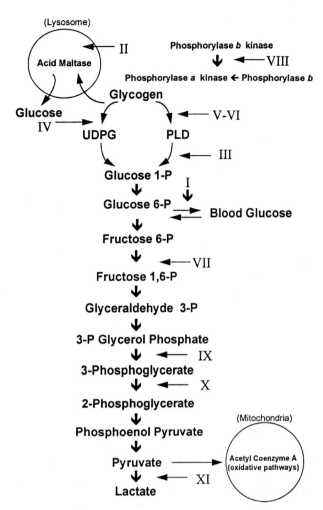

FIGURE 19.1. Metabolic pathways of muscle cell metabolism and inherited enzyme defects occurring in humans. Named glycogenoses are denoted with Roman numerals, as described in the text.

matic lysosomal enzyme, acid maltase. Despite the fact that little is known about the precise metabolic role of this enzyme, inherited deficiencies of it frequently result in clinically profound muscular abnormalities.

Type II Glycogenosis

Acid maltase deficiency (AMD) can be separated into three recognized groups: infantile, childhood, and adult AMD.[2] In the infantile form (Pompe's disease), massive quantities of glycogen (8 to 15% of the tissue wet weight) accumulate in the muscles, heart, and liver. Few patients with infantile AMD survive 1 yr, whereas patients with childhood AMD frequently survive into the second decade. Glycogen excess is less marked in the childhood form although it approaches 10% of the wet weight in severely affected muscles. Patients with adult AMD present after the age of 20, either with myopathy or

respiratory difficulties, and respiratory failure is the cause of death in most patients. Glycogen excess is milder in adult AMD than in younger patients.

The milder clinical course of childhood and adult forms apparently depends upon the absolute residual activity of the enzyme in affected tissue. Although muscle glycogen accumulation is severe and weakness pronounced, cytosolic glycogenolysis apparently proceeds normally so that clinical hallmarks of defective glycogenolysis (i.e., impaired muscle lactate production and muscle necrosis) are absent. An inexplicable feature of adult AMD is a peculiarly selective pattern of severe muscle deterioration, as delineated by cross-sectional imaging studies, described below.

Type III Glycogenosis

Muscle glycogen is the crucial source of energy during high-intensity aerobic and/or anaerobic exercise (70 to 80% V_{O_2max}). In order for glycogen degradation to proceed to completion, the enzymatic hydrolysis to glucose 1-phosphate requires the active form of the muscle enzyme phosphorylase.[3] However, phosphorylase by itself is able only to degrade about 35% of the glycogen molecule due to the fact that it cannot digest the alpha-1,6-glucosidically-linked glucose unit present at each branch point of the polysaccharide. Debrancher enzyme is required for this vital function and its absence results in type III glycogenosis (Cori-Forbes disease).

This disease is most usually a benign disease of childhood dominated by liver dysfunction and hypoglycemia. Myopathy is relatively uncommon, but when present is characterized by severe excess accumulation of partially digested glycogen. Muscles of these patients are unable to become significantly acidotic upon exercise due to the block in glycogenolysis. This accounts for the fact that during ischemic exercise, venous lactate levels fail to rise normally, that is, patients have a positive result on the "ischemic lactate test," a feature shared by other glycogenoses in which glycogenolysis is blocked. Interestingly, unlike other glycogenolytic defects, exercise intolerance, muscle cramps, and myoglobinuria are relatively uncommon whereas muscular weakness is occasionally prominent. The weakness is not explained on the basis of muscle atrophy in the few cases in which muscle imaging has been done (see below).

Type IV Glycogenosis

Just as a genetic defect can occur in the breakdown of glycogen branch points, genetic impairment of production of the branched glycogen molecule also occurs, as in glycogenosis type IV, Andersen's disease. In this disorder, absence of a transglycosylase enzyme (a.k.a. branching enzyme) results in a rapidly progressive disease of infancy dominated by liver dysfunction. Although hypotonia and muscle wasting are described, myopathy is overshadowed by the liver disease.[3]

Types V and VI Glycogenoses

Assuming an intact ability to synthesize glycogen and to degrade its branched structure, the capacity to generate energy from the glucosyl units that constitute the polysaccharide requires a series of enzymes that eventually produce adenosine triphosphate (ATP), the most fundamental unit of bioenergetics. Stores of ATP are meager in the cell and so muscle activity is highly dependent upon the ability to resynthesize ATP upon demand. Glycolysis is a critical source of substrate in this process and it begins with intracellular glucose phosphorylated at the C6 position. Although blood glucose is phosphorylated to glucose-6-phosphate by hexokinase as described above, glycogen must first be broken down to glucose-1-phosphate before being converted to glucose-6-phosphate by the action of phosphoglucomutase. Because the vast majority of substrate becomes available via glycogen metabolism, the ability to generate glucose-1-phosphate from glycogen is of obvious importance. This reaction requires an active form of the enzyme phosphorylase. Glycogenoses V and VI are named for deficiencies of the muscle and hepatic forms of phosphorylase, respectively, only the former of which interests us here. In 1951, McArdle first described a patient in whom muscle phosphorylase was inactive.[3] Hence, glycogenosis V was named after McArdle.

McArdle's patient presented with what is now recognized as characteristic signs and symptoms of muscle phosphorylase deficiency. Exercise intolerance, manifested by myalgia, early fatigue, and muscle stiffness or weakness of the exercising muscle, are the hallmarks of the disease. Two kinds of exercise are particularly poorly tolerated—brief intense work, such as isometric muscle contractions, or less intense but sustained work, such as climbing stairs. Most patients adapt to their limitations; however, when they exceed their limits, they experience painful muscle cramps, called muscle contractures, that are electrically silent on electromyography. These contractures are associated with muscle necrosis and myoglobinuria and about 25% of patients suffer renal failure at least once in their lives, as a result of rhabdomyolysis.

Fixed weakness (i.e., weakness that is present at rest), unrelated to the level of activity, is reported in approximately one-third of patients, especially in older patients. It was McArdle's observation of the inability of his patients to produce venous lactate after ischemic exercise that was the critical clue to the presence of a block in glycogen breakdown. It is now well known that a positive ischemic lactate test is not specific for glycogenosis V, but rather is an indicator of impaired glycogenolysis, and is sensitive to defects in debrancher enzyme or more "downstream" enzymes. The inability to break down glycogen is not only the basis of impaired lactate generation during exercise but also of the inability to cause a related muscle acidosis, a finding that is detectable using the noninvasive technique of ^{31}P-magnetic resonance spectroscopy (MRS) (see Chapter 9).

Histochemical study of muscle biopsy specimens shows increased accumulation of glycogen in McArdle's disease, but to a lesser extent than in other glycogenoses, accounting for less than 3% of weight in greater than two-thirds of patients. Histochemical staining of biopsied muscle shows reduced or absent phosphorylase activity. Importantly, recently injured muscle in McArdle's disease may show a small amount of phosphorylase activity due to elaboration of a "fetal" form of the enzyme, a point to remember when using imaging findings to guide the site for muscle biopsy (see below).

Type VII Glycogenosis

After glucose-1-phosphate is liberated from glycogen and transformed into glucose-6-phosphate, it next forms fructose-6-phosphate by the action of phosphohexoisomerase. Fructose-6-phosphate is then phosphorylated by the major regulatory enzyme, phosphofructokinase (PFK), to become glucose-1,6-diphosphate. PFK deficiency, or glycogenosis VII, was first recognized by Tauri in 1965.[3] Clinical features overlap with McArdle's disease in that exercise intolerance, early fatigability, and exertional muscle cramps occur. Although the latter occurs with a lesser frequency in PFK deficiency, exercise performed under ischemic conditions results in an electrically silent muscle contracture, similar to that occurring in McArdle's patients. Ischemic exercise in both conditions is associated with an inability to produce muscle lactate and acidosis upon muscle exertion. Notable differences are well recognized, however, and include that patients with PFK deficiency have an hemolytic anemia due to reduced PFK activity in the red blood cell. PFK-deficient patients have a relatively greater propensity to develop fixed weakness compared to McArdle's disease, the cause of which has remained enigmatic until recently, when selective muscle atrophy in PFK deficiency was reported using diagnostic imaging.

Although muscle biopsy shows glycogen to be increased in PFK deficiency to a similar degree as in McArdle's disease, biopsy definitively establishes the distinction from phosphorylase deficiency by use of a direct PFK stain. Interestingly, ^{31}P-MRS also reveals a striking contrast from McArdle's disease. Whereas in both diseases there is absence of the normal fall in muscle pH during exercise, in PFK deficiency, but not in McArdle's disease, glycolytic intermediates accumulate in the form of phosphorylated monoesters (PME) that are detected as a discrete peak. Absence of the PME peak in McArdle's disease is expected because of the inability to cleave glucosyl units from glycogen, as described above.[5] However, this finding alone does not distinguish PFK deficiency from other enzyme defects in which glycolysis is blocked distal to phosphorylase.

Types VIII to X Glycogenoses

Phosphorylase b kinase (PBK), phosphoglycerate kinase (PGK), and phosphoglycerate mutase (PGM) enzymes are deficient in glycogenoses VIII to X, respectively.[3] They will be discussed only very briefly here because no imaging findings have been reported to date. PBK is an important regulator of glycogen metabolism because it converts phosphorylase from the less active b form to the more active a form and, at the same time, converts glycogen synthetase from a more active dephosphorylated form to a less active phosphorylated form. Four distinct clinical syndromes of PBK are recognized, depending on the degree of hepatic or muscle involvement.[3] PGK-deficient patients may present with myopathy or hemolytic anemia, similar to patients with PFK deficiency. ^{31}P-MRS studies also resemble PFK deficiency, although a small pH drop during exercise distinguishes PGK patients. PGM deficiency has been reported in six patients.[3] Glycogen accumulation tends to be only modestly increased in muscle biopsies of patients with glycogenoses VIII to X.

Type XI Glycogenosis

Pyruvate is formed as a penultimate step in glycogenolysis, prior to oxidation and formation of acetyl coenzyme A, which enters the Krebs cycle to fuel oxidative phosphorylation. However, pyruvate has an alternative fate, which is to be reduced by the enzyme lactate dehydrogenase (LDH) to form lactate, which deficiency cannot be further metabolized in muscle and is released into the plasma. Lactate dehydrogenase deficiency has been called type XI glycogenosis.[3] The bloodstream carries it to the liver, which in turn transforms it, via a complex set of reactions (gluconeogenesis) into glucose and glycogen. The Cori cycle is complete when hepatic glycogen is again broken down into glucose for transport to the body cells, especially those of muscle.

Although deficiency of LDH is exceedingly rare, we have had the opportunity of clinically evaluating three such patients. The clinical presentation includes exercise intolerance and painful exertional cramps. Diagnosis rests upon the finding of low blood lactate and elevated pyruvate levels upon exercise.

Myoadenylate Deaminase Deficiency

Myoadenylate deaminase (MD) catalyzes the deamination of adenosine monophosphate (AMP) to inosine monophosphate (IMP), the first step in the adenine nucleotide cycle. MD deficiency is the most frequent recessively inherited metabolic myopathy. The enzyme is absent in about 1 to 2% of muscle biopsies surveyed.[6] It is associated with exertional cramps, but the majority of persons with this defect are asymptomatic.[7] Clinical findings are usually normal, although serum creatine kinase may be slightly elevated and the electromyogram slightly myopathic. During ischemic exercise, venous ammonia levels fail to rise normally. Light microscopy reveals no additional abnormalities.

Genetic Defects of Lipid Metabolism

Although glycogen breakdown is important in maintaining oxidative phosphorylation by providing 2-carbon units to the Krebs cycle, fats and free fatty acids (FFA) are far more important quantitatively, especially in the resting state and during submaximal exercise. The diversity of myopathies involving lipid metabolism exceeds the scope of this chapter, particularly in view of the paucity of reported imaging findings. Briefly, however, they span defects in the transport of FFAs into the mitochondrion and subsequent steps, including the processes of beta oxidation, the respiratory chain, and the utilization of endogenously synthesized triglyceride.[1,8]

Carnitine Palmitoyl Transferase

The transport of FFA into the mitochondria requires a special transport system involving carnitine and carnitine palmitoyl transferase (CPT).[9] The major effect of CPT deficiency on muscle is an increased dependence upon carbohydrate oxidation to support muscular work. As long as carbohydrate is available, exercise capacity is not impaired. However, when muscle glycogen is depleted (such as by fasting, prolonged exercise, or both), exertion may induce muscle pain and injury attributable to the inability to oxidize FFA. In the absence of myoglobinuria, laboratory tests are usually unremarkable. Hepatic lipid accumulation may be increased and ketogenesis upon fasting is delayed, suggesting that liver CPT is also deficient in these patients, although acute hepatic dysfunction is not a feature of the myopathy. A pure hepatic form of the disease is recognized. Muscle biopsy may reveal nonspecific changes related to previous muscle injury. Specific assays showing reduced CPT activity are required for the diagnosis.

Mitochondrial Myopathies

Mitochondrial myopathies consist of a heterogeneous group of disorders that are primarily or even solely caused by defects of mitochondrial DNA, which is maternally inherited. Most of these defects also involve tissues other than skeletal muscle. Hence, the clinical features of any specific disorder depend upon the nature of the biochemical defect and the pattern of organ involvement.

There is no consistent correlation between biochemical and clinical features. The biochemical abnormalities can be classified into defects of the substrate transport (e.g., CPT deficiency), of the utilization of substrate (e.g., carnitine deficiency syndromes), of the respiratory chain (e.g., complex I to V deficiencies), and in energy production (e.g., ATP synthase deficiency). Many mitochondrial myopathies exhibit elevated levels of lactate and pyruvate in the serum at rest and normal, or even exaggerated, exercise-induced lactate production due to a dependence upon anaerobic sources of fuel, chiefly glycogen.

The heterogeneous clinical features include variable involvement of limb and trunk muscles, predominance of central nervous abnormalities, and ophthalmoplegia. Muscle involvement may result in easy fatigability or permanent muscle weakness and wasting. Patients are distinguished from most of the glycogenoses by relative dominance of progressive weakness and by rarity of painful exertion-induced muscle cramps and myoglobinuria. Severe progressive encephalopathies (e.g., defects of pyruvate utilization) and cardiomyopathy (e.g., Kearns-Sayre syndrome) may complicate or even dominate the clinical course and result in early death. Progressive external ophthalmoplegia (PEO) is a primary feature in a variety of mitochondrial disorders and, when it occurs, the term "ophthalmoplegia plus syndrome" is sometimes used.

These diseases are classically defined by the presence of "ragged red" fibers on light microscopy, although such fibers are not obligate morphological features. They show a predominantly subsarcolemmal accumulation of abnormal mitochondria and a rim of irregular bright red or reddish-blue material in sections stained with the modified Gomori technique. Biopsy specimens may also show slight to severe muscle fibrosis and lipomatosis.

Imaging Findings

Relatively little information exists in the scientific literature regarding the distribution, etiology, and significance of focal muscle lesions in disorders of muscle energy metabolism.[10–35] This is surprising given the frequency of focal muscle atrophy in some of the disorders (e.g., AMD) and the occurrence of fixed weakness in others (e.g., PFK deficiency), which might reasonably be guessed to be due to mesenchymal deterioration of specific muscles. The authors, however, have considerable experience in imaging these disorders and a summary of our cases, together with a review of the available literature, follows in an attempt to familiarize interested individuals in the kinds, and distribution, of muscle abnormalities that may be expected in disorders of muscle energy metabolism.

Glycogenoses

To our knowledge, no studies have reported on radiographic findings in glycogenoses. Only one study described scintigraphic findings. There it was found that ^{99m}Tc pyrophosphate is avid for muscles that were damaged as a result of muscle contractures, which supported the occurrence of muscle necrosis as a result of muscle contracture.[11] This added to the long list of conditions in which the soft tissues are avid for pyrophosphates (see Chapter 1).

Type I Glycogenosis (Von Gierke's Disease)

No studies have been reported.

Type II Glycogenosis (Pompe's Disease, Acid Maltase Deficiency)

Ultrasound

In infantile AMD, Heckmatt et al.[12–14] found normal echointensities and muscle hypertrophy in one child. Hence, there are no data to promote the possibility that ultrasound is an effective tool to screen for Pompe's disease.

In a study of the adult form, Forst[15] reported increased echointensity and indistinct fasciae and septae in paraspinal and calf muscles of one patient. Reimers[16] found increased echointensities predominantly in the biceps brachii, vasti, and soleus muscles. The size of muscles, defined by fascial boundaries and not muscle content, reportedly is not altered. Abnormal echointensities, suggesting marked parenchymal changes, are presumably due to fatty deposition, as suggested by subsequent computed tomography (CT) and MRI studies (see below).

Computed Tomography

Two studies reported on findings of the paraspinal and lower extremity muscles.[17,18] In thighs, Herson et al. described prominent fatty changes in adductors, vastus medialis, and biceps femoris muscles.[17]

A relatively large CT study compared the incidence of paraspinal muscle abnormalities in types II and V glycogenoses. In that report, fatty deterioration of the psoas and erector spinae muscles was found to be very frequent in adult AMD (7 out of 9 patients). Erector spinae fatty deterioration was also common in myophosphorylase deficiency (6 out of 10 patients) but in none of those was there also atrophy of the psoas. The authors concluded with the optimistic proposition that radiologists may be able to suggest the type of myopathy present by the distribution of deteriorated muscles seen in patients whose lumbar spine MRI or CT scans disclosed selective atrophy. This conclusion does not consider that other diseases may also preferentially involve the psoas and erector spinae, including muscular dystrophies, myositis, and mitochondrial myopathies (Figure 19.2). Hence, the occurrence of a selective distribution of paraspinal muscle deterioration appears to be nonspecific in establishing

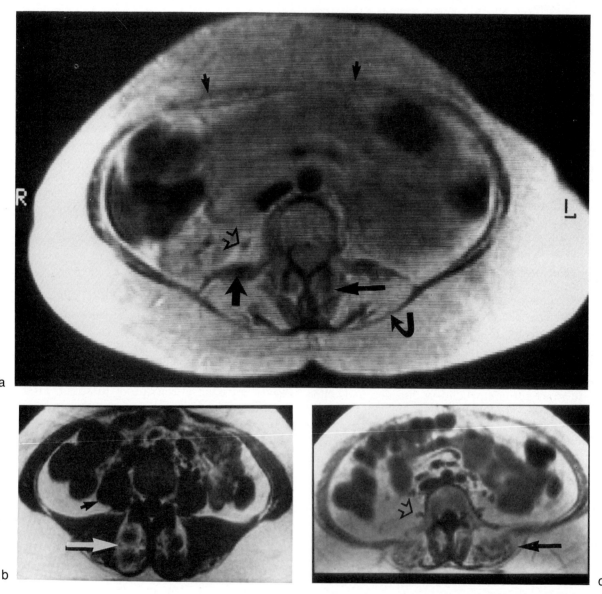

FIGURE 19.2. Trunk muscle atrophy in the unoperated back: a hint to metabolic myopathy. T_1-weighted MRI (500/30, a) of a patient with adult AMD shows marked deterioration and fatty replacement (high signal intensity) of the rectus abdominus (small arrows), psoas (open arrowhead), and erector spinae (curved arrow). Atrophy of multifidus muscles is only mild (arrow) and the quadratus lumborum is normal in appearance (thick arrow). Selective atrophy of erector spinae muscle is seen less commonly in myophosphorylase deficiency (500/30, arrow, b), although sparing of the psoas is typical (small arrow, b). Trunk muscle atrophy is a nonspecific finding, however, and may also be seen in oxidative energy defects such as in a patient with a mitochondrial myopathy, NADH-CoQ reductase deficiency, in whom the psoas is obliterated (500/30, arrowhead, c), and erector spinae atrophy is severe (arrow).

diagnoses. However, that muscle deterioration occurs in selective locations in AMD as well as other glycogenoses remains a compelling observation. Such findings offer radiologists the opportunity to suggest the presence of a significant disease in patients in whom the spine is being evaluated to search for a cause of weakness. It should be noted that paraspinal muscle atrophy is also readily apparent in a substantial percentage of patients with chronic low back pain (approximately 20% in those with previous lumbar surgery, presenting with "failed back syndrome").[19] In one of the authors' experience, the incidence of mild, diffuse fatty change in a randomly selected group of 100 patients with back pain but no previous surgery was considerably smaller, at about 5% (unpublished observations, JLF).

Magnetic Resonance Imaging

Kaiser and Schalke[20] described a 44-yr-old woman with degeneration of the quadriceps femoris and adductor magnus muscles, whereas the anteromedial and dorsal thigh muscles were less affected. Nägele and Reimers[21] found increased signal intensities, especially in the vasti and soleus muscles and in the hamstrings.

In the authors' series of MRI of the thighs in nine patients with adult AMD, severe fatty deterioration of muscles was identified in all patients, correlating with advanced muscular weakness. In all cases, involved muscles included the vastus intermedius and the short head of the biceps femoris, with more variable and milder involvement of other muscles (Figures 19.2, 19.3).

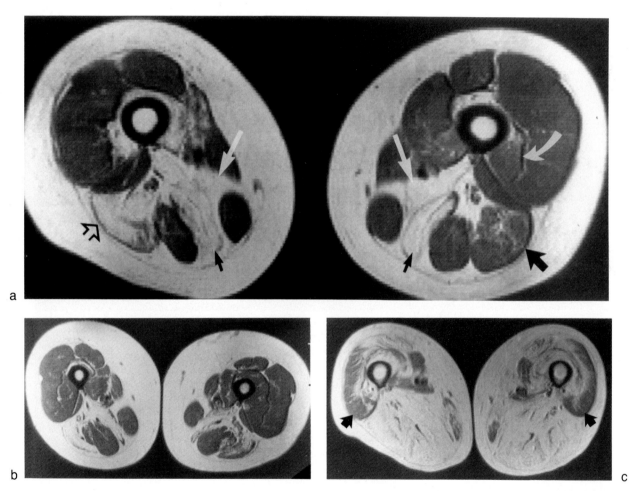

FIGURE 19.3. Thigh muscle atrophy in adult AMD in patients with proximal weakness. T_1-weighted images (500/15) in the three illustrated cases show high signal intensity (fatty degeneration) of the adductor magnus (e.g., arrows, a) and semimembranosus (e.g., small arrows, a). In the first case, fatty change is asymmetric in some muscles, such as in the long head of the biceps femoris, which is nearly obliterated on the right (open arrowhead, a) but minimal on the left (thick arrow). Also note that the vastus intermedius is partially intact on the left (curved arrow). Note a similar distribution of changes in the second patient (b). In a wheelchair-bound patient, only small volumes of muscle remain present (e.g., vastus lateralis) (arrowheads, c).

The cause of the selectivity of muscle deterioration in AMD is unknown. Possibilities include that the lysosomal content of these muscles is especially high and/or that these muscles are particularly dependent upon normal activity of acid maltase to resist deterioration.

It is interesting that in AMD although the muscle is replaced by fat, the overall configuration of the muscle is preserved without deformation of intermuscular fascia (Figure 19.3). This feature was described by Bulcke and Baert as the "filling up process," a nonspecific feature most commonly seen in muscular dystrophies.[23] The feature contrasts the appearance of other conditions, such as long-standing polymyositis, in which muscle atrophy and increased adiposity are associated with volume loss of the muscular compartment and resulting undulation of the intermuscular fasciae (see Chapter 21).

Type III Glycogenosis (Cori-Forbes Disease, Debrancher Disease)

Ultrasound

No studies have been reported.

Computed Tomography

Marbini et al.[24] reported muscle pseudohypertrophy and small, patchy foci of hypodensity diffusely distributed in the thighs of one adult patient, suspected of being composed of fat.

Magnetic Resonance Imaging

The authors' unpublished series includes two patients with glycogen debrancher deficiency. No support for fatty replacement of muscle was detected using MRI.

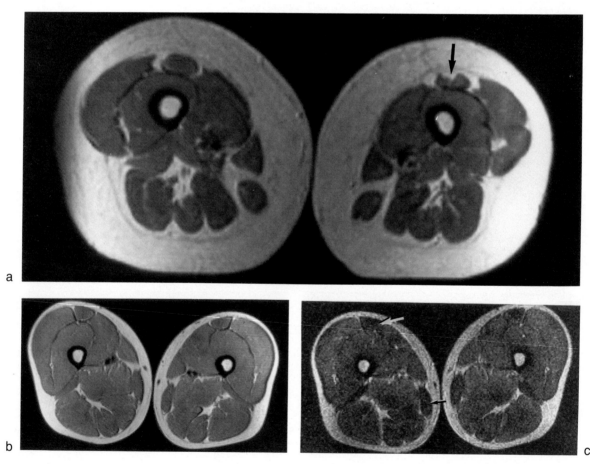

FIGURE 19.4. Thigh muscle alterations in glycogen debrancher (Forbes) disease. In the first patient, muscle signal intensity is diffusely increased on spin density image (2000/30, a), but this abnormality is not detectable subjectively because all muscles are similarly affected. The calculated T_2 times of all of this patient's muscles were markedly prolonged (approximately 40 ms, compared to normal values in the same laboratory of 28

$\pm$ 1 ms). The left rectus femoris muscle is deformed due to prior biopsy (arrow). A similar overall appearance is noted on spin density image in a second patient (2500/20, b) but prolonged T_2 times can be suspected on visual inspection of T_2-weighted image (2500/90, c) because the rectus femoris (arrow) and gracilis (small arrow) are less severely affected.

Rather a mild, diffusely increased signal intensity only on T_2-weighted images was noted, due to a prolonged T_2 time (Figure 19.4). Muscle edema is unlikely to account for the change due to absence of concomitant increases in T_1 times, increases that were found in other glycogenolytic disorders due to increased water content presumed to be related to concomitant muscle necrosis. Because muscle biopsies have shown muscles in this glycogenosis to be particularly rich in excess glycogen, the T_2 elevations are speculated to result from these alterations in some way. This is indirectly supported by the finding that T_2 times were slightly elevated in grossly normal appearing muscles in other glycogenoses, specifically myophosphorylase deficiency and PFK deficiency, in which glycogen excess is known to be less severe.[3] In any case, the finding of diffuse, mildly increased T_2 times of muscle in a patient suspected of having a myopathy is nonspecific, with similar findings noted in amyloid myopathy, among others.[25]

Type IV Glycogenosis (Andersen's Disease, Branching Enzyme Deficiency)

No imaging studies have been reported.

Type V Glycogenosis (McArdle's Disease, Myophosphorylase Deficiency)

Ultrasound

Only normal ultrasound findings were described in two reports.[16,26]

Computed Tomography

A report finding a moderately high incidence of paraspinal muscle atrophy was commented upon above.

Magnetic Resonance Imaging

Our experience with MRI of focal muscle deterioration in myophosphorylase deficiency proceeded along two routes. First, prospective evaluation of muscle contracture helped to understand the time course of pathological changes that occur as a result of brief, but intense and sustained muscular contraction. In the second, the incidence of focal muscle lesions that develop during activities of daily living as a result of contractures was assessed.

MRI of muscle contracture revealed that immediately upon development of the electrically silent cramp, no alteration in signal intensity or proton relaxation times was observed.[27] This is, in fact, an abnormal finding, because exercise normally produces a transient increase in these parameters (see Chapter 7). Given the wealth of data indicating that MRI is sensitive to muscle pathology during injury, it is noteworthy that acutely (less than 1 day) contractured muscle does not show edema-like

changes. This finding is consistent with histopathological studies indicating absence of pathological changes despite marked pain upon contracture.

When MRI was performed in two patients 24 h after contracture,[28] edematous changes of the midbellies of muscles stressed by the activity were observed, indicating a departure from the usual site of exertion-related muscle injury in otherwise healthy subjects (i.e., the muscle–tendon junction (Figure 19.5). The significance of this departure is unknown. The signal intensity characteristics were, however, identical to those seen in exertional injuries of normal subjects, including elevation of T_1 and T_2 relaxation times (Figures 19.5, 19.6). Prolonged follow-up in two patients identified to have edematous muscles within a few days of muscle contractures revealed complete recovery of the muscles by MRI criteria (Figure 19.5). The capacity to recover completely from even severe myonecrosis was supported by our observation of only normal appearing muscles in a 54-yr-old patient who participated in combat and climbed the cliffs of Normandy, France, during World War II, despite contractures and repeated episodes of myoglobinuria. Although mild fatty changes of muscle are sometimes observed on MRI in McArdle's disease, the relative frequency of normal-appearing muscles is striking in contrast to a tendency to develop severe deterioration of muscle mass in patients with other glycogenoses (e.g., types II and VII) in whom muscle contractures and pigmenturia are less common, but in whom early fatiguability and "fixed weakness" occur with greater frequency.

Of practical note, when edematous foci are identified in imaging studies of patients with undiagnosed muscle conditions, these areas should be avoided during biopsy when McArdle's disease is suspected. In such patients, relatively normal-appearing muscle is favored as a site for biopsy because necrotic muscle may produce a small amount of fetal phosphorylase.[3] This is important and contrasts the situation in inflammatory myopathy where edematous muscle is favored for biopsy (see Chapter 21).

Type VII Glycogenosis (Tauri's Disease, PFK Deficiency)

Ultrasound and Computed Tomography

No imaging studies have been reported.

Magnetic Resonance Imaging

Our experience in six patients with PFK deficiency suggests an apparent predisposition to development of focal structural lesions.[28] These include edematous foci (prolonged T_1 and T_2 relaxation times and increased spin densities) occurring in the setting of clinical evidence of

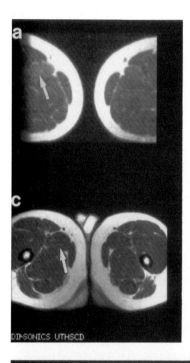

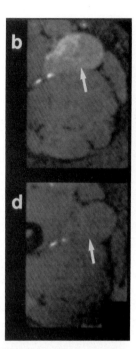

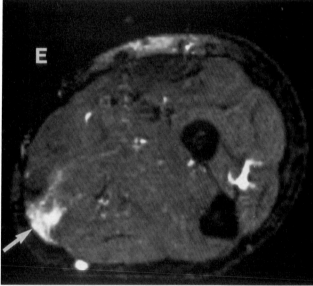

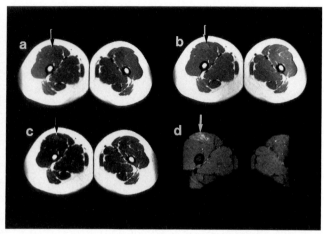

FIGURE 19.6. Relative sensitivity of pulse sequences in detecting muscle necrosis in glycogenoses. This patient with myophosphorylase deficiency had mild right thigh pain when scanned. The typical appearance of necrosis-related edema is illustrated in the right rectus femoris (arrow) by normal signal intensity using T_1 weighting (500/30, a), and visible but subtle increase in signal intensity on spin density (2000/30, b) and T_2-weighted (2000/60, c) images, which becomes obvious when a fat-suppression, edema-sensitive sequence such as STIR is used (1500/30/100, d). In the authors' experience, the rectus femoris is the muscle most frequently biopsied when image guidance is not employed. However, edematous areas such as that illustrated should be avoided during biopsy when McArdle's disease is suspected because necrotic muscle produces a small amount of fetal phosphorylase, thus providing a cause for a false-negative histopathological result. In these patients, relatively normal appearing muscle is favored as a site for biopsy.

FIGURE 19.5. Muscle contractures in myophosphorylase deficiency. One day after sustaining a "groin pull" during sexual intercourse, the patient underwent MRI evaluation. A spin density MRI sequence of the thighs shows subtle increase in signal intensity in the right adductor longus (1500/30, arrow, a). Using the highly sensitive, fat-suppression STIR sequence, the edematous abnormality is more conspicuous (1500/30/100, arrow, b). Three months later, a moderately T_2-weighted sequence showed resolution of the lesion (2000/60, arrow, c), an impression supported by a normal appearance using STIR (arrow, d). On the day of the latter examination, the patient performed handgrip exercise that was stopped at the earliest suggestion of a contracture. No MRI change was seen at that time.[27] The following day, however, a small volume of edema was seen using a STIR sequence in the midportion of the flexor digitorum superficialis (1500/30/100, arrow, e).

severe muscle injury, including contracture (Figure 19.7). Fatty deterioration of the adductor magnus without substantial edematous change was seen in two older patients (Figure 19.8). Concurrence of fatty infiltration and edema of muscles was seen in one remarkable older patient with the disease, raising the question of a causal relationship between recurrent muscle injury and fatty deterioration (Figure 19.9).

It is interesting to note that these patients report relatively fewer episodes of muscle pain and pigmenturia than do McArdle's patients.[3] Lines of speculation of what these data mean in terms of the pathogenesis of muscle loss in glycogenosis VII include the possiblity that pain limits further exertion and hence progressive injury in McArdle's disease, whereas the more subclinical pattern of progressive injury in Tauri's disease ultimately causes a more severe end-stage myopathy. An alternative viewpoint supposes that whatever determines the ultimate progression to fatty change is less dependent on the muscle injury and more related to an impaired healing response. To our knowledge, there are no additional data available to promote these or any theories. In any

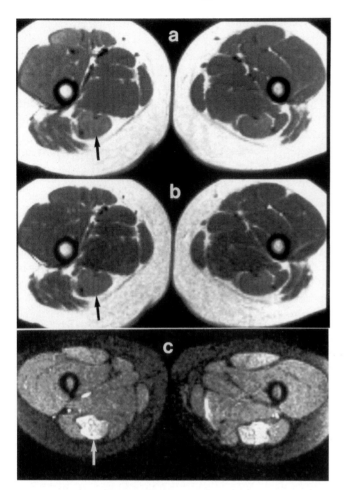

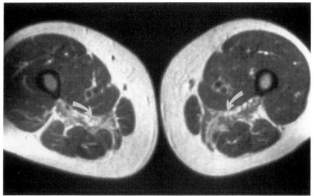

FIGURE 19.8. Fatty infiltration and atrophy in PFK deficiency. A 48-yr-old man had recurrent subclinical rhabdomyolysis and exercise intolerance. Bilateral atrophy and fatty change of the adductor magnus is evident by increased signal intensity on T_1-weighted MRI (500/30, arrows).

FIGURE 19.7. Necrosis-related edema in PFK deficiency. This patient presented for MRI with hamstring pain sustained while dancing 3 days earlier, associated with marked elevation of serum creatine kinase. Symmetrically increased signal intensity is subtle in the semitendinosi (e.g., arrow) on spin density (2000/30, a) and T_2-weighted images (2000/60, b) but is obvious using STIR (1500/30/100, c).

case, why one muscle is any more or less susceptible to injury or healing deserves careful scrutiny because it is apparently a feature of a great many myopathies of disparate etiologies.

Types VIII to X Glycogenoses (PBK, PGK, PGM)

Ultrasound, Computed Tomography, Magnetic Resonance Imaging

No imaging studies have been reported.

Type XI Glycogenosis (Lactate Dehydrogenase Deficiency)

Ultrasound and Computed Tomography

No imaging studies have been reported.

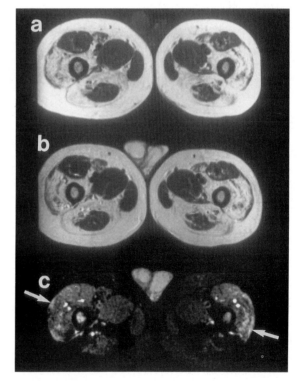

FIGURE 19.9. Coexisting intramuscular fat and edema in a patient with PFK deficiency who walked 1 to 2 miles each day as a self-prescribed treatment for his previously undiagnosed condition. T_1-weighted (500/30, a) and T_2-weighted (2000/60, b) images of the thighs demonstrate marked replacement of most thigh muscles by high signal intensity fat. STIR (1500/30/100, c) suppresses signal intensity from fat, whereas areas of high signal intensity identify regions of coexistent muscle edema in the vastus lateralis (arrows).

Magnetic Resonance Imaging

In the one patient we have scanned with LDH deficiency, a screening study of the upper and lower extremities failed to disclose an abnormality. During the course of his clinical investigation, the patient recognized his first muscle contracture. Serum muscle enzyme markers rose to markedly elevated levels. MRI showed marked edematous changes in the injured muscles 48 to 72 h after the inciting event.

Myoadenylate Deaminase Deficiency

Ultrasound

Only normal ultrasound findings were observed in one report.[16]

Computed Tomography

No studies have been reported.

Magnetic Resonance Imaging

Nägele and Reimers[21] found essentially normal findings in calf muscles. One of the authors (JLF) scanned the thighs and legs of one additional patient and no abnormality was found.

Genetic Defects of Lipid Metabolism

Muscle imaging findings are highly variable in this diverse group of disorders, paralleling the heterogeneity of the diseases themselves. Only a few reports of imaging results of the muscles are present in the literature.

Carnitine Palmitoyl Transferase Deficiency

Ultrasound and Computed Tomography

No studies have been reported.

Magnetic Resonance Imaging

In the authors' experience, muscles of 3 patients showed only normal findings. T_1 and T_2 relaxation times were normal in all cases. Use of MRI to examine the acute response of muscle to exercise (as described in Chapter 7) was normal in each case.

Mitochondrial Myopathies

Ultrasound

In two patients with carnitine deficiency, Reimers (1990)[16] found considerably increased echointensities in almost all muscles examined. Forst[15] described slightly increased echointensities in the paravertebral and thigh muscles as well as markedly increased echointensities in the calf muscles in a weak boy with ophthalmoplegia plus, whereas Heckmatt et al.[13] revealed no sonographic abnormalities in a boy with Kearns-Sayre syndrome. Reimers[16] found atrophy with slightly increased echointensities as the only abnormal finding in some mitochondrial myopathy patients, whereas the more severely affected patients presented with moderate muscle atrophy, especially of the lower extremities.

Computed Tomography

Hansman et al.[30] described bilateral atrophy of the extraocular muscles in one patient with ophthalmoplegia. Serratrice et al.[31] found diffuse muscular hypodensities in another patient, whereas Reimers[16] found normal findings or small low-density areas especially in the calf muscles of ophthalmoplegic patients.

Magnetic Resonance Imaging

In the series of Nägele and Reimers the majority of the patients with ophthalmoplegia plus revealed slight or moderate deposition of fat in the legs, and less prominent fat in thigh muscles.[22] The abnormalities were most evident in the sartorius, tibialis anterior, soleus, gastrocnemius, and hamstring muscles.

The authors studied both acute effects of exercise on muscle signal intensities and relaxation times, as well as the incidence of structural lesions in muscles of the lower extremities in a series of patients with mitochondrial defects.[32] Acute, transient effects of exercise on MRI of muscle with impaired oxidative capacity due to mitochondrial deficiencies were more variable than in patients with glycogenoses (see Chapter 7). Results ranged from exaggerated to subnormal increases in muscle T_2 times. The significance of this variability is uncertain and awaits further study but may relate to concomitant neuropathic abnormalities and/or exaggerated blood flow to active muscles in some patients (more efficient washout of lactate-mediated accumulation of extravascular water).

Our study of thigh muscles in 11 patients with mitochondrial myopathies disclosed that gross muscle structural deterioration, characterized by atrophy and a "marbling" type of fatty replacement, was common, particularly in patients with ophthalmoplegia.[32] In this subset of patients, selective deterioration of the sartorius and gracilis muscles was particularly common (Figures 19.1, 19.10 to 19.13).

Selective deterioration of the sartorius and gracilis muscles in association with weakness of the extraocular muscles raises the possibility that some feature shared by these muscles might account for their selective deterioration. This was supported by the lack of extraocular

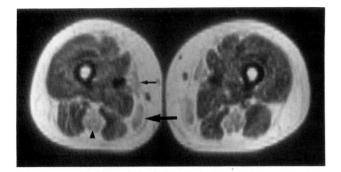

FIGURE 19.10. Typical thigh muscle abnormalities in mitochondrial myopathies. In the same patient shown in Figure 19.2c, T_1-weighted MRI shows especially severe fatty replacement in the sartorius (small arrow), gracilis (large arrow), and semitendinosus (arrowhead).

muscle weakness in patients in whom the sartorius and gracilis were selectively spared. The sartorius and gracilis muscles are known to be composed of relatively long and thin fibers, like the extraocular muscles, but how these changes would contribute to selective deterioration in defects of oxidative phosphorylation remains unknown. The fact that sartorius and gracilis are among the muscles most frequently spared in other myopathies, including dystrophinopathies,[33] congenital myopathies,[33,34] and inflammatory myopathies,[35] is similarly compelling yet inexplicable.

One possible contributing factor to muscle deterioration and weakness in patients with mitochondrial myopathy includes the genetic composition of the mitochondria, as supported by our observation of a high incidence of muscle abnormalities in patients with mitochondrial DNA deletion or point mutations. The possibility that muscle deterioration somehow results from impaired oxidative capacity appears to be refuted by observing no structural lesion of muscle by MRI or histopathologic criteria in one patient with severely limited

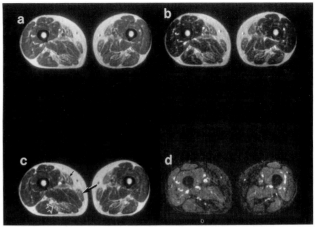

FIGURE 19.11. Tissue characterization of muscle lesions in mitochondrial myopathy. A 56-yr-old man presented with a distribution of muscle deterioration similar to the patient in Figure 19.9. Fatty infiltration of muscle is denoted by increased signal intensity on spin density (2000/30, a), T_2-weighted (2000/60, b), and T_1-weighted (500/30, c) MRI. Note in (c) particularly severe involvement of the sartorius (small arrow), gracilis (arrow), and semitendinosus (arrowhead). It is also noteworthy that edema-like changes tend to be inconspicuous in mitochondrial myopathies, despite varying degrees of muscular deterioration. This is exemplified by absence of abnormally increased muscle signal intensity using STIR (d). The small foci of very bright signal intensity in (d) are due to blood in veins.

exercise tolerance and mitochondrial cytochrome oxidase deficiency.

An interesting MRI feature of muscle abnormalities in these patients was a high incidence of fatty deterioration of muscle but a relative paucity of edema-like changes of deteriorating muscles. This feature is in contradistinction to most other muscle disorders that MRI has been employed to study. Specifically, denervation, inflammation, and myonecrosis manifest with prominent edema-like

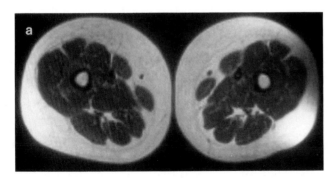

FIGURE 19.12. Progressive deterioration of thigh muscles in mitochondrial myopathy. The patient was first scanned at the age of 4 yr. T_1-weighted (500/30, a) image shows minimal abnormality. Four years later, when the patient presented with

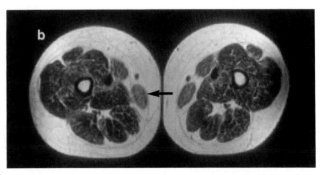

marked worsening of ophthalmoplegia, T_1-weighted image (500/30, b) shows markedly worsened appearance with diffuse, reticulated appearance of intramuscular fat. Note that specific muscles are more severely involved (e.g., gracilis) (arrow).

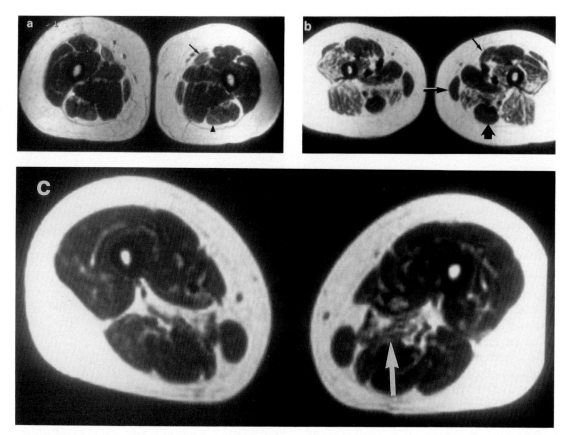

FIGURE 19.13. Muscle lesion variations in mitochondrial myopathies. The first patient presented for evaluation of ophthalmoplegia. T_1-weighted thigh image (500/30, a) shows only minimal high signal intensity intramuscular fat in the sartorius (arrow) and semitendinosus (arrowhead). A different patient's thighs reveal an unusual pattern of abnormality, with markedly reticulated fatty change on T_1-weighted image (500/30, b) in multiple thigh muscles, but selective sparing of sartorius (small arrow), gracilis (arrow), and semitendinosus (arrowhead). At the midthigh in the same patient, bilateral atrophy is restricted to the adductor magnus (500/30, arrow, c).

MRI changes, with or without associated fatty deterioration. The paucity of edematous changes correlated with only minimal histopathologic evidence of myonecrosis or inflammation, and only minimally elevated serum creatine kinase levels.

Conclusions

The mechanism(s) underlying selective muscle involvement in inherited disorders of muscle energy metabolism is unknown, but the observation that some muscles may avoid deterioration offers the hope for identification of some factor(s) that mediates resistance to myopathic alterations in these disorders. Such knowledge may advance our understanding of the pathophysiology and potential treatments of neuromuscular diseases. At the current time, the role of imaging in these disorders is therefore primarily academic. However, the recognition of patterns of muscle necrosis and fatty infiltration may eventually assist in the diagnostic evaluation, planning of rehabilitation, and assessment of prognosis and other treatments in these patients.

References

1. Haller RG, Bertocci LA. Exercise evaluation of metabolic myopathies. In: Engel AG, Franzini-Armstrong C, editors. Myology. 2nd ed. New York: McGraw-Hill, 1994:807–821.
2. Engel AG, Hirschhorn R. Acid maltase deficiency. In: Engel AG, Franzini-Armstrong C, editors. Myology. 2nd ed. New York: McGraw-Hill, 1994:1533–1553.
3. DiMauro S, Tsujino S. Nonlysosomal glycogenoses. In: Engel AG, Franzini-Armstrong C, editors. Myology. 2nd ed. New York: McGraw-Hill, 1994:1554–1576.
4. Brown DH. Glycogen metabolism and glycolysis in muscle. In: Engel AG, Franzini-Armstrong C, editors. Myology. 2nd ed. New York: McGraw-Hill, 1994:665–682.
5. Bertocci LA, Haller RG, Lewis SF, Fleckenstein JL, Nunnally RL. Phosphocreatine depletion is attenuated in human phosphofructokinase deficiency. J Appl Physiol 1991;70:2101–1207.
6. Fishbein WN. Myoadenylate deaminase deficiency: inheritance and acquired forms. Biochem. Med. 1985;33:158.

7. Layzer RB. Muscle pain, cramps, and fatigue. In: Engel AG, Franzini-Armstrong C, editors. Myology. 2nd ed. New York: McGraw-Hill, 1994:1756.
8. Morgan-Hughes JA. Mitochondrial myopathies. In: Engel AG, Franzini-Armstrong C, editors. Myology. 2nd ed. New York: McGraw-Hill, 1994:1610–1660.
9. Zierz S. Carnitine palmitoyl transferase deficiency. In: Engel AG, Franzini-Armstrong C, editors. Myology. 2nd ed. New York: McGraw-Hill, 1994:1577–1586.
10. Fleckenstein JL, Peshock RM, Lewis SF, Haller RG. Magnetic resonance imaging of muscle injury and atrophy in glycolytic myopathies. Muscle Nerve 1989;12:849–855.
11. Swift TR, Brown M. Tc-99 m pyrophosphate muscle labeling in McArdle Syndrome. J Nucl Med 1978;19:295–297.
12. Heckmatt JZ, Leeman S, Dubowitz V. Ultrasound imaging in the diagnosis of muscle disease. J Pediatr 1982;101:656–660.
13. Heckmatt JZ, Pier N, Dubowitz V. Real-time ultrasound imaging of muscles. Muscle Nerve 1988;11:56–65.
14. Heckmatt JZ, Pier N, Dubowitz V. Assessment of quadriceps muscle atrophy and hypertrophy in neuromuscular disease in children. J Clin Ultrasound 1988;16:177–181.
15. Forst R. Skelettmuskel-Sonographie bei neuromuskulären Erkrankungen. Stuttgart: Enke, 1986.
16. Reimers CD. Myosonographie. In: Pongratz DE, Reimers CD, Hahn D, Nägele M, Müller-Felber W, editors. Atlas der Muskelkrankheiten. Munich: Urban & Schwarzenberg, 1990.
17. Herson D, Larde D, Ferry M, Brunet P, Fardeau M. Apport diagnostique du scanner X en pathologie musculaire. Rev Neurol (Paris) 1985;141:482–489.
18. Cinnamon J, Slonim AE, Black KS, Gorey MT, Scuderi DM, Hyman RA. Evaluation of the lumbar spine in patients with glycogen storage disease: CT demonstration of patterns of paraspinal muscle atrophy. Am J Neuroradiol 1991;12:1099–1103.
19. Laasonen EM. Atrophy of sacrospinal muscle groups in patients with chronic, diffusely radiating lumbar back pain. Neuroradiology 1984;26:9–13.
20. Kaiser WA, Schalke BCG. Kernspintomographie bei generalisierten Skelettmuskelerkrankungen. Untersuchungsmodalitäten und Indikationsempfehlungen. Rontgenpraxis 1989;42:338–345.
21. Nägele M, Reimers CD. Kernspintomographie. In: Pongratz DE, Reimers CD, Hahn D, Nägele M, Müller-Felber W, editors. Atlas der Muskelkrankheiten. Munich: Urban & Schwarzenberg, 1990.
22. Nägele M, Reimers C. Opthalmoplegia plus and Kearns-Sayre syndrome. In Pongratz DE, editor. Atlas der Muskelkrankheiten. Munich: Urban & Schwarzenberg, 1990.
23. Bulcke JAL, Baert AL. Clinical and radiological aspects of myopathies. Berlin: Springer-Verlag, 1982:89.
24. Marbini A, Gemignani F, Saccardi F, Rimoldi M. Debrancher deficiency neuromuscular disorder with pseudohypertrophy in two brothers. J Neurol 1989;236:418–420.
25. Metzler JP, Fleckenstein JL, White CL III, Haller RG, Frenkel G, Greenlee R. MRI evaluation of amyloid myopathy. Skeletal Radiol 1992;7:463–465.
26. Fischer AQ, Carpenter DW, Hartlage PL, Carroll JE, Stephens S. Muscle imaging in neuromuscular disease using computerized real-time sonography. Muscle Nerve 1988;11:270–275.
27. Fleckenstein JL, Haller RG, Lewis SF, et al. Absence of exercise-induced MRI enhancement of skeletal muscle in McArdle's disease. J Appl Physiol 1991;71:961–969.
28. Fleckenstein JL, Peshock RM, Lewis SF, Haller RG. Magnetic resonance imaging of muscle injury and atrophy in glycolytic myopathies. Muscle Nerve 1989;12(10):849–855.
29. Fleckenstein JL, Weatherall PT, Parkey RW, Payne JA, Peshock RM. Sports-related muscle injuries: evaluation with MR imaging. Radiology 1989;172:793–798.
30. Hansman ML, Peyster RG, Heiman-Patterson T, Greenfield VL. CT demonstration of extraocular muscle atrophy. J Comput Assist Tomogr 1988;12:49–51.
31. Serratrice G, Salomon G, Jiddane M, Gastaut JL, Pellissier JF, Pouget J. Resultats du scanner X musculaire dans 145 cas de maladies neuro-musculaires. Rev Neurol (Paris) 1985;141:404–412.
32. Fleckenstein JL, Haller RG, Girson MS, Peshock RM. Focal muscle lesions in mitochondrial myopathy: MR imaging evaluation. J Magn Reson Imaging (Supp) 1992;2:121.
33. Lamminen AE. Magnetic resonance imaging of primary skeletal muscle diseases: patterns of distribution and severity of involvement. Br J Radiol 1990;63:946–950.
34. Wallgren-Pettersson, Kivisaari L, Jaaskelainen J, Lamminen A, Holberg C. Ultrasonography, CT, and MRI of muscles in congenital nemaline myopathy. Pediatr Neurol 1990;6:20–28.
35. Kuriyama M, Hayakawaa K, Konishi Y, et al. MR imaging of myopathy. Comput Med Imaging Graphics 1989;13:329–333.

20
Endocrine Myopathies

Pierre Kaminsky and Paul M. Walker

Muscular involvement is common in endocrine diseases and does not generally pose a substantial diagnostic problem. Imaging and spectroscopic techniques used in the exploration of muscle are mainly complementary to pathophysiological studies. An exception to this rule is thyroid associated ophthalmopathy (Graves' ophthalmopathy). In the evaluation of this particular disease, diagnostic imaging techniques such as ultrasound, CT, and MRI are of considerable clinical importance.

Muscle Disorders and Thyroid Hormones

Thyroid Associated Ophthalmopathy

Clinical Pattern

Thyroid associated ophthalmopathy (TAO) is characterized by swelling and thickening of the extraocular muscles and orbital fat, resulting in exophthalmos.[1,2] In Graves' disease, an orbitopathy is clinically present in 10% to 15% of the cases and in 60% to 80%, when imaging investigations are used for the diagnosis.[3,4] Graves' ophthalmopathy can precede the onset of the thyroid disease or occur anytime after treatment,[5] and is also reported in euthyroid patients or with Hashimoto's thyroiditis.[1,2]

Clinical findings in TAO include proptosis, which is commonly bilateral and sometimes asymmetrical; it may be accompanied by upper lid retraction and congestive signs (Figure 20.1). One clinical classification was proposed by Werner[6] (Table 20.1), although it is acknowledged that clinical disease does not necessarily progress from one Werner class to the next. Class 1 symptoms may be attributed to sympathetic overactivity of the levator muscle. Symptoms of classes 2 to 6 are related to retrobulbar tissue involvement. Congestive signs (class 2) are linked to venous drainage impairment. Retro-

bulbar tissue swelling is responsible for proptosis in class 3. Evolution to fibrosis progressively induces a restriction of ocular motility (class 4). The inferior and medial recti are the most frequently involved muscles, and restricted downward gaze adduction is the most frequent clinical finding. The lateral and superior recti are less frequently involved. The cornea is exposed by both exophthalmos and lid retraction in class 5. At the apex of the muscle cone, the optic nerve can be compressed (class 6).

Histology and Pathogenesis

TAO is an autoimmune disease but its pathophysiology is not clearly understood. Orbital tissue, eye muscle membrane extracts, and thyroid membrane express a 64-kDa protein recognized by serum antibodies. This suggests a cross-reactivity between eye muscle antigens and thyroid antigens. Histological analysis has been obtained only from advanced cases of TAO requiring surgical intervention. Common findings are lymphocyte infiltration, edema, and fibrosis of the muscles.[7] Accumulation of glycosaminoglycans in the retro-ocular tissues contributes to edematous swelling of the extraocular muscles and connective tissue.[1,2]

Conditions for Diagnosis

In the majority of cases, TAO can easily be diagnosed in the context of associated thyroid disease. However, this may require extensive clinical, hormonal, and immunological investigation (Table 20.2). Ophthalmological study includes investigation of the degree of proptosis (exophthalmometry), extraocular muscle motility, and potential associated visual and corneal complications (see Table 20.3). Electromyography, which can show myopathic changes, is not useful. Imaging investigations are necessary only in classes 2 to 6 and help to follow up the natural course of the disease or the effectiveness of therapy, and to detect the uncommon occurrence of optic nerve compression.

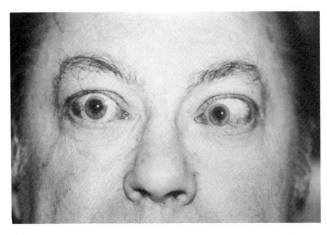

FIGURE 20.1. Graves' ophthalmopathy: bilateral orbital involvement. In the right eye, note moderate exophthalmos, eye lid retraction, stare, hypervascularity, and congestion of the conjunctival and episcleral vessels (class V). The left eye shows exophthalmos, eyelid retraction, and inferior rectus restriction (class IV).

TABLE 20.2. Clinical and biological evaluation of thyroid associated ophthalmopathy.

History	Personal history of thyroid disease and treatment
	Familial history of thyroid disease
Ophthalmological examination	Corneal examination
	Ocular motility
	Ophthalmoscopy
	Hertel's exophthalmometry
	Tonometric measurements
Systemic physical examination	
Biological investigations	
Hormone	Free thyroxine level (FT4)
	Free triiodothyronine level (FT3)
	Thyroid stimulating hormone level (TSH)
	TSH stimulation test by thyroid releasing hormone (TRH)
Immunology	TSH receptor auto-antibodies
	Antimicrosomial (thyroperoxidase) antibodies
	Antithyroglobulin antibodies

When a history of thyroid disease is absent, the diagnosis is often delayed. Bilateral proptosis with eye lid retraction and lid lag on downward gaze are characteristic.[1] When the signs are more subtle, such as unilateral proptosis, imaging investigation may be necessary.

Imaging of TAO

Imaging techniques useful in the diagnosis of TAO include ultrasound, computed tomography, and magnetic resonance imaging. The imaging diagnosis of a TAO is based on the following criteria: (1) no mass in either orbit; (2) thickening of the extraocular muscles with a variable and nonuniform distribution of involvement; (3) bilateral lesions, even in the case of clinically uniocular exophthalmos; (4) absence of involvement of the inserting tendons.

Ultrasound

Both A-scan and B-scan ultrasonography are used in orbital diagnosis and can be performed by either a contact method or a water immersion method. Transducer frequencies varying from 5 to 10 MHz are used.[8–10] A standardized 8-MHz A-scan echography (SAE), described by Ossoinig, is especially suitable for orbital diagnosis and quantitative tissue differentiation.[11,12]

SAE permits an evaluation of the internal structure and thickness of the muscles and optic nerve, with a precision of ±0.2 to 0.3 mm.[11,12] The contact B-scan is helpful in documenting gross muscle size but does not provide exact muscle measurement.[11] The main sonographic characteristic of TAO is enlargement of the extraocular muscles, with high internal reflectivity due to the inflammatory process. This high reflectivity is in contrast to all other diseases that cause extraocular muscle enlargement (Figure 20.2). Moreover, expansion of the retrobulbar fat is often seen and thickening of the optic nerve sheath may occur.

CT Scan

In order to provide substantial data, axial and coronal sectioning must be performed. Slice thickness is usually 1 to 4 mm. Despite the natural contrast provided by the orbital fat, enhancement by contrast material administration is sometimes performed. This increases the

TABLE 20.1. Classification of Graves' ophthalmopathy.

Class	Definition	Signs and symptoms
0	No symptoms	
1	Only signs	Upper lid retraction; stare; lid lag; infrequent blinking
2	Soft tissue involvement	Edema and injection of conjunctiva; edema of lids; chemosis; lacrimation
3	Proptosis	3 mm or more in excess of upper normal limit (22 mm)
4	Extraocular muscle involvement	Diplopia; limitation; restriction of motion; fixation of globe
5	Corneal involvement	Stippling; ulceration; clouding; necrosis or perforation of cornea
6	Optic nerve involvement	Sight loss; disc pallor; visual field or color defect

From Werner J. Clin Endocrinol Metab 1977;44:203–204.

TABLE 20.3. Main differential diagnoses of orbital muscle enlargement.

Mechanism	Disease	Number of enlarged muscles
Direct muscle involvement	Thyroid associated ophthalmopathy	Generally multiple and bilateral
	Acute myositis	Unique or multiple, eventually bilateral
	Chronic myositis	Generally unique
	Lymphoma	Unique or multiple, eventually bilateral
	Orbital pseudotumors	Unique or multiple, eventually bilateral
	Metastasis	Unique or multiple, unilateral
	Acromegaly	Generally multiple and bilateral
	Amyloidosis	Generally unique
Indirect muscle enlargement (venous drainage impairment)	Apex orbital tumor	
	Metastasis	Multiple unilateral
	Arterio-venous fistula or malformation	
	Superior ophthalmic vein thrombosis	

radiodensity of all the intraorbital soft tissues.[13] However, contrast agent administration could saturate the thyroid gland, and thereby render hyperthyroid treatment with radioactive iodine ineffective.

The axial section is chosen between 10° and 15° below the canthomedial line, so that the entire length of the optic nerve is seen in one scan.[14] This plane therefore visualizes the muscle cone. Coronal sections are essential to explore the superior and inferior recti and to evaluate the cross section of the muscles[14] (Figure 20.3).

In TAO, enlargement of the extraocular muscles is the most salient finding[3,13–19] (Figures 20.3 to 20.6). Muscle

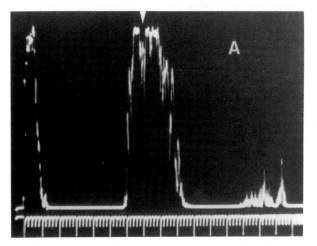

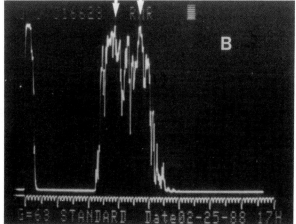

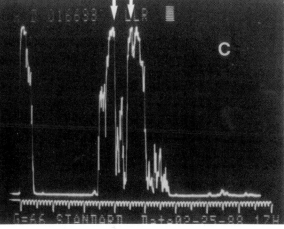

FIGURE 20.2. A-scan ultrasound in ophthalmopathies. Cross section of a normal rectus muscle shows normal reflectivity of the muscle as indicated by reduced spike heights (arrow, A). In Graves' ophthalmopathy the enlarged muscle (between arrows, B) exhibits high reflectivity. In acute myositis, the thickened muscle shows low reflectivity (between arrows, C). (From Ossoinig KC, Dev Ophthalmol 1989;20:28–37, reproduced with permission from Karger AG, Basel, Switzerland.)

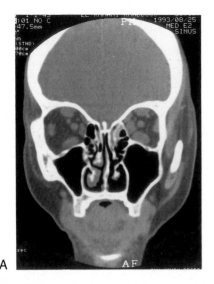

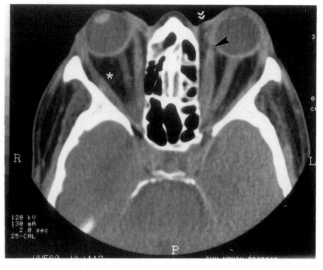

FIGURE 20.3. CT imaging of class IV Graves' ophthalmopathy. Coronal (A) and axial (B) images show bilateral exophthalmos, increased orbital fat (asterisk), and slight anterior prolapse of the orbital septum (double arrow). The bilateral muscle thickening is more readily appreciated on the coronal slice. The tendinous insertions are spared (arrowhead).

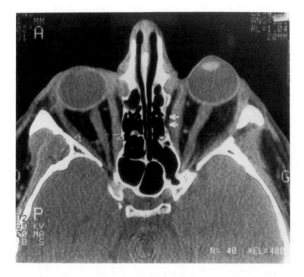

FIGURE 20.4. CT imaging of class VI Graves' ophthalmopathy. Axial image shows moderate muscle enlargement. Note prominence of orbital fat and the medial bowing of the lamina papyracea (arrows) due to increased orbital volume.

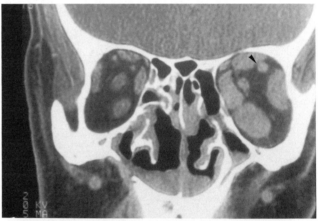

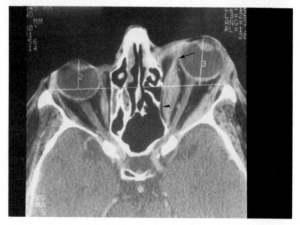

FIGURE 20.5. Class VI Graves' disease with asymmetrical involvement. Coronal (A) and axial (B) contrast-enhanced CT scans. Unilateral left exophthalmos, massive thickening of multiple rectus muscles without involvement of the tendinous insertion (arrow, B), medial bowing of the lamina papyracea (arrowhead, B). Note also slight distension of the superior ophthalmic vein (arrowhead, A). Minor involvement of the right orbit is also present.

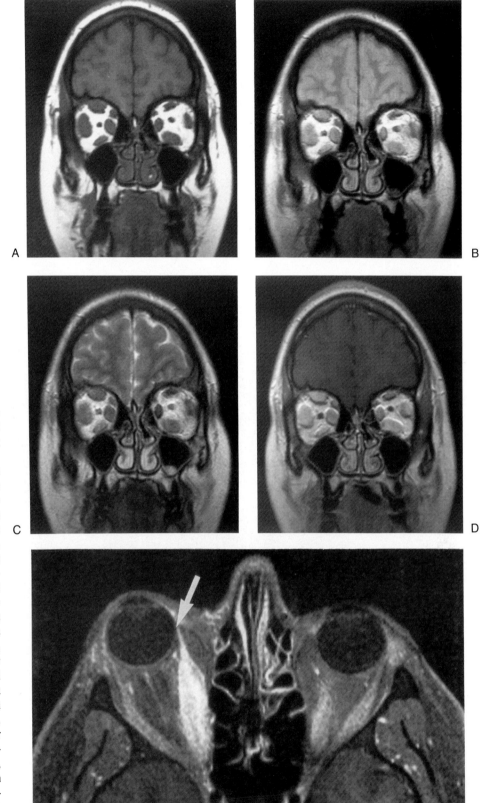

FIGURE 20.6. Graves' ophthalmo-pathy: MRI evaluation. Coronal images show variable enlargement of most of the extraocular muscles. Note that T_1-weighted image (350/15, T_R/T_E, A) is insensitive to muscle edema and shows only normal signal intensity, whereas spin density (3000/20, T_R/T_E, B) and T_2-weighted (3000/120, T_R/T_E, C) images show edematous changes by virtue of increased signal intensity, particularly in the inferior and lateral recti. Following gadolinium-DTPA infusion, signal intensity is markedly increased in all muscles on the T_1-weighted scan (350/15, T_R/T_E, D), although it is subtly greater in the inferior and lateral recti, consistent with greater edema in them. In a second patient with isolated medial rectus involvement, gadolinium enhancement is far more conspicuous when a fat sup-pression sequence is used (350/15, spectral presaturation inversion recovery, E). Note that the tend-inous attachment to the globe is uninvolved, a clue to the correct diagnosis of Graves' orbitopathy (arrow, E). (Courtesy of Dr. James L. Fleckenstein.)

radiodensity can be decreased in the case of fatty degeneration. In addition to the above-described characteristics of muscle changes, several CT scan findings are highly suggestive of TAO. Increased fat content is present in about 50% of cases[20,21] (Figure 20.3). In a few cases, this is the only finding in the orbit evaluation.[20,22] However, the fat radiodensity is normal,[16] a feature useful to distinguish thyroid ophthalmopathy from orbital pseudotumor, an idiopathic inflammatory condition that frequently causes edematous changes in the orbital fat (Figure 20.7). In thyroid ophthalmopathy, anterior displacement of the fat results in anterior prolapse of the orbital septum.[16,18,20] Medial rectus belly enlargement can induce medial bowing of the lamina papyracea (Figures 20.4, 20.5). In the case of severe Graves' disease, the enlargement of the medial rectus muscles results in a displacement of both medial orbital walls, forming a "Coca-Cola bottle" or "wasp-waist" contour. Lacrimal gland involvement and slight distension of the superior ophthalmic vein may be present[13,16,18] (Figure 20.5). Thickening of the optic nerve sheath may be detected in coronal or axial views when mechanical compression occurs at the orbital apex. CT scanning also provides evaluation of proptosis, which correlates well with exophthalmometry.

MR Imaging

Retrobulbar fat has short T_1 and intermediate T_2 relaxation times, and therefore provides a natural contrast

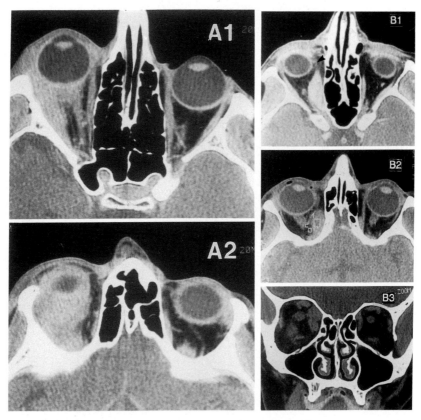

FIGURE 20.7. Differential diagnoses in thyroid associated ophthalmopathy (TAO). Muscle swelling is a feature shared by TAO and inflammatory and neoplastic orbital diseases, although unlike TAO, these other diagnoses may also extend into the adjacent orbital fat and other soft tissues. For example, in a case of orbital pseudotumor, axial CT images obtained after intravenous contrast administration (A1 and A2) not only show swelling of right lateral rectus (A1) and superior rectus (A2), but the right orbital fat also shows involvement (higher density, compared to the left). Note that the tendinous insertion of the lateral rectus is swollen (arrow, A1), in distinct contrast to the appearance of TAO. Signs and symptoms resolved after glucocorticoid therapy, thereby confirming the diagnosis of pseudotumor, a neoplastic disease could have the same pretreatment appearance. In a patient with orbital myositis, CT images (B1 to B3) show features that resemble TAO, namely increased muscle size, normal tendinous attachment of involved muscle to the globe (arrow, B1), and absence of orbital fat abnormality. However, like pseudotumor, all findings resolved upon glucocorticoid therapy, mitigating against TAO and confirming a benign disease.

for the soft tissues, such as extraocular muscles and optic nerves.[23-26] As with CT scanning, axial and coronal slices are helpful to evaluate TAO, although the flexibility of MRI allows nonorthogonal planes, as well as the sagittal plane, which can be helpful to evaluate the degree of tendinous involvement. Spatial resolution is dependent on the field strength and can be significantly improved by using special surface coils and other techniques. The usual slice thickness obtained is 3 to 7 mm. Relatively high resolution is necessary to detect optic nerve compression, and a 1.5 T field strength with the use of an adequate surface coil can provide similar spatial resolution as found in CT.[15] However, even low field strength MRI devices can provide excellent definition of soft tissue abnormalities. A limiting problem of MRI, especially at low field, is the scan time, because eye motion can degrade image quality. Because of the abundance of orbital fat, the inclusion of a fat suppression technique, such as short time inversion recovery (STIR), can be especially helpful to evaluate the presence of edema in and around muscles (Figures 20.6, 20.7).

MRI demonstrates similar results as CT, although the bony walls of the orbit are poorly seen. Measurement of muscle thickness on coronal slices, quantitation of fat content, and other details are available[1,15,24,27] (Figure 20.6). MRI can provide additional information, such as the measured relaxation times. For example, the T_2 relaxation time has been found to be increased in edematous muscles, expecially in superior and medial recti.[15,24,27] As expected, when fibrotic evolution occurs, the T_2 may be relatively short.[15] Supporting the notion that the T_2 time might serve as a guide in the choice of treatment is evidence that muscles with the longest T_2 values respond most readily to radiotherapy.[27] However, further clinical evidence is needed to corroborate this hypothesis.

Another MRI technique that may be of value in assessing Graves' orbitopathy is the use of gadolinium chelate infusion. Especially when combined with fat-suppressed T_2-weighted images, enhancement may be seen in edematous muscles (Figure 20.6). However, the efficacy of this technique remains to be established and gadolinium enhancement is prominent in normal muscles due to the unusually high capillary content of these muscles.[28]

Differential Diagnosis

A certain number of diseases present an exophthalmos and could therefore mimic a TAO.[16] However, even in the case of unilateral proptosis, TAO is the most common etiology. Although clinical correlation is very important, specific imaging findings are also pertinent. In orbital myositis, a single muscle is generally enlarged, although bilateral and multiple muscle involvement has been reported[14,16,18] (Figure 20.7). In orbital pseudotumor, the muscle enlargement tends to be less uniform than in TAO, and the inflammation generally involves the tendinous insertion and sometimes periocular tissues. The amount of orbital fat is normal but is usually edematous, visible on CT and MRI by a heterogeneous appearance of the fat (Figure 20.7). Arteriovenous fistulas and malformations (AVMs) show moderate unilateral enlargement of the extraocular muscles, with a mild proptosis. The most important feature in AVMs is the distention of the superior ophthalmic vein; the phenomenon is considerably more prominent than in TAO.[14,16,18] Muscular metastases can involve one or multiple muscles, with focal and irregular enhancement by infused contrast material (Figure 20.7). In acromegaly, muscle enlargement is generally moderate, proptosis absent, and endocrinologic findings very different.[16,29] Muscles can be infiltrated unilaterally or bilaterally by lymphoma, in which case muscle tendons are often involved. Amyloid myopathy has also been reported to involve extraocular muscle,[30] in which case a decreased T_2 time, and hence low signal intensity on a T_2-weighted image, may be seen.

Hyperthyroid Myopathy

Clinical Pattern

Patients with thyrotoxicosis may develop a proximal myopathy in 60% to 80% of cases, which usually spares bulbar muscles.[31] Muscle atrophy is common and weakness is often prominent. Distal involvement occurs but is less severe. Myalgia and pain are uncommon. More rarely, a thyrotoxic periodic paralysis can be observed, especially in Orientals. This is characterized by recurrent attacks of weakness, precipitated by a carbohydrate diet, cooling, or postexercise.

Histology

Muscle biopsy usually is normal or shows fiber atrophy. Other pathologies have been occasionally reported, including fatty infiltration, interstitial edema, focal fiber necrosis, or an increased number of sarcolemmal nuclei. Ultrastructural studies demonstrate abnormal mitochondria, myofibrillar degeneration, subsarcolemmal glycogen deposits, and tubular T abnormalities.[31] None of these findings are specific to hyperthyrodism. In the case of thyrotoxic periodic paralysis, vacuolar dilatation of the sarcoplasmic reticulum is found.

Diagnosis

Thyrotoxic myopathy must be considered in adult-onset proximal myopathy. The diagnosis is usually easy because clinical systemic signs of thyrotoxicosis are generally evident and because hormone levels in blood are always elevated. Serum creatine kinase activity is normal or low, whereas increased urinary creatinine is generally present. Electromyography shows a myopathic pattern in 84% of proximal muscles and in distal muscles in less than 20%;[32] electromyography sometimes suggests a myasthenic condition. In thyrotoxic paralysis, a decreased potassium level during the attacks is generally found.

Imaging

A CT study of seven hyperthyroid subjects showed a decreased cross-sectional area of thigh muscles (Figure 20.8) that correlated with decreased quadriceps strength.[33] A blurred and inhomogeneous appearance of the muscles was also reported using CT.[34] In MRI, a severe decrease in muscle cross section, accompanied by edema, was shown in a single case of thyrotoxic myopathy mimicking a limb girdle myopathy.[35]

Hyperthyroid myopathy was studied by a variety of investigators using ^{31}P-MR spectroscopy (MRS).[36–38] Some data suggested exaggerated phosphocreatine (PCr) depletion and acidosis during exercise,[36] abnormalities that were interpreted to illustrate a higher energetic cost of actin-myosin interaction due to transition through rapid myosin isoforms and to the activation of certain glycolytic enzymes. A different study found normal rest and exercise spectra but an increase in the PCr resynthesis rate,[37] a finding not supported by another study.[36] The discordance in findings between the studies is suspected to be due in part to variation in severity of hormone excess in the patients studied.

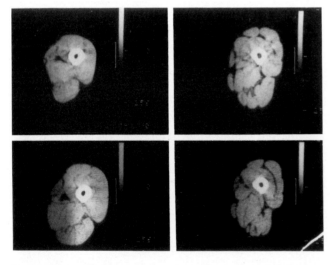

FIGURE 20.8. CT scan aspect of the thigh in hyperthyroid (left side) and hypothyroid patients (right side) before and after therapy (upper and lower, respectively). (From Zürcher R et al. J Clin Endocrinol Metab 1989;69:1082–1086, reproduced with permission from the Endocrine Society.)

Hypothyroidism

Clinical Features

Hypothyroid muscle involvement is typically characterized by slow movements, stiffness, myalgia, and myoedema.[39–41] Occasionally, proximal weakness is present. Reflex changes with delayed relaxation are common. Cramps are possible in adults. In advanced cases, muscle enlargement is present. When the hormone deficiency is less marked, clinical examination is normal although muscle fatigue and cramps are frequently observed.[31]

Histology

The percentage of type 2 muscle fibers is usually diminished whereas that of type 1 fibers is increased. Muscle biopsy can be otherwise normal or show nonspecific abnormalities. Increased numbers of nuclei, fiber necrosis, atrophy, ring fibers, glycogen accumulation, and central cores have been reported.[39–43] Ultrastructural findings include myofibrillar disorganization, glycogen and lipid accumulation, T-tubule distension, and morphological changes of mitochondria.

Diagnosis

A "hypertrophic" myopathy is typically observed in patients with a severe thyroid defect in whom systemic clinical signs of hypothyroidism are generally evident. However, it seems reasonable to evaluate for the possibility of hypothyroid myopathy in patients presenting with muscular fatiguability or cramps. This should include measurement of thyroxine and TSH levels. Creatine kinase level is commonly elevated in the serum of hypothyroid patients, even in the absence of clinical muscle involvement. Electromyography may be normal or show low-amplitude polyphasic motor unit potentials.[41,43]

Imaging

The size of muscles in cross section in hypothyroidism may be increased, and the muscle can have a swollen appearance (Figures 20.8–20.10). Zürcher et al. used CT scanning to confirm reduction of thigh muscle size in three of four patients after thyroid replacement therapy (Figure 20.8).[33] Interestingly, muscle strength increased, thereby revealing the diminished muscle efficiency of hypothyroid muscle. This also suggested that the observed changes were related to biochemical alterations or to functional changes in the bioenergetics.

In ^{31}P-MRS studies, hypothyroid muscle show decreased PCr to inorganic phosphate (P_i) ratios at rest, as well as a slower PCr resynthesis after exercise, a characteristic that reverses with hormonal replacement.[37,44] Similar features are found in mitochondrial myopathies,[45,46] which accounts for the proposal that

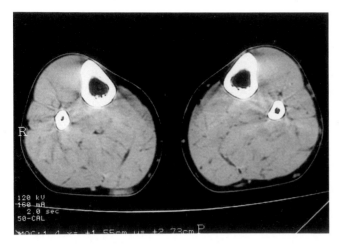

FIGURE 20.9. Hypothroid myopathy in patient with proximal weakness, stiffness, muscle hypertrophy, and markedly elevated creatine kinase levels. Axial CT scan at the midcalf level. All the muscles are enlarged, with minimal heterogeneity in muscle density probably due to edema.

impaired muscle oxidative metabolism may contribute to hypothyroid myopathy.[37,44] Moreover, exercise-induced acidosis is more marked than in normal muscle[44,47] and is slower to develop and resolve after exercise.[44,47,48] Potential mechanisms to account for these modifications would include defective pyruvate oxidation and inhibited transmembrane Na^+/H^+ exchanges. Also, an increase in the amount of muscle phosphodiesters has been noted in hypothyroidism, another finding that disappears after replacement therapy[37,48] (Figure 20.11).

Muscle Disorders and Growth Hormone

Growth Hormone Deficiency

Prepubertal hypopituitarism causes dwarfism with impaired muscle development.[31] The muscles of growth hormone (GH)-deficient children are weaker than those of age-matched or size-matched normal children.[49] Also, GH-deficient adults treated with GH improve their maximum quadriceps strength,[50] an effect that disappears after discontinuing the therapy.[51]

Imaging

CT scanning has documented that GH therapy increases muscle volume and reduces subcutaneous fat content.[50] This was associated with increased muscle strength and fiber size. The muscle density was not modified by the treatment. A recent MRI study of GH-deficient children showed that the thigh muscle cross section increased by 6% to 17% with replacement therapy, whereas subcutaneous fat decreased in similar proportion.[52] Moreover, GH treatment suspension in 12 patients demonstrated a decrease of quadriceps and forearm flexor cross sections by 5% to 8%, measured by CT.[51]

In a combined ^{31}P-MRS and [1]H-MRI study of the hindleg muscles of hypophysectomized rats treated with GH, we observed not only an augmentation of muscle cross section and of twitch tension of the gastrocnemius, but also a rise in the baseline PCr concentration and a concomitant reduction of the adenosine diphosphate (ADP) concentration.[53] In addition, the rate of ADP decline was more rapid during a subsequent postexercise

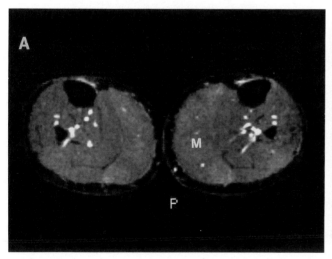

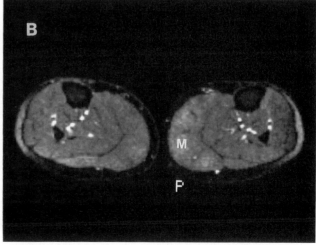

FIGURE 20.10. Hypothyroid myopathy. Axial STIR (1500/30/100) images at the midcalf level before and after thyroid replacement therapy. Note prominent size of posterior leg muscles and edema-like changes in the medial (M) head of the gastrocnemius muscles (A). Following therapy, hypertrophy and edema-like changes are less pronounced (B). (Courtesy of Drs. Ronald G. Haller and James L. Fleckenstein.)

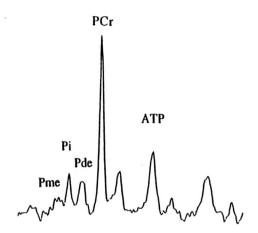

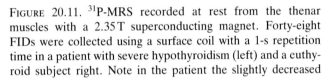

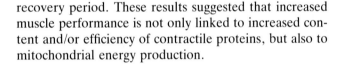

FIGURE 20.11. ^{31}P-MRS recorded at rest from the thenar muscles with a 2.35 T superconducting magnet. Forty-eight FIDs were collected using a surface coil with a 1-s repetition time in a patient with severe hypothyroidism (left) and a euthyroid subject right. Note in the patient the slightly decreased phosphocreatine peak, with diminished phosphocreatine relative to inorganic phosphate, and the abnormal peak of phosphodiesters. Abbreviations: P_i: inorganic phosphate; PCr: phosphocreatine; Pme: phosphomonoesters; Pde: phosphodiesters.

recovery period. These results suggested that increased muscle performance is not only linked to increased content and/or efficiency of contractile proteins, but also to mitochondrial energy production.

Acromegaly

GH-secreting tumors induce a proximal myopathy in 50% of acromegalic patients, especially after a long duration of GH excess.[54,55] Muscle fibers are increased in size, which contrasts with the decreased strength. The increased muscle volume, particularly of proximal muscles, was confirmed by CT measurements.[55] In four acromegalic subjects, we found a diminished concentration of PCr in gastrocnemius and thenar muscles. Potential explanations for this finding include increased muscle content of connective tissue or water;[56] a mitochondrial defect might also contribute, as supported by ultrastructural evidence of abnormal mitochondria.

Steroid Myopathy

A steroid myopathy occurs in patients treated with glucocorticoids, or with long-term endogenous glucocorticoid excess.[31] It is characterized by a severe proximal weakness and wasting. Myalgia may be present, serum creatine kinase levels are usually low or normal, and EMG findings are myopathic.

Chronic steroid excess results in muscle atrophy (Figures 20.12, 20.13), which histologically involves predominantly type 2 muscle fibers. Muscle volume was studied by CT in renal transplant patients treated with mild prednisone doses.[57] The cross section of the thigh muscles was decreased by 18% compared with control

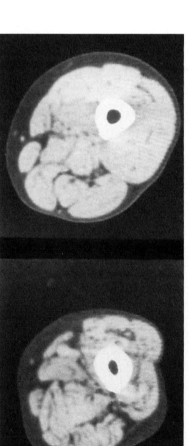

FIGURE 20.12. Steroid myopathy. CT scan at midthigh level compared with a normal control (upper figure). The lower figure illustrates a global wasting of the muscles. (Courtesy of Professor F. Frey, Medizinische Universitätspoliklinik Inselspital, Bern, Switzerland.)

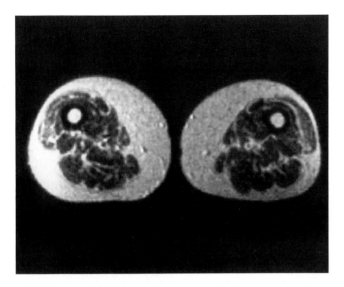

FIGURE 20.13. Steroid myopathy. After years of exogenous steroid therapy for a misdiagnosis of rheumatoid arthritis, progressive weakness was associated with atrophy and increased adiposity in the distal vastus lateralis muscles on MRI (2000/60, T_R/T_E). (Courtesy of Dr. James L. Fleckenstein.)

subjects, with an attendant decrease in strength. Muscles may have a mottled appearance and the radiodensity tends to be decreased, due to increased fat content and to increases in nonmuscular elements. Similar findings have been observed in Cushing's disease.[58]

Muscle Disorders in Osteomalacia

A proximal myopathy is possible in certain forms of osteomalacia.[31] In experimental conditions, a lack of vitamin D can induce muscular disorders independent of blood calcium. In a similar way, hypophosphatemia may alter muscle function.

Using ^{31}P-MRS, Smith et al. studied a patient with adult-onset familial hypophosphatemic myopathy and four subjects with inherited infantile-onset hypophosphatemia (vitamin D-resistant rickets) without myopathy.[59] All of these patients showed normal resting muscle ^{31}P-MRS. In phosphate-depleted rats, however, electrical stimulation of hindleg muscles induced increased acidosis and the PCr recovery after stimulation was slower than in normal rats.[60] This suggests that phosphate deficiency might impair mitochondrial oxidative phosphorylation.

Conclusions

Diagnostic imaging techniques are important in the diagnosis and the follow-up of TAO. The differentiation between fibrotic or edematous muscular changes, especially by MRI, could be helpful in choosing treatment by surgical decompression or by radiotherapy, but this needs to be confirmed by further studies. In endocrine myopathies, imaging and spectroscopic techniques could be combined with muscular strength measurements and serve as complementary methods to evaluate the pathophysiology of the diseases and systemic effects of treatment.

Acknowledgments. We wish to express our gratitude to Dr. J.L. George (Department of Ophthalmology), Drs. J. Leclere and G. Weryha (Department of Endocrinology, Centre Hospitalier Universitaire Nancy), and Dr. B. Weryha (Department of Radiology) for their generous collaboration and assistance.

References

1. Char DH. The ophthalmopathy of Graves' disease. Med Clin North Am 1991;75:97–119.
2. Gorman CA. Extrathyroid manifestations of Graves' disease. In: Ingbar SH, Braverman LE, editors. The thyroid: a fundamental and clinical text. Philadelphia: J.B. Lippincott Co, 1986:1015–1035.
3. Enzmann DR, Donaldson SS, Kriss JP. Appearance of Graves' disease on orbital computed tomography. J Comput Assist Tomogr 1979;3:815–8819.
4. Werner SC, Coleman DJ, Franzen LA. Ultrasonographic evidence of a consistent orbital involvement in Graves' disease. N Engl J Med 1974;290:1447–1450.
5. Gorman CA. Temporal relationship between onset of Graves' ophthalmopathy and diagnosis of thyrotoxicosis. Mayo Clin Proc 1983;58:583–588.
6. Werner S. Modification of the classification of the eye changes of Graves' disease: recommendations of the Ad Hoc Commitee of the American Thyroid Association. J Clin Endocrinol Metab 1977;44:203–204.
7. Trokel SL, Jakobiec FA. Correlation of CT scanning and pathologic features of ophthalmic Graves' disease. Ophthalmology 1981;88:553–564.
8. Coleman DJ, Jack RL, Franzen LA, Werner SC. High resolution B-scan ultrasonography of the orbit. Arch Ophthalmol 1972;88:465–480.
9. Coleman DJ, Woods S, Rondeau M, Silverman RH. Ophthalmic ultrasonography. Radiol Clin North Am 1992; 30:1105–1113.
10. Willinsky RA, Arenson AM, Hurwitz JJ, Szalai J. Ultrasonic B-scan measurement of the extra-ocular muscles in Graves' orbitopathy. J Can Assoc Radiol 1984;35:171–173.
11. Byrne SF, Glaser JS. Orbital tissue differentiation with standardized echography. Ophthalmology 1983;90: 1071–1090.
12. Ossoinig KC. Standardized echography: basic principles, clinical applications, and results. Int Ophthalmol Clin 1979;19:127–210.
13. Peyster RG. Computed tomography of the orbit. In: Gonzalez CF, Becker MH, Flanagan JC, editors. Diagnostic imaging in ophthalmology. New York: Springer-Verlag, 1986:19–37.

14. Hilal SK. Computed tomography of the orbit. Ophthalmology 1979;86:864–870.

15. Markl AF, Hilberts T, Mann K. Graves' ophthalmopathy: standardized evaluation of computed tomography examinations; magnetic resonance imaging. Dev Ophthalmol (Basel) 1989;20:38–50.

16. Rothfus WE, Curtin HD. Extraocular muscle enlargement: a CT review. Radiology 1984;151:677–681.

17. Sowinski J, Ziemianski A, Gembicki M. Computerized tomography in Graves' immunoophthalmopathy. Radiobiol Radiother 1984;25:749–754.

18. Trokel SL, Hilal SK. Recognition and differential diagnosis of enlarged extraocular muscles in computed tomography. Am J Ophthalmol 1979;87:503–512.

19. Wing SD, Hunsaker JN, Anderson RE, Van Dyck HJL, Osborn AG. Direct sagittal computed tomography in Graves' ophthalmopathy. J Comput Assist Tomogr 1979; 3:820–824.

20. Forbes G, Gorman CA, Brennan MD, Gehring DG, Ilstrup DM, Earnest FI. Ophthalmopathy of Graves' disease: computerized volume measurements of the orbital fat and muscle. Am J Neuroradiol 1986;7:651–656.

21. Forbes G, Gorman CA, Gehring D, Baker HL. Computer analysis of orbital fat and muscle volumes in Graves ophthalmopathy. Am J Neuroradiol 1983;4:737–740.

22. Trokel SL, Hilal SK. Submillimeter resolution CT scanning of orbital diseases. Ophthalmology 1980;87:412–417.

23. Hawkes RC, Holland GN, Moore WS, Rizk S, Worthington BS, Kean DM. NMR imaging in the evaluation of orbital tumors. Am J Neuroradiol 1983;4:254–256.

24. Hosten N, Sander B, Cordes M, Shubert CJ, Schörner W, Felix R. Graves ophthalmopathy: MR imaging of the orbits. Radiology 1989;172:759–762.

25. Li KC, Poon PY, Hinton P, et al. MR imaging of orbital tumors with CT and ultrasound correlations. J Comput Assist Tomogr 1984;8:1039–1047.

26. Roden DT, Savino PJ, Zimmerman RA. Magnetic resonance imaging in orbital diagnosis. Radiol Clin North Am 1988;26:535–545.

27. Just M, Kahaly G, Higer HP, et al. Graves ophthalmopathy: role of MR imaging in radiation therapy. Radiology 1991; 179:187–190.

28. Kaissar G, Kim JH, Bravo S, Sze G. Histologic basis for increased extraocular muscle enhancement in gadolinium-enhanced MR imaging. Radiology 1991;179:541–542.

29. Pozzo GD, Boshi MC. Extraocular muscle enlargement in acromegaly. J Comput Assist Tomogr 1982;6:706–707.

30. Gean-Marton AD, Kirsch CFE, Vezina LG, Weber AL. Focal amyloidosis of the head and neck: evaluation with CT and MR imaging. Radiology 1991;521:521–525.

31. Ruff RL. Endocrine myopathies (hyper- and hypofunction of adrenal, thyroid, pituitary and parathyroid glands and iatrogenic steroid myopathy). In: Engel AG, Banker BQ, editors. Myology. New York: McGraw-Hill Book Co., 1986:1871–1906.

32. Ramsay ID. Electromyography in thyrotoxicosis. Q J Med 1965;34:255–258.

33. Zürcher RM, Horber FF, Grünig BE, Frey FJ. Effect of thyroid dysfunction on thigh muscle efficiency. J Clin Endocrinol Metab 1989;69:1082–1086.

34. Serratrice G, Salamon G, Jiddane M, Gastaut JL, Pelissier JF, Pouget J. Results of CT examination of muscles in 145 cases of neuromuscular diseases. Rev Neurol (Paris) 1985; 141:404–412.

35. Huppert D, Witt TN, Nägele M. Chronisch-hyperthreote Myopathie. Ein Beitrag zur Differentialdiagnose des myopathischen Gliedergürtelsyndroms. Nervenarzt 1991;62: 374–377.

36. Kaminsky P, Robin-Lherbier B, Walker P, et al. Muscle bioenergetic impairment in hyperthyroid man: a study by 31P NMR spectroscopy. Acta Endocrinol (Copenh) 1991; 124:271–277.

37. Argov Z, Renshaw PF, Boden B, Winokur A, Bank WJ. Effects of thyroid hormones on skeletal muscle bioenergetics: in vivo phosphorus-31 magnetic resonance spectroscopy study of humans and rats. J Clin Invest 1988;81: 1695–1701.

38. Martin WHI, Spina RJ, Korte E, et al. Mechanisms of impaired exercise capacity in short duration experimental hyperthyroidism. J Clin Invest 1991;88:2047–2053.

39. Astrom KE, Kugelberg E, Muller R. Hypothyroid myopathy. Arch Neurol 1961;5:472–482.

40. Klein I, Parker M, Shebert R, Ayyar DR, Levey GS. Hypothyroidism presenting as muscle stiffness and pseudohypertrophy: Hoffmann's syndrome. Am J Med 1981; 70:891–894.

41. Pearce J, Aziz H. The neuromyopathy of hypothyroidism. J Neurol Sci 1969;9:243–253.

42. Khaleeli ALIA, Gohil K, McPhail G, Round JM, Edwards RHT. Muscle morphology and metabolism in hypothyroid myopathy: effects of treatment. J Clin Pathol 1983;36: 519–526.

43. Norris FH, Panner BJ. Hypothyroid myopathy. Clinical, electromyographical and ultrastructural observations. Arch Neurol 1966;14:574–589.

44. Kaminsky P, Robin-Lherbier B, Brunotte F, et al. Energetic metabolism in hypothyroid skeletal muscle, as studied by phosphorus magnetic resonance spectroscopy. J Clin Endocrinol Metab 1992;74:124–129.

45. Argov Z, Bank WJ, Maris J, Peterson P, Chance B. Bioenergetic heterogeneity of human mitochondrial myopathies as demonstrated by in vivo phosphorus magnetic resonance spectroscopy. Neurology 1987;37:257–262.

46. Arnold DL, Taylor DJ, Radda GK. Investigation of human mitochondrial myopathies by phosphorus magnetic resonance spectroscopy. Ann Neurol 1985;18:189–196.

47. Kaminsky P, Klein M, Robin-Lherbier B, et al. A 31P NMR study of different hypothyroid states in rat leg muscle. Am J Physiol 1991;262(24):E706–E712.

48. Taylor DJ, Rajagopalan B, Radda GK. Cellular energetics in hypothyroid muscle. Eur J Clin Invest 1992;22:358–365.

49. Parker DF, Round JM, Sacco P, Jones DA. A cross sectional survey of upper and lower limb strength in boys and girls during childhood and adolescence. Ann Hum Biol 1990;17:199–211.

50. Jorgensen JOL, Pedersen SA, Thuesen L, et al. Beneficial effects of growth hormone treatment in GH-deficient adults. Lancet 1989;i:1221–1225.

51. Rutherford OM, Jones DA, Round JM, Buchanan CR, Preece MA. Changes in skeletal muscle and body com-

position after discontinuation of growth hormone treatment in growth hormone deficient young adults. Clin Endocrinol 1991;34:469–475.

52. Leger J, Garel C, Legrand I, Paulsen A, Hassan M, Czernichow P. Magnetic resonance imaging of the metabolic effects of GH on muscle and fat mass in children [abstract]. Abstracts of the Ninth International Congress of Endocrinology, Nice, France, August 30–September 5, 1992:292.

53. Kaminsky P, Klein M, Walker PM, Straczek J, Forrett MC, Duc M. GH effects on muscle bioenergetics in-vivo [abstract]. Abstracts of the Ninth International Congress of Endocrinology, Nice, France, August 30–September 5, 1992:292.

54. Mastiglia FL, Barwick DD, Hall R. Myopathy in acromegaly. Lancet 1970;ii:907–909.

55. Pickett JBE, Layser RB, Levin SR, Schneider V, Campbell MJ, Sumner AG. Neuromuscular complications of acromegaly. Neurology 1975;25:638–645.

56. Bigland B, Jehring B. Muscle performance in rats, normal and treated with growth hormone. J Physiol (Lond) 1952; 116:129–136.

57. Horber FF, Scheidegger JR, Grünig BE, Frey FJ. Evidence that prednisone-induced myopathy is reversed by physical training. J Clin Endocrinol Metab 985;61:83–87.

58. Khaleeli AA, Betteridge DJ, Edwards RHT, Round JM, Ross EJ. Effect of treatment of Cushing's syndrome on skeletal muscle structure and function. Clin Endocrinol 1983;19:547–556.

59. Smith R, Newman RJ, Radda GK, Stokes M, Young A. Hypophosphataemic osteomalacia and myopathy: studies with nuclear magnetic resonance spectroscopy. Clin Sci 1984;67:505–509.

60. Bollaert PE, Gimenez M, Robin-Lherbier B, et al. Respective effects of malnutrition and phosphate depletion on endurance swimming and muscle metabolism in rats. Acta Physiol Scand 1992;144:1–7.

21
Inflammatory Myopathies

Carl D. Reimers and Thomas J. Vogl

Clinical Features

Inflammatory myopathies encompass a heterogeneous group of acquired muscle disorders caused by infectious agents or autoimmune processes. *Infectious myositis* can be subclassified into bacterial, viral, fungal, and parasitic forms. Bacterial myositis may be purulent (e.g., in staphylococcal or streptococcal myositis) or not (e.g., in clostridial or tuberculous myositis). Parasites causing inflammatory reaction of skeletal muscles are protozoa (e.g., toxoplasma), tapeworms (e.g., cysticercus or teania echinococcus), and nematodes (e.g., trichinella spiralis). Worldwide, staphylococcal myositis is the most frequent inflammatory myopathy. In industrialized countries, *autoimmune myositis* is much more common than infectious myositis. Autoimmune myositides are subclassified according to Bohan et al.[1] into the idiopathic polymyositis in adults (type 1), dermatomyositis (type 2), myositis with malignancy (type 3), myositis in childhood (type 4), myositis associated with other autoimmune disorders (e.g., rheumatoid arthritis, lupus erythematosus, mixed connective tissue disease) (type 5), and other types (e.g., granulomatous, eosinophilic, focal, and inclusion body myositis) (type 6).

The hallmark of the diagnosis is inflammatory lymphohistiocytic infiltrates in muscle biopsy specimens. However, the presence of all of the following criteria is commonly accepted for the definite diagnosis of a *polymyositis*:[2] (1) clinical features consistent with an inflammatory myopathy (i.e., usually proximal and symmetric muscle weakness with or without myalgia), (2) increased activity of serum creatine kinase, (3) a multifocal myopathic pattern in the electromyogram, and (4) fiber necrosis and regeneration as well as mononuclear cell infiltrates with or without perifascicular atrophy in muscle biopsy samples. Myositis is the probable diagnosis if three out of the four criteria are fulfilled. *Dermatomyositis* requires an additional criterion, a permanent or transient exanthema on the face, chest, or extensor surfaces of the extremities.

Inclusion body myositis (IBM) often cannot be diagnosed by these criteria, because distal muscles are frequently predominantly affected, serum creatine kinase activity sometimes lies within the normal range, and inflammatory changes in the muscle biopsy sample may be absent. However, a number of histopathological findings support the probability of IBM, such as abnormal filamentous inclusions and rimmed vacuoles. Serum Mi-2, Jo-1, and other autoantibodies are infrequent in IBM but are strongly associated with other myositidies. Hence, when they are present they are valuable aids in making the correct diagnosis. Ultimately, the diagnosis depends on the correlation of the biopsy findings with the clinical and EMG data.[3]

Eosinophilic polymyositis is a very rare myositis, mainly affecting men. It is part of the so-called hypereosinophilic syndrome consisting of eosinophilia of the blood, bone marrow, and other organs. The most frequent clinical features are myalgia, cramps, muscle tenderness, and swelling. Muscle weakness is relatively seldom seen. Involvement of joints and the heart as well as Raynaud's phenomenon may appear. Erythrocyte sedimentation rate (ESR) and serum creatine kinase levels are usually increased.

The diagnostic evaluation includes the history, physical examination, measurement of the serum creatine kinase activity, electromyography, and muscle biopsy. If infectious myositis is suspected, aspiration and culture or serological examinations are indicated. In autoimmune-mediated myositis, testing for autoantibodies (rheumatoid factor, antinuclear antibodies, etc.) may be helpful for refining the diagnosis.

Focal myositis, initially described by Cumming et al.[5] and Heffner et al.,[6] is a benign inflammatory pseudotumor of skeletal muscle of unknown origin, presenting as a localized painful swelling within the soft tissue of an extremity. Histopathology reveals lymphocytic infiltration, scattered muscle fiber necrosis and regeneration, and interstitial fibrosis. Complete recovery may follow surgical removal of the lesion.[7]

Proliferative myositis is another rare, benign, "pseudosarcomatous," quickly expanding lesion of skeletal muscle. The coarse swelling may be painful or not. The histopathological hallmarks of this myositis are a diffusely spreading mass of fibroblasts and basophilic giant cells.[8]

Diagnostic Imaging in Inflammatory Myopathies

Radiography

Plain soft tissue roentgenograms are extremely limited in diagnosing myositis. Minor exceptions are swelling[9,10] and increased radiodensity[11] of the soft tissue in pyomyositis and calcifications in childhood dermatomyositis[12-14] and parasitic myositis.[15]

Scintigraphy

Scintigraphy by [99m]technetium chelates, and [67]gallium citrate can be used for localizing *pyomyositis*[11,16-26] and for documenting the activity and extent of *autoimmune-mediated inflammatory muscle disorders.*[27-34] In those studies that included at least six patients with active autoimmune-mediated myositis,[27,28,30,31,34] the sensitivity of scintigraphy was 88%. However, Renwick and Ritterbusch[35] found normal technetium scans in each of their four patients with pyomyositis. Scintigraphy is not generally accepted as a routine diagnostic procedure in suspected inflammatory myopathy, probably due to radiation effects and superior sensitivity of other imaging techniques such as MRI.

Ultrasound

Infectious Myositis

In *pyomyositis*, intramuscular echo-poor regions indicating focal inflammation can be found.[9,11,17,19,36-42] The hypoechoic collection may show septa.[11] The muscle increases in diameter.[38,40,43] The subcutaneous fat may sometimes be thickened and hyperechoic.[40] More rarely diffuse inflammation in the muscles is visible, resulting in extensive low[36] or high echointensities.[38] Ultrasound also may show areas of both increased and decreased echogenicity.[43] In a woman with *Lyme myositis*, ultrasound revealed slightly increased echogenicity of the rectus femoris muscles.[44] In a patient with muscular *echinococcosis*, confluent abscesses could be detected.[45]

Autoimmune-Mediate Myositis

Poly- and *dermatomyositis* in childhood result in slight, focal, homogeneous[46,47] areas of increased muscle echogenicity. The bone edge may be diminished,[46] and the fasciae and septae obscure.[48] In childhood, von Rohden et al. found decreased muscle diameters in myositis associated with mixed connective tissue disease and increased muscle size in poly- and dermatomyositis.[47] Heckmatt et al.[49] reported a marked alteration in relative echogenicity of the rectus femoris and vastus intermedius muscles when the transducer is angulated in the transverse plane. It was assumed that this alteration in echointensity relates to perifascicular atrophy and infiltration of the connective tissue. Subcutaneous and intramuscular calcifications can be visualized by ultrasound.[13,50] In chronic polymyositis, ultrasound shows atrophy and increased echointensity, predominantly of lower extremity muscles due to fat infiltration (Figure 21.1), whereas in dermatomyositis, clear muscle atrophy is rare and echointensities are highest in forearm muscles. Echointensities are less abnormal in dermatomyositis as compared to poly- and granulomatous myositis.[51] Hofman et al.[52] found hyperechogenicity in the gastrocnemius of one patient with myositis due to polyarteritis nodosa.

In the *nodular type of sarcoid myositis*, ultrasound shows hypoechoic areas.[53] *Diffuse chronic granulomatous myositis* is characterized by high echointensities due to fatty infiltration and a tendency towards true hypertrophy or pseudohypertrophy. The triceps brachii and the calves often show pseudohypertrophy.[51] In *inclusion body myositis*, severe muscle atrophy is the most impressive feature in the majority of patients (Figure 21.2).[51]

Computed Tomography

Infectious Myositis

In *pyomyositis*, increased muscle volume[9,18,39,54] with one or more low-density areas may be identified.[9,19,24,29,35,37,39,55-59] After application of contrast-media, ring enhancement can sometimes result.[29,37,58] Identification of visible subcutaneous edema was rare until recently.[9,18] In 1995, from a large CT and MRI series of pyomyositis, it was reported that subcutaneous fat edema was the rule, rather than the exception.[60] This conflicted with a previous MRI report describing minimal subcutaneous fat changes in pyomyositis.[16] Because the latter study was restricted to patients infected with the human immunodeficiency virus, a difference in the immune status of the patients was speculated to account for the disparate results. In a separate report of a patient with HIV-associated myositis, contrast-enhanced CT showed normal findings.[61] However, in the larger series of patients, contrast infusion was suggested as a helpful way to identify some cases of pyomyositis,

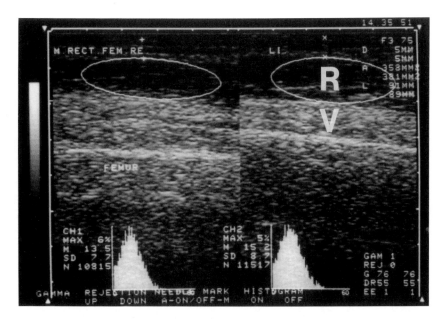

FIGURE 21.1. Chronic polymyositis: ultrasound findings. Longitudinal scans (3.75 MHz; left side of the figure = right thigh and vice versa) show normal echointensities of the rectus femoris (R) and high echointensities of the vastus intermedius (V), indicating bilateral replacement of muscle fibers by fat. Ellipses denote regions of interest for gray-scale echointensity analyses (histograms in figure bottoms).

particularly in MRI.[60] CT was insensitive in detecting disease in two patients with *Lyme myositis*.[44,62]

In *cysticercosis*, multiple 4 to 7 mm wide intramuscular hypodense foci can be found.[63,64] The scolices were depicted as small hyperdense, contrast enhancing foci.[64]

Autoimmune-Mediated Myositis

In *polymyositis*, CT discloses symmetric muscle wasting of the pelvic muscles and lower extremities, particularly in the thighs, which in early stages is associated with

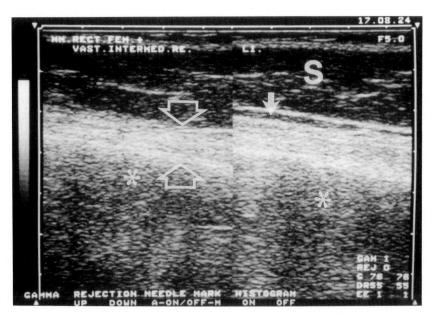

FIGURE 21.2. Chronic inclusion body myositis: ultrasound findings. Longitudinal thigh scans (5.0 MHz; left side of the figure = right thigh and vice versa) do not enable the distinction of the rectus femoris and vastus intermedius muscles (between open arrows). Both muscles show marked atrophy (diameter less than 1 cm) and high echointensities due to severe fatty change. The femur shadows exhibit abnormally high echointensity (asterisks). S indicates subcutaneous fat, arrow indicates thin layer of fat between two of the fascial sheets.

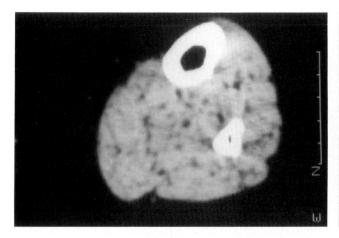

FIGURE 21.3. Chronic polymyositis: computed tomography findings. Transverse image of left leg shows small, low-density patches distributed diffusely throughout multiple muscles due to areas of "marble-like," "moth-eaten," or "vermiform" fatty replacement of muscle.

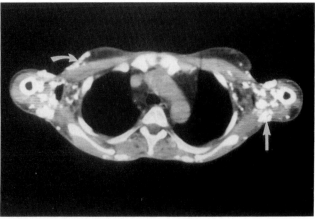

FIGURE 21.4. Late sequelae of childhood-onset dermatomyositis: computed tomography findings. Transverse image of arms and chest show numerous high-density areas in the subcutaneous fat (curved arrow) and muscles (arrow), indicating calcium deposits. The muscles show no definite hypodensity to suggest fatty change or edema.

small areas of hypodensity, giving the muscle a trabecular or spotted ("worm- or moth-eaten") appearance[63,65–68] (Figure 21.3). Low-density areas indicating fat are more apparent in the vastus lateralis compared to the semimembranosus and biceps femoris muscle.[69]

In *childhood dermatomyositis*, CT can identify subcutaneous and intramuscular calcifications[14,50] (Figure 21.4). Coackley et al.[70] observed one adult patient with polymyositis exhibiting muscle calcifications, which were reversible after treatment.

Maruyama et al. described one patient with a histopathologically proven, chronic multifocal myositis exhibiting asymmetrical muscle atrophy and patchy low-density foci in skeletal muscles.[71]

In the *nodular type of granulomatous myositis*, CT demonstrates normal findings[53,72] or shows areas of low attenuation with a rim of contrast enhancement.[73] In the *chronic myopathic type of granulomatous myositis*, CT findings may be normal,[72,73] but more typically show marked fatty change[74] (Figure 21.5). As in polymyositis,

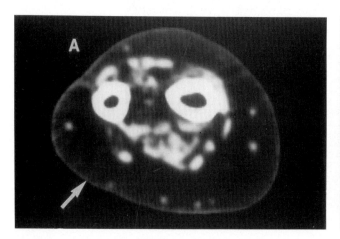

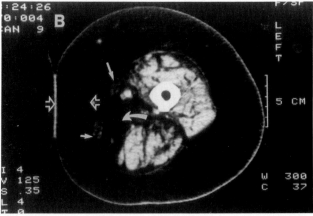

FIGURE 21.5. Chronic granulomatous polymyositis: computed tomography findings. (A) Only a few islands of muscle parenchyma are visible in the forearm. Note prominence of the subcutaneous fat (arrow). (B) Axial image of the same patient's left thigh shows the subcutaneous fat to be extremely increased (between open arrows). The thigh muscles are atrophic. In particular, the sartorius (long arrow), gracilis (shortest arrow), and adductor magnus/semimembranosus (curved arrow) are totally replaced by fat. In the remaining muscles small, low-density areas indicating fat infiltrations are depicted.

a "moth-eaten" appearance of the muscles can be seen.[67]

In *focal myositis*, CT reveals diffuse homogeneous enlargement with fatty infiltration of the affected muscles[54,75] or without[76] abnormality of the muscular radiodensity. In *proliferative myositis*, Flury et al.[8] found a muscular mass with inhomogeneous radiodensity and marked contrast enhancement.

Magnetic Resonance Imaging

Infectious Myositis

In three of six HIV patients with *pyomyositis*, Fleckenstein et al.[16] found a rim of high signal intensity separating a central region isointense with the surrounding muscle or regions of slightly increased signal intensity on T_1-weighted images. T_2-weighted and short tau inversion recovery (STIR) images showed very high signal intensity in the central portion of the abscesses (see Chapter 22). Ahrens et al.,[43] Barlier et al.,[77] and Reutter-Simon et al.[11] report one patient each with pyomyositis showing a small center of low signal intensity with a large surrounding area of increased signal intensity on the T_1-weighted image. On the T_2-weighted image in pyomyositis, the diseased area presents with high signal intensities.[11,35,43,77,78] Walling and Kaelin[59] also report one patient with staphylococcal pyomyositis presenting with high signal intensity on the T_1-weighted image. On the other hand, high signal intensity on proton and T_2-weighted images in pyomyositis may be associated with normal or only slightly abnormal appearances on T_1-weighted images.[9,18,79,80] Intravenous injection of gadolinium-DTPA causes enhancement around central foci of purulent necrosis/pus.[60,79,81]

In one volunteer with an experimental *postvaccinial myositis*, edema was visible, characterized by focally increased signal intensity on T_2-weighted and normal signal intensity on T_1-weighted images.[63]

In one patient with *Lyme myositis*, visual assessment revealed slightly higher signal intensity in the medial head of the gastrocnemius muscles on T_2-weighted compared to the T_1-weighted images, indicating edema.[44]

Autoimmune-Mediated Myositis

In acute *poly- and dermatomyositis* of children and adults, MRI shows muscle edema. This is characterized by a normal or nearly normal appearance on T_1-weighted images and focally or diffusely increased signal intensity on T_2-weighted and/or STIR sequences (Figures 21.6 to 21.8).[72,82–87] Functional disability[86,88] and disease activity[82–84,88,89] correlate strongly with increased T_2 and STIR signal intensity. MRI is more sensitive, but less specific, than the muscle biopsy in detecting pathological changes and disease activity.[83,84] Fraser et al.[82–84] additionally found a correlation between the presence of inflammation and myopathy at muscle biopsy on the one hand and increased T_2 and STIR signal intensity on the other hand, whereas Reimers et al.[89] did not. One MRI study employing exclusively T_1-weighted images suggested a correlation between MRI abnormalities and disease activity.[90]

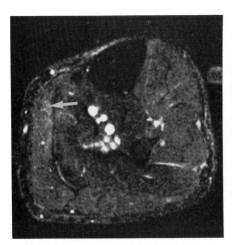
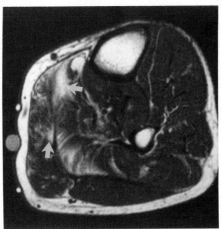
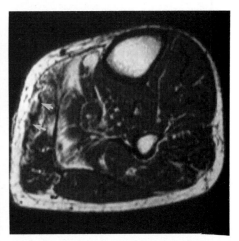

A   B   C

FIGURE 21.6. MRI documentation of biopsy site in dermatomyositis. (A) Prebiopsy STIR image shows edema-like high signal intensity in the medial head of the left gastrocnemius (arrow). (B) A T_1-weighted image at the same level shows (266/11) a few "moth-eaten" foci of fatty change (arrowheads).

(C) Repeat imaging with the T_1-weighted sequence after the site biopsied was marked by undiluted intramuscular gadolinium-DTPA; the muscle tract is denoted by the linear region of T_2^* shortening (short arrows).

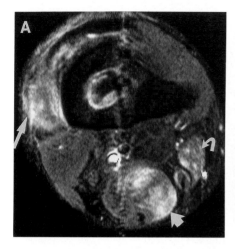
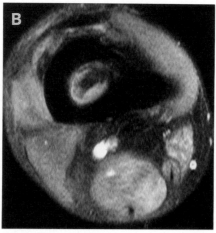
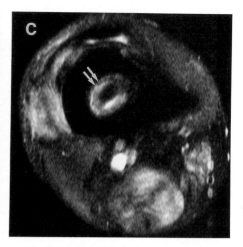

FIGURE 21.7. Relative sensitivity of fat-suppression sequences in detecting muscle edema in polymyositis. (A) Axial STIR image (2500/30/150, $T_R/T_E/T_I$) of the right thigh shows edematous changes in vastus lateralis (arrow), semimembranosus (arrowhead), and sartorius (curved arrow). (B) When the same slice is studied with a fat-specific suppression pulse at the same T_R and T_E, but no inversion pulse, the conspicuity of edema is much reduced. (C) Trial and error identified that an echo time (T_E) of 70 ms was needed to provide similar contrast to noise as the STIR image. Bone marrow edema (double small arrow) was from a bone infarct, related to glucocorticoid treatment.

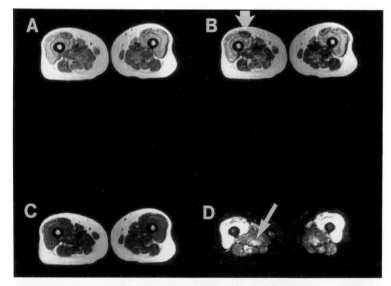

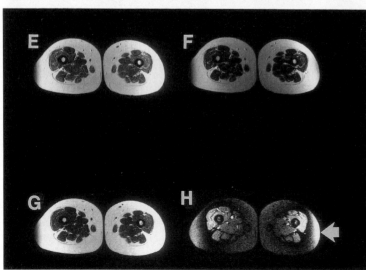

FIGURE 21.8. Acute dermatomyositis: pre- and posttherapy MRI findings. (A) Proton density (2000/30) image shows moderately increased signal intensity of multiple thigh muscles. (B) With greater T_2 weighting (2000/60), the contrast of abnormal muscles is greater. Note, for example, that each of the quadriceps muscles are abnormal, with the right rectus femoris less involved (arrowhead). (C) That the signal intensity changes are due to edema, and not to fat, is evident by normality of signal intensity with T_1 weighting (500/30). (D) Edematous change is most conspicuous using STIR (1500/30/100), even in sites where it was difficult to identify without fat suppression (arrow). MRI support of improvement in this case was provided by repeat MRI performed after 60 days of treatment with corticosteroids. (E-H) Using the same MRI sequences as on the pretreatment study, only mild atrophy and minimal signal intensity alteration remains in the quadriceps. High signal intensity in the lateral aspect of the subcutaneous fat (arrow) is due to radiofrequency field inhomogeneity, a well-recognized artifact using STIR. (Reprinted from Pitt et al.[101]).

In contrast to a nearly normal appearance of muscle edema on T_1-weighted images, fatty infiltration of muscle, as frequently occurs in *chronic poly- or dermatomyosits*,[89] shows increased signal intensity on T_1-weighted images. The T_2-weighted appearance alone does not allow distinction between fat and edema because both of these muscle alterations cause increases in the T_2 time and hence a hyperintense appearance on T_2-weighted images. This is a clinically relevant technical point, because relying upon only these two sequences to characterize chronic myositis may underestimate active muscle inflammation because the edema may be masked by concurrent fatty change. In this situation, fat-suppressed edema-sensitive sequences are ideal, with the STIR sequence being used most often.[82,84,91] Just as increased muscle adiposity was more typical of *chronic poly- or dermatomyositis* than of acute myositis, the size of the residual muscle mass also correlated with the duration of the disease[84] (Figures 21.6, 21.9).

The utility of intravenous contrast was also assessed in autoimmune-mediated myositis.[89] Contrast-enhanced T_1-weighted images did not provide more information than T_2-weighted images alone and it was concluded that the routine use of contrast could not be recommended.

The distribution of muscle lesions has been addressed in autoimmune-mediated myositis. In general, abnormalities are symmetric[78,84,89] and most marked in proximal muscles.[78,92] Exceptions to both generalizations are well documented, however.[89,92] Interestingly, the muscles that are the most abnormal are very variable in the literature. These include the vasti,[78,87,89,92,93] adductors,[85,86] hamstrings,[85] tibialis anterior,[89] gastrocnemius,[92,93] and soleus muscles.[92] The importance of this variability in distribution includes that there is not a pathognomonic pattern that can be sought on imaging studies in hopes of noninvasively securing a specific diagnosis. On the other hand, knowledge of the distribution of changes in a given patient can aid in individualizing invasive procedures, such as EMG and biopsy. In so doing, a reduction in the number of falsely negative biopsies can be expected. This advantage has been documented to result in an overall reduction in health care costs.[92]

MRI has also been used as an approach to monitor the response of myositis to therapy. For example, it was shown that signal intensity normalizes after successful treatment.[52,85,86,88,89] More work needs to be conducted to determine the value of MRI in this application relative to the clinical parameters of muscle strength and serum creatine kinase, however.[94]

Occasionally, increased signal intensity indicating edema can also be depicted adjacent to muscles[88] and in the subcutaneous fat tissue, particularly in dermatomyositis.[84,86,88,95] Chronic myositis may be indistinguishable from muscular dystrophies (Figures 21.9 to 21.11), although pseudohypertrophy has not been described as a feature of polymyositis. While Beese et al.[78] were unable to find any significant difference between poly- and dermatomyositis, Reimers et al.[89] found edema-like abnormalities to be more common, and muscle atrophy less common, in dermato- compared to polymyositis. However, differentiation between the two can be difficult in any given case.

In *inclusion body myositis*, no specific MRI finding has been reported. Signal intensity characteristics of single or several muscles on T_1- and T_2-weighted images suggest the presence of fat, edema-like change, or both.[78,89] The majority of patients show predominant involvement of the anterior muscle compartment of the thigh[84,89] (Figure 21.10). Focal and diffuse patterns of MRI abnormalities occur with similar frequencies.[84]

In a patient with *eosinophilic myositis*, Kaufman et al.[4] described nonspecific edematous changes on T_2-weighted images in the vastus medialis and vastus intermedius muscles. The *nodular type of sarcoid myositis* has a more peculiar MRI appearance. MRI reportedly shows a center of low signal intensity on T_1-weighted images,[73] surrounded by a zone of higher signal intensity that is more prominent with progressive T_2 weighting.[73,96] In the *myopathic type of sarcoid myositis*, MRI findings may be normal,[73] but more frequently show nonspecific increases in signal intensity on T_1- and T_2-weighted images, indicating fatty change[72,74,89] (Figure 21.11). A

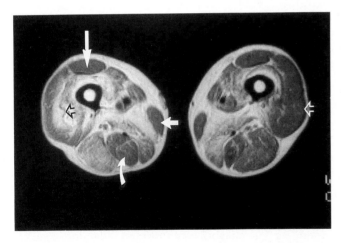

FIGURE 21.9. Chronic polymyositis: magnetic resonance imaging findings. Proton density spin echo sequence (T_R 1600 ms/T_E 30 ms) reveals high signal intensity in all muscles except the rectus femoris (arrow), gracilis (short arrow), semitendinosus (curved arrow), and the left vastus lateralis (open arrows). The signal intensities were equal to those of fat on more T_2-weighted images (not shown here). The curved epimysium between the right vastus lateralis and intermedius muscle (black open arrow) indicates loss of muscle volume and is frequently seen in inflammatory myopathies, although it is not a specific finding.

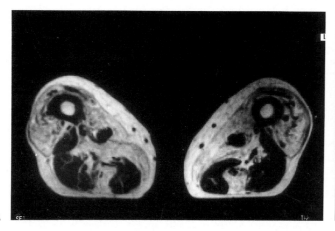

A

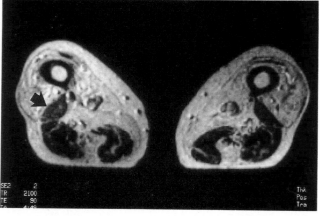

B

FIGURE 21.10. Inclusion body myositis: magnetic resonance imaging findings of chronic atrophy. (A) T_1-weighted spin echo image (T_R 750 ms/T_E 15 ms) shows high signal intensity, indicating fatty replacement, in all muscles except both heads of the biceps femoris muscles and the semimembranosus muscles. The quadriceps femoris muscles are severely atrophic. (B) A

T_2-weighted spin echo image (T_R 2100 ms/T_E 90 ms) at the same level shows similar findings to that in (A). However, minimally increased signal intensity in the short head of the biceps femoris on the right (arrow) indicates additional edema-like abnormality.

few patients present predominantly with muscle edema, indicated by much higher signal intensity on T_2- compared to T_1-weighted images.[89]

Focal myositis is relatively rare in the imaging literature. Colding-Jorgensen et al.[7] reported that MRI of focal myositis reveals a localized muscular lesion, but it was not described in detail. Beese et al.[78] and Schedel et al.[79] found edema-like abnormalities in two of five patients

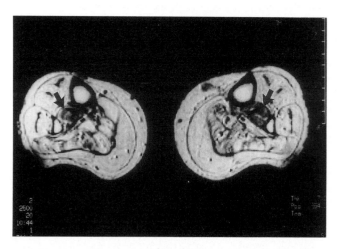

FIGURE 21.11. Chronic granulomatous myositis: magnetic resonance imaging findings of chronic atrophy. Proton density-weighted spin echo sequence (T_R 2500 ms/T_E 20 ms) shows the signal intensity of all muscles, except part of the tibialis posterior (arrows) to be very high. A T_2-weighted spin echo sequence (not shown) showed the same result, indicating fatty degeneration without associated edema of the muscles. Note that the fascial contours are normal, denoting the "filling up" process characteristic of a very longstanding, slowly progressive disease.

with focal myositis. Flaisler et al.[97] described a heterogeneous signal in affected muscle with increased signal around the soft tissue mass on T_1- and T_2-weighted images, suggesting a malignant tumor. Finally, Noel et al.[98] found no abnormality on T_1- and T_2-weighted images.

Impact on the Diagnosis and Management of Inflammatory Myopathies

Muscle imaging has proven useful in noninvasively characterizing the distribution and mesenchymal changes that occur in infectious and autoimmune-mediated myositis. In pyomyositis, imaging facilitates percutaneous needle aspiration[17,23,25,26,36,39,59,80,99,100] or surgical treatment.[40,41,81] In autoimmune-mediated myositis, imaging, especially MRI, can insure that the muscle biopsy is selected from diseased tissue.[86,90,91,101] Edema-sensitive images that indicate muscle edema or inflammation permit assessment of disease activity and potentially can help monitoring the progression of disease and may guide therapeutic decisions.[84,86] Although MR imaging is currently an expensive examination, preoperative MR imaging may substantially reduce medical costs by reducing the need for repeat biopsies.[92] Ultrasound and computed tomography are much less sensitive than MRI in detecting signs of muscle edema,[18,72,80,102] and the cost effectiveness of them has yet to be rigorously studied. Imaging, particularly MRI, may be helpful in distinguishing myositis from fibromyalgia, which exhibits normal images.[103] In the future, detection of fat replacement and edema or inflammation by MRI might be an important tool for assessment of the disease activity in clinical or scientific treatment studies.

References

1. Bohan A, Peter JB, Bowman RL, Pearson CM. A computer-assisted analysis of 153 patients with polymyositis and dermatomyositis. Medicine 1977;56:255–286.
2. Hudgson P, Peter JB. Classification. Clin Rheum Dis 1984;10:3–8.
3. Mikol J, Engel AG. Inclusion body myositis. In: Engel AG, Franzini-Armstrong C, eds. Myology, 2nd ed. New York: McGraw Hill, 1994:1533–1553.
4. Kaufman LD, Kephart GM, Seidman RJ, et al. The spectrum of eosinophilic myositis. Clinical and immunopathogenic studies of three patients, and review of the literature. Arthritis Rheum 1993;36:1014–1024.
5. Cumming W, Weiser R, Teoh R, et al. Localized nodular myositis: a clinical and pathological variant of polymyositis. Q J Med 1977;46:531–546.
6. Heffner RR, Armbrustmacher VW, Earle KM. Focal myositis. Cancer 1977;40:301–306.
7. Colding-Jorgensen E, Laursen H, Lauritzen M. Focal myositis of the thigh: report of two cases. Acta Neurol Scand 1993;88:289–292.
8. Flury D, von Hochstetter AR, Landolt U, Schmid S. Proliferative Myositis—eine wenig bekannte pseudomaligne Läsion. Schweiz Med Wochenschr 1993;123:29–34.
9. González-Gay MA, Sánchez-Andrade A, Cereijo MJ, Pulpeiro JR, Armesto V. Pyomyositis and septic arthritis from Fusobacterium nucleatum in a nonimmunocompromised adult. J Rheumatol 1993;20:518–520.
10. Singer J. Neonatal psoas pyomyositis simulating pyathrosis of the hip. Pediatr Emerg Care 1993;9:87–89.
11. Reutter-Simon G, Schwarzer U, Reither M. "Tropische" Pyomyositis im Kindesalter. Monatsschr Kinderheilk 1993;141:293–296.
12. Blane CF, White SJ, Braunstein EM, et al. Patterns of calcification in childhood dermatomyositis. AJR 1984;142:397.
13. Hesla RB, Karlson LK, McCauley RG. Milk of calcium fluid collection in dermatomyositis: ultrasound findings. Pediatr Radiol 1990;20:344–346.
14. Randle HW, Sander HM, Temple T. Early diagnosis of calcinosis cutis in childhood dermatomyositis using computed tomography. JAMA 1986;256:1137–1138.
15. Burgener FA, Kormano M. Differential diagnosis in conventional radiology. 2nd ed. Stuttgart: Thieme, 1991:114–116.
16. Fleckenstein JL, Burns DK, Murphy FK, et al. Differential diagnosis of bacterial myositis in AIDS: evaluation with MR imaging. Radiology 1991;179:653–658.
17. Datz FL, Lewis SE, Conrad MR, et al. Pyomyositis diagnosed by radionuclide imaging and ultrasonography. South Med J 1980;73:649–651.
18. Fam AG, Rubenstein J, Saibil F. Pyomyositis: early detection and treatment. J Rheumatol 1993;20:521–524.
19. Flory P, Brocq O, Euller-Ziegler L, Ziegler G. Pyomyositis: cervical localization. J Rheumatol 1993;20:1411–1413.
20. Hirano T, Srinivasan G, Janakiraman N, et al. Gallium 67 citrate scintigraphy in pyomyositis. J Pediatr 1986;97:596–597.
21. Howman-Giles R, McCauley D, Brown J. Multifocal pyomyositis. Diagnosis on technetium-99m MDP bone scan. Clin Nucl Med 1984;9:149–151.
22. Lamki L, Willis RB. Radionuclide findings of pyomyositis. Clin Nucl Med 1982;7:465–467.
23. Rao R, Gerber FH, Greaney RB, et al. Gallium-67 citrate imaging in pyomyositis. J Nucl Med 1981;22:836–837.
24. Tumeh SS, Butler GJ, Maguire JH, et al. Pyogenic myositis: CT evaluation. J Comput Assist Tomogr 1988;12:1002–1005.
25. Wolf RF, Sprenger HG, Mooyaart EL, et al. Nontropical pyomyositis as a cause of subacute, multifocal myalgia in the acquired immunodeficiency syndrome. Arthritis Rheum 1990;33:1728–1732.
26. Yousefzadeh DK, Schumann EM, Mulligan GM, et al. The role of imaging modalities in diagnosis and management of pyomyositis. Skeletal Radiol 1982;8:285–289.
27. Brown MW, Swift TR, Spies ST. Radioisotope scanning in inflammatory muscle disease. Neurology 1976;26:517–520.
28. Buchpiquel CA, Roizenblatt S, Lucena-Fernandes MF, et al. Radioisotopic assessment of peripheral and cardiac muscle involvement and dysfunction in polymyositis/dermatomyositis. J Rheumatol 1991;18:1359–1363.
29. Hall RL, Callaghan JJ, Moloney E, et al. Pyomyositis in a temperate climate. J Bone Joint Surg 1990;72-A:1240–1244.
30. Kula RW, Line BR, Siegel BA, et al. ^{99m}Tc-diphosphonate scanning of soft-tissue in neuromuscular diseases. Neurology 1976;26:370.
31. Messina C, Bonanno N, Baldari S, et al. Muscle uptake of ^{99m}technetium pyrophosphate in patients with neuromuscular disorders. A quantitative study. J Neurol Sci 1982;53:1–7.
32. Patel N, Krasnow A, Sebastian JL, et al. Isolated muscular sarcoidosis causing fever of unknown origin: the value of gallium-67 imaging. J Nucl Med 1991;32:319–321.
33. Steinfeld JR, Thorne NA, Kennedy TF. Positive ^{99m}Tc-pyrophosphate bone scan in polymyositis. Radiology 1977;122:168.
34. Yonker RA, Webster EM, Edwards NL, et al. Technetium pyrophosphate muscle scans in inflammatory muscle disease. Br J Rheumatol 1987;26:267–269.
35. Renwick SE, Ritterbusch JF. Pyomyositis in children. J Pediatr Orthop 1993;13:769–727.
36. Belli L, Reggiori A, Cocozza E, et al. Ultrasound in tropical pyomyositis. Skeletal Radiol 1992;21:107–109.
37. Gyssens IC, Timmermans UM. Tropical pyomyositis. Netherlands J Med 1989;34:205–209.
38. Holsbeeck van M, Introcaso JH. Musculoskeletal ultrasound. St. Louis: Mosby Year Book, 1991:39–40.
39. Piper C, Henrich R, Wendt B, et al. Nichttropische Pyomyositis in Deutschland. Med Klinik 1990;85:707–714.
40. Quillin SP, McAlister WH. Rapidly progressive pyomyositis. Diagnosis by repeated sonography. J Ultrasound Med 1991;10:181–184.
41. Weinberg WG, Dembert ML. Tropical pyomyositis: delineation by gray scale ultrasound. Am J Trop Hyg 1984;33:930–932.

42. Yagupsky P, Shazak E, Barki Y. Non-invasive diagnosis of pyomyositis. Clin Pediatr 1988;27:299–301.

43. Ahrens P, Gross-Fengels W, Bovelet K. Zur Differentialdiagnose maligner Weichteiltumoren: Pyomyositis. Akt Radiol 1991;1:40–42.

44. Reimers CD, Pongratz DE, Neubert U, et al. Myositis caused by Borrelia burgdorferi: report of four cases. J Neurol Sci 1989;91:215–226.

45. Meyer E, Adam T. Über ungewöhnliche Manifestationen der Echinokokkose. Radiologe 1989;29:245–249.

46. Fischer AG, Carpenter DW, Hartlage PL, et al. Muscle imaging in neuromuscular disease using computerized real-time sonography. Muscle Nerve 1988;11:270–275.

47. Rohden L von, Wiemann D, Köditz H. Ist die Ultraschalldiagnostik (B-Bild) bei Kollagenosen im Kindesalter nützlich? Kinderarzt 1985;16:1345–1350.

48. Forst R. Skelettmuskel-Sonographie bei neuromuskulären Erkrankungen. Stuttgart: Enke, 1986.

49. Heckmatt JZ, Pier N, Dubowitz V. Real-time ultrasound imaging of muscles. Muscle Nerve 1988;11:56–65.

50. Reimers CD, Naegele M, Fenzl G, et al. Entzündliche Myopathien: Diagnostische Wertigkeit bildgebender Verfahren an der Skelettmuskulatur. Therapiewoche 1989;39:560–565.

51. Reimers CD, Fleckenstein JL, Witt TN, et al. Muscular ultrasound in idiopathic inflammatory myopathies of adults. J Neurol Sci 1993;95:82–92.

52. Hofman DM, Lems WF, Witkamp TD, et al. Demonstration of calf abnormalities by magnetic resonance imaging in polyarteriitis nodosa. Clin Rheumatol 1992;11:402–404.

53. Kayanuma K, Uono M. A case of muscular sarcoidosis of palpable nodules type with pseudohypertrophy—comparison of computerized tomography and ultrasound imaging of skeletal muscles. Clin Neurol 1987;27:760–766.

54. Liefeld PA, Ferguson AB Jr, Fu FH. Focal myositis: a benign lesion that mimics malignant disease. A case report. J Bone Joint Surg 1982;64A:1373–1373.

55. Chaitow J, Martin HCO, Knight P, et al. Pyomyositis tropicans: a diagnostic dilemma. Med J Aust 1980;2:512–513.

56. Gaut P, Wong PK, Meyer RD. Pyomyositis in a patient with the acquired immunodeficiency syndrome. Arch Intern Med 1988;148:1608–1610.

57. Lachiewicz PF, Hadler NM. Spontaneous pyomyositis in a patient with Felty's syndrome: diagnosis using computerized tomography. South Med J 1986;79:1047–1048.

58. Schlech WF III, Moulton P, Kaiser AB. Pyomyositis: tropical disease in a temperate climate. Am J Med 1981;71:900–902.

59. Walling DM, Kaelin WG. Pyomyositis in patients with diabetes mellitus. Rev Infect Dis 1991;13:797–802.

60. Collins AJ. Pyomyositis: Characteristics at CT and MR imaging. Radiology 1995;197:279–286.

61. Scott JA, Palmer EL, Fischman AJ. HIV-associated myositis detected by radionuclide bone scanning. J Nucl Med 1989;30:556–558.

62. Atlas E, Novak SN, Duray PH, et al. Lyme myositis: muscle invasion by Borrelia burgdorferi. Ann Intern Med 1988;109:245–246.

63. Rodiek S-R. CT, MR-Tomographie und MR-Spektroskopie bei neuromuskulären Erkrankungen. Stuttgart: Enke, 1987.

64. Wadia N, Desai S, Bhatt M. Disseminated cysticercosis. New observations, including CT scan findings and experience with treatment by praziquantel. Brain 1988;111:597–614.

65. Konagaya Y, Konagaya M, Mano Y. Quadriceps myositis. Intern Med 1992;31:926–929.

66. Laroche M, Rousseau H, Mazières B, et al. Intérèt de la tomodensitométrie dans la pathologie musculaire. Rev Rhum 1989;56:433–439.

67. Serratrice G, Acquaviva P, Schiano A, et al. Apport du scanner musculaire dans la polyarthrite et en rhumatologie. Rev Rhum 1985;52:313–315.

68. Serratrice G, Salamon G, Jiddane M, et al. Résultats du scanner X musculaire dans 145 cas de maladies neuromusculaires. Rev Neurol 1985;141:404–412.

69. Schwartz MS, Swash M, Ingram DA, et al. Patterns of selective involvement of thigh muscles in neuromuscular disease. Muscle Nerve 1988;11:1240–1245.

70. Coackley JH, Smith PEM, Jackson MJ, et al. Myositis ossificans non-progressiva reversible muscle calcification in polymyositis. Br J Rheumatol 1989;28:443–445.

71. Marayuma T, Kondo K, Tabata K, Yanagisawa N. A case of chronic multifocal myositis. Rinsho Shinkeigaku 1992;32:1294–1298.

72. Kurashima K, Shimizu H, Ogawa H, et al. MR and CT in the evaluation of sarcoid myopathy. J Comput Assist Tomogr 1991;15:1004–1007.

73. Otake S, Banno T, Ohba S, et al. Muscular sarcoidosis: findings at MR imaging. Radiology 1990;176:145–148.

74. Reimers CD, Naegele M, Hübner G, et al. Fasziitis bei granulomatöser Myositis—eine atypische Manifestation einer Sarkoidose? Klin Wochenschr 1990;68:335–341.

75. Moskovic E, Fisher C, Westbury G, Parsons C. Focal myositis, a benign inflammatory pseudotumor: CT appearances. Br J Radiol 1991;64:489–493.

76. Isaacson G, Chan KH, Heffner RR. Focal myositis. A new cause for the pediatric neck mass. Arch Otolaryngol Head Neck Surg 1991;117:103–105.

77. Barlier A, Berrut G, Chameau AM, et al. Pyomyosite du vaste externe chez une diabetique. Ann Med Interne Paris 1993;144:137–138.

78. Beese MS, Winkler G, Nicolas V, et al. Diagnostik entzündlicher Muskel- und Gefäßerkrankungen in der MRT mit STIR-Sequenzen. Fortschr Geb Röntgenstrahlen Neuen Bildgeb Verfahr 1993;158:542–549.

79. Schedel H, Vogl T, Reimers CD, et al. Diagnostik akuter Myositiden. Kernspintomographie mit Gd-DTPA. Fortschr Röntgenstr 1991;155:370–372.

80. Yuh WTC, Schreiber AE, Montgomery WJ, et al. Magnetic resonance imaging in pyomyositis. Skeletal Radiol 1988;17:190–193.

81. Schedel H, Reimers CD, Vogl T, et al. Ultrasound and MR imaging of acute myositis. Eur Radiol 1992;2:70–72.

82. Fraser DD, Frank JA, Dalakas MC. Inflammatory myopathies: MR imaging and spectroscopy. Radiology 1991;179:341–344.

83. Fraser DD, Frank JA, Dalakas M, et al. Magnetic resonance imaging (MRI) demonstrates muscle inflammation in idiopathic inflammatory myopathies (IIM). Arthritis Rheum 1989;32:S125.

84. Fraser DD, Frank JA, Dalakas M, et al. Magnetic resonance imaging in the idiopathic inflammatory myopathies. J Rheumatol 1991;18:1693–1700.

85. Fujino H, Kobayashi T, Goto I, Quitsuka M. Magnetic resonance imaging of the muscles in patients with polymyositis and dermatomyositis. Muscle Nerve 1991;14:716–720.

86. Hernandez RJ, Keim DR, Sullivan DB, et al. Magnetic resonance imaging appearance of the muscles in childhood dermatomyositis. J Pediatr 1990;117:546–550.

87. Park JH, Vansant JP, Kumar NG, et al. Dermatomyositis: correlative MR imaging and P-31 MR spectroscopy for quantitative characterization of inflammatory disease. Radiology 1990;177:473–479.

88. Hernandez RJ, Sullivan DB, Chenevert TL, Keim DR. MR imaging in children with dermatomyositis: musculoskeletal findings and correlation with clinical and laboratory findings. AJR 1993;161:359–366.

89. Reimers CD, Schedel H, Fleckenstein JL, et al. Magnetic resonance imaging of skeletal muscles in idiopathic inflammatory myopathies of adults. J Neurol 1994;241:306–314.

90. Kaufman LD, Gruber BL, Gerstman DP, Kaell AT. Preliminary observations on the role of magnetic resonance imaging for polymyositis and dermatomyositis. Ann Rheum Dis 1987;46:569–572.

91. Hernandez RJ, Keim DR, Chenevert TL, et al. Fat-suppressed MR imaging in myositis. Radiology 1992;182:217–219.

92. Schweitzer ME, Fort JG. Polymyositis: MR findings, utility, and cost-effectiveness of MR imaging as a biopsy guide. AJR 1995;165:1469–1471.

93. Lamminen AE. Magnetic resonance imaging of primary skeletal muscle diseases: patterns of distribution and severity of involvement. Br J Radiol 1990;63:946–950.

94. Beese MS, Winkler G, Krupsy G, Steiner P, Nicolas V. Usefulness of T_2 relaxation times in monitoring therapeutic effects in neuromuscular diseases. Radiology 1994;193:259.

95. Braunschweig R, Sieberth HG, Neuerburg J, Bohndorf K. Polymyositis bei Sharp-Syndrom. Kernspintomographische, licht- und elektronenmikroskopische Befunde. Fortschr Röntgenstr 1989;151:754–756.

96. Senju R, Sakito O, Fukushima K, et al. MRI findings of muscular sarcoidosis. Jpn J Clin Radiol 1990;35:703–708.

97. Flaisler F, Blin D, Asencio G, et al. Focal myositis: a localized form of polymyositis? J Rheumatol 1993;20:1414–1416.

98. Noel E, Tebib J, Walch G, et al. La myosite focale: une forme pseudotumorale de la polymyosite. Rev Rhum Mal Osteoartic (in press).

99. McLoughlin MJ. CT and percutaneous fine-needle aspiration biopsy in tropical myositis. AJR 1980;134:157–158.

100. Radvaui MG, Chandnani VP. Tropical pyomyositis. Australas Radiol 1993;39:78–79.

101. Pitt AM, Fleckenstein JL, Greenlee RG Jr, et al. MRI-guided biopsy in inflammatory myopathy: initial results. Magn Reson Imaging 1993;11:1093–1099.

102. Schalke BCG, Kaiser WA, Schindler G, Rohkamm R. Einsatz von bildgebenden Verfahren (Computertomographie/CT und Kernspintomographie/NMR) bei entzündlichen Muskelerkrankungen (Poly/Dermatomyositis—PM/DM): Möglichkeiten in Diagnwostik und Therapiekontrolle. In: Poeck K, Hacke W, Schneider R, eds. Verhandlungen der Deutschen Gesellschaft für Neurologie 4. Berlin: Springer, 1987:84–85.

103. Kravis MM, Munk PL, McCain GA, et al. MR imaging of muscle and tender points in fibromyalgia. J Magn Reson Imaging 1993;3:669–670.

22
Muscle Disease in the Acquired Immunodeficiency Syndrome (AIDS)

James L. Fleckenstein and David P. Chason

Weakness is a common feature of AIDS that is often incorrectly assumed to result from a number of common and uncommon AIDS-related central nervous system complications.[1-9] This misconception contributes to the difficulty in diagnosing treatable causes of weakness that are due to disorders of the peripheral nervous system and/or skeletal muscle. A broad variety of pathological alterations of muscle have been reported in both biopsy[1,10] and autopsy series[11] of patients with AIDS. In these series, the range of pathological conditions spanned from nonspecific findings such as angulated fibers and fiber atrophy to specific etiologies such as *Mycobacterial avium intracellulare* myositis and *Cryptococcus neoformans* myositis. Because diagnostic imaging techniques have the ability to detect and characterize lesions of muscles, imaging modalities may be helpful to clinicians in evaluating weakness of an unclear etiology in AIDS patients.

Muscle abnormalities in AIDS which can be expected to be visible on imaging studies include myopathies that are drug-related,[12-18] autoimmune (e.g., polymyositis,[1-4,11,19-22] and infections.[2,11,23-27] Neuropathies,[3,5-7,10,11,28-33] lymphedema,[23] and other conditions[11,34,35] are also prevalent. This chapter will review the spectrum of muscle disease in AIDS and associated imaging fingings.

Drug-Related Myopathy

A myopathy induced by the commonly prescribed antiviral drug zidovudine (also referred to as azidothymidine, AZT) is recognized in AIDS patients.[12-18] Histopathology in such cases reveals "ragged red" fibers and paracrystalline inclusions, indicative of abnormal mitochondria.[12] An associated inflammatory myopathy, indistinguishable from polymyositis, may also be observed in patients with drug-related mitochondrial alterations.[12,13] Cessation of zidovudine treatment is associated with marked histo-pathological and clinical improvement. Although there are no reported cases of proven AZT-related myopathy in the imaging literature, one could speculate that imaging modalities would reveal findings typical of mitochondrial myopathy (selective deterioration of the sartorius and gracilis)[36] and/or polymyositis (selective sparing of the sartorius and gracilis).[37]

Myositidies

The incidence of bacteremia and fungemia is far greater in AIDS compared to the general population.[38] This likely contributes to the high incidence of myositis in AIDS.

Infectious myositis in AIDS may be caused by multiple organisms including bacteria, fungi, and parasites.[1,10,11,23-27] Viral myositis caused by HIV itself appears to be extremely rare, if it exists at all,[1] although myositis due to coinfection with Human T-Cell Leukemia Virus Type 1 (HTLV-1) in AIDS is recognized.[19] Idiopathic polymyositis, an autoimmune disorder, is well documented in AIDS and may precede the onset of signs and symptoms of AIDS in the HIV+ patient.[2,20,21,24]

Pyogenic Bacterial Myositis (Pyomyositis)

Pyogenic bacterial myositis (pyomyositis), usually caused by *Staphylococcus aureus*, is very common in the tropics, and is typically diagnosed in otherwise healthy males.[39] However, in nontropical zones, where pyomyositis is rare, afflicted patients tend to be malnourished or are immunodeficient for other reasons.[23-26,40-45] A high index of suspicion is required because clinical signs of inflammation are mild in the early stages; fever and leukocytosis are typically low grade, if present, and physical examination is characterized by a nonspecific "wooden" stiffness without fluctuance. In the more advanced stages, the skeletal muscle may be almost totally destroyed and replaced by pus.[39]

Recognition of bacterial myositis in AIDS is important because it represents a readily curable condition that may be fatal if not recognized. A few case reports have documented the utility of scintigraphy studies to detect pyomyositis in AIDS and other immunocompromised states. These include [67]gallium[40–45] and [111]indium-tagged white blood cell techniques.[40] By identifying increased nuclide accumulation, foci of inflammation can be roughly localized to the muscles. Using [99m]technetium phosphate scintigraphy, evidence of pyomyositis may be detected if immediate and "blood pool" images are obtained, due to hyperemia associated with the inflammatory process causing relative "hot spots" in the muscles. Delayed scintigrams, on the other hand, typically show no abnormal nuclide accumulation and hence are insensitive in the detection of pyomyositis.[40–43,46,47] This is important because pyomyositis may go undiagnosed if only a delayed study is performed. In addition, Kaposi's sarcoma of the muscle may share the appearance of pyomyositis on three-phase [99m]technetium bone scans (see below). Finally, other pathologic conditions of muscle, such as myositis ossificans[51] or polymyositis,[22] may concentrate radiounclide tracers in the muscles of AIDS patients, simulating pyomyositis.

Ultrasound and CT can be useful to localize pyomyositis and may be able to detect the presence of drainable fluid, although both have limitations. Early in pyomyositis, ultrasound may demonstrate a normal echogenic pattern; this becomes progressively hypoechoic as fluid-filled cavities develop.[40,43,47,48] CT can occasionally detect drainable fluid in abscesses, particularly if iodinated contrast material is infused.[40,42,44–47,49] However, CT is inherently insensitive to muscle edema, is further hindered by beam-hardening artifacts, and the use of intravenous contrast media poses additional potential health risks.

MRI can reveal muscle edema in the early stages of bacterial myositis by increased signal intensity on long TR sequences, especially STIR.[23,24,40,50] This edema is frequently not apparent on T_1-weighted images. As abscess cavities form in muscle, a well-defined central zone of marked signal hyperintensity, denoting drainable fluid, appears on edema-sensitive sequences, bounded by a thin, hypointense rim that separates the abscess cavity from surrounding phlegmonous tissue. On T_1-weighted images, the rim of the abscess is curiously hyperintense (Figures 22.1, 22.2). Although the physical basis of the MRI appearance of abscess capsules has not been studied, a similar appearance has been reported in cerebral abscesses.[52] In that study, the T_1-weighted appearance was attributed to the likely presence of paramagnetic material in the abscess capsule. However, several such substances, including methemoglobin and bacterial or macrophage sequestration of iron, were excluded histopathologically.

It was concluded that free radicals might be responsible for the apparent shortening of the T_1 time of abscess capsules. It should be noted that muscle abscesses may show no abnormality on T_1-weighted images or may be diffusely hyperintense.[23,24] In an animal model, abscess capsules that were isointense with muscle on T_1-weighted images enhanced after intravenous infusion of gadolinium chelates, corresponding to hypervascular peripheral zones.[53] Hence, gadolinium infusion may increase the accuracy of MRI in defining drainable abscesses in bacterial myositis.

Abscesses are multiple in approximately 30% of cases[23,24,39,40,43,44] (Figures 22.1, 22.3). Therefore, whole-body scintigraphic studies are a practical method for screening the entire body for additional lesions.[45,46] MRI is an alternative method to screen for additional lesions due to its high sensitivity.[23,24,40] Because the muscle–tendon junction may be the site of abscess formation, the ability of MRI to accurately delineate this structure can faciliate localizing such lesions (Figure 22.3).

Yuh et al. reported MRI findings in two non-AIDS patients with bacterial myositis. They emphasized that disproportionate edematous involvement of muscles in comparison to subcutaneous tissue favored the diagnosis of bacterial myositis over cellulitis.[50] The differential diagnosis of soft tissue edema is actually more extensive, however, because subcutaneous edema also occurs when lymphatic obstruction develops in AIDS, such as in lymphoma or Kaposi's sarcoma.[23] Therefore, the finding of subcutaneous edema is not specific for cellulitis and careful clinical correlation is imperative so that a relatively benign process (cellulitis) is not assumed when a more ominous disease is present.

Mycobacterial Myositis

Mycobacterial infection is very common in AIDS, accounting for the most frequent cause of sepsis in AIDS patients.[38] Hence, it is not surprising that mycobacterial myositis has been reported in AIDS.[11,23,24] In one well-documented case of tuberculous myositis, the lesion was readily identified scintigraphically and on MRI but the nonspecific imaging features could not distinguish mycobacterial from pyogenic infection (Figure 22.4).

Fungal and Parasitic Myositis

The appearances of fungal or parasitic myositis on imaging studies have yet to be reported despite the fact that such cases have been observed using histopathological means.[11,27]

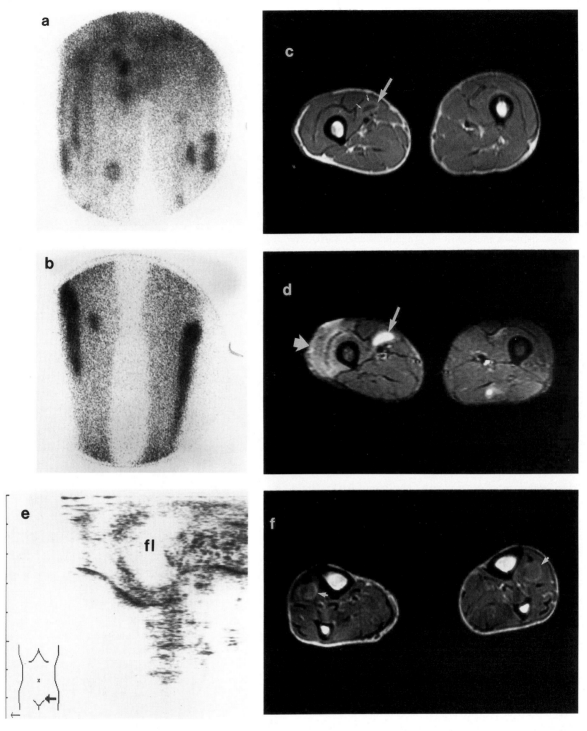

FIGURE 22.1. Pyomyositis in AIDS. The patient presented with a fluctuant mass in the left thigh that was aspirated, yielding frank pus and *Staphylococcus aureus*. Despite drainage and intravenous antibiotics, the patient continued to be febrile. [63]Gallium citrate scintigraphy over the thighs (a) and legs (b) demonstrates multiple regions of increased tracer accumulation. T_1-weighted image of the thighs reveals a lesion in the right adductor longus (arrow, 500/30, c). The lesion is characteristic of pyomyositis by exhibiting a rim of increased signal intensity (small arrows) surrounded by a relatively hypointense area of drainable pus. At the same level, STIR image shows the pus pocket to be markedly intense (arrow, 1500/30/100, d).

Other abnormalities are more sensitively identified with STIR, including edema in the right vastus lateralis (arrowhead), inferior to the site of the previously drained abscess. Axial ultrasound scan performed prior to aspiration of a different thigh lesion shows a rounded focus of decreased echogenicity without increased through-transmission, consistent with a complicated fluid (fl) collection (e). Pus was aspirated but was culture-negative, presumably due to concurrent antibiotic therapy. In the legs, T_1-weighted image reveals bilateral lesions characteristic of pyomyositis in the anterior compartments (arrows, 500/30).

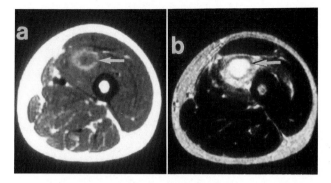

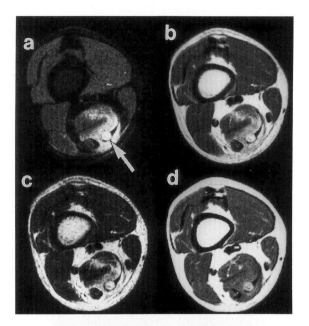

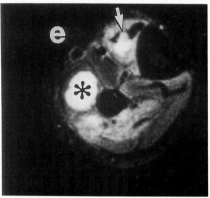

FIGURE 22.2. Pyomyositis in AIDS. Note hyperintense rim in the left vastus medialis muscle on T_1-weighted image (arrow, 500/30, a) and closely associated hypointense band on T_2-weighted image (arrow, 2000/90, b). The T_2-weighted image shows a central focus of extremely high signal intensity (light bulb sign), corresponding to drainable pus. Note that muscle edema surrounds the pus on T_2 weighting (b). Culture of aspirated fluid yielded *Staphylococcus aureus*. (Steinbach LS, Tehranzadeh J, Fleckenstein JL, Vanarthos W, Pais MJ. Musculoskeletal manifestions of human immunodeficiency virus (HIV) infection. Radiology 1993;186:833–838.)

Autoimmune Myositis (Polymyositis)

Idiopathic inflammatory myositis (polymyositis) is a well-recognized cause of muscular weakness and serum creatine kinase elevation in HIV-infected patients, occurring in some before the classical signs of AIDS become manifest.[5,20,21] Interestingly, polymyositis occurs in 50% of primates with experimentally induced AIDS.[54] Because of the high sensitivity of MRI to muscle edema,[55] it is not surprising that MRI has been employed to aid in the diagnosis of polymyositis in HIV⁺ patients. Ths is exemplified by a case in which MRI documented edematous changes in the posterior leg muscles of a patient not previously known to be HIV⁺ (Figure 22.5). Needle biopsy performed in the MRI suite confirmed the presence of lymphocytic infiltration of muscle, corroborating the clinical suspicion of polymyositis.[24] Although the mechanism underlying the association between HIV⁺ serology and polymyositis has not been elucidated, the association should be remembered by clinicians who biopsy patients with polymyositis so that appropriate caution is employed.

FIGURE 22.3. Tendon and muscle abscesses in an HIV⁺ patient without AIDS. A focal area of increased signal intensity is visible in the semimembranosus tendon on STIR (arrow, 1500/30/100, a), 2000/30 (b), 2000/90 (c), and 500/30 (d) sequences. Less intense changes are easily visible in the adjacent muscle on edema-sensitive sequences (a–c) but with difficulty on T_1-weighted image (d). STIR image of the lower leg in the same patient shows foci of varying degrees of signal hyperintensity (1500/30/100, e), including a well-circumscribed focus in the peroneus longus (*) and one involving the anterior tibialis tendon (arrow). Blood cultures grew group B *Streptococcus pyogenes* and appropriate antibiotic treatment was associated with complete resolution of MRI abnormalities. (Fleckenstein JL, Burns D, Murphy K, Jayson H, Bonte F. Differential diagnosis of bacterial myositis in AIDS: MRI evaluation. Radiology 1991;179:653–658.)

Neurogenic Muscle Disease in AIDS

Peripheral neuropathy is common in AIDS, being suspected in up to 40% of patients. Biopsy and autopsy studies reveal an inflammatory neuropathy with variable demyelination and axonal loss. Although evidence of direct nerve infection by HIV is scant, cytomegalovirus is a well-established direct cause of polyradiculop-

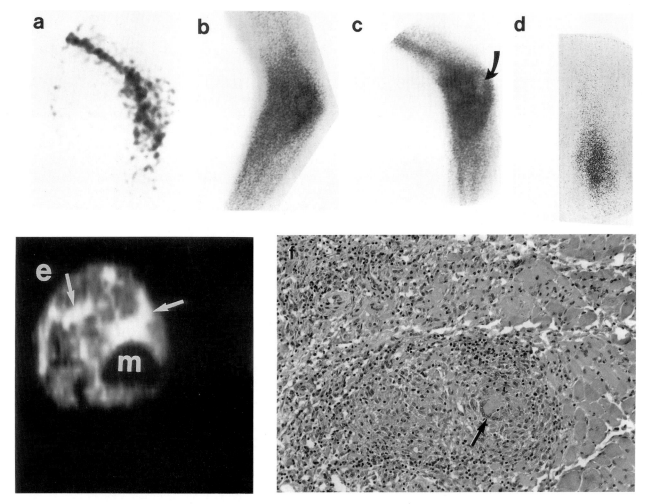

FIGURE 22.4. Tuberculous myositis in AIDS patient presenting with tuberculous sacroiliitis and a soft tissue mass near the elbow. Triple-phase [99m]technetium pyrophosphate muscle scintigrams reveal increased tracer delivery to the proximal forearm, as shown on 7-s (a) and "blood pool" (b) scintigrams. After a 2-h delay, increased tracer activity is seen adjacent to a focal photopenic area (arrow, c). [111]Indium-labelled white cell accumulation is visible in the same region 24 h after injection (d). Due to agitation, only a low resolution, 1-min fast STIR MRI was obtained (1500/30/100, e). It reveals markedly increased signal intensity in muscles (arrows) but only normal, fat-suppressed signal intensity in the marrow (m) of the adjacent humerus, indicating absence of osteomyelitis. Postmortem examination of the forearm revealed multinucleated giant cells (hematoxylin and eosin 100×, arrow, f). Muscle tissue culture was positive for *Mycobacterium tuberculosis*. (Fleckenstein JL. Diagnostic Imaging of Muscle Manifestations in the Acquired Immunodeficiency Syndrome (AIDS). In: Tehranzadeh J, ed., *Diagnostic Imaging of Musculoskeletal System in the Acquired Immunodeficiency Syndrome (AIDS)*. Warren H. Green, Inc., St. Louis, MO 1994.)

FIGURE 22.5. Polymyositis in patient diagnosed as HIV[+] after presenting with marked muscle weakness. MRI was requested to localize site for muscle biopsy. Axial T_1-weighted image shows streaky foci of increased signal intensity, consistent with increased fat deposition in the left medial gastrocnemius (arrow, 500/30, a). STIR shows signal suppression in the same region, due to the fat content, but also shows signal hyperintensity in other muscles, including the left lateral gastrocnemius muscle (arrowhead, 1500/30/95, b), which was biopsied in the MRI suite using a needle biopsy "gun." Histopathology showed lymphocytic infiltration of the muscle, securing the diagnosis of polymyositis. (Steinbach LS, Tehranzadeh J, Fleckenstein JL, Vanarthos W, Pais MJ. Musculoskeletal manifestions of human immunodeficiency virus (HIV) infection. Radiology 1993;186:833–838.)

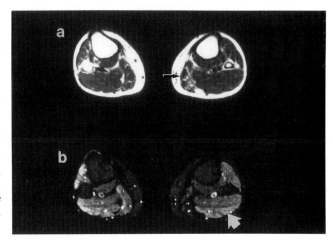

athy.[5,10,11,28–33] Although no imaging study of muscle change related to neuropathy in AIDS has been reported, the high sensitivity of MRI in detecting denervation (see Chapter 14) predicts that neuropathies in AIDS would be detectable on muscle MRI by having an appearance similar to polymyositis.[56] Therefore, denervation should be remembered as a differential diagnostic possibility in the patient whose MRI study shows edema-like changes of the muscles. It remains to be established whether disuse atrophy of muscle, as occurs in the wasting syndrome of AIDS, may cause changes similar to denervation on MRI.

Muscle Neoplasms in AIDS

Little data exist in the literature regarding the incidence of skeletal muscle neoplasms in AIDS. Anecdotal reports of Kaposi's sarcoma of skeletal muscle include a patient presenting with a painful neck mass (Figure 22.6).[23] Given the hypervascular nature of this sarcoma, flow-sensitive imaging studies, such as triple-phase [99m]technetium pyrophosphate scintigraphy, would be expected to identify the lesion. This was in fact observed in the patient, although delayed scintigrams did not show an abnormality, resulting in an appearance indistinguish-

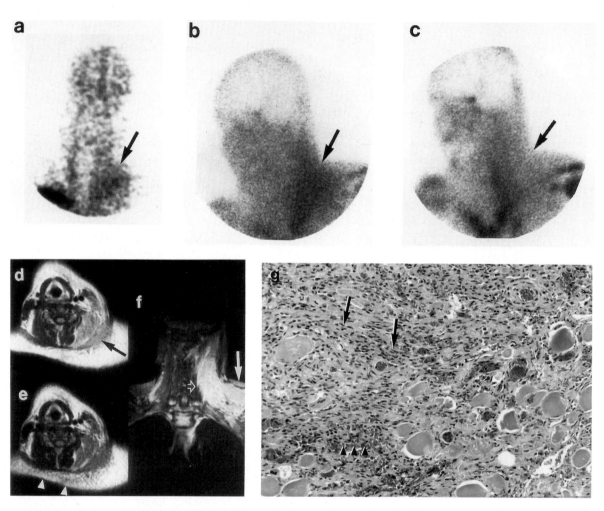

FIGURE 22.6. MRI of Kaposi's sarcoma of muscle in AIDS. The patient presented with painful swelling in the left neck, clinically suspicious for lymphoma. [99m]Technetium pyrophosphate muscle scintigraphy reveals increased tracer delivery to the site (arrow), as shown on 7-s (a) and "blood pool" (b) images. After a 2-h delay, only normal tracer activity is seen (c). [63]Gallium citrate scintigrams demonstrated no abnormality (not shown). Axial T_2-weighted MRI of the neck, performed for prebiopsy localization, shows increased signal intensity in specific neck muscles (arrow, 2000/90, d). Streaky hypointensities of subcutaneous tissue are evident on T_1-weighted image (arrowheads, 500/30, e), suggesting lymphatic involvement. Coronal STIR image reveals the longitudinal extent of the muscle lesion (open arrowhead, 1500/30/95, f) as well as edematous alteration of the subcutaneous tissue (arrow). Postmortem specimen demonstrated spindle-shaped cells (arrows) in a highly vascular stroma, with extravasated red blood cells (arrowheads, hematoxylin and eosin 100×, g), consistent with Kaposi's sarcoma. (Fleckenstein JL, Burns D, Murphy K, Jayson H, Bonte F. Differential diagnosis of bacterial myositis in AIDS: MRI evaluation. Radiology 1991;179:653–658.)

able from pyomyositis. MRI in the same case revealed edema-like changes in specific neck muscles as well as signal abnormality in the adjacent subcutaneous fat. Primary muscular lymphoma has yet to be reported in AIDS and in fact is exceedingly rare in non-AIDS patients. However, muscular lymphoma reportedly has a lower signal intensity on T_2-weighted images than does normal fat.[57] This contrasts with what was observed in our patient with Kaposi's sarcoma in whom the T_2 time was greatly prolonged, due in part to the high blood content of the lesion.

Muscle Edema in the Setting of Edematous Subcutaneous Tissues

One study employing MRI to evaluate swollen extremities in AIDS reported a pattern of soft tissue changes in lymphedema that is distinct from myositis.[23] Whereas in myositis, edema-like changes are primarily restricted to the muscles themselves, in lymphedema, edematous change of subcutaneous tissues also occurs and in a bilateral, asymmetric distribution. As already emphasized, the subcutaneous edema in lymphedema may mimic cellulitis, but dermal infection was present in only one of seven AIDS patients in whom MRI showed subcutaneous edema (Figure 22.7). Also, despite reports that the combination of muscle and subcutaneous edema

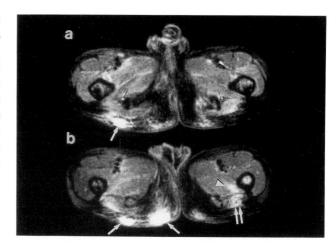

FIGURE 22.7. Carbunculosis in AIDS. Contiguous axial STIR images (1500/30/100, a, b) of the proximal thighs shows foci of markedly increased signal intensity, not only in the subcutaneous fat (arrows) but also in the gluteus (double arrow) and adductor muscles (e.g., arrowhead), indicating edematous changes. (Fleckenstein JL, Burns D, Murphy K, Jayson H, Bonte F. Differential diagnosis of bacterial myositis in AIDS: MRI evaluation. Radiology 1991;179:653–658.)

is usually associated with venous thrombosis,[58–60] venography was normal in each of the AIDS patients with this pattern of edema (Figures 22.8 to 22.10).[23] Two of the patients with lymphedema had clear etiologies for lym-

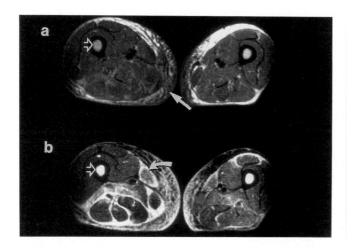

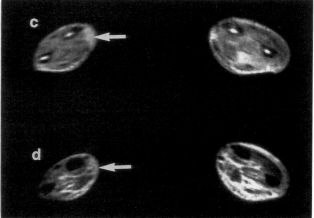

FIGURE 22.8. Lymphoma-associated lymphedema in AIDS patient presenting with asymmetric swelling of the extremities. Axial T_1-weighted images of the thighs show skin thickening and a "honeycomb" pattern of low signal intensity streaks in the subcutaneous tissue (arrow, 500/30, a). STIR image at the same level shows abnormally increased signal intensity in the subcutaneous fat and a variable degree of increased signal intensity in and around muscles, for example, the right sartorius (curved arrow, 1500/30/100, b). Signal intensity in the femoral bone marrow is abnormally low on T_1-weighted image (arrow-

head, a) and high on STIR (arrowhead, b), suggesting marrow infiltration. Axial T_1-weighted MRI of the forearms is centered on a palpable mass, which was subsequently found to contain high-grade lymphoma (arrow, 500/30, c). STIR image at the same level shows increased signal intensity in the palpable nodule (arrow, 1500/30/100, d) as well as in subcutaneous and intermuscular perifascial regions. (Fleckenstein JL, Burns D, Murphy K, Jayson H, Bonte F. Differential diagnosis of bacterial myositis in AIDS: MRI evaluation. Radiology 1991; 179:653–658.)

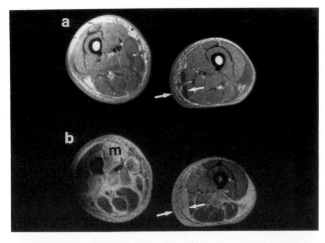

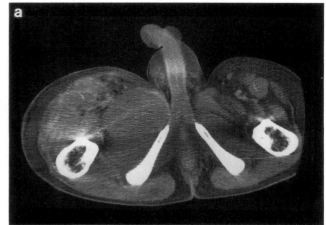

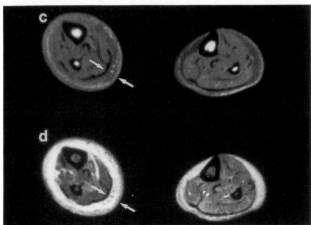

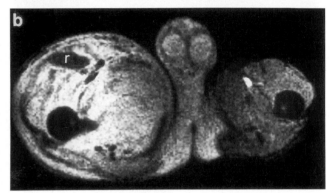

FIGURE 22.9. Lymphedema pattern in disseminated Kaposi's sarcoma and slowly progressive, asymmetric "brawny" edema of the lower extremities. Subcutaneous edema is easily visible in the thighs on T_1-weighted image by skin thickening, a subcutaneous "honeycomb" appearance, and perifascial fluid collections (between arrows, 500/30, a) and on STIR by diffuse hyperintensity (between arrows, 1500/30/100, b). Variable involvement of muscles is best appreciated using STIR. For example, the right vastus medialis (m) appears markedly abnormal (b). In the legs, subcutaneous abnormalities (between arrows) are also conspicuous on T_1-weighted (500/30, c) and STIR images (1500/30/95, d). (Fleckenstein JL, Burns D, Murphy K, Jayson H, Bonte F. Differential diagnosis of bacterial myositis in AIDS: MRI evaluation. Radiology 1991; 179:653–658.)

FIGURE 22.10. Lymphedema pattern in AIDS. Enhanced CT scan of the proximal thighs reveals swelling of the right thigh (a). STIR (1500/30/100, b) demonstrates to better advantage the subcutaneous and muscle edema on the right as well as apparent sparing of the right rectus femoris muscle (r). It also shows absence of abnormality of the left thigh muscles and ipsilateral subcutaneous fat. Venography excluded deep venous thrombosis (not shown). Blindly performed aspiration of swollen tissues yielded only negative cultures and puncture sites oozed serous fluid. The patient died without a diagnosis, but the case demonstrates the superior depiction of soft tissue edema using MRI compared to CT in AIDS. (Fleckenstein JL. Diagnostic Imaging of Muscle Manifestations in the Acquired Immunodeficiency Syndrome (AIDS). In: Tehranzadeh J, ed., *Diagnostic Imaging of Musculoskeletal System in the Acquired Immunodeficiency Syndrome (AIDS)*. Warren H. Green, Inc., St. Louis, MO 1994.)

phatic obstruction, including Kaposi's sarcoma (Figure 22.8) and lymphoma (Figure 22.9). These cases suggest that, at least in AIDS, muscle edema may indeed accompany subcutaneous edema in the setting of lymphedema. Possible explanations for the apparent discrepancy between studies include reliance of some of the studies on the limited sensitivity of CT to mild muscle edema and to the fact that the MRI studies did not use fat-suppression sequences to search for muscle edema. It is also possible that in AIDS, the rapidity with which lym-

phatics become engorged may contribute to a tendency to produce lymphatic stasis in muscles, visible by MRI as muscle edema.

Conclusions

Many muscle diseases occur in AIDS. Imaging studies have only begun to be applied to this important group of conditions. What is currently clear is that imaging can be extremely helpful in guiding invasive procedures, including biopsy and histopathological evaluation, and in noninvasively monitoring the response of the disease to therapy.

References

1. Simpson D, Bender A. HIV-associated myopathy: analysis of 11 patients. Ann Neurol 1988;24:79–84.

2. Berman A, Espinoza L, Diaz J, et al. Rheumatic manifestations of human immunodeficiency virus infection. Am J Med 1988;85:59–64.

3. Gabuzda D, Hirsch M. Neurologic manifestations of infection with human immunodeficiency virus. Clinical features and pathogenesis. Ann Intern Med 1987;107:383–391.

4. Kaye B. Rheumatologic manifestations of infection with human immunodeficiency virus (HIV). Ann Intern Med 1989;111:158–167.

5. Dalakas M, Illa I, Pezeshkpour G, et al. Neuromuscular diseases associated with human immunodeficiency virus infection. Ann Neurol 1988;(Suppl):S38–S48.

6. Dalakas M. Neuromuscular complications of AIDS. Muscle Nerve 1986;9:92.

7. Britton C, Miller J. Neurologic complications in the acquired immunodeficiency syndrome (AIDS). Neurol Clin 1984;2:315–339.

8. Lange D, Britton C, Younger D, Hays A. The neuromuscular manifestations of human immunodeficiency virus infections. Arch Neurol 1988;45:1084–1088.

9. Simpson D, Bender A, Farraye J, Mendelson S, Wolfe D. HIV wasting syndrome may represent a treatable myopathy. Neurology 1990;40:535–538.

10. Gabbai A, Schmidt B, Castelo A, Oliveira A, Lima J. Muscle biopsy in AIDS and ARC: analysis of 50 patients. Muscle Nerve 1990;13:541–544.

11. Wrzolek M, Sher J, Kozlowski P, Rao C. Skeletal muscle pathology in AIDS: an autopsy study. Muscle Nerve 1990;13:508–515.

12. Dalakas M, Illa I, Pezeshkpour G, et al. Mitochondrial myopathy caused by long-term zidovudine therapy. N Engl J Med 1990;322:1098–1105.

13. Bessen L, Greene J, Louie E, Seitzman P, Weinberg H. Severe polymyositis-like syndrome associated with zidovudine therapy of AIDS and ARC [letter]. N Engl J Med 1988;318:708.

14. Gertner E, Thurn J, Williams D, et al. Zidovudine-associated myopathy. Am J Med 1989;86:814–818.

15. Chariot P, Gherardi R. Partial cytochrome c oxidase deficiency and cytoplasmic bodies in patients with zidovudine myopathy. Neuromuscul Dis 1991;1:357–363.

16. Gorard D, Henry K, Guiloff R. Necrotising myopathy and zidovudine. Lancet 1988;1:1050.

17. Helbert M, Fletcher T, Peddle B, Harris J, Pinching A. Zidovudine-associated myopathy. Lancet 1988;2:689–690.

18. Chalmers AC, Greco CM, Miller RG. Prognosis in AZT myopathy. Neurology 1991;41:1181–1184.

19. Wiley C, Nerenberg M, Cros D, Soto-Aguilar M. HLTV-I polymyositis in a patient also infected with the HIV virus. N Engl J Med 1989;320:992–995.

20. Dalakas M, Pezeshkpour G, Gravell M, Sever J. Polymyositis associated with AIDS retrovirus. JAMA 1986;256:2381–2383.

21. Nordstrom D, Petropolis A, Giorno R, Gates R, Reddy V. Inflammatory myopathy and acquired immunodeficiency syndrome. Arth Rheum 1989;32:475–479.

22. Scott J, Palmer E, Fischman A. HIV-associated myositis detected by radionuclide bone scanning. J Nucl Med 1989;30:556–558.

23. Fleckenstein J, Burns D, Murphy F, Jayson H, Bonte F. Differential diagnosis of bacterial myositis in AIDS: Evaluation with MR imaging. Radiology 1991;179:653–658.

24. Steinbach L, Tehranzadeh J, Fleckenstein J, Vanarthos W, Pais M. Musculoskeletal manifestations of human immunodeficiency virus (HIV) infection. Radiology 1993;186:833–838.

25. Vartian C, Septimus E. Pyomyositis in an intravenous drug user with human immunodeficiency virus [letter]. Arch Int Med 1988;148:2689.

26. Watts R, Hoffbrand B, Paton D, Davis J. Pyomyositis associated with human immunodeficiency virus infection. Br Med J Clin Res 1987;294:1524–1525.

27. Ledford D, Oveman M, Gonzalvo A, Cali A, Mester S, Lockey R. Microsporidiosis myositis in a patient with the acquired immunodeficiency syndrome Ann Int Med 1985;102:628–630.

28. Cornblath D. Treatment of the neuromuscular complications of human immunodeficiency virus infection. Ann Neurol 1988;23(Suppl):S88–S91.

29. Cornblath D, McArthur J, Kennedy P, Witt A, Griffin J. Inflammatory demyelinating peripheral neuropathies associated with human T-cell lymphotropic virus type III infection. Ann Neurol 1987;21:32–40.

30. De LaMonte S, Gabuzda D, Ho D, et al. Peripheral neuropathy in acquired immune deficiency syndrome. Ann Neurol 1988;23:485–492.

31. Eidelberg D, Sotrel A, Vogel A, et al. Progressive polyradiculopathy in acquired immune deficiency syndrome. Neurology 1986;36:912–916.

32. Grage M, Wiley C. Spinal cord and peripheral nerve pathology in AIDS: the roles of cytomegalovirus and human immunodeficiency virus. Ann Neurol 1989;25:561–566.

33. Parry G. Peripheral neuropathies associated with human immunodeficiency virus infection. Ann Neurol 1988;23(Suppl):S49–S53.

34. Dalakas M, Pezeshkpour G, Flaherty M. Progressive nemaline (rod) myopathy associated with HIV infection [letter]. N Engl J 1987;317:1602–1603.

35. Gonzalez M, Olney R, So Y, et al. Subacute structural myopathy associated with human immunodeficiency virus infection. Arch Neurol 1988;45:585–587.

36. Fleckenstein J, Haller R, Girson M, Peshock R. Focal muscle lesions in mitochondrial myopathy: MR imaging evaluation [abstract]. JRMI 1992;2(Suppl):121.

37. Lamminen A. Magnetic resonance imaging of primary skeletal muscle diseases: Patterns of distribution and severity of involvement. Br J Radiol 1990;63:946–950.

38. Whimbey E, Gold J, Polsky B, et al. Bacteremia and fungemia in patients with the acquired immunodeficiency syndrome. Ann Int Med 1986;104:511–514.

39. Chiedozi L. Pyomyositis: a review of 205 cases in 112 patients. Am J Surg 1979;137:255–259.

40. Applegate G, Cohen A. Pyomyositis: early detection utilizing multiple imaging modalties. Magn Reson Imag 1991; 9:187–193.

41. Lamki L, Willis B. Radionuclide findings of pyomyositis. Clin Nucl Med 1982;10:465–467.

42. Datz F, Lewis S, Conrad M, Maravilla A, Parkey R. Pyomyositis diagnosed by radionuclide imaging and ultrasonogaphy. South Med J 1980;73:649–651.

43. Moore D, Delage G, Labelle H, Gauthier M. Peracute streptococcal pyomyositis: report of two cases and review of the literature. J Pediatr Orthop 1986;232–235.

44. Tumeh S, Butler G, Maguire J, Nagel J. Pyogenic myositis: CT evaluation. J Comput Assist Tomogr 1988;12:1002–1005.

45. Bouvier J, Bocquet B, Lahneche B. Gallium-67 studies in a patient with multiple muscular abscesses. Clin Nucl Med 1986;11:807–808.

46. Howman-Giles R, McCauley D, Brown J. Multifocal pyomyositis diagnosis on technetium-99m MDP bone scan. Clin Nucl Med 1984;12:149–151.

47. McLoughlin M. CT and percutaneous fine-needle aspiration biopsy in tropical myositis. AJR 1980;134:167–168.

48. Weinberg W, Dembert M. Tropical pyomyositis: delineation by gray-scale ultrasound. Am J Trop Med Hyg 1984; 33:930–932.

49. Lachiewicz P, Hadler N. Spontaneous pyomyositis in a patient with Felty's syndrome: diagnosis using computerized CT. South Med J 1986;79:1047–1048.

50. Yuh W, Schreiber A, Montgomery W, Ehara S. Magnetic resonance imaging of pyomyositis. Skeletal Radiol 1988; 17:190–193.

51. Drane W, Tipler B. Heterotopic ossification (myositis ossificans) in acquired immune deficiency syndrome. Clin Nucl Med 1987;12:433–434.

52. Haimes AB, Zimmerman RD, Morgello S, et al. MR imaging of brain abscesses. AJNR 1989;10:279–291.

53. Paajanen H, Grodd W, Revel D, Engelstad B, Brasch RC. Gadolinium-DTPA enhanced MR imaging of intramuscular abscess. Mag Reson Imag 1987;109–115.

54. Dalakas M, Gravel M, London W, Cunningham G, Sever J. Morphological changes of an inflammatory myopathy in Rhesus monkeys with simian acquired immunodeficiency syndrome. Proc Soc Exp Biol Med 1987;185:368–376.

55. Fujino H, Kobayashi T, Goto I, Onitsuka H. Magnetic resonance imaging of the muscles in patients with polymyositis and dermatomyositis. Muscle Nerve 1991;14:716–720.

56. Fleckenstein J, Watumull D, Conner K, et al. Denervated human skeletal muscle: MR imaging evaluation. Radiology 1993;187:213–218.

57. Metzler JP, Fleckenstein JL, Vuitch F, Frenkel P. Skeletal muscle lymphoma: MRI evaluation. Magn Reson Imaging 1992;10:491–494.

58. Duewell S, Hagspiel K, Zuber J, von Schulthess G, Bollinger A, Fuchs W. Swollen lower extremity: role of MR imaging. Radiology 1992;184:227.

59. Musumeci R, Balzarini L, Ceglia E, et al. MRI in the evaluation of the swollen lower limb: a new diagnostic tool. In: Partsch H, editor. Progress in lymphology, vol. 11. Amsterdam: Excerpta Medica, 1988:387–390.

60. Hadjis N, Carr D, Banks L, Pflug J. The role of CT in the diagnosis of primary lymphedema of the lower limb. AJR 1985;144:361–364.

23
Eosinophilic Fasciitis

Luc S. DeClerck, R. Ceulemans, A.M. De Schepper, and W.J. Stevens

Eosinophilic fasciitis, first described by Shulman in 1974,[1] is a rare disease characterized by scleroderma-like skin changes and eosinophilia: the skin is initially edematous and tender, but later in the course of the disease, indentations and induration become evident (Figure 23.1).

Histopathology

A deep biopsy, which must include tissue from the epidermis to skeletal muscle and deep fascia, is the mainstay for the diagnosis of eosinophilic fasciitis.[2,3] In eosinophilic fasciitis, epidermis and upper dermis are usually spared (in contrast with scleroderma), and the myositis along with the fasciitis in the superficial muscle fibers—if present—is much milder than seen in polymyositis (Figure 23.2). Most importantly, eosinophilic fasciitis is characterized by clear inflammation and thickening of the fasciae. The initial changes include edema and infiltration by lymphocytes, macrophages, plasma cells, and eosinophils, followed by fibrosis.

Diagnosis

History

History reveals complaints of tender swelling of arms and legs, sometimes following an episode of strenuous exertion. One should always question the patient about intake of L-tryptophan, an over-the-counter remedy for a variety of problems including depression, insomnia, and chronic pain. Indeed, recently there have been increasing reports of L-tryptophan-induced "eosinophilia-myalgia syndrome," some cases of which closely resemble eosinophilic fasciitis.[4]

Physical Examination

Cutaneous manifestations are the dominant presenting feature: initially edematous swelling of arms and/or legs are present, evolving to "peau d'orange" (dimply skin) and indurations. Diffuse or patchy hyperpigmentation and loss of hair are common in the late phase of the disease, resembling localized scleroderma (Figure 23.1). Differences with scleroderma include the absence of Raynaud's phenomenon, normal nailfold capillaroscopy, and infrequent visceral involvement.[5]

Myalgias, arthralgias or arthritis, joint contractures, and carpal tunnel syndrome are other common features of eosinophilic fasciitis.[5,6]

Laboratory Findings

The laboratory findings include often marked blood eosinophilia, although this feature can be transient and the diagnosis should not be dismissed because of a normal number of peripheral blood eosinophils (the same holds true for the tissue eosinophilia).

Creatine phosphokinase (CPK) levels are usually normal, although low-grade myositis on biopsy can be found as well as abnormal electromyograms showing nonspecific changes of motor unit potentials of reduced amplitude and duration.[5]

Antinuclear antibodies, often characteristic for systemic sclerosis (anticentromere antibodies, anti-Scl70 antibodies), are absent in eosinophilic fasciitis.

Imaging

Fascia

A fascia is a collagenous lamellar sheath or blade that peripherally and circumferentially envelops the musculotendinous, nervous and vascular structures of each limb, the trunk, and the head and neck region. A larger circumferential rim of subcutaneous fatty tissue separates the fascia from the cutaneous surface. The fascia adheres to bony structures, blending with the periosteum. It

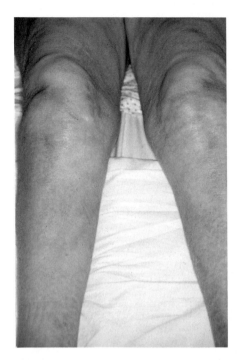

FIGURE 23.1. Clinical involvement of the lower extremities in eosinophilic fasciitis showing induration and indentation of skin, hyperpigmentation, and loss of hair.

may septate and enwrap a single or usually a group of functionally identical muscles. For example, the crural fascia of the lower leg gives rise to (a) an anterior and (b) a posterior intermuscular septum, (c) a septum separating the superficial and deep flexor muscles (= deep crural fascia) and also shows (d) a limited, focal duplication around the smaller saphenic vein and sural nerve. The anterior intermuscular septum separates the anterior extensor muscles from the peroneal muscles; the poste-

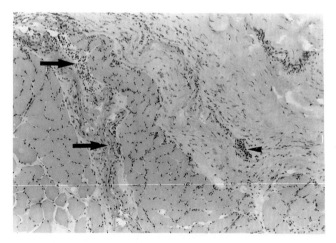

FIGURE 23.2. Inflammatory infiltrates in thickened epimysial (arrowhead) and perimysial (arrows) fascia (HE staining, ×100).

rior intermuscular septum separates the peroneal muscles from the posterior flexor muscles.

Focal, anatomical reinforcements of the fascia exist. For instance, the iliotibial tract in the upper leg, the superior and inferior extensor retinaculum of the ankle, the palmar aponeurosis, the flexor retinaculum of the wrist (= transverse carpal ligament), etc.

Radiographically the fascia can only be individualized if a sufficient, small amount of fat is interposed between the muscular belly on the one hand and the adjacent fascia on the other hand. This usually is not the case in the upper arm and forearm. In contradistinction, the crural fascia of the lower leg is quite consistently visualized in CT and MRI investigations over the whole of its circumference.

Conventional Radiography

Conventional radiography in eosinophilic fasciitis usually shows no musculoskeletal alterations, but it may reveal soft tissue swelling, infiltration or obliteration of subcutaneous fat planes, or osteopenia.

Sometimes there is a symmetrical polyarthritis resembling rheumatoid arthritis with erosions in the hand and wrist.[6]

With extensive fascial and subcutaneous inflammation or fibrosis, joint contractures of elbows, wrists, ankles, and knees may occur. Severe truncal involvement may result in extrapulmonary thoracic restriction ("hidebound chest"): chest plain film will demonstrate small lung volumes due to hypoventilation, which may be associated with plate-like atelectasis.[7]

Ultrasound

Ultrasound has not been applied as an imaging modality in eosinophilic fasciitis. However, fasciitis as a result of repetitive mechanical overload at the level of the plantar aponeurosis has been studied by high-resolution linear array ultrasound[8,9] with excellent results.

The normal fascia is a hyperechogenic lamellar structure, superficial to muscular tissue, with a visible, small amount of fat in between them. With inflammation, the fascia thickens focally or diffusely. In the affected area, hyperechogenicity is lost and replaced by hypoechogenicity.[8,9]

Interstitial myositis in the neighboring muscle can result in a hyperechogenic pattern, whereas the intramuscular fibroadipose septations turn hypoechogenic due to an inflammation-induced increase in water content.[10]

The cutis is visualized as a hyperechogenic layer, which in normal circumstances can easily be differentiated from the subcutaneous hypoechogenic fatty tissue. With marked inflammation, however, the delineation between cutis and subdermal fat is lost as the subcutis also becomes hyperechogenic.[10] Moreover, hypoechogenic and thickened fibrous septa may be identified when cross-sectioning the subcutis and associated fat lobules.

Computed Axial Tomography

Computed axial tomography (CT) is routinely conducted perpendicular to the longitudinal axis of the trunk and extremities. This axial imaging plane is very appropriate to visualize fascial thickening.

The fascia can be individualized if a sufficient, small amount of fat is present between the muscle belly and fascia—which is usually the case in the posterior and medial portion of the upper leg and circumferentially in the lower leg—and if a slice thickness of 5 mm or less is selected. In soft tissue window settings, the fascia can be identified as a thin linear striation wth intermediate density paralleling the muscle belly contour. In eosinophilic fasciitis, the fascial thickening may be regular or irregular in width, nodular, limited to only a portion of the fascial circumference, or completely circumferential (Figure 23.3).[11,12]

Although to a lesser extent, subcutis and adjacent striated muscle can be involved in eosinophilic fasciitis. Streaky, linear, or branching soft tissue densities may smudge the subcutaneous hypodense fatty tissue in case of moderate subcutaneous inflammation; they correspond to enlarged fibrous septa interspersing the subcutaneous fat lobules.[10]

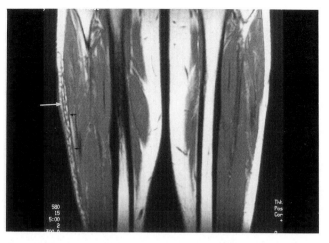

FIGURE 23.4. Coronal T_1-weighted SE image (T_R 580/T_E 15) of the lower legs, at the doral aspect of the tibial diaphysis. Notice again inflammatory thickening and intermediate signal intensity of the right sided subcutaneous fibrous septa (white arrow), intersecting the hyperintense, subcutaneous fatty lobules. Thickening of the crural fascia (black arrows) superficial to the peroneal compartment is visualized in the distal half of the lower leg. There is loss of normal low signal intensity of the fascia, with replacement by intermediate signal intensity on T_1-weighted image.

With extensive subcutaneous inflammation, there is total obliteration of subcutaneous hypodense fatty tissue. This results in loss of distinction between cutis-subcutis on the one hand and subcutis-fascia on the other.[10,13]

Without intravenous water-soluble iodine contrast administration, a possible associated inflammation of striated muscle adjacent to the fascial thickening will certainly go undetected. When contrast medium is administered, the area of inflammation could display relative hypodensity in relation to the homogeneously, slightly enhancing skeletal muscular tissue.

Hyperemia of the inflamed subcutaneous tissue and slight contrast enhancement of the inflamed fascia may also be noted after intravenous contrast administration (Figure 23.3).

Magnetic Resonance Imaging

Of the available imaging modalities, magnetic resonance imaging (MRI) most distinctly and accurately depicts the tissues affected by eosinophilic fasciitis, their alterations, and the inflammatory activity (Figures 23.4 to 23.6).

Normal fascia (Figure 23.4) appears as a regular, thin, band-like structure exhibiting low signal intensity on T_1-weighted, T_2-weighted, and proton density spin echo (SE) images as well as on gradient echo images. The low signal intensity is due to the lack of mobile protons as a result of its high collagen content and relatively low cellularity.

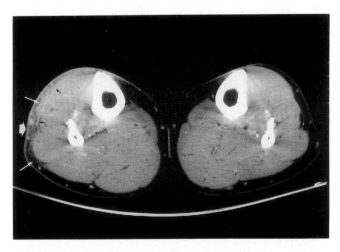

FIGURE 23.3. CT scan of the lower leg (mid-diaphyseal level) after intravenous contrast medium administration. Notice on the right side, skin thickening (arrowhead), streaky soft tissue densities in the subcutaneous fatty tissue (white arrows) with principal orientation parallel to the skin surface, and focal, regular thickening of the crural fascia (black arrows) superficial to the extensor compartment. There is slight contrast enhancement at this level of the crural fascia.

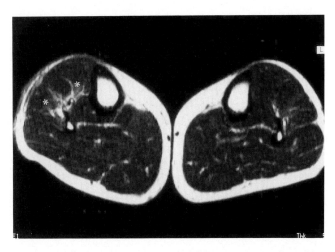

FIGURE 23.5. Axial T_2-weighted Turbo SE images (T_R 4700/T_E 90) demonstrate an asymmetric, more prominent aspect of the tibialis anterior artery and its branches on the right. Also visualized are areas of increased signal intensity (asterisks) in the extensor compartment, deep within the muscle, adjacent to the arborization of the tibialis anterior vessels.

Muscular tissue has an intermediate signal intensity (SI) on T_1- and T_2-weighted SE images and fat has a high SI.[14] On gradient echo sequences both structures display an intermediate, almost equal SI (see Chapter 3).

Both the pattern (regular, irregular, nodular) and extent (partial or complete) of fascial thickening are optimally visualized by MRI.

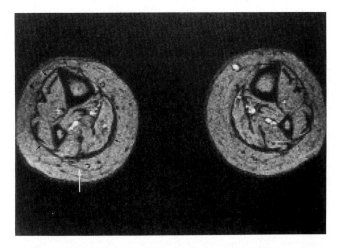

FIGURE 23.6. Axial gradient echo image (T_R 350/T_E 15/flip angle 22°) of the distal lower limb in a patient with chronic eosinophilic fasciitis (clinical involvement in this patient is shown in Figure 23.1). Note bilateral, symmetrical, irregular, and circumferential thickening of the crural fascia (black arrows). Low signal intensity linear striations are seen within the subcutaneous fatty tissue, correlating with thickening of the fibrous, interadipose septa (white arrow).

Normal fascial hypointensity on T_1-weighted images may be lost and replaced by intermediate signal intensity (Figure 23.4).

In the early stage of the disease, active inflammation either of the subcutis or the skeletal muscle (Figure 23.5) can be depicted by high SI on T_2-weighted SE sequences, gradient echo sequences, or other T_2-weighted sequence variables.[11,12,15–17]

Another imaging sequence advocated to accentuate the increased signal intensity in acutely inflamed, edematous muscle is the short inversion time inversion recovery sequences (STIR) in idiopathic inflammatory myopathies[18] and T_2-weighted hybrid fat-suppression techniques in dermatomyositis, viral myositis and vasculitis.[19]

In the advanced, chronic stage of eosinophilic fasciitis (Figure 23.6) no residual elevation of intramuscular SI can be visualized on T_2-weighted or gradient echo images. The subcutaneous, enlarged fibrous septa appear as low SI strands on T_1- and T_2-weighted images. In this stage of the disease process this gradient echo sequences may even depict focal duplication of the fascia, enclosing an area of high SI.[11,12]

Other Types of Fasciitis

Plantar fasciitis investigated by MRI presents with diffuse or focal fascial thickening. T_1-weighted images show hypointensity or intrasubstance intermediate signal intensity.[20] T_2-weighted SE and STIR images show high signal intensity with active inflammation, but the T_2 appearance may remain hypointense in less acute situations.[20] Biopsy in this condition reveals collagen necrosis and angiofibroblastic hyperplasia.[21,22] The high SI may extend within the soft tissues surrounding the plantar fascia.

Nodular fasciitis (= *pseudosarcomatous fasciitis* = *proliferative fasciitis*) is a posttraumatic reparative, pseudotumoral process involving in decreasing order of frequency, interlobular subcutaneous septa, myofascial planes, or the fascia. It occurs most often in the forearm and shoulder and less frequently in the thigh, trunk, head, and neck region. Ultrasound demonstrates a solid soft tissue mass with hypoechogenic or mixed echogenic texture.[23,24] CT demonstrates a subcutaneous/fascial well-defined, or an intramuscular ill-defined, soft tissue mass with intermediate density. In case of a fascial subtype, CT[25] or MRI may depict continuity between the soft tissue mass on the one hand and the fascia on the other hand. MRI characteristics vary according to the histology, being hyperintense on T_1- and T_2-weighted SE images when mucoid or cellular and hypointense when fibrous in composition. The lesion is well defined on MRI.[23,24]

Conclusion

Imaging modalities, especially MRI, can clearly demonstrate thickening and inflammation-related changes of the fascia in eosinophilic fasciitis. The number of imaging cuts during a CT study is limited due to radiation exposure, offering the dilemma of a selective investigation of a small area versus a nonselective coverage of a large area and the possible result of a false negative investigation or under-estimation of the disease extent.

MR is superior in its anatomic display, facilitating fascial identification. By using sagittal or coronal imaging planes, MR can screen a broad area (e.g., lower leg) and then, in the same imaging session, precisely direct the axial imaging sections to that region showing the most marked subcutaneous/fascial alterations on coronal and/or sagittal images.

MR depicts the activity of fascial and, subcutaneous inflammation and depicts the muscular component of eosinophilic fasciitis, when present, to its best advantage. MR also omits radiation exposure during the initial investigation and in the long-term follow-up. These characteristics make MRI the superior noninvasive imaging technique in the diagnosis of eosinophilic fasciitis and can guide biopsy of selected abnormal areas.

References

1. Shulman LE. Diffuse fasciitis with hypergammaglobulinemia and eosinophilia: a new syndrome? J Rheumatol 1974;(Suppl)1:46.
2. Barnes L, Rodnan GP, Medsger TA. Eosinophilic fasciitis: a pathological study of twenty cases. Am J Pathol 1979;96:493–507.
3. De Jonge-Bok JM, Steven MM, Eulderink F. Diffuse (eosinophiic) fasciitis. A series of six cases. Clin Rheumatol 1984;3:365–373.
4. Belongia EA, Mayeno AN, Osterholm MT. The eosinophilia-myalgia syndrome and tryptophan. Annu Rev Nutr 1992;12:235–256.
5. Lakhanpal S, Ginsburg WW, Michet CJ. Eosinophilic fasciitis: clinical spectrum and therapeutic response in 52 cases. Semin Arthritis Rheum 1988;17:221–231.
6. Pressly TA, Treadwell AL, Ansbacker LE, et al. Eosinophilic fasciitis with porphyria cutanea tarda and progressive destructive arthritis. J Rheumatol 1989;16:390–393.
7. Chalker RB, Dickey BF, Rosenthal NC, Simms RW. Extrapulmonary thoracic restriction complicating eosinophilic fasciitis. Chest 1991;100(5):1453–1455.
8. Van Holsbeeck M, Introcaso J. Musculoskeletal ultrasound. St. Louis: Mosby Year Book, 1991:313.
9. Gibbon WW. Letter to the editor. Plantar fasciitis: US imaging. Radiology 1992;182:285.
10. Van Holsbeeck M, Introcaso J. Musculoskeletal ultrasound. St. Louis: Mosby Year Book, 1991:207–210.
11. De Clerck LS, Degryse HR, Wouters E, et al. Magnetic resonance imaging in the evaluation of patients with eosinophilic fasciitis. J Rheumatol 1989;16:1270–1273.
12. Montane de la Roqe P. Apport de l' IRM dans l'évaluation de la fasciite avec éosinophilie due au L-tryptophane. Rev Rhum 1991;58:887–889.
13. Yeh HC, Rabinowitz JG. Ultrasonography of the extremities and pelvic girdle and correlation with computed tomography. Radiology 1982;143:519–525.
14. Murphy WA, Totty WG, Carroll JE. MRI of normal and pathologic skeletal muscle. AJR 1986;146:565–574.
15. Park JH, Vansant JP, Kumar NG, et al. Dermatomyositis: correlative MR imaging and P-31 MR spectroscopy for quantitative characterization of inflammatory disease. Radiology 1990;177:473–479.
16. Park JH, Gibbs SJ, Price RR, Partain CL, James AE. Reply 2. Radiology 1991;179:343–344.
17. Fujino H, Kobayashi T, Goto I, Onitsuka H. Magnetic resonance imaging of the muscles in patients with polymyositis and dermatomyositis. Muscle Nerve 1991;14:716–720.
18. Fraser DD, Frank JA, Dalakas MC. Inflammatory myopathies: MR imaging and spectroscopy. Radiology 1991;179:341–344.
19. Hernandez RJ, Keim DR, Chenevert TL, Sullivan DB, Aisen AM. Fat-suppressed MR imaging in myositis. Radiology 1992;182:217–219.
20. Kier R, McCarthy S, Diets MJ, Rudicel S. MR appearance of painful conditions of the ankle. RadioGraphics 1991;11:407–408.
21. Berkowitz JF, Kier R, Rudicel S. Plantar fasciitis: MR imaging. Radiology 1991;179:665–667.
22. Deutsch AL, Mink JH, Kerr R. MRI of the foot and ankle. New York: Raven Press;1992:356–360.
23. Frei S, de Lange EE, Fechner RE. Case report 690: nodular fasciitis of the elbow. Skeletal Radiol 1991;20:468–471.
24. Meyer CA, Kransdorf MJ, Jelinek JS, Moser RP. MR and CT appearance of nodular fasciitis. J Comput Assist Tomogr 1991;15(2):276–279.
25. Hermans R. A case of nodular fasciitis of the zygomatic arch. Journal Belge de Radiologie-Belgisch Tijdschrift voor Radiologie 1990;73:493–495.

24
Pediatric Muscle Ultrasound

John Heckmatt

Pediatric applications of ultrasound imaging of muscle dates from 1980 when we reported increased echogenicity in dystrophic muscle.[1] Until that time, ultrasound imaging was used successfully to measure cross-sectional area in healthy subjects,[2,3] and Young et al. used it to measure quadriceps wasting secondary to disorders of the knee joint.[4] Ultrasound is now quite a sophisticated tool for assessing muscle disease as demonstrated throughout the chapters of this book and elsewhere.[5-12] Ultrasound imaging answers the need for a simple, potentially widely available, noninvasive screening tool for the primary diagnosis of muscle disease, which can be easily applied in the pediatric clinic.

Background

Most muscle disorders of childhood are associated with pathological changes in muscle tissue. This is especially true in muscular dystrophies, where there is progressive replacement of muscle tissue by adipose and connective tissue, and is also true of the chronic neuropathies and congenital myopathies where there is usually adipose tissue infiltration and proliferation of perimysial connective tissue in addition to the characteristic changes affecting the muscle fibers. This infiltration disrupts the normal, regular architecture of muscle and gives rise to innumerable interfaces within the muscle that act as a source of specular and nonspecular reflection of the ultrasound beam.

Technique

Only a brief review of ultrasound techniques of imaging muscles is necessary here due to its thorough discussion in Chapter 2. Recall that pathological muscle tissue is abnormally echogenic. There is a corresponding reduction of the echo reflected from the underlying bone surface as the muscle echo increases. Ultrasound diagnosis of muscle disease therefore places a strong reliance on the assessment of relative echo intensities. For this reason, a consistent imaging technique is fundamental. This primarily depends upon scanning normal muscle to determine machine gain settings to clearly delineate all the major anatomical structures. These gain settings should be adhered to when scanning children with diseased muscle. Consistency of hard copy can also be a problem, hence a normal scan is included with most of the figures in this chapter.

The thigh is the most suitable muscle for routine imaging, as many muscle disorders are proximal in distribution. When scanning over the anterior thigh, strong echoes are reflected from the outline of the rectus femoris, the midthigh aponeurosis, which covers the contiguous surfaces of that muscle and the underlying vastus intermedius, and the bone surface. Although gain is adjusted so that muscle appears almost black, low-intensity echoes are reflected from the boundaries of the muscle fascicles within the muscle.

Initial studies were done with a static B-scanner[13] and attention quickly turned to real-time scanning due to greater speed, portability, and convenience. The most suitable type of real-time scanner is the linear array, because the parallel beams give a strong bone image and a consistent muscle echo. Sector scanners have divergent beams, and give a poor or nonexistent bone image and inconsistent muscle echo, and are therefore unsuitable (Figure 24.1). A Toshiba SAL20A with a 5-MHz transducer, and a 3.5-MHz transducer in older patients, were used in most cases shown here. In some cases, higher resolution scanners are desireable.

The technique of scanning is as follows. When assessing muscle thickness, care is taken to standardize the child's position, the exact site of the scan, and the pressure of the transducer on the skin surface. The child is seated, as relaxed as possible, with the knee extended and the scan performed at midthigh level (half way from the greater

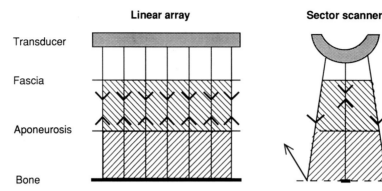

FIGURE 24.1. Schematic comparison of real-time linear array and sector transducers for imaging muscle of the thigh (longitudinal image). The linear array gives a good bone echo over the whole image, and the parallel ultrasound beams strike the muscle fascicles (represented as diagonal lines) at a consistent angle. The sector scanner gives an acceptable bone echo over only a small portion of the image, and the diverging ultrasound beams strike the muscle fascicles at variable angles. See Chapter 2 for greater technical detail.

trochanter to the joint line of the knee). The transducer is applied transversely across the thigh using a generous amount of gel. Tissue compression is avoided by observing the outline of the skin echo on the screen, the aim being to maintain this as a semicircle and to avoid flattening it. When assessing muscle thickness only the middle few transducer elements are in contact with the skin surface. To get a more complete image in order to assess muscle echogenicity, it is necessary to press slightly harder to ensure skin contact across most of the array. Attenuation of the ultrasound beam within the thigh muscle is assessed by the proportion of anterior surface of the femur imaged on the transverse scan. This normally appears as a full semicircle and is reduced to a line or blip when muscle echo intensity is increased.[14]

Appearance of Ultrasound Scans in Various Diseases

The various abnormalities are illustrated in Figures 24.2 to 24.7 and are summarized in Table 24.1. In a study of

Duchenne (4 years)

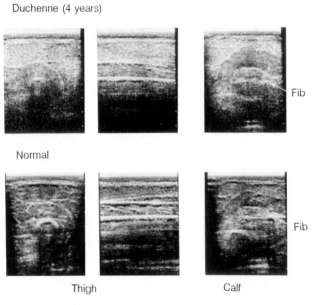

Normal

Thigh   Calf

FIGURE 24.2. Ultrasound scans (5 MHz) of the thigh and calf in Duchenne muscular dystrophy showing the uniform increase in echogenicity of the muscle. On the transverse scan of the thigh (first image), the bone echo is reduced from a semicircle to a line, as a result of attenuation of the ultrasound beam. ("fib" = fibula)

Congenital muscular dystrophy (3 years)

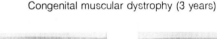

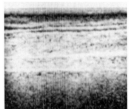

Ataxia

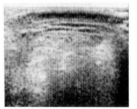

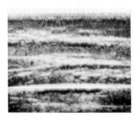

FIGURE 24.3. Ultrasound scans (5 MHz) of the thigh in an ambulatory girl with congenital muscular dystrophy. There is marked muscle echogenicity and bone echo is absent on the transverse (first) scan. The control patient has ataxia but no neuromuscular disease.

Spinal muscular atrophy (2 years)

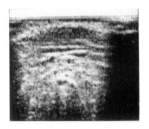 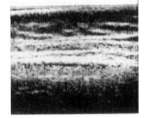

Lax ligaments

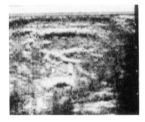 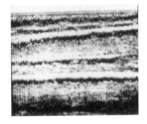

FIGURE 24.4. Ultrasound scan (5 MHz) of the thigh in an ambulatory boy with spinal muscular atrophy. The muscle subcutaneous tissue ratio is 1:1 compared with >2:1 for the control. Muscle echogenicity is moderately increased and bone echo is reduced but present. The control has lax ligaments, which is a benign cause of delayed motor development, but normal ultrasound scans.

222 consecutive new patients referred to the pediatric muscle clinic, we assessed the diagnostic value of real-time ultrasound imaging.[14] The ultrasound scan was done "blindly" (i.e., without knowledge of the history or examination). The sensitivity of ultrasound scanning was 68% and the specificity was 97%. This compared favorably with needle electromyography performed on the same patients, where the same figures were 69% and 96%, respectively (Table 24.2).

It is important to be aware of the limitations of the technique. Disorders that are associated with purely intracellular changes, such as mitochondrial myopathy, glycogenoses, and congenital myopathies in young infants, are associated with normal scans. The same is true of the severe type of spinal muscular atrophy when the history is brief (this also often coincides with "prepathological" change on the muscle biopsy) and in Duchenne muscular dystrophy under the age of 3 years, when there is little adipose tissue infiltration to which the ultrasound is most sensitive. We have found ultrasound scanning of muscle of limited use in the neonatal unit, because adipose tissue infiltration of muscle at that age is uncommon and connective tissue proliferation is mainly around the muscle fibers and difficult to resolve on ultrasound scanning.

Normal (3 years)   Duchenne (4 years)

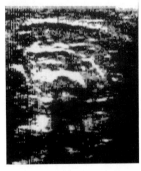 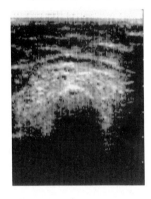

Congenital dystrophy (3 years)   Spinal atrophy (5 years)

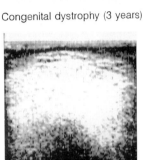 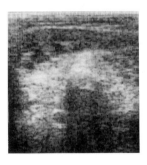

FIGURE 24.5. Comparison of transverse ultrasound scans (5 MHz) of the thigh in four ambulatory children. In Duchenne muscular dystrophy, there is increased muscle echogenicity, but at this advanced age (4 years old), bone echo is present but reduced. In congenital muscular dystrophy, the muscle echo is so intense that bone echo is lost. In spinal muscular atrophy there is marked "muscle atrophy," subcutaneous tissue thickness is increased, and muscle is echogenic, but bone echo is still present.

Emery Dreifuss syndrome

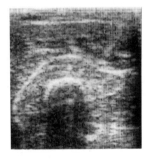

Left   Right

FIGURE 24.6. Selective muscle involvement in an 18 year old with Emery-Dreifuss muscular dystrophy. Ultrasound scans show increased echogenicity of the vastus intermedius muscle adjacent to the bone on both sides. His calves showed selective involvement of the medial heads of the gastrocnemius (not shown) (3.5-MHz transducer).

Transverse ultrasound scans of the thigh

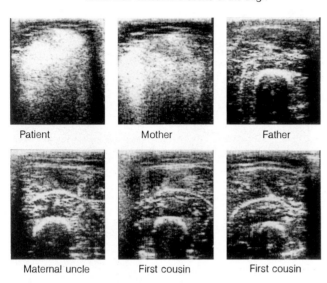

Patient   Mother   Father

Maternal uncle   First cousin   First cousin

FIGURE 24.7. Transverse ultrasound scans (3.5 MHz) of the thigh in a 16 year old with Emery-Dreifuss muscular dystrophy and his family. Ultrasound scanning showed marked echogenicity in his and his mother's muscles. Both had mild weakness and Achilles tendon contractures. Needle biopsy of the thigh confirmed mild dystrophic changes in the muscles of both patient and mother.

TABLE 24.1. Ultrasound scanning of muscle in children: summary of typical findings in various disorders at initial presentation.

Disease	Principal findings on ultrasound imaging of the thigh	Comments and cautions
Duchenne muscular dystrophy	Increased echogenicity in all quadriceps muscles giving a "ground glass" appearance.[14] Muscle may appear bulky.	No or subtle change under 3 years of age. Consistent technique essential.
Becker muscular dystrophy	As Duchenne, but sometimes some selective involvement.	Normal when no weakness (e.g., muscle cramps on exertion only symptom).
Emery-Dreifuss muscular dystrophy	Striking selective involvement typical.[18]	Other areas (arm/calf) may also show selective involvement.
Congenital muscular dystrophy.	Muscle very echogenic, bone echo absent, and sometimes selective involvement.[5,18]	A very sensitive test, except for neonatal presentation.
Congenital myopathy	Selective or mild generalized muscle echogenicity.[13,18]	Except for neonatal presentation.
Juvenile dermatomyositis (polymyositis)	Variable echogenicity according to angulation of the transducer in the transverse plane.[14]	Standardize carefully. Normal scan does not exclude acute diagnosis.
Spinal muscular atrophy, (a) severe, (b) intermediate, and (c) mild	Muscle atrophic and echogenic, but bone echo usually weak but present.[13,14]	(a) Normal when brief history of weakness; (b) and (c) always abnormal.
Peroneal muscular atrophy	Distal muscles echogenic (and atrophic).	Peripheral nerve conduction test essential.

The myotonic and myasthenic disorders are most appropriately investigated by electrodiagnostic studies.
For a full clinical account of these disorders, see Dubowitz.[22]
"Selective involvement" refers to involvement of the quadriceps femoris with sparing of the rectus femoris relative to the vasti.

TABLE 24.2. Sensitivity of ultrasound scanning and needle EMG.

Disorder	Ages	Number	Ultrasound imaging	EMG
		1. Myopathies		
Duchenne muscular dystrophy (early and "preclinical" cases)	2–30 months	7	0%	43%
Duchenne muscular dystrophy (clinical presentation)	3–7 years	22	95%	90%
Becker (and limb girdle) muscular dystrophy	2–18 years	18	68%	79%
Congenital muscular dystrophy	5 days to 3 years	14	86%	86%
Emery-Dreifuss muscular dystrophy	16–21 years	4	100%	100%
Others	11 days to 14 years	18	55%	56%
Subtotal		84	71%	76%
		2. Neuropathies		
Spinal muscular atrophy (severe)	11 days to 9 months	15	47%	47%
Spinal muscular atrophy (intermediate and mild)	18 months to 14 years	13	100%	85%
Others	8 months to 14 years	19	47%	42%
Subtotal		47	62%	57%
Total		133	68%	69%

EMG data not previously published. Ultrasound data from Heckmatt et al.[14]

Specificity in 94 patients who did not have neuromuscular disease (but had similar symptoms, e.g., floppy infant, delayed motor development) was 97% for ultrasound and 96% for EMG.

The 7 "early and preclinical" cases of Duchenne muscular dystrophy presented as follows: + family history 3, hypotonia during intercurrent infection 2, delayed walking 1, incidentally noted elevation of serum CK 1.

Clinically, central nervous system disorders are often the chief differential diagnosis of myopathy, and they are rarely associated with increased muscle echogenicity.[13,14] In fact, increased muscle echogenicity in a child is strongly suggestive of primary muscle disease despite only mild disability. An example is "minimal change myopathy" (a congenital myopathy), which often selects out the respiratory muscles and yet is associated with marked echogenicity of the thigh muscle.

Muscle "Atrophy"

In spinal muscular atrophy and some of the other neurogenic disorders (e.g., peroneal muscular atrophy) there is "muscle atrophy." Here, this is defined as a reduction in muscle thickness associated with an increase in subcutaneous tissue thickness so that the muscle subcutaneous tissue ratio at midthigh level is 1:1 or less, rather than the usual 2:1 or more. This 2:1 ratio is only broken in obesity and at 1 year of age, when the healthy infant becomes covered temporarily by a "wave of fat." We have published normal values for thigh muscle and subcutaneous tissue thickness,[15,16] but assessment of the ratio is usually sufficient. Muscle may be atrophic in central nervous system disorders but without increased echogenicity.

Selective Muscle Involvement

One of the most interesting and important findings on ultrasound scanning is differential involvement of the various components of a muscle group such as the quadriceps femoris. The usual pattern in the thigh is sparing of the rectus femoris in relation to the vasti, with vastus intermedius often the most affected (Figure 24.6). Exceptionally, we have seen the reverse pattern, for example in facioscapulohumeral muscular dystrophy. These ultrasound findings were verified by selective needle biopsies.[17,18]

Selective muscle involvement is important diagnostically because normal muscle may be hypertrophic and diseased muscle atrophic. Thus, biopsy over a normal hypertrophic muscle may miss the diseased muscle.[17] We view muscle biopsy without prior ultrasound as analogous to renal biopsy without prior imaging. It is usually difficult to predict selective involvement clinically or by electromyography. Most children with selective involvement have only mild clinical disability because of compensation by less diseased muscles.

Selective muscle involvement may arise for a number of reasons. Different muscles do different types of work (eccentric versus concentric work) and thus may be liable to different rates of damage.[18] There may be variable gene expression and, in female carriers of X-linked muscle disorders, different degrees of Lyonization. A different proportion of the two fiber types in the various muscles is an additional but less likely factor.

Carriers

Ultrasound scanning of potential female carriers of the allelic X-linked recessive Duchenne and Becker muscular dystrophies is unrewarding as a means of routine detection. This is mainly because too few carriers manifest (only about 5% of Duchenne muscular dystrophy carriers are clinically manifesting). Molecular techniques have generally taken over carrier detection. It is always worth scanning any potential female carrier of Emery-Dreifuss muscular dystrophy (same mode of inheritance, different gene) who has physical signs (e.g., Achilles tendon contractures, cardiac involvement) (Figure 24.7). For more on this topic see Chapter 16.

Future Developments

It is possible to improve the quality of images and to increase the sensitivity of the technique by using higher-frequency transducers than 5 MHz. The modern wide-frequency transducers (e.g., from 7.5 to 10 MHz) are capable of giving excellent images. Ultrasound imaging can be used to follow disease progress in controlled clinical trials, such as in Duchenne muscular dystrophy in which there is sufficient change in 1 year to be quantitated on sequential scans.[19,20]

One of the drawbacks of this diagnostic technique is the difficulty in quantitating the changes, although it should be realized that in many patients the abnormality is obvious. Recent advances using high resolution transducers, however, indicate an increase in perimysial septa per unit depth in muscular dystrophics.[7] Such advances are highly promising and require further investigation.

We measured echo strength from raw radiofrequency data bypassing user-controlled time–gain–compensation (TGC) settings. This improved objectivity but the diagnostic yield was small, perhaps because our implementation of the technique at the time was crude; powerful personal computers had not yet been invented![21] A few manufacturers allow measurement of pixel strength from the video freeze frame image (see Chapter 2). The usefulness of this approach depends upon the ability to precisely control TGC. Nonlinear compression of the dynamic range of the original radio frequency signal may be an additional drawback.

Conclusion

Ultrasound imaging of muscle is an invaluable tool for the noninvasive diagnosis of neuromuscular disease. It is particularly useful in the evaluation of young children who are unable or reluctant to cooperate with physical examination. In the author's opinion, it is an essential first step before muscle biopsy to evaluate the most suitable muscle for sampling, especially in patients with mild degrees of weakness. Modern digital technology should allow future development of effective techniques of quantitation.

References

1. Heckmatt JZ, Dubowitz V, Leeman S. Detection of pathological change in dystrophic muscle with B-scan ultrasound imaging. Lancet 1980;i:1389–1390.
2. Dons B, Bollerup K, Bonde-Peterson F, Hancke S. The effects of weight-lifting exercise related to muscle fibre composition and muscle cross-sectional area in humans. Eur J Appl Physiol 1979;40:95–98.
3. Ikai M, Fukunaga T. Calculation of muscle strength per unit cross-sectional area of human muscle by means of ultrasonic measurement. Int Z Angew Physiol Einschl Arbeitsphysiol 1968;26:26–30.
4. Young A, Hughes I, Russell P, Parker MJ, Nichols P Jr. Measurement of quadriceps muscle wasting by ultrasonography. Rheumatol Rehabil 1980;19:141–145.
5. Topaloglu H, Gucuyener K, Yalaz K, et al. Selective involvement of the quadriceps muscle in congenital muscular dystrophies: an ultrasonographic study. Brain Dev 1992;14:84–87.
6. Gunreben G, Bogdahn U. Real-time sonography of acute and chronic muscle denervation. Muscle Nerve 1991;14:654–664.
7. Dock W, Happak, Grabenwoger F, Toifl K, Bittner R, Gruber H. Neuromuscular diseases: evaluation with high-frequency sonography. Radiology 1990;177:825–828.
8. Lamminen A, Jaaskelainen J, Rapola J, Suramo I. High-frequency ultrasonography of skeletal muscle in children with neuromuscular disease. J Ultrasound Med 1988;7:505–509.
9. Fischer AQ, Carpenter DW, Hartlage PL, Carroll JE, Stephens S. Muscle imaging in neuromuscular disease using computerized real-time sonography. Muscle Nerve 1988;11:270–275.
10. Fischer AQ, Stephens S. Computerized real-time neuromuscular sonography: new application techniques and methods. J Child Neurol 1988;3:69–74.
11. Stern L. New techniques in diagnosis, assessment of progression and research in muscular dystrophy. Aust Paediatr J 1988;24 Suppl 1:34–36.
12. Aspelin P, Ekberg O, Thorsson O, Wilhelmsson M, Westlin N. Ultrasound examination of soft tissue injury of the lower limb in athletes. Am J Sports Med 1992;20:601–603.
13. Heckmatt JZ, Leeman S, Dubowitz V. Ultrasound imaging in the diagnosis of muscle disease. J Pediatr 1982;101:656–660.
14. Heckmatt JZ, Pier N, Dubowitz V. Real-time ultrasound imaging of muscles. Muscle Nerve 1988;11:56–65.
15. Heckmatt JZ, Pier N, Dubowitz V. Measurement of quadriceps muscle thickness in normal children by real-time ultrasound imaging. J Clin Ultrasound 1988;16:177–181.
16. Heckmatt JZ, Pier N, Dubowitz V. Assessment of quadriceps muscle atrophy and hypertrophy in neuromuscular disease in children. J Clin Ultrasound 1988;16:171–176.
17. Heckmatt JZ, Dubowitz V. Diagnostic advantage of needle muscle biopsy and ultrasound imaging in the detection of focal pathology in a girl with limb-girdle dystrophy. Muscle Nerve 1985;8:705–709.
18. Heckmatt JZ, Dubowitz V. Ultrasound imaging and directed needle biopsy in the diagnosis of selective involvement in neuromuscular disease. J Child Neurol 1987;2:205–213.

19. Heckmatt JZ, Hyde SA, Gabain A, Dubowitz V. Therapeutic trial of isaxonine in Duchenne muscular dystrophy. Muscle Nerve 1988;11:836–847.

20. Manzur AY, Hyde SA, Rodillo E, Heckmatt JZ, Bentley G, Dubowitz V. A randomised controlled trial of early surgery in Duchenne muscular dystrophy. Neuromuscul Dis 1992;2:379–87.

21. Heckmatt JZ, Doherty M, Leeman S, Willson K. Quantitative muscle sonography. J Child Neurol 1989;4:S101–S106.

Part V
Orthopaedic Muscle Disorders

25
The Role of Muscle Imaging in Orthopaedics

Russell C. Fritz and John V. Crues III

Magnetic resonance imaging (MRI) is gradually emerging as the premier method of depicting muscle pathology. In this chapter we will examine the role of this technique in modern orthopaedic practice by presenting current clinical applications of MRI. We will also speculate about the potential of MRI to provide more economical diagnostic information in the future through decreases in imaging time and cost.

Technique

Normal muscle has intermediate to long T_1 and short T_2 relaxation times relative to surrounding soft tissues, and thus is gray on most pulse sequences. Most muscle pathology is associated with increases in T_2 relaxation time that are conspicuous on T_2-weighted and STIR sequences. Fat-saturated T_2-weighted and STIR sequences have the added benefit of fat suppression, which further increases the conspicuity of muscle pathology. Accordingly, most current protocols emphasize these sequences to detect and characterize orthopaedic disorders that affect muscles (see Chapter 3).

The axial plane is often the plane that images the muscle in cross section, thereby minimizing potential partial volume artifacts. Consequently, axial T_2-weighted or STIR sequences are usually the most important and diagnostic for imaging muscle pathology.[1–3] The T_2-weighted sequence has the advantage of a greater number of slices and a greater length of coverage relative to the STIR sequence. Fast spin echo (FSE) T_2-weighted sequences with or without radiofrequency fat suppression offer increased speed as well as greater flexibility in design and may be substituted for the conventional spin echo sequences if available. Fat-suppressed T_2-weighted images are most easily obtained at high magnetic fields (1.0 to 1.5 T) because of the increased separation of the fat and water peaks at higher fields. These sequences are often used by the authors on high field scanners.

Fast STIR sequences have also been developed and greatly decrease the acquisition time for STIR sequences.[4] In our experience the fast STIR sequences maintain the high sensitivity of standard STIR acquisitions, but are more practical in clinical practice. The STIR sequence is an excellent sequence for midfield imaging (0.35 to 1.0 T) because this technique does not depend upon the fat-water peak separation, but does depend upon both long T_1 and T_2 relaxation, which are often present in muscle pathology. The authors tend to use the STIR sequence predominately when imaging muscle pathology using midfield scanners.

Sagittal or coronal images are useful for illustrating the longitudinal extent of muscle pathology relative to adjacent bony landmarks. A sagittal sequence best delineates abnormalities that lie anteriorly or posteriorly whereas a coronal sequence best depicts abnormalities that lie medially or laterally. Longitudinal imaging planes are especially helpful in detecting musculotendinous avulsions, which can be difficult to detect on axial imaging. Consequently, imaging in two orthogonal planes is often necessary for accurate delineation of the full extent of muscle disease. A T_1-weighted sequence in the same plane as the STIR sequence is useful for visualizing fat in chronic muscle atrophy or hemorrhage in relatively acute trauma. A T_2^*-weighted sequence, because of its sensitivity to paramagnetic effects, is occasionally helpful to detect hemosiderin from a remote bleed or calcification in myositis ossificans. Computed tomography, however, is a more accurate method of identifying the presence and distribution of calcification in myositis ossificans.

Gadolinium-enhanced images may provide additional information regarding muscle disorders. T_1-weighted images with fat suppression provide the greatest contrast for enhancement and are the most helpful images after intravenous administration of gadolinium.[5–7] STIR images should not be used as the primary imaging sequence after administration of paramagnetic contrast agents because these agents induce tissue contrast by decreasing tissue T_1 relaxation times. If the contrast agent decreases a tissues T_1 relaxation time to that of fat, then the enhancement may become inconspicuous because it will be suppressed along with fat when using a STIR sequence.

The selection of an appropriate receiver coil is often critically important for optimal image quality in musculoskeletal imaging. A large receiver coil, such as a body coil, is usually required to image the large muscles of the torso and thighs. A head coil may be used to image both lower legs. A small coil designed for imaging the extremities may be used to image the arm or leg if comparison with the opposite side is not necessary. Patients can be imaged in the supine position for most applications. Prone positioning should be considered for posterior pathology involving the gluteal, hamstring, or calf regions in which compression may cause mild distortion of these structures. Supplemental scans performed during muscle contraction may be useful in demonstrating fascial herniation or retraction of torn muscles, which may produce palpable soft tissue masses.[8] A surface skin marker, such as a vitamin E capsule, should be placed on a palpable mass or focal area of tenderness to ensure that the area of concern was imaged; this is especially helpful when no abnormalities are seen on the images.

Pathology

Trauma accounts for the majority of muscle disorders seen by orthopaedic surgeons. Acute muscle injury is most often due to indirect trauma from excessive stretch of a muscle–tendon unit. Such strain injuries typically occur in response to powerful contraction combined with forced lengthening of a muscle.[9] Strain injuries also frequently occur in muscles that typically function in an eccentric fashion to regulate motion. Muscles whose origin and insertion span more than one joint as well as muscles with the highest proportion of type II (fast-twitch) fibers are also prone to strain injury.[9,10] Examples of muscles that meet these criteria are the hamstrings, rectus femoris, and gastrocnemius (Figures 25.1 to 25.3).

A simple clinical grading system is commonly used to characterize muscle strain injury. In mild (first-degree) strains there is no loss of strength or range of motion. Low-grade inflammation without substantial tissue disruption is noted pathologically.[10] MRI demonstrates mild signal alteration, which may only be conspicuous on STIR sequences (Figure 25.4).[3] Moderate (second-degree) strains are characterized by loss of strength secondary to partial muscle tearing. MRI demonstrates more prominent signal alteration within muscles, which is usually obvious on both the STIR and T_2-weighted sequences (Figure 25.5).[11] Perifascial fluid is often identified in grade II strains on MRI.[1,12] In severe (third-degree) strains there is complete disruption of some portion of the muscle–tendon unit. MRI reveals the site of rupture as well as the degree of separation of the components of the muscle–tendon unit.[11,13,14] A hematoma is often present in grade III strains at the site of rupture (Figure 25.6).

Clinically and experimentally, the normal muscle–tendon unit typically fails within the muscle near the

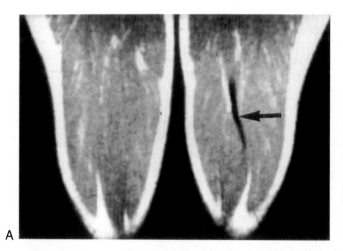

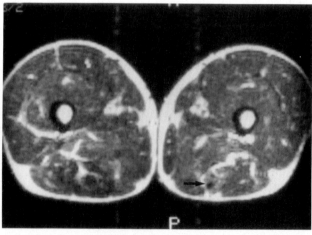

A   B

FIGURE 25.1. Hamstring tendon tear. This 18-year-old high school football player presented to his family physician with a palpable, tender mass on the posterior aspect of his thigh. (A) T_1-weighted (T_R 800/T_E 20) coronal image reveals a black serpiginous lesion (arrow), initially thought to be a draining vein. (B) An intermediately weighted (T_R 2000/T_E 20) axial image reveals a round, low signal lesion and focal atrophy in the region of the palpable mass (arrow). In retrospect the patient had a history of hamstring injuries. These findings represent a tear of a portion of the hamstring tendon with proximal retraction of the tendon and associated muscle atrophy.

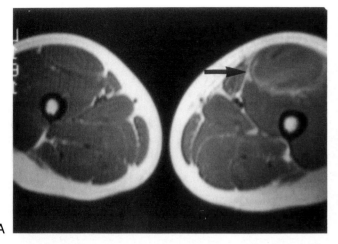

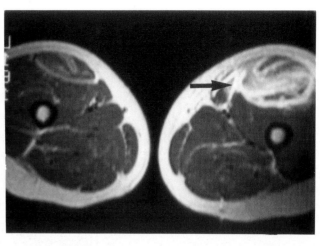

A

B

FIGURE 25.2. Bilateral rectus femoris muscle tears. This young woman began jogging with an experienced companion. After the third day of prolonged jogging, the patient presented with left quadriceps pain and a flaccid knee. (A) Intermediately weighted (T_R 2000/T_E 20) and (B) T_2-weighted (T_R 2000/T_E 80) images reveal diffuse, increased signal intensity within the myotendinous junction.[10] Chronic tendon degeneration, however, not uncommonly leads to rupture within a tendon in response to an acute strain rather than at the theoretical weak link in the unit (Figure 25.7).[15,16] Failure of the muscle–tendon unit may occur at various sites: within the belly of the muscle, at the myotendinous junction, within the tendon, at the tendon–bone junction, within the attached bone, or within an unfused apophyseal growth plate. Furthermore, the injury may occur either proximally (Figure 25.8) or distally (Figure 25.9) within the muscle–tendon unit at any of the above sites, or may involve multiple different muscles. In skeletally

left rectus femoris muscle (arrows). Lesser signal abnormalities were also detected in the right rectus femoris muscle. The muscle fibers, however, appeared contiguous on MRI. Based upon MRI findings, surgical repair was canceled. The patient did well on conservative follow-up.

immature individuals, the unfused apophyseal growth plate may be the weakest link in the muscle–tendon unit, which may fail before the myotendinous junction (Figure 25.10).[17–19]

Treatment of most strains is conservative with management directed towards relief of symptoms and protection from further injury. Grade III injuries, however, may require early surgery as retraction and scarring of the ruptured tissue compromises later attempts at repair.[9] Accurate clinical diagnosis may be impeded by recruitment of synergists when only a portion of a group of muscles is completely torn. Also, a complete rupture

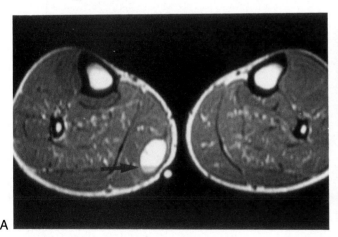

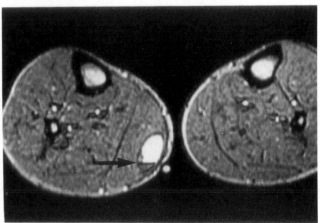

A

B

FIGURE 25.3. Gastrocnemius traumatic hematoma. This young male presented with acute onset of calf pain while jogging. (A) Posttraumatic muscle hematomas often appear sharply demarcated with fluid levels on intermediately weighted (T_R 2000/T_E 20) images (arrow). (B) The fluid level is better seen on gradient echo images (FA [flip angle] 30°, T_R 50/T_E 15) because of the magnetic susceptibility changes from the intact red cells that layer dependently (arrow).

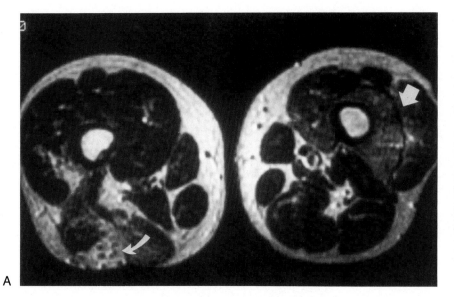
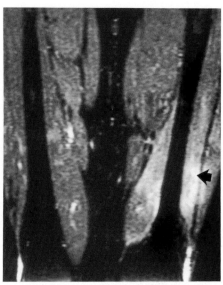

FIGURE 25.4. Acute grade I left quadriceps strain and old right hamstring rupture. (A)T_2-weighted (2000/80) axial image shows mild increased signal in the left vastus intermedius and vastus lateralis (arrow). Fatty replacement of the right semitendinosus muscle with central foci of low signal intensity scarring is noted from an old complete rupture (curved arrow). (B) STIR (2000/43/160) coronal image reveals edema within the distal left vastus medialis, intermedius, and lateralis (arrow), which is much more conspicuous.

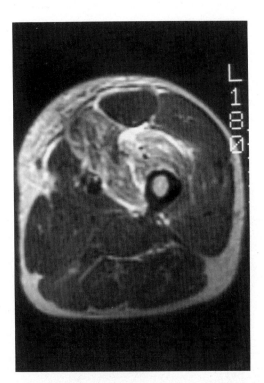

FIGURE 25.5. Grade II quadriceps strain in a soccer player. T_2-weighted (2000/80) axial image shows increased signal throughout the vastus medialis and vastus intermedius muscles as well as a thin, high signal intensity rim of perifascial fluid.

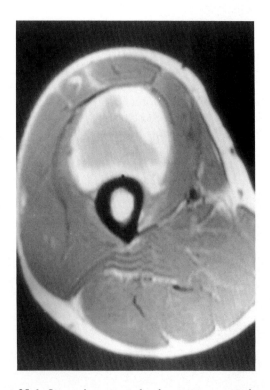

FIGURE 25.6. Large intramuscular hematoma secondary to a grade III strain in a soccer player. Proton density (2000/20) image of the left thigh reveals a hematoma within the substance of the disrupted vastus intermedius muscle. This acute hematoma has peripheral high signal intensity and central low signal intensity.

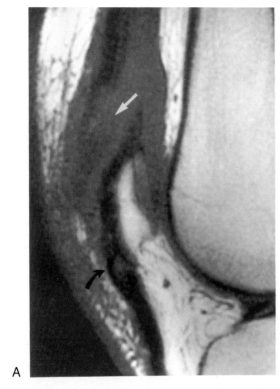

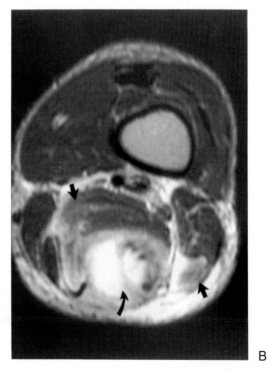

FIGURE 25.7. Complete quadriceps tendon tear in a 55-year-old man. (A) T_1 (600/15) and (B) T_2^*-weighted gradient echo (600/20/15°) sagittal images show fluid outlining a complete rupture of the quadriceps tendon from its insertion on the superior pole of the patella (arrows). Focal degeneration of the proximal patellar tendon is also identified (curved arrows).

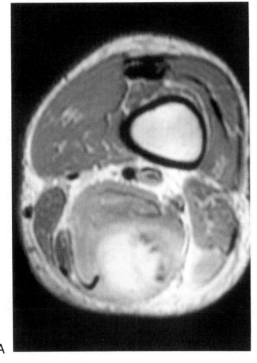

FIGURE 25.8. Acute hamstring strain in a soccer player. (A) Proton density (2000/20) and (B) T_2-weighted (2000/80) axial images of the distal thigh reveal increased signal within the long head of the biceps and semimembranosus muscles (arrows). A hematoma (curved arrows) delineates a complete tear of the semitendinosus at the musculotendinous junction.

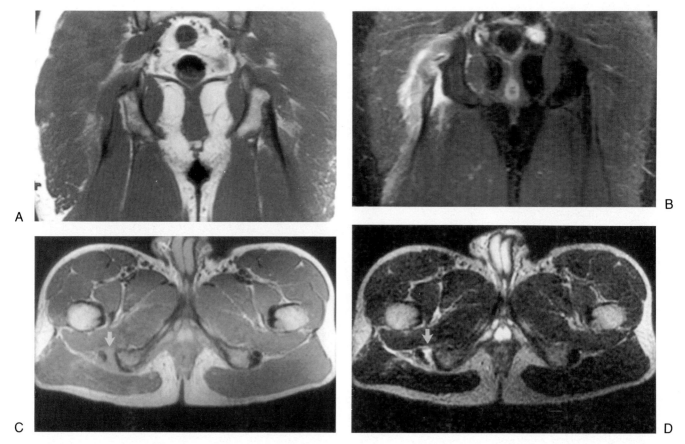

FIGURE 25.9. Rupture of the origin of the hamstring tendon ischial tuberosity. (A) T_1-weighted (600/15) and (B) STIR (2000/43/160) coronal images of the pelvis demonstrates detachment of the right hamstring tendons from the ischial tuberosity. (C) Proton density (2000/20) and (D) T_2-weighted (2000/80) axial images of the pelvis reveal fluid separating the semimembranosus, biceps femoris, and semitendinosus tendons from the ischial tuberosity (arrows).

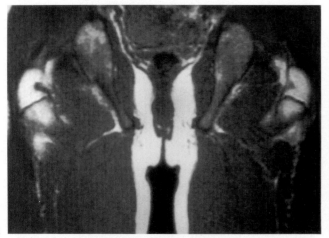
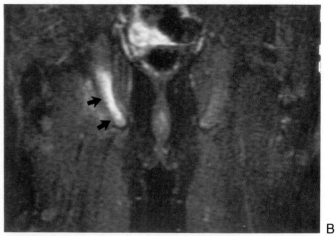

FIGURE 25.10. Stress response of the ischial tuberosity in a 13-year-old hurdler with a suspected hamstring tear. (A) T_1-weighted (600/15) and (B) STIR (2000/43/160) coronal images reveal no evidence of hamstring strain. Marrow edema is noted on the STIR sequence within the ischial tuberosity (arrows), which was not conspicuous on the T_1-weighted sequence due to the presence of normal intermediate signal intensity red marrow.

may be difficult to detect clinically when it lies deep to intact muscles. The evaluation of trauma to the muscle–tendon unit with MRI allows *better* delineation of the site and degree of injury, which should result in greater understanding and more rational treatment.[20] These advantages are especially important when an injury is severe and early surgery is being considered.

MRI may also be useful when there is diagnostic uncertainty after the clinical examination and standard x-rays have been performed (Figure 25.11), or when the working diagnosis is in question due to failure to respond to a course of treatment. An example of the latter is a world-class track and field athlete who was diagnosed with a grade II strain of the vastus medialis obliquus (VMO) muscle and suffered from worsening anteromedial knee pain (Figure 25.12). The MRI study confirmed the clinical impression of a high-grade partial tear at the myotendinous junction of the VMO and excluded internal derangement of the knee as a contributing factor.

MRI may provide objective evidence of injuries that are thought to be unusual or controversial. An example of such an injury is a strain of the plantaris muscle, which may result in posterior knee or leg pain (Figure 25.13). Plantaris strain, despite being a common clinical diagnosis, is thought by many sports medicine experts to not occur as there are no reported cases proved by surgery or autopsy.[21] Evidence of plantaris rupture with ultrasound and MRI has been recently reported in two cases.[22] We have also seen cases of plantaris rupture with MRI or with ultrasound in patients that presented with calf pain and suspected deep venous thrombosis. An intramuscular hematoma in the plane between the soleus and medial gastrocnemius muscles may be associated with rupture of the plantaris (Figure 25.14). In such cases, a retracted plantaris muscle will be evident on the images posterior to the knee due to rupture at the distal myotendinous junction.

In our experience, the clinical syndrome of "tennis leg" is characterized by injury to the posterior muscles of the leg. MRI may demonstrate involvement of the soleus (Figure 25.15) or plantaris muscles in the minority of cases; however, the gastrocnemius muscle is involved in the majority of cases. The typical case of "tennis leg" or calf strain involves the medial head of the gastrocnemius muscle at the myotendinous junction (Figure 25.16).[23] Follow-up MRI may provide clinically useful information regarding the degree of remaining signal alteration prior to resuming intense activity (Figure 25.17).[3,12] Serial imaging may reveal fatty infiltration and atrophy or a return to normal, depending on whether the muscle–

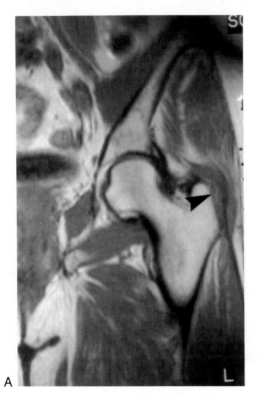
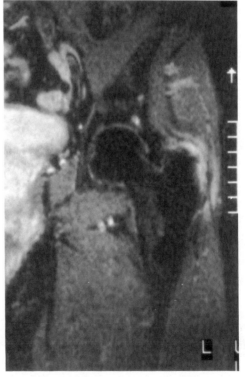

FIGURE 25.11. Strain of the gluteus minimus and medius muscles at their insertion on the greater tuberosity in a 65-year-old woman with a suspected hip fracture following a fall. (A) T_1 (600/15) and (B) STIR (1800/30/110) coronal images of the left hip reveal increased signal in the distal gluteus minimus and medius muscles at their insertion on the greater tuberosity (arrowhead).

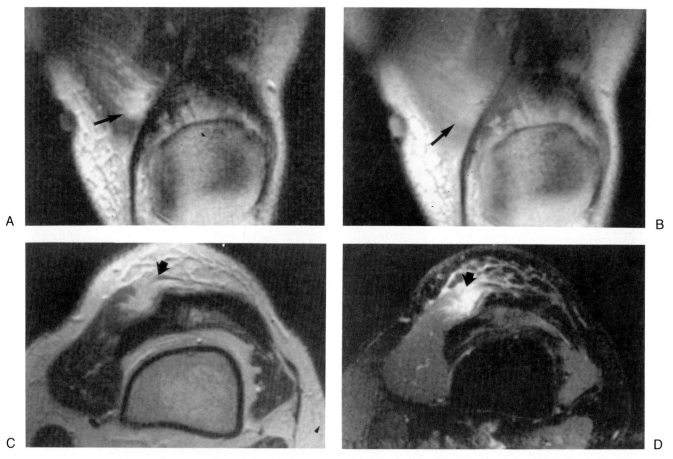

FIGURE 25.12. Tear of the vastus medialis obliquus (VMO). (A) Proton density (2000/20) and (B) T_2-weighted (2000/80) coronal images through the patella reveal a focal gap (arrows) within the fibers of the VMO at the musculotendinous junction.

This fiber disruption is further delineated on the (C) T_2-weighted (2000/80) and (D) STIR (1800/30/110) axial images through the musculotendinous junction. The fluid filled gap is conspicuous on the STIR sequence (arrowheads).

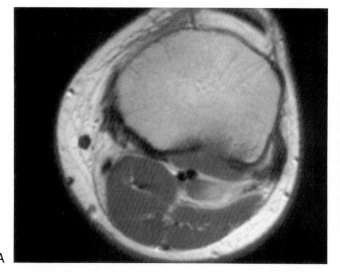

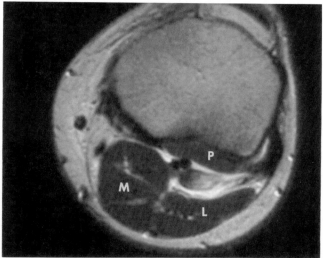

FIGURE 25.13. Isolated strain of the plantaris muscle in a basketball player with posterior knee pain. (A) Proton density (1800/20) and (B) T_2-weighted (1800/80) axial images of the knee reveal focal increased signal within the plantaris muscle with perifascial fluid. The medial (M) and lateral (L) heads of the gastrocnemius muscle superficially, and the popliteus muscle (P) deep to the plantaris, are uninvolved.

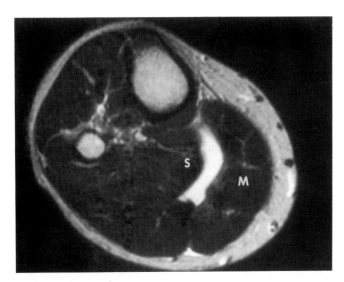

FIGURE 25.14. Rupture of the plantaris muscle with an intermuscular hematoma between the soleus and medial head of the gastrocnemius in a 35-year-old tennis player with sudden calf pain. A focal fluid collection is noted between the soleus (S) and medial head of the gastrocnemius (M) in the proximal calf on this T_2-weighted (2000/80) image. The plantaris tendon normally lies in the plane between the soleus and medial head of the gastrocnemius. The plantaris is not visualized due to a complete tear at the musculotendinous junction with superior retraction of the muscle belly.

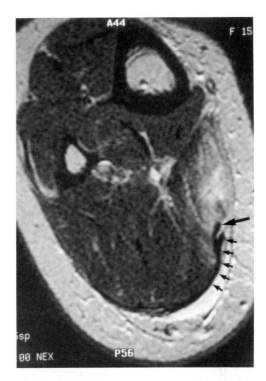

FIGURE 25.15. Acute medial calf pain that occurred during an aerobics workout. Increased signal is noted throughout the medial soleus muscle within the lower part of the middle third of the leg on this T_2-weighted (2000/80) image. The adjacent plantaris tendon (arrow) and adjacent gastrocnemius aponeurosis (small arrows) appear intact. Fluid is noted superficial to the fascia.

tendon unit is intact.[14] Associated findings such as hematomas, fascial tears, and muscle herniation through fascial defects may be seen with MRI.[8,24]

Hematomas may be characterized as *intra*muscular (Figure 25.6) or *inter*muscular (Figure 25.14) with MRI.[25] Intramuscular hematomas are only half as common as

intermuscular hematomas, but may take three times as long to resolve.[26,27] Hematomas have variable and complex signal depending on the age of blood degradation products and the field strength of the MRI system (Figure

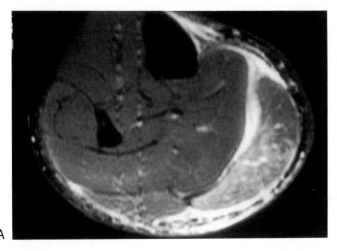

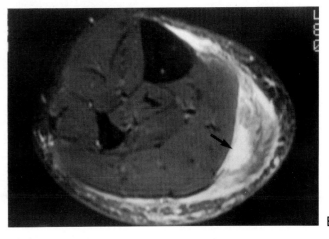

A   B

FIGURE 25.16. Tennis leg. STIR (2000/43/155) axial images of the midcalf reveal increased signal throughout the medial gastrocnemius muscle in the middle third of the leg (A). A focal fluid filled gap (arrow) at the musculotendinous junction is identified more distally (B).

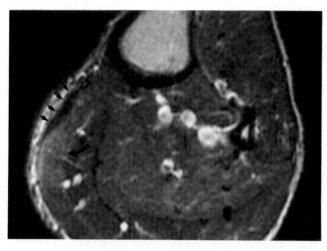

FIGURE 25.17. A 20-year-old tennis player with complete resolution of symptoms 6 weeks following a medial gastrocnemius strain. T_2-weighted (2000/80) axial image of the midcalf reveals mild increased signal within the medial gastrocnemius muscle (curved arrow) with low signal intensity thickening of the adjacent crural fascia (small arrows), compatible with scar formation.

25.18).[13,28] On T_1-weighted images, increased signal is typically seen within subacute hematomas due to methemoglobin (Figures 25.18, 25.19). On T_2-weighted images, central low signal intensity is seen in acute hematomas at high field strength secondary to deoxyhemoglobin within intact red blood cells (Figure 25.6). Fluid levels may also be present in acute muscle hematomas (Figure 25.3). The dependent fluid may be rich in intact red cells containing deoxyhemoglobin and methemoglobin, which causes signal loss on spin echo and gradient echo images from magnetic susceptibility effects. A low signal intensity rim is typically seen in chronic hematomas secondary to hemosiderin-laden macrophages. This low signal intensity rim is most prominent at high field strength and with T_2^*-weighted sequences. Low signal intensity rims may also be seen secondary to surrounding fibrosis, especially when it is seen in association with a tear of a component of the musculotendinous unit that becomes retracted. Fibrosis and focal fluid collections have been reported to be associated with delayed healing in athletes and may require more aggressive surgical management.[3]

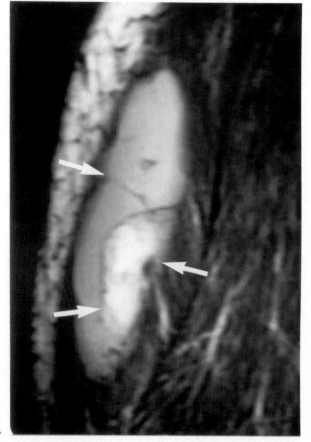

A

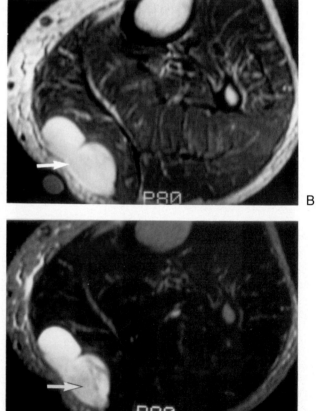

B

C

FIGURE 25.18. Medial gastrocnemius muscle hematoma. The patient presented with a palpable mass in the medial calf after "pulling my muscle." (A) A coronal T_1-weighted (T_R 800/T_E 17) image reveals regions of septations and differing signal intensity due to different ages of maturing oxidative denatura-

tion of the hemoglobin in different segments of the hematoma (arrows). These are characteristic findings in muscle hematomas. The signal inhomogeneity is more subtly seen on (B) intermediately weighted (T_R 2000/T_E 17) and (C) T_2-weighted (T_R 2000/T_E 80) images (arrows).

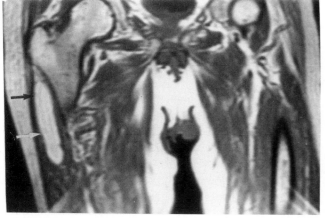

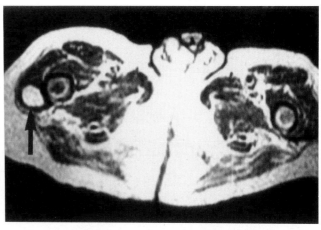

A

B

FIGURE 25.19. Vastus lateralis hematoma. This patient presented with a subacute onset of right hip pain over 6 weeks. This MR scan was performed to evaluate for possible osteonecrosis of the right femoral head. (A) The T_1-weighted (T_R 500/T_E 20) coronal image reveals sharply demarcated, uniformly bright signal in the vastus lateralis muscle (arrows). (B) The T_1-weighted (T_R 800/T_E 20) axial images also show uniform increased signal within the subacute hematoma (arrow).

Deep hematomas may be difficult to distinguish from swollen, edematous muscles on physical exam. The detection and characterization of hematomas with MRI or ultrasound may guide clinical management and prompt consideration of evacuation in selected cases.

In addition to the frequently seen injuries of the thigh and calf, MRI is also helpful in evaluating less common sites of muscle strain injury. For example, muscle strains and tears of the adjacent plantar fascia may be seen in athletes and dancers (Figure 25.20). MRI allows distinction from tenosynovitis, ligamentous injury, and stress fractures of the foot, which may have a similar clinical presentation but different treatment. A common clinical presentation is pain in the region of the heel of the foot. The clinical differentiation between plantar fascitis, enthesopathy at the attachment of the plantar fascia to the calcaneus (often called the "heel pain syndrome"), and stress fracture of the calcaneus is unreliable. MRI, however, is a reliable diagnostic technique in this condition.[29,30]

Abdominal and chest wall strains occur commonly in major league baseball players (Figure 25.21). MRI may delineate the location of these injuries and provide objective information regarding the status of recovery. These muscle injuries typically follow a clinical course similar to hamstring strains, which are characterized by

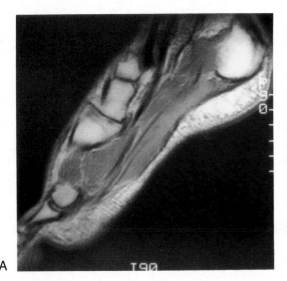

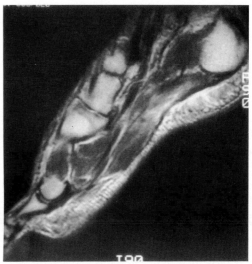

A

B

FIGURE 25.20. Recurrent plantar foot strain in a professional ballet dancer. (A) Proton density (2000/20) and (B) T_2-weighted (2000/70) sagittal images of the foot reveal a strain of the flexor digitorum brevis muscle. The overlying plantar fascia appears subtly irregular but intact.

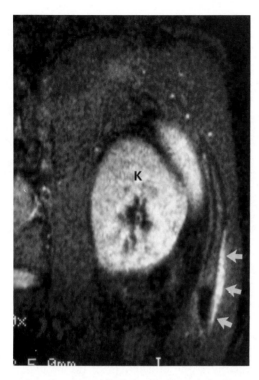

FIGURE 25.21. Recurrent abdominal wall strain in a professional baseball player. STIR (1500/30/100) oblique coronal images at the level of the left kidney (K) reveals increased signal within the external abdominal oblique muscle adjacent to the costochondral junction of the left 11th rib (arrows). This seemingly small strain of the abdominal wall was recurrent and resulted in 10 weeks of missed playing time during the baseball season.

frequent recurrence of injury and absence from competition. MRI signal alteration, which persists in strained muscles despite the resolution of symptoms, may define a period of vulnerability to reinjury.[3,12,31,32] Whether or not persistent MRI signal alteration will be a useful marker for ongoing muscle repair is not yet known and requires further study.

Arthrography, arthroscopy, and other invasive procedures may be avoided by identifying a muscle strain with MRI. A deltoid strain was detected in a professional baseball player with a suspected rotator cuff tear (Figure 25.22). This finding allowed early conservative therapy and rehabilitation rather than further invasive tests. This case also introduces a potential pitfall in that signal alteration within muscles, although commonly secondary to strain injury, is nonspecific and may be entirely on the basis of local injections.[33,34] Lidocaine and corticosteroid injections are commonly administered about the shoulder and may result in a false positive diagnosis of muscle pathology or bursitis if the radiologist is unaware of this intervention. Signal alteration secondary to an intramuscular injection may persist for several weeks.[33] Iatrogenic complications of multiple injections can be

identified by MRI, such as postinjection abscesses (Figure 25.23). Gymnasts may experience significant forces through the muscles of the upper extremities. Tears of the triceps (Figure 25.24) or other upper extremity muscles may, if not aggressively treated with rest, result in chronic symptoms that can lead to the clinical suspicion of malignancy. MRI is often able to confirm the benign condition.

In severe injuries for which surgery is being considered, MRI may be useful to plan the approach and decrease the amount of operative exploration required. For example, preoperative information was accurate and helpful in a high-grade partial tear of the pectoralis major in which the physical examination was limited by tenderness and a large hematoma at the site of rupture (Figure 25.25).[35]

Acute muscle injury may also be due to direct trauma that results in laceration or contusion, depending on whether the force is penetrating or blunt. Severe contusions usually result in extensive edema, interstitial hemorrhage, and swelling, which may result in compartment syndrome (see Chapter 28) (Figure 25.26).[13,25] Compartment syndromes occur when pressure increases within a confined fascial space and perfusion decreases below levels needed for tissue viability.[36] MRI may be useful in acute compartment syndromes to detect asso-

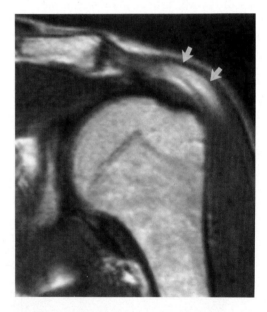

FIGURE 25.22. Deltoid strain in a professional baseball player with a suspected rotator cuff tear. T_2-weighted (1800/80) oblique coronal image reveals increased signal within the origin of the deltoid muscle in an outfielder with persistent shoulder pain in his throwing arm (arrows). A similar appearance could be seen following local injection with corticosteroids. No injections were administered in this case, however. The underlying rotator cuff appeared completely normal.

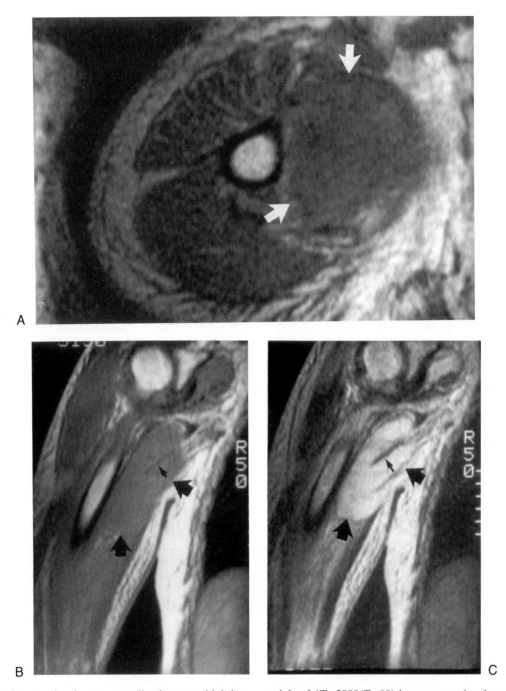

FIGURE 25.23. Iatrogenic abscess complicating steroid injections. This gentleman presented complaining of 18 months of right shoulder pain and 6 weeks of increasing pain, swelling, and redness in his medial proximal right arm. He had been given greater than 20 steroid injections during the past 18 months. (A) A T_1-weighted (T_R 500/T_E 20) axial image reveals a homogeneous mass medial to the proximal humerus (arrows). (B) The intermediately weighted (T_R 2000/T_E 20) and (C) T_2- weighted (T_R 2000/T_E 80) images reveal a sharply demarcated mass (large arrows) with uniform high signal on the T_2-weighted image, except for the brachial vessels (small arrows). Additional high resolution images of the shoulder revealed a rotator cuff tear as the etiology of the patient's symptoms. After the abscess was treated, the patient underwent a rotator cuff repair, instead of additional steroid injections!

ciated hematomas preoperatively or to evaluate the results of fasciotomy on muscle perfusion.[1] MRI may also be useful to assess chronic exercise-induced compartment syndromes.[37]

Deep lacerations may be evaluated with MRI for surgical planning or may be followed to assess for denervation within portions of the lacerated muscle (Figure 25.27).[8] The information provided by MRI may be com-

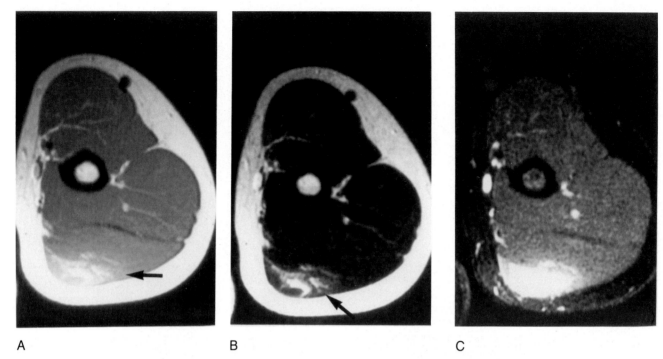

A   B   C

FIGURE 25.24. Triceps muscle tear. This gymnast suffered from chronic recurring triceps pain after exercise. Symptoms gradually increased over the course of a year with a palpable swelling in the region of the pain, arousing the suspicion of malignancy. (A) Intermediately weighted (T_R 2000/T_E 17) and (B) T_2-weighted (T_R 2000/T_E 80) axial images reveal increased signal in the triceps muscle (arrows). (C) Contrast is increased on the fast STIR images. The lack of a defined mass and the "interstitial pattern" of the increased signal confirms a muscle tear and not a neoplastic mass.

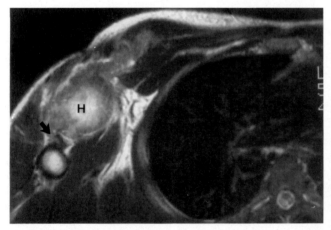

FIGURE 25.25. High grade partial tear of the right pectoralis major muscle in a professional rodeo cowboy following violent abduction of the arm. T_2-weighted fast spin echo (4000/102) axial image of the right anterior chest wall reveals a large hematoma (H) separating the muscular fibers of the pectoralis major from a remaining stump of tendon on the humerus (arrow). A high grade tear involving approximately 85% of the musculotendinous junction was found at surgery and repaired.

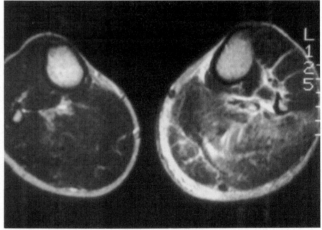

FIGURE 25.26. Compartment syndrome secondary to a contusion of the posterior calf in a football player. Axial T_2-weighted (2000/80) image reveals swelling of the left calf and increased signal throughout the muscles of the superficial and deep posterior compartments secondary to a direct blow. The anterior and lateral compartments show only mild perifascial edema.

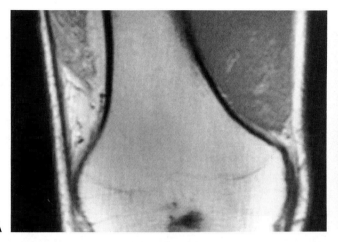

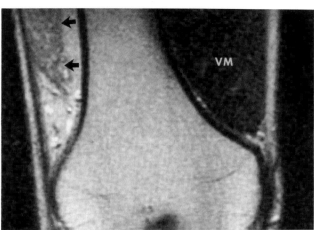

A   B

FIGURE 25.27. Denervation atrophy of the vastus lateralis secondary to a deep laceration of the thigh. (A) Proton density (2000/20) and (B) T_2-weighted (2000/80) coronal images of the distal thigh reveal fatty infiltration, decreased bulk, and increased signal intensity of the vastus lateralis muscle (arrows) relative to the normal vastus medialis (VM).

plementary to clinical and electrophysiologic data in complex cases (Figure 25.28).[20]

MRI may also be complementary to EMG and nerve conduction studies in cases of peripheral nerve entrapment.[38,39] In subacute denervation the affected muscles have prolongation of T_1 and T_2 relaxation times secondary to muscle fiber shrinkage and associated increases in extracellular water (Figure 25.29).[40] These changes may be followed to resolution or progressive atrophy and fatty infiltration (Figure 25.30).[20] The site and cause of entrapment may also be discovered with MRI by following the nerve implicated from the distri-

bution of abnormal muscles on MRI (Figure 25.31). Entrapment of the suprascapular nerve in the shoulder by ganglion cysts is currently being diagnosed with greater frequency due to detection with MRI.[38,41] Ganglion cysts typically arise from the posterosuperior shoulder capsule in association with labral tears. Entrapment of the distal suprascapular nerve occurs in the spinoglenoid notch and results in isolated denervation of the infraspinatus muscle. Anterior extension of a ganglion along the proximal suprascapular nerve may result in denervation of the supraspinatus as well (Figure 25.30).

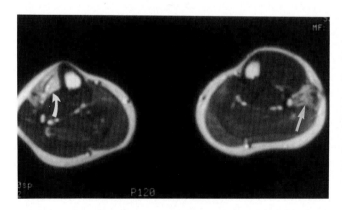

FIGURE 25.28. Denervation changes in both legs secondary to muscle lacerations in a child who fell through a plate glass window. Fast spin echo T_2-weighted (4300/102) axial image reveals increased signal in the anterior compartment of the right leg (curved arrow) and increased signal in the lateral compartment of the left leg (arrow) secondary to a laceration which interrupted the innervation to the more proximal muscle fibers in these compartments.

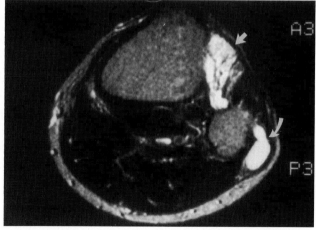

FIGURE 25.29. Entrapment of the deep peroneal nerve with denervation changes in the anterior compartment of the leg. T_2-weighted (2000/80) axial image in the proximal leg reveals edema-like changes in the anterior compartment (arrow). A ganglion cyst (curved arrow) was found compressing the deep peroneal nerve at surgery.

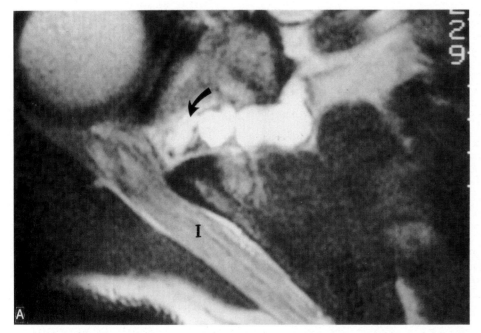

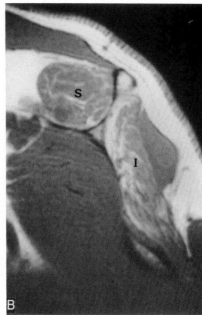

FIGURE 25.30. Suprascapular nerve entrapment resulting in chronic shoulder pain and atrophy of the supraspinatus and infraspinatus muscles. (A) T_2-weighted (2000/60) axial image reveals increased signal and decreased bulk of the left infraspinatus muscle (I). A ganglion cyst (curved arrow) was found arising from the posterosuperior joint capsule at surgery and extending anteriorly along the suprascapular nerve. (B) T_1-weighted (600/20) oblique sagittal image reveals fatty infiltration of the supraspinatus (S) and infraspinatus (I) secondary to suprascapular nerve entrapment.

Hypertrophy of the pyriformis muscle may occasionally result in extraspinal sciatica secondary to compression of the sciatic nerve at the greater sciatic notch.[42] Enlargement of the pyriformis muscle resulting in the "pyriformis syndrome" is well characterized with MRI (Figure 25.32).[43]

Compensatory hypertrophy due to denervation (Figure 25.31) or rupture (Figure 25.33) of an adjacent muscle can be identified with MRI. Such compensatory hypertrophy of a muscle can occasionally present as an enlarging soft tissue mass, which may mimic a neoplasm (Figure 25.33).[8] Finally, MRI may be useful to assess the degree and distribution of deep muscle atrophy in complex cases (Figure 25.34). Clinical findings and EMG data may underestimate the extent of muscle injury.[20]

Infections

Infections of the muscle are more completely discussed in Chapters 21 and 22. Muscle infections and neoplasms involving the muscles can appear similar to muscle injuries on MRI. Consequently, a short review of MRI of these conditions is included in this chapter.

Acute suppurative infections are usually bacterial in origin with *Staphylococcus aureus* and *Streptococcus* organisms being most common. Muscle infections are usually secondary to direct extension of infection from external wounds, but may also occur secondary to direct extension from adjacent structures, such as a bone in osteomyelitis, hematogenous spread, or iatrogenic complication (Figure 25.23). Acute infections are usually depicted on MRI as irregularly marginated edematous regions in the muscle with inhomogeneous low signal on T_1-weighted and high signal intensity on T_2-weighted and STIR images.[44-46] Close correlation of MRI findings with patient history and clinical signs and symptoms is often necessary to obtain an accurate diagnosis. Abscesses present as sharply marginated, mostly homogeneous, regions of similar signal intensity (Figure 25.23).

Chronic infections may present differently depending upon the organism. Tuberculosis often presents with prominent abscess, especially around the spine.[47,48] Chronic fungal disease or infections due to actinomycoses may present as masses without prominent high signal intensity on T_2-weighted images.[49] Because chronic infections typically are sharply defined lesions, they less frequently mimic acute muscle injuries than acute suppurative muscle infections. These lesions, however, may be difficult to distinguish from other masses within the musculoskeletal system.

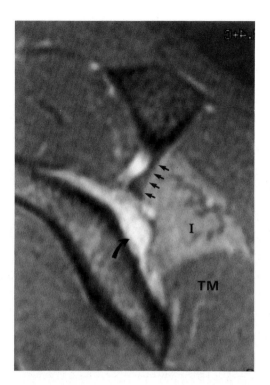

FIGURE 25.31. Entrapment of the distal suprascapular nerve secondary to a thickened inferior transverse scapular ligament in a collegiate volleyball player. T_1-weighted (800/20) oblique sagittal image of the shoulder with fat suppression following IV administration of gadolinium reveals prestenotic dilatation of enhancing veins (curved arrow) secondary to a thickened inferior transverse scapular ligament (small arrows). Mild enhancement of the infraspinatus muscle (I) is noted secondary to denervation. There is compensatory hypertrophy of the teres minor (TM) muscle. EMG and nerve conduction velocities were also compatible with distal suprascapular nerve entrapment.

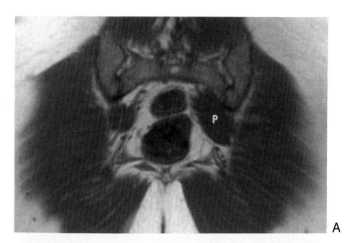

A

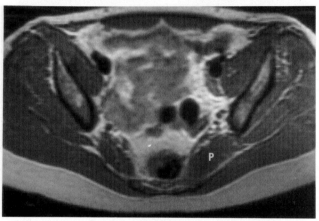

B

FIGURE 25.32. Piriformis syndrome in a 25-year-old woman with left sciatica and normal MRI of the lumbar spine. (A) T_1-weighted (800/20) coronal and (B) proton density (2000/20) axial images of the pelvis reveal hypertrophy of the left piriformis muscle (P), which decreased the volume of the greater sciatic notch and caused entrapment of the exiting left sciatic nerve.

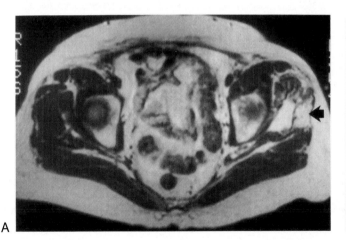

A

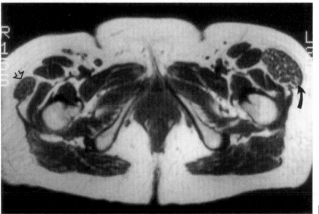

B

FIGURE 25.33. A 65-year-old woman with left hip pain and a palpable anterior thigh mass. MRI was obtained to exclude a soft tissue sarcoma. T_1-weighted (800/20) axial images (A) at the level of the acetabulum reveal fatty replacement of the gluteus minimus and medius muscles secondary to an old tear (arrow). A distal T_1-weighted axial image (B) reveals compensatory hypertrophy of the left tensor fascia lata muscle (curved arrow) accounting for the patient's palpable left thigh mass. The hypertrophied left muscle is several times the size of the right tensor fascia lata muscle (open arrow).

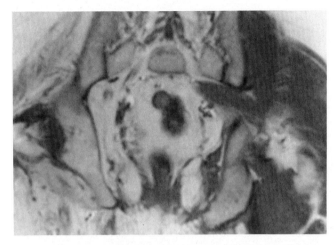

FIGURE 25.34. Disuse atrophy of the right-sided pelvic muscles in a 40-year-old man secondary to long-standing ankylosis of the right hip from remote trauma. A T_1-weighted (800/15) coronal image of the pelvis reveals severe fatty replacement of the muscles about the right hip. This information was useful in deciding against a total hip arthroplasty due to the lack of muscular support for the right hip.

Neoplastic Disease

MRI can differentiate between most benign and malignant masses within the musculoskeletal system.[50] Muscle malignancies are more completely discussed in Chapter 31. Most benign masses are relatively uniform in signal intensity with sharp, well-defined margins. The more common benign lesions include cysts, neural tumors, joint effusions, bursal fluid collections, and traumatic muscle tears. Most malignant masses have variable internal signal intensity and irregular margins.[50] MRI is usually excellent in differentiating between common cystic lesions and solid neoplasms, though occasionally gadolinium may be helpful in distinguishing between joint effusions and synovitis, and between ganglion cysts and neurofibromas as each of these may be uniformly bright on T_2-weighted images.[5-7] MRI, however, is not reliable in differentiating benign from malignant solid soft tissue masses.[51-57]

Muscle tears may present similarly to malignant masses if they present with central hemorrhage (Figure 25.35).

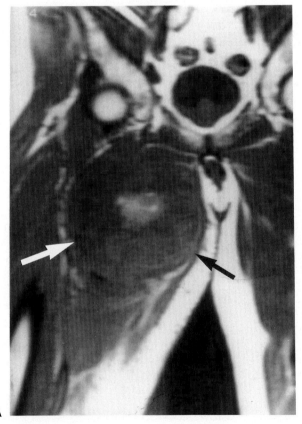

A

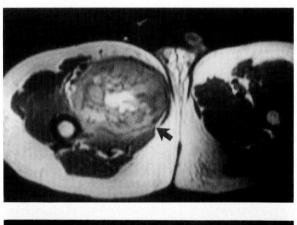

B

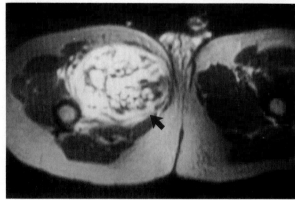

C

FIGURE 25.35. Adductor muscle tear. This middle-aged male developed acute onset on groin pain while reaching for a backhand on the tennis court. (A) Coronal T_1-weighted (T_R 500/T_E 20) image reveals a large groin mass (arrows) with central high signal intensity consistent with hemorrhage. (B) Intermediately weighted (T_R 2000/T_E 20) and (C) T_2-weighted (T_R 2000/T_E 80) images reveal a mass with indistinct posterior margins and marked internal signal inhomogeneity, characteristically associated with malignancy (arrows).[50] This patient did well with conservative treatment.

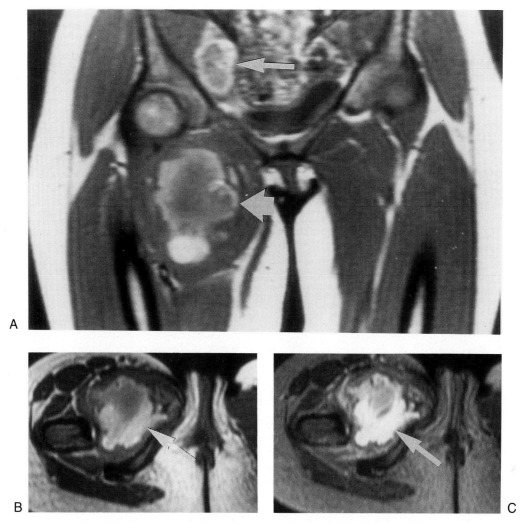

FIGURE 25.36. Synovial sarcoma. This patient presented with a rapidly increasing mass and right hip and groin pain. (A) T_1-weighted (T_R 500/T_E 20) image shows high signal intensity masses proximal (arrows) and distal (fat arrow) to the right hip. These signal changes are characteristic of tissue hematomas. (B) Axial intermediately weighted (T_R 2000/T_E 20) and (C) T_2-weighted (T_R 2000/T_E 80) images reveal irregularly marginated masses with inhomogeneous high signal intensity (arrows). Synovial sarcomas, such as shown here, frequently present as hemorrhagic masses on either side of a major joint and can be misinterpreted as benign hematomas if the irregularity and typical locations are not noted.[50]

Rarely, muscle tears may occur from weakening of the muscle from other muscle pathology, such as malignancy. In older patients with muscle tears and history of only minor trauma, it may be prudent to follow the muscle injury to complete resolution as the underlying neoplasm may be obscured by hemorrhage and edema on the initial MRI scan.[2] Synovial sarcomas characteristically present with MRI findings that can masquerade as benign hematoma or muscle tear on MRI.[50] Synovial sarcomas are often hemorrhagic masses on either side, or at the margins, of major joints (Figure 25.36). By recognizing both the signal characteristics and locations, synovial sarcoma can usually be differentiated from muscle trauma.

Future Application of MRI in Orthopaedics

Currently, the number of MRI systems worldwide continues to grow. Competition and increased supply are contributing to price reduction for MRI in the United States. Newer pulse sequences and hardware modifications are resulting in improved images that require shorter acquisition times. All of these factors will likely result in faster examinations at decreased cost in the near future. More economic MRI coupled with further improvements in technology should lead to increased utilization for orthopaedic applications. Follow-up MRI evaluation of muscle injuries should become more practical and cost-effective. MRI of muscle injuries will likely be used in a manner analogous to current x-ray imaging of fractures in which serial assessment clearly provides additional information regarding the adequacy of therapy and healing. The additional diagnostic precision provided by MRI should result in more efficacious therapy and improved outcome.

References

1. Fleckenstein JL, Shellock FG. Exertional muscle injuries: magnetic resonance imaging evaluation. Top Magn Reson Imaging 1991;3:50–70.
2. Fleckenstein JL, Weatherall PT, Bertocci LA, et al. Locomotor system assessment by muscle magnetic resonance imaging. Magn Reson Q 1991;7(2):79–103.
3. Greco A, McNamara MT, Escher MB, Trifilio G, Parienti J. Spin-echo and STIR MRI of sports-related muscle injuries at 1.5T. J Comput Assist Tomogr 1991;15:994–999.
4. Fleckenstein JL, Archer B, Barker B, Vaugh T, Parkey RW, Peshock RM. Fast, short tau inversion recovery imaging. Radiology 1991;179:499–504.
5. Pettersson H, Ackerman N, Kaude J, et al. Gadolinium-DTPA enhancement of experimental soft tissue carcinoma and hemorrhage in magnetic resonance imaging. Acta Radiol 1987;28:75–78.
6. Pettersson H, Eliasson J, Egund N, et al. Gadolinium-DTPA enhancement of soft tissue tumors in magnetic resonance imaging—preliminary clinical experience in five patients. Skeletal Radiol 1988;17:319–323.
7. Reiser MF, Naegele M. Inflammatory joint disease: static and dynamic gadolinium-enhanced MRI. J Magn Reson Imaging 1993;3(1):307–310.
8. DeSmet AA, Fisher DR, Heiner JP, Keene JS. Magnetic resonance imaging of muscle tears. Skeletal Radiol 1990; 19:283–286.
9. Garrett WEJ. Injuries to the muscle-tendon unit. Instr Course Lect 1988;37:275–282.
10. Noonan TJ, Garrett WEJ. Injuries of the myotendinous junction. Clin Sports Med 1992;11:783–806.
11. Speer KP, Lohnes J, Garrett WEJ. Radiographic imaging of muscle strain injury. Am J Sports Med 1993;21:89–96.
12. Fleckenstein JL, Weatherall PT, Parkey RW, Payne JA, Peshock RM. Sports related muscle injuries: evaluation with MRI. Radiology 1989;172:793–798.
13. Deutsch AL, Mink JH. Magnetic resonance imaging of musculoskeletal injuries. Radiol Clin North Am 1989; 27:983–1002.
14. Ehman RL, Berquist TH. Magnetic resonance imaging of musculoskeletal trauma. Radiol Clin North Am 1986; 24:291–319.
15. Crues JV, Ryu R. The shoulder. In: Stark D, Bradley WG, editors. Magnetic resonance imaging. St. Louis: Mosby, In press.
16. Crues JV, Fareed DO. Magnetic resonance imaging of shoulder impingement. Top Magn Reson Imaging 1991; 3(4):39–49.
17. Jaramillo D, Hoffer FA, Shapiro F, Rand F. MRI of fractures of the growth plate. AJR 1990;155:1261–1265.
18. Jaramillo D, Shapiro F, Hoffer FA, et al. Post-traumatic growth-plate abnormalities: MRI of bony-bridge formation in rabbits. Radiology 1990;175:767–773.
19. Jaramillo D, Hoffer FA. Cartilaginous epiphysis and growth plate: normal and abnormal MRI findings. AJR 1992;158:1105–1110.
20. Fleckenstein JL, Watumull D, Conner KE, Ezaki M, Purdy PD. Denervated human skeletal muscle: MRI evaluation. Radiology 1993;187:213–218.
21. Severance HWJ, Bassett FHI. Rupture of the plantaris—does it exist? J Bone Joint Surg 1982;64A:1387–1388.
22. Allard JC, Bancroft J, Porter G. Imaging of plantaris muscle rupture. Clin Imaging 1992;16:55–58.
23. Menz MJ, Lucas GL. Magnetic resonance imaging af a rupture of the medial head of the gastrocnemius muscle. J Bone Joint Surg 1991;73A:1260–1262.
24. Zeiss J, Ebraheim NA, Woldenberg LS. Magnetic resonance imaging in the diagnosis of anterior tibialis muscle herniation. Clin Orthop 1989;244:249–253.
25. Whitehouse GH. Magnetic resonance imaging in the diagnosis of muscle and tendon injuries. Imaging 1992;4:95–105.
26. Lewin G. The incidence of injury in an English professional soccer club during one competitive season. Physiotherapy 1989;75:601–605.
27. Muckle DS. Injuries in professional football. Br J Sports Med 1981;15:77–79.
28. Dooms GC, Fischer MF, Hricak H, Higgins CB. MRI of intramuscular hemorrhage. J Comput Assist Tomogr 1985;9:908–913.
29. Kumar R, Matasar K, Stansberry S, et al. The calcaneus: normal and abnormal. RadioGraphics 1991;11(3):415–440.
30. Berkowitz JF, Kier R, Rudicel S. Plantar fasciitis: MRI. Radiology 1991;179(3):665–667.
31. Shellock FG, Fukunaga T, Mink JH, Edgerton VR. Exertional muscle injury: evaluation of concentric versus eccentric actions with serial MRI. Radiology 1991;179:659–664.
32. Taylor DC, Dalton JD, Seaber AV, Garrett WE Jr. Experimental muscle strain injury. Early functional and structural deficits and the increased risk for reinjury. Am J Sports Med 1993;21(2):190–194.
33. Huber DS, Sumers E, Klein M. Soft tissue pseudotumor following intramuscular injection of "DPT": a pitfall in magnetic resonance imaging. Skeletal Radiol 1987;16:469–473.
34. Resendes M, Helms CA, Fritz RC, Genant HK. MR appearance of intramuscular injections. AJR 1992;158:1293–1294.
35. Liu J, Wu J, Chang C, Chou Y, Lo W. Avulsion of the pectoralis major tendon. Am J Sports Med 1992;20:366–368.
36. Murbarak SJ, Hargens AR. Acute compartment syndromes. Surg Clin North Am 1983;63:539–552.
37. Amendola A, Rorabeck CH, Vellet D, Vezina W, Rutt B, Nott L. The use of magnetic resonance imaging in exertional compartment syndromes. Am J Sports Med 1990;18:29–34.

38. Fritz RC, Helms CA, Steinbach LS, Genant HK. Suprascapular nerve entrapment: Evaluation with MRI. Radiology 1992;182(2):437–444.
39. Shabas D, Gerard G, Rossi D. Magnetic resonance imaging of denervated muscle. Comput Radiol 1987;11:9–13.
40. Polak JF, Jolesz FA, Adams DF. Magnetic resonance imaging examination of skeletal muscle prolongation of T1 and T2 subsequent to denervation. Invest Radiol 1988;23:365–369.
41. Zeiss J, Woldenberg LS, Saddemi SR, Ebraheim NA. MRI of suprascapular neuropathy in a weight lifter. J Comput Assist Tomogr 1993;17(2):303–308.
42. Vandertop WP, Bosma NJ. The piriformis syndrome. J Bone Joint Surg 1991;73A:1095–1097.
43. Jankiewicz JJ, Hennrikus WL, Houkom JA. The appearance of the piriformis muscle syndrome in computed tomography and magnetic resonance imaging. Clin Orthop 1991;262:205–209.
44. Fleckenstein JL, Burns DK, Murphy FK, Jayson HT, Bonte FJ. Differential diagnosis of bacterial myositis in AIDS: evaluation with MRI. Radiology 1991;179(3):653–658.
45. Kransdorf MJ, Meis JM, Jelinek JS. Myositis ossificans: MRI appearance with radiologic-pathologic correlation. AJR 1991;157:1243–1248.
46. Hernandez RJ, Keim DR, Chenevert TL, Sullivan DB, Aisen AM. Fat-suppressed MRI of myositis. Radiology 1992;182(1):217–219.
47. Sharif HS, Clark DC, Aabed MY, et al. Granulomatous spinal infections: MRI. Radiology 1990;177(1):101–107.
48. Sharif HS. Role of MRI in the management of spinal infections. AJR 1992;158:1333–1345.
49. Sharif H, Clark DC, Aabed MY, et al. Mycetoma: comparison of MRI with CT. Radiology 1991;178:865–870.
50. Berquist TH, Ehman RL, King BF, Hodgman CG, Ilstrup DM. Value of MRI in differentiating benign from malignant soft-tissue masses: study of 95 lesions. AJR 1990;155:1251–1255.
51. Wetzel LH, Levine E. Soft-tissue tumors of the foot: value of MRI for specific diagnosis. AJR 1990;155:1025–1030.
52. Binkovitz LA, Berquist TH, McLeod RA. Masses of the hand and wrist: detection and characterization with MRI. AJR 1990;154:323–326.
53. Morton MJ, Berquist TH, McLeod RA, Unni KK, Sim FH. Pictorial essay. MRI of synovial sarcoma. AJR 1991;156:337–340.
54. Hanna SL, Fletcher BD, Parham DM, Bugg MF. Muscle edema in musculoskeletal tumors: MRI characteristics and clinical significance. J Magn Reson Imaging 1991;1(4):441–449.
55. Murphy WD, Hurst GC, Duerk JL, Feiglin DH, Christopher M, Bellon EM. Atypical appearance of lipomatous tumors on MRI: high signal intensity with fat-suppression STIR sequences. J Magn Reson Imaging 1991;1(4):477–480.
56. Biondetti PR, Ehman RL. Soft-tissue sarcomas: use of textural patterns in skeletal muscle as a diagnostic feature in postoperative MRI. Radiology 1992;183:845–848.
57. Crim JR, Seeger LL, Yao L, Chandnani V, Eckardt JJ. Diagnosis of soft-tissue masses with MRI: can benign masses be differentiated from malignant ones? Radiology 1992;185:581–586.

26
Rhabdomyolysis

Antti Lamminen

Rhabdomyolysis, or myonecrosis, is a condition characterized by diffuse injury and destruction of skeletal muscle fibers. When muscle cells are disrupted, the sarcoplasmic contents, including myoglobin, are released into the extracellular fluid and plasma. This leads to myoglobinemia, which often results in myoglobinuria.[1] The histopathological features in muscle tissue include myocyte swelling, hyaline degeneration, and varying degrees of degeneration and regeneration of the muscle fibers.[2] Rhabdomyolysis can be focal, often involving the deep musculature and sparing the superficial muscles,[3] or it can be diffusely distributed.[4] Especially in dehydrated subjects, marked rhabdomyolysis with myoglobinuria may lead to acute renal failure, often requiring temporary dialysis treatment. Renal damage may be prevented by adequate hydration of the patient and by alkalinization of the patient's urine, but, particularly in cases of delayed diagnosis, the syndrome may have a fatal outcome. In clinical practice, the most important manifestation of rhabdomyolysis is myoglobinuria, producing reddish-brown discoloration of urine. A markedly elevated level of serum creatine kinase is the most prominent laboratory finding; others include hyperkalemia, metabolic acidosis, and hypocalcemia.[1]

Mechanisms of Myonecrosis

The clinical syndrome of rhabdomyolysis was first described among trauma casualties during the second world war.[5] Because the first clinical reports described patients with muscle injuries due to massive extrinsic trauma and compression, rhabdomyolysis was long known as the crush syndrome. At the present day, other etiological factors are more important.[1,6,7] These factors may be either idiopathic or extrinsic, including drug or alcohol abuse, prolonged muscular compression, ischemic muscle injury, excessive muscular activity, and various metabolic disorders (Table 26.1). In many studies, alcoholism has been found as the most common etiology, but multiple factors are usually involved in the majority of individual cases.[1,7] Rhabdomyolysis and acute renal failure have also been described in chronic alcoholics without acute alcohol ingestion and coma,[8] and ethanol itself appears to be a direct toxin.[9] Intravenous heroin and certain pharmaceuticals may also have a directly toxic effect on muscle tissue.[10,11] In cases of acute overdose, however, the pathogenesis often appears to be mechanical: the patient lies comatose on a hard surface, and the weight of the body on a limb produces a markedly elevated pressure in muscle compartments, sufficient to cause muscle ischemia and necrosis by local obstruction to the circulation.[12] The muscles become edematous, further raising intracompartmental pressure. Thus, a vicious cycle of increasing pressure and ischemia is established. The peculiar susceptibility of deep-lying muscles, with a tendency to sparing of the superficial musculature, is a recognized phenomenon.[3] This may imply that the biomechanical pressure gradients are different in the deeper parts of the extremities, or that some other selective susceptibility factors are involved.

Local symptoms and signs in the musculature may be absent;[1] often, however, the acute muscle compartment syndrome described above may lead to irreversible muscle necrosis and peripheral nerve injury. Percutaneous measurement of intracompartmental pressure is a valuable aid in the clinical evaluation of these patients. If the pressure exceeds 40 mm Hg, fasciotomy is usually recommended within 8 h.[13] This is considered necessary not only to prevent further damage to the limb,[14] but also to reduce the systemic effects of myonecrosis.[12,15]

Exact identification and delineation of damaged muscle tissue is important to avoid extensive fasciotomies with the risk of secondary wound infection.[15] Also, because local symptoms and signs in the musculature may sometimes be minor and misleading,[6] the monitoring of appropriate muscle compartments by unguided pressure measurements may prove difficult. Noninvasive methods

TABLE 26.1. Causes of rhabdomyolysis.

Direct muscle injury
  Trauma (Crush syndrome)
  Burns
  Electric shock
Ischemia
  Arterial occlusion
  External compression
  Cardiopulmonary bypass surgery
Excessive muscular activity
  Muscular exercise
  Status epilepticus
  Status asthmaticus
Myositis
  Polymyositis and dermatomyositis
  Viral and bacterial infections
Drugs and toxins
  Ethanol
  Heroin
  Cocaine
  Lovastatin
  Sedatives
  Salicylates
  Carbon monoxide
Metabolic disorders
  Hypokalemia
  Hypophosphatemia
  Diabetic ketoacidosis
  Metabolic myopathies

for the localization of affected muscles are thus needed.

Radiologic imaging methods, especially the cross-sectional imaging techniques, offer significant advantages for mapping involved muscles and muscle compartments in patients with clinical rhabdomyolysis, but their clinical use has been sporadic, and very few comparative imaging studies have been published.

Nuclear Scintigraphy

As technetium-99m phosphorus compounds were introduced for bone imaging in the early 1970s, it was soon recognized that these radiopharmaceutical agents would also accumulate in tissues other than bone (see Chapter 1). A number of studies have described their use for the evaluation of muscle injury in several disease states. Most reports deal with clearly traumatic conditions or with rhabdomyolysis and muscle necrosis due to either traumatic or nontraumatic causes.[4,16,17] Although the mechanisms underlying the uptake of technetium-99m phosphates in injured muscle tissue have not been thoroughly clarified, experimental and clinical evidence suggests that adsorption onto soft tissue calcium is the most likely alternative.[18] This hypothesis is supported by the frequent clinical observation of profound hypocalcemia in the early stages of rhabdomyolysis, which is explained by precipitation of calcium into the damaged muscle.[19]

In particular, technetium-99m pyrophosphate appears promising for the localization of muscle injury. However, problems have been encountered with nonspecificity of the tracer uptake; technetium-99m pyrophosphate will localize in muscle also after strenuous muscular excercise, and diffuse muscle uptake has been found without overt evidence of muscle injury.[16] Because nuclear scintigraphy is usually performed without cross-sectional tomographic imaging and because of the limited spatial resolution of whole-body gamma cameras, accurate delineation of the injured tissue has also been problematic.[17] Confident discrimination between injured and unaffected muscle compartments in the extremities is difficult with scintigraphy.

Ultrasonography

Modern high-frequency ultrasound (US) transducers give good spatial and contrast resolution in the superficial soft tissues, thus affording adequate possibilities for noninvasive tissue characterization. However, the interpretation of real-time US studies is operator dependent, and the identification of individual muscles and muscle compartments may present difficulties. The use of an echo-free standoff pad is strongly recommended in high-frequency US studies for the reduction of near-field reverberation artifacts.

Studies on US imaging of muscles in patients with rhabdomyolysis have mostly been published as case reports.[3,20-22] The largest collection of cases comprised five patients with rhabdomyolysis.[3] In the first documentation of acute rhabdomyolysis by US, the finding was reported as an area of decreased echogenicity and this appearance was mostly attributed to inflammation and fluid within and surrounding necrotic muscle.[20] Later reports described findings with more mixed echogenicity: predominantly hypoechoic areas interspersed with inhomogeneous regions of increased echogenicity.[3,22] Differential diagnosis in regard to nonspecific muscle edema is mostly based on the disruption of muscular architecture seen in rhabdomyolysis. Intramuscular hematomas may be indistinguishable from myonecrosis, and these two conditions may coexist.[21] Clinically, rhabdomyolysis in an extremity may be confused with deep vein thrombosis; these two entities are usually quite confidently differentiated by US.

A prospective, comparative study performed in our institution[23] with 12 cases of clinical, acute rhabdomyolysis studied by US showed abnormal changes in muscle structure and echogenicity in five patients; these findings consisted of foci of decreased echogenicity in muscles and a locally disorganized fascicular architecture

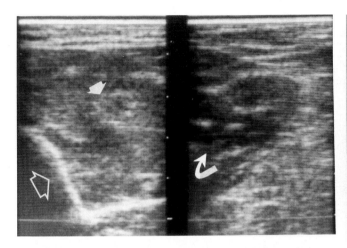

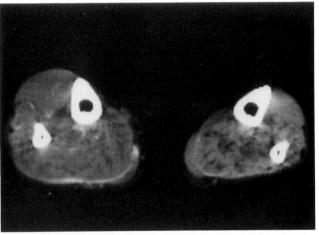

FIGURE 26.1. Ultrasound findings in rhabdomyolysis: two views of the adductor muscles of the right thigh in a 36-year-old male patient with rhabdomyolysis due to drug overdose. The fascicular architecture is disturbed, and both hypoechoic areas (curved arrow) and regions of increased echogenicity (filled arrowhead) are seen. The femoral bone shadow is marked with an open arrowhead.

FIGURE 26.2. CT of legs in a 28-year-old man with bilateral leg edema after severe alcohol intoxication. Myonecrosis is seen in both calves and in the right anterior and peroneal muscle compartments as diffuse and patchy hypodense regions. Widespread muscle necrosis was found at surgery in the corresponding compartments.

(Figure 26.1); in two patients, regions of increased muscle echogenicity were also found. Compared with magnetic resonance imaging and computed tomography, US was the least sensitive modality in the evaluation of muscle necrosis. Problems were encountered especially in recognizing compartmental boundaries, and thus the identification of individual muscle compartment was not accurate enough for planning fasciotomy.

Computed Tomography

Computed tomography (CT) has been more extensively utilized for the evaluation of rhabdomyolysis than US.[3,24–29] The major CT features of acute myonecrosis include diffuse regions of low attenuation in muscle and muscular swelling corresponding to muscle edema, and more sharply defined intramuscular hypodense foci corresponding to areas of necrotic muscle (Figure 26.2). Abnormal patchy hyperdensity consistent with muscle calcification has also been described; this finding correlated with antecedent hypocalcemia and with renal insufficiency,[28] and seemed to develop during the subacute stage of rhabdomyolysis.[27] Muscle calcification in association with acute renal failure has been described as characteristic of nontraumatic rhabdomyolysis.[30] Fatty degeneration in necrotic muscle has also been described by CT.[31]

Differential diagnosis of the CT findings includes deep venous thrombosis, which usually shows a pattern of diffuse swelling of all tissue layers and less pronounced muscular hypodensity.[3] The initially hyperdense intramuscular hematomas may become hypodense with resolution, and may be mistaken for foci of rhabdomyolysis.

In some CT studies,[3,24,29] intravenous contrast medium has been administered; this was reported to provide better demarcation of lesions and to confirm the avascularity of the necrotic areas. However, other reports strongly suggest that the use of intravenous contrast media should be avoided in patients with rhabdomyolysis, in order to avoid aggravating the renal failure that often is part of the clinical picture.[32,33]

In our prospective series,[23] noncontrast CT was performed on 13 patients with acute rhabdomyolysis. In eight patients, abnormal muscle findings were seen, consisting of hypodense intramuscular foci, muscle swelling, and fascial thickening due to edema. These lesions were not as conspicious as they were in the corresponding magnetic resonance images, and especially in the thighs, the evaluation of muscle hypodensity in CT images was sometimes complicated by beam-hardening artifacts from the dense femoral cortex (Figure 26.3A).

Magnetic Resonance Imaging

Clinical rhabdomyolysis was first studied with magnetic resonance (MRI) by Zagoria et al.,[34] who described two patients in whom the signal intensities of muscles in T_2-weighted spin echo (SE) images were clearly increased; differentiation of damaged muscle from surrounding fat was somewhat difficult due to the relatively high fat signal at the low field strength (0.15 T) used in the study.

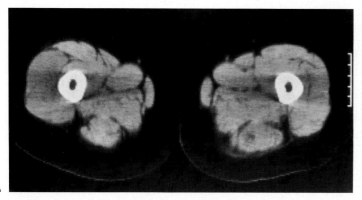
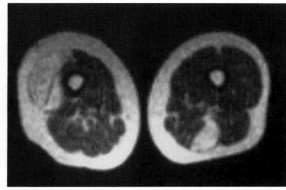

A B

FIGURE 26.3. Corresponding CT (A) and T_2-weighted MRI (B) images of thighs of a 52-year-old female with biopsy-proven focal rhabdomyolysis due to ergotamine overdose. Selective involvement of the right vastus lateralis and the left semitendinosus muscles is seen with MRI, whereas the CT findings are inconspicuous and the image is hampered by artifact from the femoral cortex. (From Lamminen AE, Hekali PE, Tiula E, et al. Acute rhabdomyolysis: evaluation with MRI compared with CT and US. Br J Radiol 1989;62:326–331.)

With T_1-weighted inversion recovery (IR) imaging, the corresponding muscles had decreased signal intensity, and better demarcation of affected muscles from fat was seen. In one case, MRI provided greater detail of the damaged muscles than did technetium-99m pyrophosphate scanning. The signal changes were assumed to be due to tissue inflammation and edema. In both cases, however, MRI was done 3 to 4 days after surgical intervention to the affected muscle compartments.

In an experimental model of acute muscle necrosis performed with MRI at 0.35 T, infarcted muscles of rats had significantly longer T_1 and T_2 values at 24 h after vascular occlusion than intact muscles. The muscle signals were clearly increased in T_2-weighted images. These changes corresponded to a significant increase in the water content of the infarcted muscles.[35] In clinical rhabdomyolysis and muscle compartment syndrome, the pathophysiological phenomena also include muscle necrosis, increased intramuscular water content, and tissue edema.[12,13] Thus, the majority of MRI signal intensity changes may be attributed to these features. The signal contribution of intrinsic macromolecular changes in damaged muscle is difficult to evaluate.

Changes of similar type have been described in patients with glycolytic myopathies, who have a tendency to recurrent idiopathic rhabdomyolysis.[36] Focal areas of prolonged T_1 and T_2 appeared in the forearm muscles after muscular exertion lead to contractures. These changes did not represent fully developed myonecrosis, as complete recovery was the rule. Apparently, the MRI signal changes seen in muscle injury are unspecific, representing a continuum between mild postexertional muscle abnormalities and definite rhabdomyolysis. This was also found in normal volunteers, when delayed effects of strenuous exercise on MRI signal were evaluated and correlated with serum creatine kinase values.[37,38] A

recent study utilized MRI-guided muscle biopsy to correlate muscle signal intensity changes with ultrastructural muscle fiber abnormalities after muscular exercise.[39] A high correlation was found between the degree of MRI signal intensity increase 48 h after exercise and the degree of ultrastructural muscle fiber injury.

In a prospective study to compare different cross-sectional imaging modalities in the evaluation of acute rhabdomyolysis, we performed MRI in 15 patients. Comparative studies were done with CT in 13 patients and with US in 12 patients.[23] Surgical confirmation was available in nine cases. In addition to standard T_2-weighted sequences, we utilized short TI inversion recovery (STIR) sequences, which displayed good contrast between normal and abnormal muscles and also better differentiation of the damaged muscle from adjacent fat, due to suppression of the fat signal. MRI detected abnormal muscles in all of the 15 patients (100%) with an established clinical diagnosis of rhabdomyolysis, whereas CT demonstrated abnormal muscles in 8 of the 13 patients studied (62%), and US in 5 of 12 (42%). Thus, when compared to US and CT, MRI was the best technique for visualizing affected muscles and muscle compartments (Figure 26.3). In most cases, fasciotomy or muscle biopsy confirmed that increased signal intensity represented necrotic and/or edematous muscle tissue.

The distribution and magnitude of pathological muscle signals in rhabdomyolysis varies from a slight and diffuse increase in signal intensity to very intense, clearly demarcated focal lesions (Figures 26.4, 26.5). These areas of high signal intensity reflect increased water content and increased mobility of water molecules due to an inflammatory reaction in the injured and necrotic muscles. In the extremities, deep muscles like the soleus are often affected, whereas superficial muscles of the

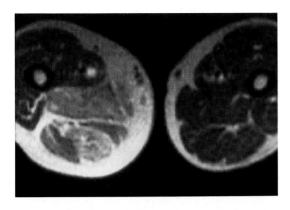

FIGURE 26.4. Diffuse abnormal signal intensity of the adductor and semitendinosus muscles in a 39-year-old male with acute rhabdomyolysis due to an overdose of sedatives and alcohol. T_2-weighted low-field (0.02 T) MR image of thighs.

same region, like the gastrocnemius, may be spared (Figure 26.5). In the acute stage, abnormal signal intensity is usually associated with an increase in the cross-sectional diameter of the affected muscle or muscle compartment. In follow-up examinations, a decrease in pathological signals coincides with clinical improvement and a decrease in serum creatine kinase values, but the signal abnormalities may persist longer than the creatine kinase elevations.[38] Also, the diameter of the affected

limb returns towards normal. The most frequent complication of fasciotomy is wound infection, which may spread deep into the necrotic muscle tissue of the extremities. In these cases, follow-up MRI reveals increasing and more widespread areas of abnormal signal intensity.

Conclusion

In patients with a clinical diagnosis of rhabdomyolysis, MRI is the method of choice to effectively evaluate the distribution of the muscle lesions. The imaging findings are nonspecific, but considered alongside the clinical and laboratory data, they confirm the diagnosis. The precise identification of affected muscles and muscle compartments is especially valuable when fasciotomy is considered for treatment. The operation can be applied to the compartments with clearly abnormal muscles, thus facilitating relief of edema and pressure-related ischemia in the appropriate areas. Extensive fasciotomies with an increased risk of secondary wound infection can be avoided.

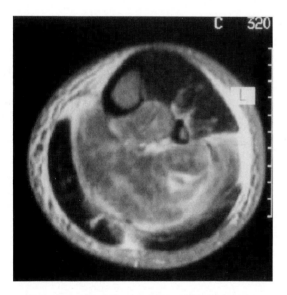

FIGURE 26.5. T_2-weighted high-field MRI of right leg in a 25-year-old male with rhabdomyolysis. Clearly abnormal signal intensity is seen in the deep muscles. The soleus and tibialis posterior muscles were confirmed to be edematous and partly necrotic at surgery. The superficially situated gastrocnemius was only mildly edematous. The anterior and peroneal muscle compartments were unaffected.

References

1. Gabow PA, Kaehny WD, Kelleher SP. The spectrum of rhabdomyolysis. Medicine 1982;61:141–152.
2. Armbrustmacher VW. Skeletal muscle. In: Rubin E, Farber JL, eds. Pathology. Philadephia: J.B. Lippincott, 1988:1394–1415.
3. Vukanovic S, Hauser H, Curati WL. Myonecrosis induced by drug overdose: pathogenesis, clinical aspects and radiological manifestations. Eur J Radiol 1983;3:314–318.
4. Haseman MK, Kriss JP. Selective, symmetric, skeletal muscle uptake of Tc-99m pyrophosphate in rhabdomyolysis. Clin Nucl Med 1985;10:180–183.
5. Bywaters EGL, Beall D. Crush injuries with impairment of renal function. Br Med J 1941;i:427–432.
6. Grossman RA, Hamilton RW, Morse BM, et al. Nontraumatic rhabdomyolysis and acute renal failure. N Engl J Med 1974;291:807–811.
7. Haapanen E, Pellinen TJ, Partanen J. Acute renal failure caused by alcohol-induced rhabdomyolysis. Nephron 1984; 36:191–193.
8. Saltissi D, Parfrey PS, Curtis JR, et al. Rhabdomyolysis and acute renal failure in chronic alcoholics with myopathy, unrelated to acute alcohol ingestion. Clin Nephrol 1984; 21:294–300.
9. Song SK, Rubin E. Ethanol produces muscle damage in human volunteers. Science 1972;175:327–328.
10. deGans J, Stam J, van Wijngaarden GK. Rhabdomyolysis and concomitant neurological lesions after intravenous heroin abuse. J Neurol Neurosurg Psychiatry 1985;48: 1057–1059.
11. Pierce LR, Wysowski DK, Gross TP. Myopathy and rhabdomyolysis associated with lovastatin-gemfibrozil combination therapy. JAMA 1990;264:71–75.

12. Owen CA, Mubarak SJ, Hargens AR, et al. Intramuscular pressures with limb compression: clarification of the pathogenesis of the drug-induced muscle compartment syndrome. N Engl J Med 1979;300:1169–1172.

13. Rorabeck CH, Clarke KM. The pathophysiology of the anterior tibial compartment syndrome: an experimental investigation. J Trauma 1978;18:299–304.

14. Schreiber SN, Liebowitz MR, Bernstein LH. Limb compression and renal impairment (Crush syndrome) following narcotic and sedative overdose. J Bone Joint Surg 1972;54-A:1683–1692.

15. Better OS, Stein JH. Early management of shock and prophylaxis of acute renal failure in traumatic rhabdomyolysis. N Engl J Med 1990;322:825–829.

16. Patel R, Mishkin FS. Technetium-99m pyrophosphate imaging in acute renal failure associated with nontraumatic rhabdomyolysis. AJR 1986;147:815–817.

17. Timmons JH, Hartshorne MF, Peters VJ, et al. Muscle necrosis in the extremities: evaluation with Tc-99m pyrophosphate scanning—a retrospective review. Radiology 1988;167:173–178.

18. Buja LM, Tofe AJ, Kulkarni PV, et al. Sites and mechanisms of localization of technetium-99m phosphorus radiopharmaceuticals in acute myocardial infarcts and other tissues. J Clin Invest 1977;60:724–740.

19. Knochel JP. Calcium in acute renal failure. In: Brenner BM, Lazarus JM, eds. Acute renal failure. New York: Chuchill Livingstone, 1988:685–688.

20. Kaplan GN. Ultrasonic appearance of rhabdomyolysis. AJR 1980;134:375–377.

21. Auerbach DN, Bowen AD. Sonography of leg in posterior compartment syndrome. AJR 1981;136:407–408.

22. Fornage BD, Nerot C. Sonographic diagnosis of rhabdomyolysis. J Clin Ultrasound 1986;14:389–392.

23. Lamminen AE, Hekali PE, Tiula E, et al. Acute rhabdomyolysis: evaluation with magnetic resonance imaging compared with computed tomography and ultrasonography. Br J Radiol 1989;62:326–331.

24. Vukanovic S, Hauser H, Wettstein P. CT localization of myonecrosis for surgical decompression. AJR 1980;135:1298–1299.

25. Farmlett EJ, Fishman EK, Magid D, Siegelman S. Computed tomography in the assessment of myonecrosis. J Can Assoc Radiol 1987;38:278–282.

26. Barloon TJ, Zachar CK, Harkens KL, Honda H. Rhabdomyolysis: computed tomography findings. CT 1988;12:193–195.

27. Towers MJ, Downey DB, Poon PY. Psoas muscle calcification and acute renal failure associated with nontraumatic rhabdomyolysis: CT features. J Comput Assist Tomogr 1990;14:1027–1029.

28. Russ PD, Dillingham M. Demonstration of CT hyperdensity in patients with acute renal failure associated with rhabdomyolysis. J Comput Assist Tomogr 1991;15:458–463.

29. Rosenkranz K, Zwicker C, Langer R, et al. Rhabdomyolyse in der Computertomographie. Fortschr Röntgenstr 1992;156:601–603.

30. Clark JG, Sumerling MD. Muscle necrosis and calcification in acute renal failure due to barbiturate intoxication. Br Med J 1966;i:214–215.

31. von Rottkay P. CT signs of ischemic muscle necrosis. J Comput Assist Tomogr 1985;9:833–834.

32. Winearls CG, Ledingham JGG, Dixon AJ. Acute renal failure precipitated by radiographic contrast medium in a patient with rhabdomyolysis. Br Med J 1980;281:1603.

33. Mangano FA, Zaontz M, Pahira JJ, et al. Computed tomography of acute renal failure secondary to rhabdomyolysis. J Comput Assist Tomogr 1985;9:777–779.

34. Zagoria RJ, Karstaedt N, Koubek TD. MRI of rhabdomyolysis. J Comput Assist Tomogr 1986;10:268–270.

35. Herfkens RJ, Sievers R, Kaufman L, et al. Nuclear magnetic resonance imaging of the infarcted muscle: a rat model. Radiology 1983;147:761–764.

36. Fleckenstein JL, Peshock RM, Lewis SL, Haller RG. Magnetic resonance imaging of muscle injury and atrophy in glycolytic myopathies. Muscle Nerve 1989;12:849–855.

37. Fleckenstein JL, Canby RC, Parkey RW, Peshock RM. Acute effects of exercise on MRI of skeletal muscle in normal volunteers. AJR 1988;151:231–237.

38. Fleckenstein JL, Weatherall PT, Parkey RW, Payne JA, Peshock RM. Sports-related muscle injuries: evaluation with MRI. Radiology 1989;172:793–798.

39. Nurenberg P, Giddings CJ, Stray-Gundersen J, et al. MRI-guided muscle biopsy for correlation of increased signal intensity with ultrastructural change and delayed-onset muscle soreness after exercise. Radiology 1992;184:865–869.

27
Myositis Ossificans

Matthias Nägele, Michaela Hamann, and Walter F. Koch

Skeletal muscle ossification was first reported as a complication of traumatic spinal paraplegia over a century ago.[1] The frequency and severity of this complication among military veterans with spinal cord injuries stimulated futher interest following the first world war.[2]

Soule coined the term "neurogenic ossifying fibro-myositis" and was the first to recognize that the condition was primarily due to alteration of perimysial connective tissue and not of myocytes themselves.[3] It is now generally agreed that perimysial tissue inducible osteo-progenitor cells (IOPCs) constitute the source of hetero-topic bone characteristic of myositis ossificans.[4–6] The IOPC is a ubiquitous component of stromal connective tissue. Under the influence of a variety of local and systemic factors. IOPCs can undergo chondro-osseous differentiation.[7] They are nonfixed cells, which can migrate via the bloodstream or lymphatics.[8]

IOPCs have been demonstrated in lymph nodes, skin, thymus, and spleen. They were initially considered undifferentiated cells because under normal physiologic conditions they are morphologically and functionally indistinguishable from other connective tissue cells.[6,7] However, when appropriately stimulated, their ability to differentiate along chondro-osseous lines demonstrated a degree of differentiation that clearly distinguished them from other "undifferentiated" connective tissue cells of the human body. As yet, the relative contributions of local IOPC and blood-borne IOPC in the differentiation of osteoblasts at ectopic sites are unknown.

The following pages focus on various imaging findings in the evaluation of muscle ossification. Individual characteristics that might be anticipated on conventional radiographs, scintigraphy, CT, and MRI are discussed and the appropriate utilization of them in the detection of disease in various stages, as well as in discriminating differential diagnostic clues, will be described.

Six clinical variations of heterotopic (muscle) ossification will be discussed in detail:

1. Myositis ossificans traumatica (MOT);
2. Calcific myonecrosis;
3. Ossification of muscle in cerebral injury, paraplegia, and burns;
4. Myositis ossificans circumscripta (MOC);
5. Myositis (fibrodysplasia) ossificans progressiva (MOP);
6. Surgical trauma, including joint implants.

Myositis Ossificans Traumatica (MOT)

There are no recorded statistics on the incidence of MOT; however, 60% to 75% of patients with localized soft tissue ossification are reported to have had a single or repeated trauma history.[9,10] It is also recognized that the frequency of MOT is highest in young adults, but is also high in adolescents and younger children.[11–16]

The muscles affected are variable, with any injured region subject to involvement with MOT. The lesion consists of bone and cartilage, and may not only occur in muscles, but also in tendons, ligaments, fasciae, aponeuroses, and joint capsules. The most common muscles affected are the quadriceps femoris and brachialis.[17] MOT has even been described in the face, spine, and hand.[18,19]

In has been proposed that the development of MOT requires a trauma that is sufficient to cause proliferative repair.[20] Initially, the lesion presents clinically as a localized inflammatory reaction with redness, heat, pain, mass-like tumor, and loss of function. The term "inflammation" is arguably invalid since inflammation is not the dominant feature histopathologically. The characteristic histopathological features are reactions of the IOPC that manifest as migration, proliferation, and differentiation into cartilage and bone.

Three zones can be distinguished microscopically in the early phases of MOT.[21] Centrally, the lesion is made up of proliferating cells with mitotic figures as well as necrosis and hemorrhage. An intermediate zone is composed of osteoblasts and immature osteoid. Biopsies taken from these two zones may lead to the incorrect diagnosis of osteosarcoma. The third zone reveals the benign characteristics of MOT. This resembles mature bone, histopathologically, and is well delineated from the surrounding tissue. The IOPCs transform to osteoblasts which produce collagen that subsequently mineralizes. The proliferation characteristically begins in the periphery of the lesion and progresses towards the center. Within 6 to 8 weeks, the new bone encloses a central soft tissue lesion that gradually undergoes cystic degeneration. Five to six months after the trauma, clinical signs suggesting inflammation regress and a palpable, shrunken and painless mass results.

Differential Diagnosis

Patients with osteosarcoma present clinically with progressive pain and progressive enlargement of the lesion. In contrast, MOT masses decline in size and pain over time. Osteosarcoma is predominantly located near metaphyses of the long bones whereas MOT prefers

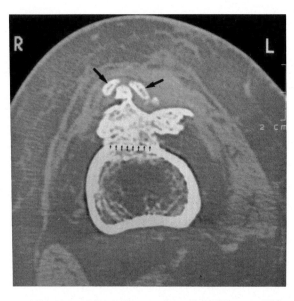

FIGURE 27.2. Myositis ossificans traumatica: 37-year-old female patient. History of a strike of a metal bar to right thigh. Computed tomography of distal diaphysis of right femur shows posttraumatic ossification anterior to femur. Large arrows = nonattached fragments, small arrows = cortical fixation of bulky, ossified mass.

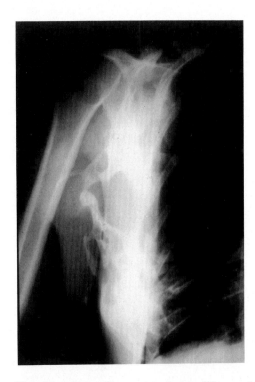

FIGURE 27.1. Myositis ossificans traumatica: 45-year-old male patient. History of severe chest contusion following a car accident. Conventional radiograph of right thorax and humerus, anteroposterior view, shows new bone formation along right lateral chest wall.

diaphyses. In contrast to osteosarcoma, MOT does not lead to destruction of bone (see Figures 27.1 and 27.2).

MOT shows mature bone components at the periphery of the lesion whereas osteosarcoma develops dystrophic calcifications in the center. Differential diagnostic considerations include periosteal osteosarcoma, intra- and extraosseous osteosarcoma, calcified subperiosteal hematoma, osteochondroma, osteoma, juxtacortical chondroma and pseudotumorous calcinosis with secondary hyperparathyroidism.[20,22]

Therapy

Therapy of MOT includes conservative measures and surgery. Conservative therapy prevents the formation of extraosseous ossification by strict rest of the injured extremity.[20] Additional treatment includes ice pads, compression bandages, and massage. Further damage may delay the healing process and this includes the trauma of surgery. For this reason, the maturity of the lesion must be ensured before surgery is elected.

Surgery of large lesions is performed to reduce the risk of reinjury of the traumatized location. After surgical treatment, a 2-week period of immobilization is followed by active range-of-motion therapy which is in turn followed by passive range-of-motion therapy for 5 to 6 months.[17] The role of medical treatment of heterotopic ossification is controversial.[23]

Calcific Myonecrosis

Calcific myonecrosis is a rare late posttraumatic condition in which an entire muscle of the calf is replaced by a fusiform mass with central liquefaction and peripheral calcification.[24] Calcific myonecrosis is related to fractures with ischemic paralysis of limbs, peripheral nerve injury, or laceration of the supplying arteries.[25,26] Open excision should be avoided because of the danger of chronic infection with sinus formation. The radiologic appearance of the lesion, combined with a history of previous trauma and peripheral nerve damage, allows a confident diagnosis and obviates surgical biopsy or excision (see Chapter 33).[24]

Ossification of Muscle in Cerebral Injury, Paraplegia, and Burns

Soft tissue ossification occurs in approximately 30% of patients with spinal cord injuries and can complicate a variety of other paralyzing central nervous system diseases, often leading to extensive and debilitating

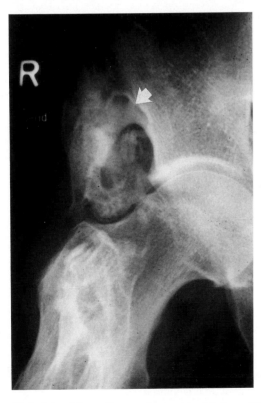

FIGURE 27.3. Myositis ossificans after cerebral injury: 64-year-old male patient. History of cerebral injury after a bicycle accident. Conventional radiograph of right hip joint, shows characteristic peripheral ossification at the origin of the rectus femoris muscle (arrow).

contractures.[27–32] Heterotopic bone formation (Figure 27.3) typically occurs below the level of damage of the spinal cord lesion.[33]

The specific factors responsible for the transformation of these ossifying cells in paralyzed muscle remain unclear. Paraplegic patients frequently develop ossification without any inflammatory symptoms or history of trauma whatsoever, suggesting that local inflammatory changes or trauma are not prerequisites for osseous differentiation of perimysial IOPCs.[11,29,32,34,35]

Myositis Ossificans Circumscripta (MOC)

In a subset of patients with heterotopic ossification, no history of trauma can be elicited. Extraosseous non-neoplastic localized development of bone without a history of trauma is termed MOC or pseudomalignant osseous tumor of soft tissue.[36] Patients with MOC tend to be adolescents or young adults, whereas those with extraosseous osteosarcomas are usually in the sixth decade of life.[36] The pain associated with nonneoplastic heterotopic bone formation is most severe early in the course of the lesion and gradually diminishes, a pattern that is not characteristic of malignancies.

Blood chemistry studies are normal.[10] Microscopically, MOC is isolated from the host muscle by a fibrous connective tissue capsule and is organized into three zones similar to MOT: an inner zone of proliferating spindle-shaped cells, a middle zone of osteoblasts and osteoid, and an outer zone of lamellar bone that may include bone marrow. Most areas of nonneoplastic heterotopic bone formation arise in the large muscle groups of the thighs, buttocks and upper arms, frequently in close proximity to the shaft of a bone.[37]

The roentgenographic appearance of MOC on serial images reflects the maturation of the lesion. Initially there is soft tissue swelling with or without periosteal reaction. This proceeds to flocculated calcification, which is finally replaced by mature bone (see Figure 27.4).[37]

Myositis (Fibrodysplasia) Ossificans Progressiva (MOP)

A generalized progressively disabling disease characterized by heterotopic ossification in the paravertebral soft tissue, shoulder, pelvic girdle (see Figure 27.5), jaw and head musculature, and congenital malformations of the great toes is known as MOP.[38] Extraocular muscles, cardiac muscle, tongue, larynx, esophagus, diaphragm, intestines, sphincter muscles, skin, and facial muscles

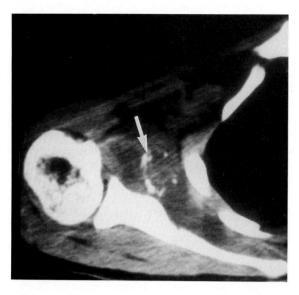

FIGURE 27.4. Myositis ossificans circumscripta: 43-year-old female patient, no history of trauma. CT of the right shoulder Note circumscribed ossification in the subscapularis muscle (arrow).

are usually not involved.[39,40] Although the lifespan is reduced in patients with MOP, most patients reach adulthood. The most common cause of death is pneumonia.[38] Routine laboratory tests are normal.[41]

The condition develops from an autosomal dominant mutation. The most significant feature of MOP is the genetic predisposition of the connective tissue cells to differentiate into cartilage and bone at the site of injections, injuries, surgery, or even spontaneously.[39] Progressive heterotopic ossification usually begins during the first decade of life.[23,39] Microscopically, muscle fibers degenerate, calcify, and are replaced by connective tissue, bone, and bone marrow. The mature heterotopic bone in patients with MOP is morphologically indistinguishable from mature skeletal bone.[38,40] In general, the local pathologic changes are very simlar to MOT.[40,41]

Surgical Trauma, including Joint Implants

Para-articular ossification occurs very commonly after implantation of metallic devices for fixation and artificial joint components (see Figure 27.6). The incidence of heterotopic ossification after hip arthroplasty has been reported to range from 2% to 90%, the variance of which is probably due to differences in surgical methods and in grading techniques.[42,43] After total knee replace-

ment, however, ectopic bone formation is usually not observed.[44]

In the histopathologically similar conditions, MOT, para-articular ossification following artificial hip replacement, and heterotopic ossification following sepsis, the necroinflammatory tissue environment is believed to constitute an important predisposing factor for the development of ossification. In these conditions, uncharacterized inflammatory mediators may play a role, but nonspecific physicochemical alterations in the traumatized tissue milieu, in particular, chronically decreased tissue pH consequent to inflammatory cell infiltration and vascular disruption—are also argued to contribute.[28]

The efficacy of radiation therapy in the prevention of myositis ossificans is well documented. Doses ranging from 2000 cGy administered over 10 sessions to 700 cGy administered in a single fraction have been shown to be effective schedules in prevention of heterotopic ossification in patients with risk factors[45–48] (i.e., active ankylosing spondylitis, hypertrophic osteoarthritis, posttraumatic degenerative joint disease, multiple hip surgeries, diffuse idiopathic skeletal hyperostosis,

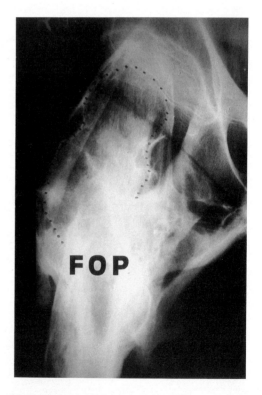

FIGURE 27.5. Myositis (fibrodysplasia) ossificans progressiva: conventional radiograph of right hip joint, anteroposterior view. Note dense ossification of gluteus minimus, gluteus maximus, quadratus femoris, and iliopsoas. Dots: original outline of femoral head and neck.

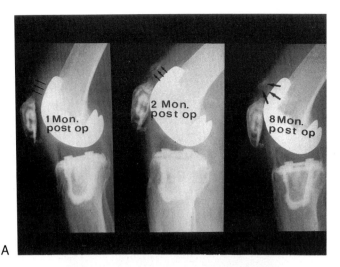

A

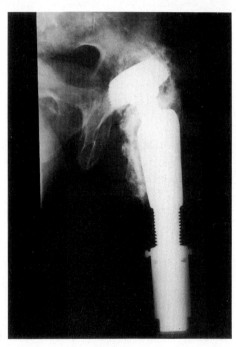

B

FIGURE 27.6. Myositis ossificans after surgical trauma and joint implant operation. (A) Prosthesis of the right knee joint: follow-up study 1, 2, and 8 months postimplantation. Note heterotopic bone formation in the quadriceps tendon (arrows). (B) Prosthesis of left hip joint: observe web-like new bone formation along proximal stem.

etc.).[45,49,50] The outcome of aggressive treatment of heterotopic ossification depends upon residual ossification after surgery, adequacy of radiation therapy coverage, and timing of radiation therapy after surgery.[51] Surgical removal of all heterotopic ossification should be undertaken whenever possible, radiation portals should cover an adequate field, including all potentially involved soft tissue, and radiation therapy should be initiated within 3 days after surgery.[51] Prophylaxis of heterotopic bone by means of preoperative irradiation is a new idea that is gaining momentum, although animal studies indicated no difference in overall bone formation in rats irradiated 1 h before surgery compared to postoperative irradiation.[52]

Imaging Modalities

Conventional Radiography

Conventional radiographs are the method of first choice for the diagnostic workup of heterotopic ossifications (see Figures 27.1 and 27.3). Overall, they provide the most complete information about the lesion in early, middle, and late phases, of heterotopic ossification and at the least expense (see Figure 27.6). In the first 10 days following soft tissue injury, radiographs can detect heterotopic ossification by soft tissue swelling. By the third to fourth week, flocculated densities may arise, sometimes associated with periosteal reactions. At 6 to 8 weeks, a lacy pattern of new bone is sharply circumscribed about the periphery of the cortex. In the end stage, a calcified eggshell-like mass is formed. Maturity of the ossified mass is reached after 5 to 6 months and initial mass effects disappear.[9] A radiolucent zone of soft tissue often separates the lesion from the underlying periosteal reaction and cortex, and thereby assists in the radiological differentiation from juxtacortical osteosarcoma, which lacks this characteristic (Figure 27.3).[9]

The differential diagnosis includes osteosarcoma, hematoma, osteochondroma, and pseudotumorous calcinosis which can frequently be distinguished on conventional radiographs alone. Radiographs have been advocated as a means to classify the severity of heterotopic ossification.[53]

Scintigraphy

Like any other osteoblastic activity, heterotopic bone formation results in increased uptake of bone-avid radionuclides (see Chapter 1). Although ^{99m}Tc-pyrophosphate studies were shown to detect MOT prior to observable roentgenographic changes,[54] the use of this agent has not yet been extended to early diagnosis and follow-up of MOT because of inconsistent results. However, serial bone scans that show a progressive decrease in radiotracer accumulation in late stages of heterotopic bone followed by a steady state over a period of at least two to three consecutive monthly examinations correlate well with inactive disease.[55] Definitive management of heterotopic bone in some cases requires surgical intervention; however, if the bone is not fully mature at the time of surgery, recurrence will develop, often more extensively than before and a second operation may be necessary.[55] Therefore, quantitative and qualitative bone scintigraphic data can be helpful to assist in planning the correct timing of the surgical intervention.

Computed Tomography (CT)

In the early phase, the lesion is hypodense compared to muscle and with mass effect on the surrounding fasciae. Peripheral edema is less distinctly depicted compared to MRI. The dominant CT feature of the intermediate to late phase of myositis ossificans is the mineralized ossification and calcification in the peripheral zone of the lesion (Figures 27.2 and 27.4), which starts about 2 weeks after the trauma.[9] These dense formations can be ringlike or small and punctate in shape. The zonal pattern of calcification helps to distinguish heterotopic ossification from malignant tumors such as paraosteal osteosarcoma, which have denser central calcification, and from extraosseous osteosarcoma, which presents with amorphous calcification.[56] Bone window settings help to accentuate the zonal patterns of calcification. The lack of a prominent soft tissue mass at the stage when calcification occurs improves the differentiation between heterotopic ossification and malignant tumors.[57]

Magnetic Resonance Imaging

In the early and intermediate phases, the lesion shows inhomogeneously increased signal intensity on T_2-weighted images.[58-61] The inhomogeneity is due to the proliferating cells as well as necrosis and hemorrhage of the lesion. An edematous peripheral zone can be delineated up to 8 weeks after injury.[62,63] On T_1-weighted images the lesions are isointense to muscle and so may be inconspicuous or only detected by the mass effect on the displaced fasciae of the surrounding muscles. Clear-cut differentiation of the borders of edematous zone and margin of the lesion on T_2-weighted images is often impossible. Administration of paramagnetic contrast agents (i.e. gadolinium chelates) may show inhomogeneous enhancement of the center of the lesion on T_1-weighted images. The outer margins of the mass may stay low in signal intensity due to the formation of mature bone. Small spotted calcification or new bone formation is frequently missed on MRI scans. Fluid–fluid levels are consistent with previous hemorrhage, and are not an uncommon finding in the innermost immature portion of the lesion (see Figure 27.7). However, they are nonspecific, being seen in aneurysmal bone cysts and other lesions.[64]

Correlating the high signal intensity on T_2-weighted images with histological specimens, Kransdorf et al. found highly cellular areas of proliferating fibroblasts and myofibroblasts within a myxoid stroma of extracell-

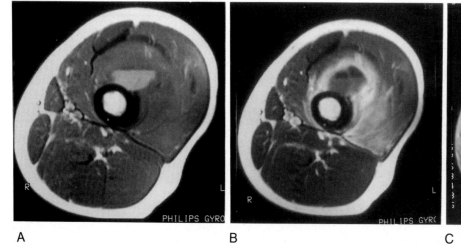
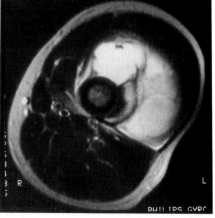

A   B   C

FIGURE 27.7. MRI of myositis ossificans traumatica in early phase: 51-year-old patient with a history of skiing accident. (A) T_1-weighted axial scan of left thigh (SE T_R/T_E: 500/25 ms) shows subacute hemorrhage with fluid level in vastus intermedius. High signal intensity region of sediment is caused by methemoglobin. (B) When same sequence is performed after intravenous gadolinium bolus injection (0.1 mmol/kg), note increased signal intensity in the rim of the lesion and in the edematous zone of the vastus lateralis muscle. (C) T_2-weighted image (SE T_R/T_E: 1800/90 ms) shows high signal intensity of the cystic lesion and the edematous zone.

ular matrix.[63] Similar correlations were found by Meyer et al. in nodular fasciitis.[65]

In the end stage of the disease, signal intensity is intermediate to high on T_1- and T_2-weighted sequences (see Figure 27.8). The high signal intense areas on both sequences reflect fatty infiltrations between trabeculae.[63] The outer rim of the lesion stays low in signal on all sequences. These areas constitute trabeculae and/or hemosiderin deposits from associated hemorrhage and concomitant fibrosis. The overall lesion size diminishes over time. The edematous rim of the early phase disappears gradually. Due to its high soft tissue contrast, MRI complements conventional radiographs for follow-up studies of heterotopic ossification.

Conclusion

Conventional radiographs are the method of first choice in evaluating ossification of muscle. CT and MRI complement radiographic studies by adding the relevant cross-sectional anatomy, contrast-enhanced dynamics, and detailed observation of the internal and peripheral composition of calcifications, new bone formation, and soft tissue components of the tumor. Also, quantitative and qualitative ^{99m}Tc-pyrophosphate bone scans, contrast-enhanced CT, and MRI can help in the planning of surgical interventions by classifying the maturity and activity of bone formation.

All of the described imaging modalities provide valuable information about the differential diagnosis of myositis ossificans.

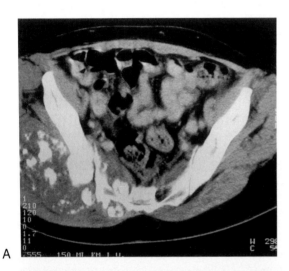

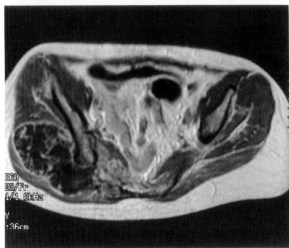

FIGURE 27.8. Myositis ossificans traumatica: late phase. (A) Computed tomography: Note posttraumatic stippled calcifications of gluteus medius on the right. (B) Modestly T_1-weighted image (SE T_R/T_E: 860/23 ms) shows high signal intense areas that reflect fatty infiltrations between the trabeculae of the heterotopic bone. Low signal intensity areas correspond to heterotopic bone formation, hemosiderin deposits from hemorrhage, and/or concomitant fibrosis.

References

1. Riedel B. Demonstration eines durch achttägiges Umhergehen total destruierten Kniegelenkes von einem Patienten mit Stichverletzung des Rückens. Verh Dtsch Ges Chir 1883;12:93–96.
2. Dejerine J, Ceillier A, Dejerine Y. Paraosteoarthropathies des paraplegiques par lesion medullaire. Rev Neurol 1919;34:399–407.
3. Soule AB. Neurogenic ossifying fibromyopathies. A preliminary report. J Neurosurg 1945;2:485–497.
4. Friedenstein AY. Determined and inducible osteogenetic precursor cells. In: Hard tissue growth, repair and remineralization. Ciba Foundation Symposium II. New York: Elsevier, 1973:169–181.
5. Friedenstein AY. Precursor cells of mechanocytes. Int Rev Cytol 1976;47:327–355.
6. Urist MR. Fundamental and clinical bone physiology. Philadelphia: J.B. Lippincott Company, 1980:331–368.
7. Friedenstein AY. Osteogenic stem cells in the bone marrow. In: Heersche JNM, Kanis JA, editors. Bone and mineral research. Amsterdam: Elsevier Science Publishers B.V., 1990:243–272.
8. Koch FW, Messler HH, Kaden B, v. Deimling U, Rüther W. Die in vivo-Transformation der induzierbaren Osteoprogenitorzelle zum Osteoblasten in alkalischer Biokeramik. In: Reiser M, Heuck M, editors. Osteologie VIII. In press.
9. Norman A, Dorfman HD. Juxtacortical circumscribed myositis ossificans: evolution and radiographic features. Radiology 1970;16:301–306.
10. Paterson DC. Myositis ossificans circumscripta: a report of 4 cases without a history of injury. J Bone Joint Surg 1970;52B:296–301.
11. Gilmer WS, Anderson LD. Reactions of soft somatic tissue which may progress to bone formation: circumscribed

(traumatic) myositis ossificans. South Med J 1959;52: 1432–1438.

12. Ray MJ, Bassett RL. Myositis ossificans. Orthopedics 1984;7:532–535.

13. Weinstein I, Fraerman S. Difficulties in early diagnosis of myositis ossificans. JAMA 1954;154:994–996.

14. Clapton WK, James CL, Morris LL, Davey RB, Peacock MJ, Byard RW. Myositis ossificans in childhood. Pathology 1992;24:311–314.

15. Dickerson RC. Myositis ossificans in early childhood. Report of an unusual case. Clin Orthop Rel Res 1971; 79:42.

16. Hughton J, Whatley G, Stone M. Myositis ossificans traumatica. South Med J 1962;55:1167–1170.

17. Hait G, Boswick JA, Stone NH. Heterotopic bone formation secondary to trauma (myositis ossificans traumatica): an unusual case and a review of current concepts. J Trauma 1970;10:405–411.

18. Arima R, Shiba R, Hayashi T. Traumatic myositis ossificans in the masseter muscle. J Oral Maxillofac Surg 1984;42:512.

19. Mourad KA, Grant RW. Unusual post traumatic ossification within the intertransversarius muscle. Br J Radiol 1983;56:55.

20. Cushner FD, Morwessel RM. Myositis ossificans traumatica. Orthop Rev 1922;21(11):1319–1326.

21. Ackerman LV. Extraosseous localized non-neoplastic bone and cartilage formation (so-called myositis ossificans). J Bone Joint Surg 1958;40A:279.

22. Schutte HE, van der Heul RO. Pseudomalignant, nonneoplastic osseous soft-tissue tumors of the hand and foot. Radiology 1990;176:149.

23. Rogers JG, Geho WB. Fibrodysplasia ossificans progressiva: a survey of forty-two cases. J Bone Joint Surg AM 1979;61A:909–914.

24. Janzen DL, Conell DG, Vaisler BJ. Calcific myonecrosis of the calf manifesting as an enlarging soft-tissue mass: imaging features. AJR 1993;160:1072–1074.

25. Broder MS, Worell RV, Shafi NQ. Cystic degeneration and calcification following ischemic paralysis of the leg. Clin Orthop 1977;122:193–195.

26. Viau MR, Pedersen HE, Salciccioli GG, Manoli A. Ectopic calcification as a late sequela of compartment syndrome. Clin Orthop 1983;176:178–180.

27. Blane CE, Perkash I. True heterotopic bone in paralysed patients. Skeletal Radiol 1981;7:21–25.

28. Hardy AG, Dickson JW. Pathological ossification in traumatic paraplegia. J Bone Joint Surg 1963;45B:76–87.

29. Hernandez AM, Forner JV, De la Fuente T, Gonzalez C, Miro R. The paraarticular ossification in our paraplegics and tetraplegics: a survey of 704 patients. Paraplegia 1978; 16:272–275.

30. Miller LF, O'Neill CJ. Myositis ossificans in paraplegics. J Bone Joint Surg 1949;31A:283–294.

31. Stover SL, Hataway CJ, Zieger HE. Heterotopic ossification in spinal cord injured patients. Arch Phys Med Rehabil 1975:56:199–204.

32. Wharton GW, Morgan TH. Ankylosis in the paralyzed patient. J Bone Joint Surg 1970;52A:105–112.

33. Kewalramani LS. Ectopic ossification. Am J Phys Med 1977;56:99.

34. Garland DE, Blum CE, Waters R. Periarticular heterotopic ossification in head injured adults. J Bone Joint Surg 1980;62A:1143–1146.

35. Koch FW, v. Deimling U, Messler H. Das Verhalten des Knochens auf künstliche Matrix ohne biochemischen Einfluß. In: Pesch HJ, Stöß H, editors. Osteologie aktuell VII. Berlin: Springer-Verlag, 1992.

36. Fine G, Stout AP. Osteogenic sarcoma of the extraskeletal soft tissues. Cancer 1956;9:1027–1042.

37. Goldmann AB. Myositis ossificans circumscripta: a benign lesion with a malignant differential diagnosis. AJR 1976; 126:32–40.

38. McKusick VA. Heritable disorders of connective tissue. 4th ed. St. Louis: The C.V. Mosby Co., 1972:687–702.

39. Connor JM, Evans DAP. Fibrodysplasia ossificans progressiva: clinical features and natural history of 34 patients. J Bone Joint Surg Br 1982;64B:76–83.

40. Lutwak L. Myositis ossificans progressiva. Am J Med 1964;37:269–293.

41. Smith R, Russel RGG, Woods CG. Myositis ossificans circumscripta. J Bone Joint Surg 1976; 58B:48.

42. Kjaersgaard-Andersen P, Hougaard K, Linde F, Christiansen SE, Jensen J. Heterotopic bone formation after total hip arthroplasty in patients with primary or secondary coxarthrosis. Orthopedics 1990;13:1211–1217.

43. Lindholm TS, Viljakka T, Popov L, Lindholm TC. Development of heterotopic ossification around the hip. Arch Orthop Trauma Surg 1986;105:263–267.

44. Koch FW, Messler H, Puls P, Münzenberg KJ. Die periartikuläre Ossifikation nach Kniegelenksendoprothetik: Eine Studie an 331 Fällen. In: Werner E, Matthiass HH, editors. Osteologie interdisziplinär. Berlin: Springer-Verlag, 1991.

45. Ayers DC, Evarts CM, Parkinson JR. The prevention of heterotopic ossification in high-risk patients with low-dose radiation therapy after total hip arthroplasty. J Bone Joint Surg Am 1986;68:1423– 1429.

46. Bosse MJ, Poka A, Reinert CM, Ellwanger F, Slawson R, McDevitt ER. Heterotopic ossification as a complication of acetabular fracture: prophylaxis with low-dose irradiation. J Bone Joint Surg Am 1988;70:1231–1237.

47. Parkinson JR, Evarts CM, Hubbard LF. Radiation therapy in the prevention of heterotopic ossification after total hip arthroplasty. In: Nelson JP, editor. The hip. Proceedings of the Tenth Open Scientific Meeting of the Hip Society. St. Louis, MO: Mosby, 1982:211–227.

48. van der Werf GJIM, van Hasel NGM, Tonino AJ. Radiotherapy in the prevention of recurrence of paraarticular ossification in the total hip protheses. Arch Orthop Trauma Surg 1985;104:85–88.

49. Jowsey J, Coventry MB, Robins PR. Heterotopic ossification: theoretical consideration, possible etiologic factors, and a clinical review of total hip arthroplasty patients exhibiting this phenomenon. In: The hip. Proceedings of the Fifth Open Scientific Meeting of the Hip Society. St. Louis, MO: Mosby, 1977:210–221.

50. Ritter MA, Vaughan RB. Ectopic ossification after total hip arthroplasty: predisposing factors, frequency, and effect on results. J Bone Joint Surg Am 1977;59:345–351.

51. DeFlitch CJ, Stryker JA. Postoperative hip irradiation in prevention of heterotopic ossification: causes of treatment failure. Radiology 1993;188:265–270.

52. Kantorowitz DA, Miller GJ, Ferrara JA, Ibott GS, Fisher R, Ahrens CR. Preoperative versus postoperative irradiation in the prophylaxis of heterotopic bone formation in rats. Int J Radiat Oncol Biol Phys 1990;19:1413–1438.

53. Brooker AF, Bowermann JW, Robinson RA, Riley LH. Ectopic ossification following total hip replacement: incidence and a method of classification. J Bone Joint Surg Am 1973;55:1629–1632.

54. Szuki Y, Hisada K, Takeda M. Demonstration of myositis ossificans by 99mTc pyrophosphate bone scanning. Radiology 1974;111:663–664.

55. Tanaka T, Rossier AB, Hussey RW, Ahnberg BA, Treves S. Quantitative assessment of para-osteo-arthropathy and its maturation on serial radionuclide bone images. Radiology 1977;123:217–221.

56. Edeiken J, Hodes PJ. Diagnosis of diseases of bone. 2nd ed. Baltimore: Williams & Wilkins, 1973:1145–1148.

57. Heinrich SD, Zembo MM, MacEen GD. Pseudomalignant myositis ossificans. Orthopedics 1989; 10:599.

58. Berquist TH, Ehmann RL, King BF, Hodgman CG, Ilstrup DM. Value of MR imaging in differentiating benign from malignant soft-tissue masses: study of 95 lesions. AJR 1990;155:1251.

59. De Smet AA, Norris MA, Fisher DR. Magnetic resonance imaging of myositis ossificans: analysis of seven cases. Skeletal Radiol 1992;21:503–507.

60. Oestreich AE. Imaging of the skeleton and soft tissues in children. Curr Opin Radiol 1992;4:VI: 55–61.

61. Sundarm M, McLeod RA. MR Imaging of tumor and tumorlike lesions of bone and soft tissue. AJR 1990;155: 817.

62. Hanna SL, Magill HL, Brooks MT, Burton EM, Boulden TF, Seidel FG. Case of the day. Pediatric myositis ossificans circumscripta. Radiographics 1990;10:945–949.

63. Kransdorf MJ, Meis JM, Jelinek JS. Myositis ossificans: MR appearance with radiologic-pathologic correlation. AJR 1991;157:1243.

64. Tsai JC, Dalinka MK, Fallon MD, Zlatkin MB, Kressel HY. Fluid-fluid level: a nonspecific finding in tumors of bone and soft tissue. Radiology 1990; 175:779–782.

65. Meyer CA, Kransdorf MJ, Jelinek JS, Moser RP. Radiologic appearance of nodular fasciitis with emphasis on MR and CT. J Compu Assist Tomogr 1991;15:276–279.

28
Compartment Syndrome

Marga B. Rominger and Christian J. Lukosch

Definitions, Pathophysiology, and Clinical Findings

In 1881, Volkmann described a contracture state related to ischemia caused by trauma, tight bandaging, and swelling; in short, the late state of an ischemic compartment syndrome.[1] Strictly speaking, a Volkmann's contracture is confined to the forearm and occurs most commonly after supracondylar fracture of the humerus in children. However, some authors use Volkmann's contracture as a synonym for a compartment syndrome regardless of the location.[2] In 1941, Bywaters and Beall reported on the crushed limbs of civilian victims of London's wartime air raids.[3] When massive limb swelling, ischemic muscle necrosis, myoglobinuria, and renal failure complicated such injuries they recognized it as a clinical entity—Crush syndrome. Crush syndromes or rhabdomyolysis (lysis of skeletal muscle cells) can be a cause or complication of compartment syndrome (see Chapter 26). The formal notion of compartment syndrome was introduced in 1963 by Reszel.[4]

Matsen defines the compartment syndrome as a condition in which increased pressure within a limited space compromises the circulation and function of the tissues within that space.[5] The tolerance of muscle and nerve tissue for increased tissue pressure depends on the time course and the relationship of the mean arterial pressure to tissue pressure (arteriovenous gradient). A decrease in the arteriovenous gradient causes a lowering of tissue PO_2 and a subsequent metabolic deficit. A variety of etiologies are described that either expand the compartment volume (edema, hematoma, exertion, intoxication, neoplasm) or restrict the compartment size (constrictive dressings and casts, closure of fascial defects, positioning during surgery).[6] More than 70% have a traumatic origin.

A compartment syndrome may arise in any area of the body that has little or no capacity for tissue expansion,[5] for example, the orbit,[7] scapula,[8] forearm and hand,[9] spine,[10] pelvis,[11] thigh,[12] and foot.[13] The most common affected site is the lower leg.[5] Clinically, compartment syndromes can be classified into an imminent and manifest compartment syndrome.[14] In an imminent compartment syndrome there is severe pain (disproportional to the trauma), no neurological symptoms, moderate disturbances of muscular perfusion, and increasing tissue pressure. Neurological symptoms, pathological tissue pressures, compromised circulation, and loss of tissue function are found in the manifest compartment syndrome. Besides compartment syndromes of traumatic origin there are functional compartment syndromes after exercise that can occur with an acute (manifest) and chronic form. The functional compartment syndromes most commonly happen in the anterior compartment of the leg.[14] To terminate a compartment syndrome and avert irreversible tissue injury and associated sequelae, fasciotomy is necessary. The untreated manifest compartment syndrome will result in muscular fibrosis, nerve injury, and possible amputation.[14]

Diagnostic Imaging

Compartment syndrome is a clinical diagnosis.[15] However, symptoms and signs of a compartment syndrome at times may be sufficiently ambiguous that a definite diagnosis cannot be made on clinical grounds alone. Tissue pressure measurements, especially in conjunction with the mean arterial pressure, are helpful and are routinely used to confirm the diagnosis of compartment syndromes.[5,16–18] Although compartment syndrome is a clinical diagnosis, imaging can be helpful for diagnosis when there is an uncommon site (e.g., the orbit) or cause (e.g., tumor infiltration), for guiding catheters for tissue pressure measurements, when tissue pressures are ambiguous, for preoperative assessment of extent of abnormality, to assess muscle viability, and for follow-up.

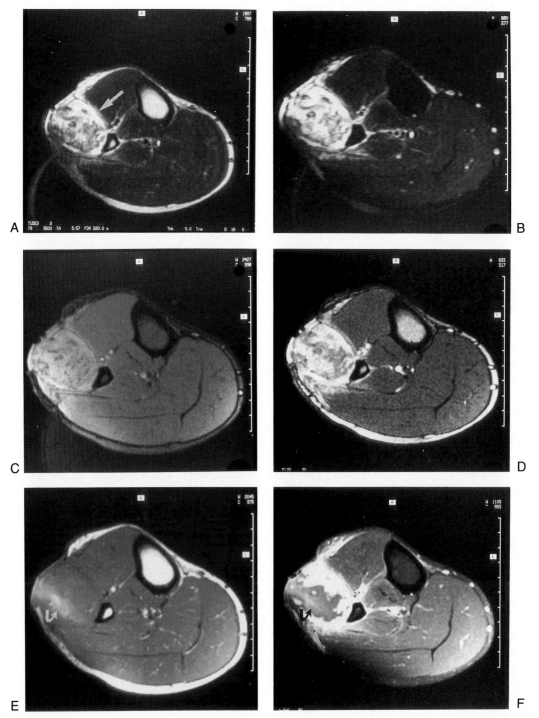

FIGURE 28.1. MRI pulse sequences in manifest compartment syndrome after minor trauma and subsequent fasciotomy. T_2-weighted image shows markedly edematous tissue by virtue of increased signal intensity (arrow, T_R 3500/T_E 90, A), which is even more conspicuous by including a fat-saturation pulse (T_R 3500/T_E 90, B). High signal intensity is also evident within the edematous muscle by using a proton density-weighted gradient echo sequence (T_R 400, T_E 12, flip 20°) without (C) and with (D) a magnetization transfer saturation pulse. The image with the saturation pulse (D) has more of a T_2-like appearance. T_1-weighted MRI performed without contrast material shows swelling and loss of muscle architecture as well as high signal intensity due to hemorrhage from the injury (curved arrow, T_R 500/T_E 12, E). Fat-saturated, gadolinium-enhanced T_1-weighted image shows strong enhancement peripheral to the central hemorrhagic necrosis (curved arrow) (F). Cross-sectional and longitudinal sections of muscle (hematoxylin-eosin stains) show edema around muscle fibers (magnification ×100, G), a necrotic muscle fiber (arrow, magnification ×400, H), and replacement by granulation tissue (arrow, magnification ×100, I).

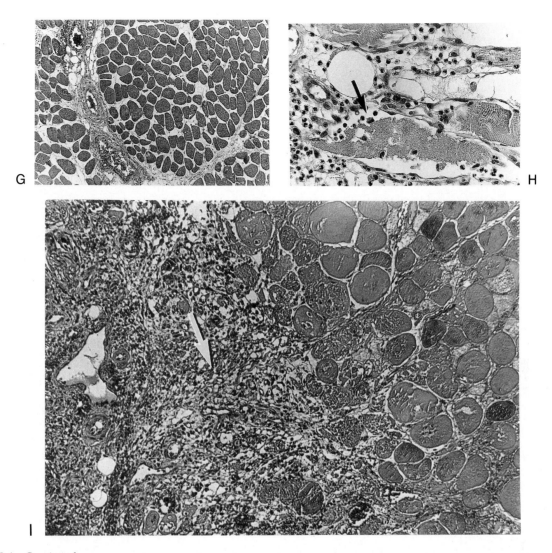

FIGURE 28.1. *Continued*

Roentgenograms are not helpful in the modern era but are of historical interest in that they were used to study Volkmann's contracture. The radiological picture of Volkmann's contracture of the forearm revealed flexion in the wrist and in the interphalangeal joints and hyperextension (or rarely, flexion) of the metacarpophalangeal joints associated with soft tissue atrophy. Trophic changes were revealed by variably severe osteoporosis, growth disturbances, as well as alterations of ossification rates of epiphyses and apophyses of tubular and carpal bones.[19] Nuclear medicine has been tried but its application is limited. Technetium-99m phosphate compounds can identify lesions of rhabdomyolysis as positive lesions and thus could conceivably be useful to show the location of compartment syndromes[20] (see Chapters 1 and 30).

Ultrasound can show and quantify muscle swelling, demonstrate a loss of muscle architecture, and reveal echo-dense and/or echo-poor areas depending on the degree of edema and liquefaction.[21,22] To avoid nerve and vascular injury during tissue pressure measurement in the deep posterior compartment, safe placement of the catheter and documentation of the catheter tip can be achieved with ultrasound.[23]

CT scans can show location, extent, and the densitometric features of muscle infarction.[24,25] Landi et al. distinguished two groups of CT patterns of compartment syndromes.[25] A group with diffuse hypodensity of the muscular sheaths and unclear borders typically has coefficient of attenuation values of approximately 30 to 40 Hounsfield units (H.U.) (according to Wegener, normal muscle has approximately 50 H.U.).[26] At surgery this group corresponded to diffuse fibrosis. A second group with localized hypodensity of various muscle groups equal to 10 to 20 H.U. corresponded to infarction. This range of density values is nonspecific, however, as partial fatty replacement of muscles can result in similar Hounsfield values (see below).

The authors have used a large variety of MRI sequences in patients with manifest compartment syndromes.[27] T_1-weighted MR images of the affected site typically showed swollen compartments and loss of the normal muscular architecture. In some cases, high signal intensity regions were noted that likely represent foci of hemorrhage.[28] T_2-weighted MR images show inhomogeneous hyperintense areas, which are typically more conspicuous when combined with a fat-suppression pulse sequence. Two additional techniques that may improve the diagnostic yield of the MRI examination include the use of intravenous gadolinium-DTPA infusion and magnetization transfer contrast (MTC).

We find gadolinium-DTPA to improve the distinction of subvolumes of necrotic muscle compartments on T_1-weighted sequences, particularly when combined with fat-suppression pulses. We have observed not only that affected compartments strongly enhance, but also that within enhancing compartments, areas of liquefaction necrosis, hemorrhage, and normal muscle can be readily identified (Figure 28.1). This is similar to the findings of Fleckenstein[29] (Chapter 30), who found gadolinium useful to characterize edema as either enhancing (perfused and therefore potentially viable) or nonenhancing (nonperfused and therefore nonviable). The presence and extent of nonviable muscle tissue presents valuable preoperative information to plan muscle resection.

Magnetization transfer contrast MRI refers to a novel form of image contrast (see Chapter 3). It depends on a variety of factors related to the saturation of macromolecule-bound water present, for example, in muscle. Briefly, a saturation pulse induces an observable decrease in the proton signal intensity due to selective saturation of water that is bound to macromolecules. When there is a substantial decrease in the content of macromolecules and membranes and an increase in free water, such as occurs in edematous muscle, these saturation pulses cause a net loss in signal intensity that is quantitatively less than in neighboring normal muscle. This increases the visual conspicuity of the damaged muscle on proton-weighted gradient echo images and results in images having a more T_2-weighted appearance[27] (Figure 28.1). In our study, MTC ratios were calculated from SI measurements made from sequences without and with the saturation pulses. These ratios were significantly lower in affected compartments of manifest syndromes than in normal muscle. When used in conjunction with T_1-weighted spin echo sequences after infusion of gadolinium-DTPA, MTC can increase the contrast between normal muscle and enhancing areas by suppressing the signal intensity of the nonenhancing tissue and increasing the signal intensity of the enhancing tissue due to synergistic effects with gadolinium.[30]

Despite the plethora of MRI techniques that can be used to evaluate compartment syndromes, no imaging technique is yet capable of measuring the pressure within the muscle and so the MRI appearance should be considered nonspecific for compartment syndrome. Clinical resemblance to compartment syndromes is encountered in patients presenting with painful, swollen extremities due to other causes. In patients with deep venous thrombosis, for example, skin thickening and subcutaneous fat edema are associated with muscle edema and swelling, particularly of the posterior compartment. In these cases, it is useful to recall that MRI allows evaluation of the patency of veins and so flow-sensitive sequences can be critical to distinguish between these entities. Patients with lymphedema may also present with swollen painful limbs. This condition is usually distinguished by the clinical situation but the MRI and CT appearances have been characterized. Prominent subcutaneous edema and skin thickening is usually associated with muscles having normal signal intensity and no swelling.[31] An exception was reported in rapidly progressive lymphatic congestion such as in lymphoma, in which muscle swelling and edema may be marked (see Chapter 22).[32] In manifest compartment syndrome, muscle swelling and edema are the predominant features, with subcutaneous tissue edema being relatively less conspicuous.

The swelling of muscle in compartment syndrome is thus not a feature that is specific, diagnostically. Because neoplastic diseases may also cause swelling and edema of muscle, careful consideration to the clinical history should help avoid perilous misdiagnoses. Another look-alike of compartment syndrome is the condition of crush syndrome, which also sometimes causes dangerous elevations of compartment pressures (see Chapter 26). The MRI features may not allow distinction between a crush injury in which pressures are elevated from those in which pressures are not pathological. In serial MRI studies of crush syndrome, Shintani et al.[33] showed that the high-intensity areas seen on T_2-weighted MR images resolve in parallel with the clinical course. This reversibility of the MRI findings suggests that the high-intensity areas do not reflect permanent myopathic changes, but at least in part represent transient edema in the acute phase of rhabdomyolysis, similar to that seen in sports injuries.[34] The crush syndrome can lead to increased pressure, muscle cell damage and thus to further edema, and finally to a manifest compartment syndrome (Figure 28.2).

Patients with an imminent compartment syndrome after surgery for trauma are especially clinically challenging when the only symptom is disproportionately strong pain and ambiguous tissue pressures. In our group of imminent compartment syndromes three of four patients did not show any imaging changes before or after gadolinium-DTPA and MTC. The fourth patient showed small subfascial areas of increased signal intensity on T_2-weighted images which enhanced with gadolinium-

FIGURE 28.2. Patient with a crush syndrome developed a manifest compartment syndrome of the right lower leg. T_1-weighted MRI (T_R 650/T_E 15) shows swelling and loss of muscle architecture of all four compartments. Note fasciotomy defects in the subcutaneous tissues (arrows).

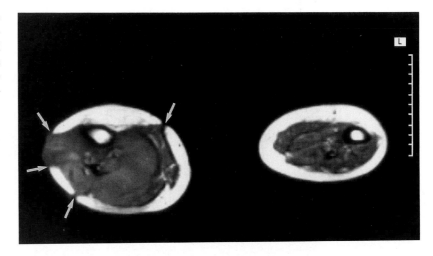

DTPA on T_1-weighted images (Figure 28.3). At surgery these areas showed reduced viability. The histopathologic study of these areas showed pressure damage similar to those within a manifest compartment syndrome.[27]

In cases of imminent compartment syndromes, functional MRI may also be useful, as suggested in a preliminary study by Amendola. They report failure of T_1 relaxation time to return to baseline in four out of five patients with a chronic compartment syndrome.[35] Such a finding would be expected to cause a prolonged increase in the normal exercise-induced signal intensity changes using a short TI inversion recovery (STIR) sequence (Figure 28.4).

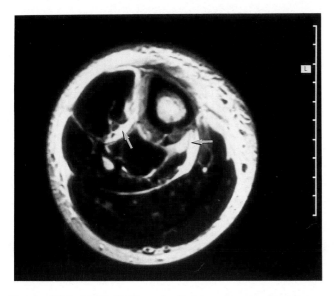

FIGURE 28.3. MRI fiindings in imminent compartment syndrome. T_2-weighted MRI shows perifascial edema as hyperintense areas in the anterior tibial and deep posterior compartments (T_R 3500/T_E 90, arrows).

Except for the use of x-ray studies of fibrous contractures following supracondylar fractures in children (Volkmann) and limited CT data,[25] little information exists on the long-term sequelae of muscle composition in compartment syndrome. We used CT to document diffuse fatty replacement in one case 1 year after a manifest compartment syndrome. In the same patient, MRI was used acutely and for follow-up 1 year after. This case demonstrated the reversibility of gadolinium enhancement (Figure 28.5).

The extent of cellular damage due to ischemia can be quantitatively assessed by noninvasive ^{31}P-MRS.[36,37] In resting skeletal muscle, the cytosolic pH and intracellular phosphorylation state do not fluctuate directly with tissue blood flow or tissue oxygen tension. In the compartment syndrome an abnormal cell bioenergetic state results. Anaerobic metabolism becomes predominant and the high-energy phosphocreatine compounds are consumed, altering the ^{31}P-MRS spectra according to severity of the ischemia. Thus, ^{31}P-MRS might be able to quantify the severity of compartment syndrome and predict the potential for recovery.

Conclusion

A compartment syndrome presents an emergency situation and diagnostic imaging should not delay surgery. However, ultrasound is a convenient technique that allows safe placement of the catheter tip into the deep posterior compartment for tissue pressure measurement. Because of its high contrast, spatial resolution, choice of imaging planes, and tissue characterization, MRI is the imaging method of choice for diagnosis, evaluation of the extent, follow-up, and functional studies. MRI can serve as a map for tissue pressure measurements and can provide the surgeon with the information necessary to optimize the choice of a selective split of fascias. Gado-

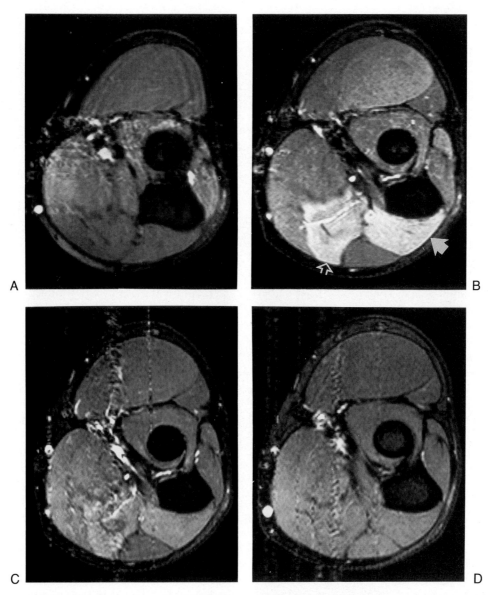

FIGURE 28.4. Functional MRI in laborer with recurrent pain while hammering and clinical suspicion of chronic compartment syndrome. Sequential axial STIR images (2500/30/150, $T_R/T_E/T_I$) were obtained to assess the time course of signal intensity changes following 2 min of handgrip exercise. Prior to exercise, the study shows no abnormal signal intensity to support compartment syndrome (A). In the first 4 min after exercise, activated superficial finger flexor (open arrowhead, B) and deep finger flexor (arrowhead, B) show expected physiological increases in signal intensity (see Chapter 7). Successive 4-min images show normal rapid "washout" of accumulated tissue edema (C,D). Such rapid return to normal argues against chronic compartment syndrome, based on the report of Amendola.[35] Subsequently, pressure was measured during a similar exercise in the deep flexor and confirmed only normal pressure changes. (Case provided by Dr. Marybeth Ezaki, M.D., Dallas, Texas.)

linium-DTPA offers the ability to distinguish between potentially viable and nonviable muscle. Functional MRI appears promising in the detection of relaxation time abnormalities in chronic functional compartment syndromes. Finally, MRI spectroscopy may be able to quantify the severity of disease. Ultimately, MRI and spectroscopy may clarify the need for fasciotomy in cases with ambiguous clinical signs and tissue pressure measurements and help predict the prognosis following surgery.

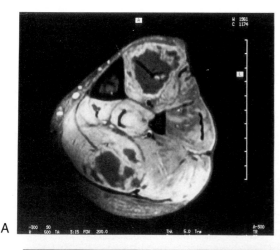
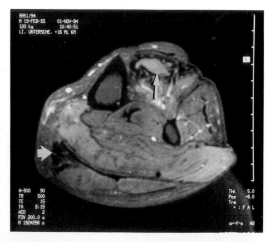

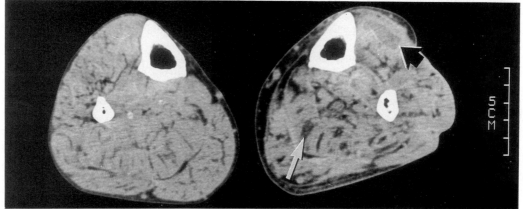

FIGURE 28.5. Delayed findings of manifest compartment involving all four compartments. Fat-suppressed, T_1-weighted image of the midleg at the time of the manifest compartment syndrome shows a few islands of normal muscle surrounded by enhancement in all four compartments following gadolinium-DTPA (T_R 500/T_E 15, A). The same sequence as in (A) obtained at a slightly more cephalad level 1 year later shows the reversibility of enhancement characteristics. Decreased signal intensity in the medial gastrocnemius represents a fibrotic healing response (arrowhead, B). Nonenhancing intermediate signal in the anterior compartment (arrow, B) corresponds to a complicated cystic region on axial CT (36 H.U., arrowhead, C) performed at the time of the second MRI. CT also shows diffuse fatty replacement in the posterior compartment reflected by decreased attenuation (20 H.U., arrow, C).

References

1. Volkmann R von. Die ischämischen Muskellähmungen und Kontrakturen. Zentralbl Chir 1881;51:801–803.
2. Oestern HJ, Echtermeyer V, Tscherne H. The compartment syndrome. Orthopäde 1983;12:34–46.
3. Bywaters EGL, Beall D. Crush injuries with impairment of renal function. Br Med J 1941;1:427–434.
4. Reszel PA, Janes JM, Spittell JA. Ischemic necrosis of the peroneal musculature, a lateral compartment syndrome: report of a case. Proc Staff Med Mayo Clin 1963;38:130–137.
5. Matsen FA. Compartmental syndromes. New York: Grune & Stratton, 1980.
6. Oestern HJ. Compartment syndrome. Definiton, etiology and pathophysiology. Unfallchirurg 1991;94:210–215.
7. Kratky V, Hurwitz JJ, Avram DR. Orbital compartment syndrome. Direct measurement of orbital tissue pressure: first technique. Can J Ophthalmol 1990;25:293–297.
8. Landi A, Schoenhuber R, Funicello R, Rasio G, Esposito M. Compartment syndrome of the scapula. Ann Hand Surg 1992;11:383–388.
9. Naidu SH, Heppenstall RB. Compartment syndrome of the forearm and hand. Hand Clin 1994;10:13–27.
10. DiFazio FA, Barth RA, Frymoyer JW. Acute lumbar paraspinal compartment syndrome: a case report. J Bone Joint Surg Am 1991;73:1101–1103.
11. Bosch U, Tscherne H. The pelvic compartment syndrome. Arch Orthop Trauma Surg 1992;111:314–317.
12. Schwartz JT Jr, Brumback RJ, Lakatos R, Poka A, Bathon GH, Burgess AR. Acute compartment syndrome of the thigh. A spectrum of injury. J Bone Joint Surg Am 1989; 71:392–400.
13. Myerson MS. Management of compartment syndromes of the foot. Clin Orthop 1991;271:239–248.
14. Echtermeyer V. The compartment syndrome. Berlin: Springer-Verlag, 1985.

15. Reschauer R. The diagnosis of compartment syndrome. Unfallchirurg 1991;94:216–219.
16. Heckmann MM, Whitesides TE Jr, Grewe SR, Judd RL, Miller M, Lawrence JH III. Histologic determination of the ischemic threshold of muscle in the canine compartment syndrome model. J Orthop Trauma 1993;7:199–210.
17. Royle SG. The role of tissue pressure recording in forearm fractures in children. Injury 1992;23:549–552.
18. Scola E. Pathophysiology and pressure monitoring in compartment syndromes. Unfallchirurg 1991;94:220–224.
19. Fishchenko PIa, Tsyretorov STs. Clinico-roentgenological characteristics of the changes in ischemic Volkmann's contracture. Ortop Travmotol Protez 1990;11:49–53.
20. Kawamura Y, Waki K, Torigoshi Y, et al. A case of rhabdomyolysis demonstrated by Tc-99m methylene diphosphate scintigraphy. Kaku Igaku 1990;27:267–271.
21. Lamminen AE, Hekali PE, Tiula E, Suramo I, Korhola OA. Acute rhabdomyolysis: evaluation with magnetic resonance imaging compared with computed tomography and ultrasound. Br J Radiol 1989;62:326–330.
22. Reimers CD, Haider M, Mehltretter G, Kääb S, Wunderer B, Pongratz DE. Rectus abdominis syndrome. Dtsch Med Wschr 1992;117:1474–1478.
23. Wiley JP, Short WB, Wiseman DA, Miller SD. Ultrasound catheter placement for deep posterior compartment pressure measurements in chronic compartment syndrome. Am J Sports Med 1990;18:74–79.
24. Strohmaier A, Friedrich M. A nontraumatic compartment syndrome of both lower legs resulting from acute rhabdomyolysis. Fortschr Röntgenstr 1991;155:277–279.
25. Landi A, De Santis G, Sacchetti GL, Ciuccarelli C, Luchetti R, Bedeschi P. The use of CT scan in evaluating Volkmann's syndrome in the limbs. Ital J Orthop Traumtol 1989;15:521–533.
26. Wegener OH. Ganzkörpercomputertomographie. Berlin: Blackwell Wissenschaft, 1992.
27. Lukosch CJ, Rominger MB, Hausmann R, Kunze K. Compartment syndrome: value of MRI. Proceedings of the Society of Magnetic Resonance. 2nd Meeting, 1994: 250.
28. Fleckenstein JL, Shellock FG. Exertional muscle injuries: MRI evaluation. Top Magn Reson Imaging 1991;3:50–70.
29. Fleckenstein JL, Chason DP, Bonte FJ, et al. High-voltage electric injury: assessment of muscle viability with MRI and Tc-99m pyrophosphate scintigraphy. Radiology 1995; 195:205–210.
30. Wolff SD, Balaban RS. Magnetization transfer imaging: practical aspects and clinical applications. Radiology 1994; 192:593–599.
31. Haaverstad R, Nilsen G, Myhre HO, Saether OD, Rinck PA. The use of MRI in the investigation of leg oedema. Eur J Vasc Surg 1992;6:124–129.
32. Fleckenstein JL, Burns D, Murphy K, Jayson H, Bonte F. Differential diagnosis of bacterial myositis in AIDS: MRI evaluation. Radiology 1991;179:653–658.
33. Shintani S, Shiigai T. Repeat MRI in acute rhabdomyolysis: correlation with clinicopathological findings. J Comput Assist Tomogr 1993;17:786–791.
34. Fleckenstein JL, Parkey RW, Peshock RM. Sports-related muscle injuries: evaluation with MRI. Radiology 1989; 172:793–798.
35. Amendola A, Rorabeck CH, Vellett D, Vezina W, Rutt B, Nott L. The use of magnetic resonance imaging in exertional compartment syndromes. Am J Sports Med 1990;18:29–34.
36. Heppenstall RB, Sapega AA, Izant T, et al. Compartment syndrome. A quantitative study of high-energy phosphorus compounds using 31P-magnetic resonance spectroscopy. J Trauma 1989;29:1113–1119.
37. Wilke N, Landsleitner B. The investigation of an acute compartment syndrome of unusual etiology using MRI (magnetic resonance imaging) and 31P-MRS (magnetic resonance spectroscopy). Handchir Mikrochir Plast Chir 1990;22:255–260.

29
Congenital Muscular Deformations

Marybeth Ezaki

Congenital muscular deformation is a category into which fall all of the developmental structural abnormalities of the musculoskeletal system. These deformations include absent, hypoplastic, enlarged, accessory, duplicated, and anomalous muscles found incidentally, or associated with congenital limb differences. The spectrum of these conditions includes isolated, clinically evident diagnoses, such as congenital absence of the sternal head of the pectoralis muscle, known as Poland syndrome (Figure 29.1),[1,2] or may involve complicated, atypical limb anomalies, such as the phocomelic or intercalary deficiencies.

This group of congenital muscular deformations is distinguished from congenital myopathies and muscular dystrophies because the physiologic, histologic, and biochemical characteristics of skeletal muscle in these conditions are normal. This category also excludes secondary deformities related to upper motor neuron diseases.

Exceptions to this group of congenital muscular deformations, although arbitrary, are the arthrogrypotic conditions. Patients with arthrogryposis have musculoskeletal deformities that are secondary to undefined neuromuscular insults to the developing limbs. Muscle quality is abnormal in that fibrous replacement of muscle occurs to a variable degree.[3] Individual muscle fibers that remain may be histologically normal. Failure of differentiation of insertional tendons, poor quality and quantity of residual muscle, and associated limb deformities are features shared with congenital muscular deformations.

Diagnostic imaging is important in the surgical planning of patients with congenital muscle deformities when it is impossible to assess the physiological quality of muscle by other means.

Developmental Background

A brief review of the embryological development of the musculoskeletal system is in order to understand the nature of the problem in imaging limb anomalies and in considering reconstructive alteration of these limbs.

During normal limb development, all connective tissue, including the skeletal structures and muscles, derive from the mesoderm. Normal function of a muscle–tendon unit, acting across a joint to move a skeletal segment, results from a carefully orchestrated series of developmental events. Differentiation occurs as the limb bud forms from proximal to distal. Muscles require innervation by nerves that derive from neurectoderm. Appropriately timed muscle contraction and appropriate location and orientation of movement are crucial to joint development as skeletal differentiation proceeds.[4] Potential errors in this sequence are many. The anterior horn cell may be defective (as is suspected to occur in some forms of arthrogryposis);[3] the muscle itself may be hypoplastic, absent, duplicated, or accessory; the muscle–tendon unit may not span the joint, or may insert incorrectly, or the joint may fail to cavitate and provide a mobile articulation.

A knowledge of the normal developmental sequence allows the examiner to make certain assumptions. If a patient is able to actively move a joint through a range of motion, one may assume that the muscle has formed, that it is innervated and under volitional control, that the tendon of insertion crosses the joint that it moves, and that the size and strength of the muscle are also appropriate for that motion segment. If this is not the case, specific investigation may define the muscle and limb status and suggest reconstructive options.

Standard Evaluation Techniques

Standard assessment of the musculoskeletal system relies upon the physical diagnostic techniques of palpation of the muscle to assess bulk, tone, and strength of contraction, measurement of active and passive joint range of motion, and assessment of stretch reflexes. Functional electrical stimulation with surface contact electrodes may add information about the contractility of a muscle and

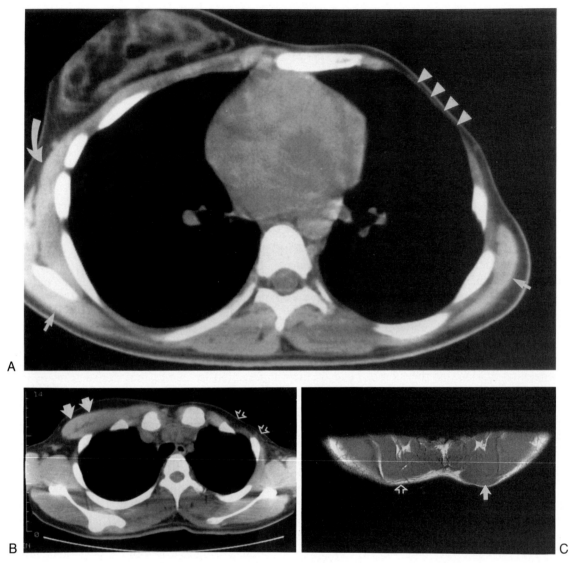

FIGURE 29.1. Congenital absence of muscles. Poland syndrome is characterized by deficient unilateral development of chest wall tissues. In a female with this condition, CT scanning was performed to aid planning of cosmetic surgery for absence of the left breast. Axial CT at the level of the heart (A) shows absence of mammary tissue and intercostal muscles on the left (arrowheads). Note that whereas the serratus anterior is present on the right (curved arrow), it is absent on the left, whereas the latissimus dorsi is present bilaterally (arrows). This informa-tion facilitated operative management in that the left latissimus dorsi was transferred as a pedicle flap for creation of an axillary fold. At a higher level, CT shows presence of normal right-sided pectoralis muscles (arrowheads, B) but absence of the same muscles on the left (open arrowheads). In a different patient, axial T_1-weighted MRI shows presence of the normal left trapezius (500/15, arrowhead, C) but absence of the same muscle on the right (open arrowhead).

whether or not joint motion can be elicited. Electrodiag-nostic techniques such as needle electromyography are rarely indicated in the congenital muscle deformations. Most congenital muscle deformations do not require sophisticated imaging techniques.

Muscle Imaging

Congenital anomalies present a different set of challenges to the imaging specialist. Reference atlases of normal anatomy often are not helpful. Image interpretation in congenital muscle deformations relies upon a knowledge of the characteristic appearance of tissue types and is independent of normal spatial relationships. In general, the imaging modality that best defines the skeletal mus-cle, myotendinous junctions, and tendon insertions is most helpful.

Imaging studies are indicated to answer specific basic questions about the morphology of muscles in congenital abnormalities. Is muscle present? From what does it originate and onto what does it insert? What is the cross-sectional area of muscle belly, as this relates directly to the potential strength of contraction?[5] Is muscle composition normal?

Standard radiographs suggest the presence of muscle by its characteristic shape and density, which may correlate with clinical findings. They do not resolve important details of origin and insertion of the relevant anatomy. Information obtained about muscular anatomy, even with soft tissue views or subtraction techniques, is often insufficient for surgical decision making.

Ultrasonography can provide information about the dimensions of muscle, but details of muscle quality, and resolution of origin, insertion, and anatomy are frequently hazy. Real-time ultrasonography can provide information about differential motion between structures.

Computerized tomography of muscle deformations provides better three-dimensional orientation than radiographs or ultrasound do, albeit at a higher cost and greater radiation dosage. Computerized tomography plays a much more important role in the evaluation of bony structures than in the study of muscle abnormality.

Muscular Variations: Isolated

Normal variations in the presence or absence, size, configuration, origin and insertion, and innervation of muscles are common. Probably the best known variable muscle is the palmaris longus, absent in 11.2% of the population,[6] but more noticeable muscular absences such as the pectoralis major[1,2] or trapezius[7] also occur (Figure 29.1).

Accessory and anomalous muscles are often found incidentally at surgical procedures for other conditions, by antomists in their dissection, and by imaging radiologists. They are frequently of no clinical significance, representing variations on an otherwise broadly normal theme, but may present as palpable masses simulating neoplasms.[8] Named examples of these muscles are numerous, particularly in the leg and ankle, and include accessory calf and popliteal muscles (Figure 29.2).[5,9–12]

Another example of isolated muscular variations offers an alternative for reconstruction when it is found. The extensor carpi radialis intermedius is an extra muscle with a definable origin and insertion, making it available as a donor for tendon transfer. The extensor carpi radialis accessorius, however, is an additional tendinous slip arising from either the extensor carpi radialis longus or brevis and is not a separate muscle.[13] Variability in numbers of muscles within a functional group is not uncommon, other examples of which include the peroneus tertius and quartus.[7,14,15]

Relative contributions of component parts of complex muscles may vary, as in the variable vasti and rectus configuration of the quadriceps mechanism.[16] Confluence of usually separate muscles may be clinically evident, as in the lack of independence of the flexor pollicis longus from the index profundus muscle.

At times, secondary deformity may occur either due to, or in conjunction with, aberrant muscles. An anomalous muscle can produce skeletal deformity by exerting its pull on an immature skeleton. An example is camptodactyly, a flexion deformity of the proximal interphalangeal joint of the finger, where the deforming force may be the anomalous insertion of the small finger intrinsic or superficialis muscle. An example of an anomalous muscle's presence in a more dramatic condition occurs in Madelung's deformity. The pronator quadratus muscle is often enlarged in this progressive deformity of the distal radius.[17] The radius bows with radial and dorsal convexity, and growth of the ulnar and volar distal radial physis is disturbed (Figure 29.3).

MRI has recently confirmed anatomic descriptions of surgeons and has replaced dissection as the primary means of defining these interesting variations. It is highly attractive as a diagnostic tool because of its ability to characterize the composition of soft tissue. It is specific enough in diagnosing muscular variation to preclude the need for exploration and biopsy when anomalous muscles present as soft tissue masses.[8]

Muscular Variations with Associated Anomalies

Muscle deformities are a part of nearly all the limb anomalies. Aberrant formation, differentiation, migration, or segmentation of the developing limb will also affect muscles. The muscular component of the limb difference may be the primary functional impediment but often is only part of a larger morphologic challenge. An example of a complex malformation is Sprengel's deformity, characterized by abnormal formation and subsequent failure of descent of the scapula from its origin as a cervical structure to its normal position on the dorsal chest wall (Figure 29.4). Other examples are cases of limb hypertrophy with generalized unilateral muscle enlargement. Idiopathic cases are rare and poorly understood; imaging is necessary to diagnose possible underlying vascular or neoplastic conditions (Figure 29.5). Multimodality imaging studies are often needed to adequately evaluate anatomy in planning surgery in children with complex congenital limb deformities. (Figures 29.6, 29.7).

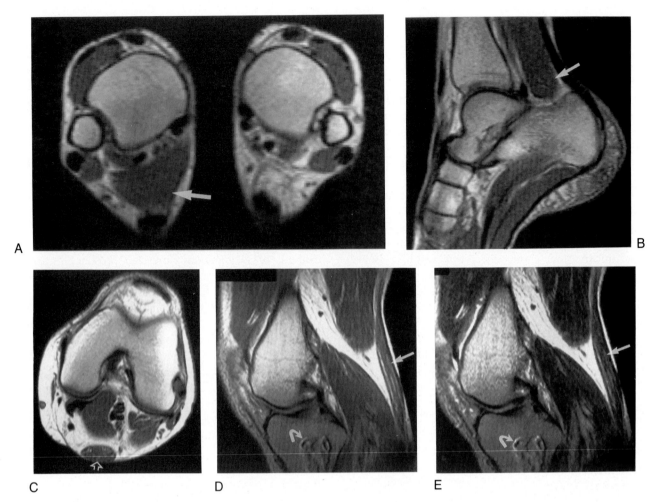

FIGURE 29.2. Accessory muscles. MRI was performed in these two patients for palpable soft tissue "masses." In the first patient, axial (A) and sagittal (B) MRI reveals an accessory soleus muscle on the right, deep to the Achilles tendon (500/20, arrows). The muscle showed signal intensity equal to other muscles on all imaging sequences (not shown). MRI of a second patient, who presented with a popliteal "mass," simi-larly shows the "mass" to consist of normal muscle. Axial T_1-weighted image reveals a superficially located, smoothly marginated muscle (C, 500/15, arrowhead) whereas sagittal spin density (D, 2500/30) and T_2-weighted (E, 2500/80) images reveal the longitudinal configuration of the accessory muscle, tensor fascia suralis (arrows). (C-E republished from AJR 1995;165:1220–1221).

FIGURE 29.3. Madelung's deformity. Anteroposterior radiograph shows deformity, including notching of ulnar aspect of distal radius (A, arrow). Oblique, longitudinal CT hints at enlarged pronator quadratus palmar and ulnar to radius, particularly by visibility of bowed pronator fat plane (B, arrows). Bony metaphyseal notch (arrowhead) represents site of abnormal attachment of fibrous volar capsule.

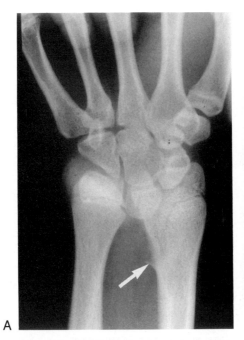

A

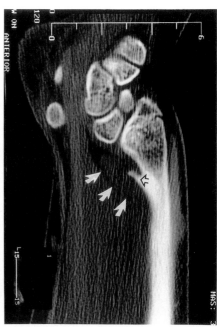

B

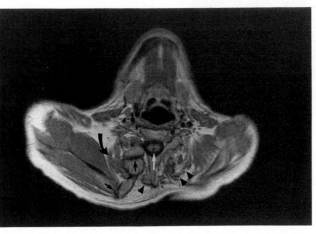

A

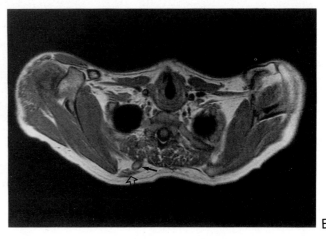

B

FIGURE 29.4. Sprengel's deformity. Axial T_1-weighted MRI at lower cervical level (A, 500/15) shows two articulations of omovertebral bone (black arrows) and spinal cord diaschisis (small white arrow). Note atrophic paraspinal muscles (black arrowheads) and unnamed anomalous muscle (curved arrow). More caudal image shows inferior aspect of omovertebral bone (B, arrow) and associated unnamed superficial muscle (arrowhead).

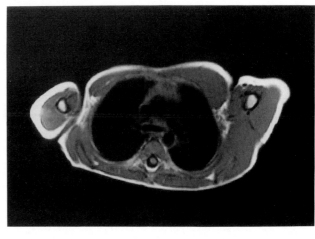

FIGURE 29.5. Idiopathic muscle hypertrophy. Unilateral prominence of left upper arm strength was associated with diffusely enlarged left-sided chest, arm, and back muscles on MRI (500/15). MRI supported the clinical impression of absence of associated abnormalities.

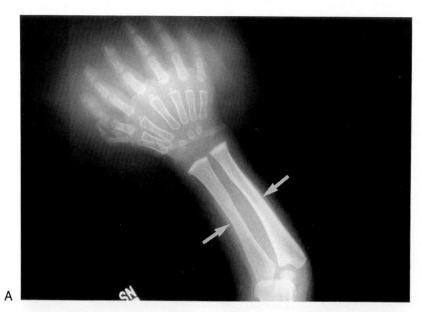

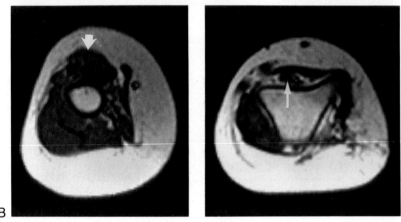

FIGURE 29.6. Complex limb deformity: ulnar dimelia. Anteroposterior radiograph shows "mirror hand," polydactyly, and two ulnae (arrows, A). Electrically responsive muscle was present volar to the humerus but elbow flexion was not elicited. Axial T_1-weighted MRI confirms the presence of normal appearing muscle at the midhumerus level (B, 500/15, arrow) that tapered to a tendon proximal to the anomalous elbow (C, 500/15, arrow). The tendon was surgically transferred to a proximal ulna to provide elbow flexion.

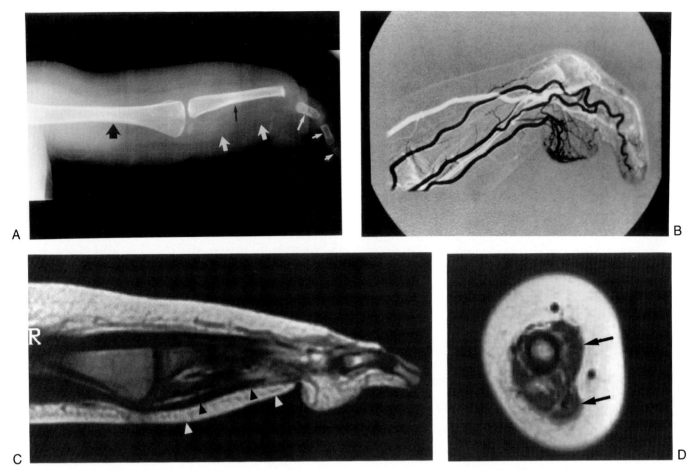

FIGURE 29.7. Complex congenital limb deformities. This infant presented with proximal absence of right upper limb, clinical evidence of left humeroradial synostosis in extension, and a single nonfunctional segmented digit with passive motion only. Longitudinal radiograph of left upper limb (A) reveals well-formed humerus (black arrowhead), and single forearm bone (black arrow), metacarpal (white arrow), and phalanges (small arrows). Note subtle appearance of forearm muscles (white arrowheads). Digital subtraction arteriogram of left forearm and hand (B) reveals the relevant arteries (black) and veins (white). Sagittal T_1-weighted MRI (500/15, C) in orientation similar to radiograph shows superior contrast resolution between subcutaneous fat (white arrowheads) and flexor muscles (black arrowheads). Axial T_1-weighted MRI 2 cm distal to humeroradial junction (500/15, arrows, D) confirms presence of forearm flexor muscles (500/15, arrows, D). These imaging studies facilitated surgical planning of prolongation tendon graft performed to motor the single digit. Flexion osteotomy of the distal humerus was performed during the same operation.

Summary

A brief review of the development of the limb musculoskeletal system has been provided in the context of how it relates to planning for reconstructive procedures in conditions of congenital musculoskeletal deformation. Standard clinical modalities for assessment of the musculoskeletal system usually suffice in guiding preoperative decision making. Specific cases that illustrate how imaging plays a role in surgical planning are discussed. MRI provides a versatile tool in defining congenital muscular deformations. Muscle quality, size, cross-sectional area, orientation, and specifics of origin and insertion are well imaged by MRI. MRI also offers the advantage of a high degree of safety, an issue of particular importance in pediatrics, the patient group in which operative management of these deformities is most often contemplated.

References

1. Poland A. Deficiency of the pectoralis major muscles. Guy's Hosp Rep 1841;6:191.
2. Wright AR, Milner RH, Bainbridge LC, Wilson JB. MRI and CT in the assessment of Poland syndrome. J Comput Assist Tomogr 1992;16:442–447.
3. Swinyard CA, Bleck EE. The etiology of arthrogryposis (multiple congenital contractures). Clin Orthop Rel Res 1985;194:15–27.
4. Uhthoff HK. The embryology of the human locomotor system. Berlin: Springer-Verlag, 1990.
5. Boyes JH. Selections of a donor muscle for tendon transfer. Bull Hosp Jt Dis 1961;21:97–105.
6. Bergman RA, Thompson SA, Afifi AK, et al. Compendium of human anatomic variation. Text, atlas, world literature. Baltimore: Urban & Schwarzenberg, 1988.
7. Selden BR. Congenital absence of trapezius and rhomboideus major muscles. J Bone Joint Surg 1935;17:1058–1059.
8. Paul MA, Imansc J, Golding RP, Loomen AR, Meijer S. Accessory soleus muscle mimicking a soft tissue tumor. Acta Orthop Scand 1991;62:609–611.
9. Bejjani FJ, Jahss MH (translators). Le Double's study of muscle variations of the human body. Part I: Muscle variations of the leg. Foot Ankle 1985;6:111–134.
10. Bejjani FJ, Jahss MH (translators). Le Double's study of muscle variations of the human body. Part II: Muscle variations of the foot. Foot Ankle 1986;6:157–176.
11. Bonnell J, Cruess RL. Anomalous insertion of soleus muscle as a cause of fixed equinus deformity. A case report. J Bone Joint Surg 1969;51A:999–1000.
12. Eckstrom JE, Shuman WP, Hack LA. MRI of accessory soleus muscle. J Comput Assis Tomogr 1990;14:239–242.
13. LeClerq C. Are the radial supernumerary muscles suitable for transfer? Presented at Fourth International Congress on Upper Extremity Reconstruction in Tetraplegia. Palo Alto, CA, 1991.
14. Buschmann WR, Cheung Y, Jahss MH. Magnetic resonance imaging of anomalous leg muscles: accessory soleus, peroneus quartus and the flexor digitorum longus accessorius. Foot Ankle 1991;12:109–116.
15. Krammer EB, Lischka MF, Gruber H. Gross anatomy and evolutionary significance of the human peroneus III. Anat Embryol 1979;155:291–302.
16. Willan PLT, Mahon M, Golland JA. Morphological variations of the human vastus lateralis muscle. J Anat 1990;168:235–239.
17. Linscheid RL. Madelung's deformity. Correspondence Newsletter No 24. American Society for Surgery of the Hand, 1979.

30
Muscle Viability

James L. Fleckenstein, David P. Chason, Robert W. Parkey, John L. Hunt, Gary F. Purdue, and Dennis K. Burns

Muscle viability is an important clinical issue confronting surgeons who manage severe muscle injury. This is because nonviable muscle, aside from being nonfunctional, is at high risk for infection. Because the determination of tissue viability is so important in patients with severe muscle necrosis, they may be subjected to multiple operations in vigilance of avoiding sepsis.

High-voltage electrical injuries of the extremities are perhaps the most difficult for a surgeon to deal with because the path of the electrical current is so destructive and unpredictable, frequently coursing through electrically conductive vascular, neural, and muscular pathways, coagulating blood and impeding oxygen delivery to tissues in the process. Rhabdomyolysis, from severe muscle necrosis, may itself be life-threatening, due to associated hyperkalemia, myoglobinuria, and acute renal failure.[1,2]

Another situation in which muscle viability is important to surgeons is when muscle–tendon units are employed as flaps for coverage in plastic procedures or when they are transferred in patients with congenital or posttraumatic musculotendinous dysfunction.[3] A third example where muscle viability may be critical to determine is in the setting of compartment syndromes of the extremities (see Chapter 28). Finally, assessment of muscle viability in vascular insufficiency is potentially important.[4–6]

Diagnostic imaging in these situations, as in other muscle disorders, allows the surgeon to noninvasively probe beyond the relatively bland surface of the skin to assess the extent and quality of underlying skeletal muscle. The ability of imaging to localize severe muscle injury and characterize the degree of perfusion, and hence viability, of muscle can have obvious importance in the clinical management of these patients.

Skeletal Muscle Viability: Scintigraphic Evaluation

Pioneering attempts to detect nonviable muscle in situations of severe myonecrosis and electrical injuries employed a radionuclide method of quantitating myocardial necrosis following infarction.[7,8] The mechanism of the technique was shown to occur via irreversibly injured ischemic muscle cells accumulating ^{99m}technetium-labeled pyrophosphates (^{99m}Tc-PYP) through cell membrane disruption and subsequent mitochondrial chelation.[9–11] Triple-phase ^{99m}Tc-PYP scintigraphy has since become a critical element in the preoperative management of patients with electrical injuries of the extremities by both assessing tissue perfusion and localizing necrotic muscle prior to surgical exploration of the traumatized tissue.

Limitations of scintigraphic evaluation of muscle damage include poor spatial resolution, restricted number of body regions that can be studied dynamically, and difficulty in discriminating injured but viable tissue from injured, nonviable tissue. Although the technique is clearly valuable in high-voltage electrical injuries, there remains a need for a method that is more specific in identifying nonviable tissue and that provides optimal anatomic localization of damaged muscle.

Skeletal Muscle Viability: MRI Evaluation

MRI is sensitive to muscle necrosis,[12,13] thermal burns,[14] and can assess tissue perfusion.[15] Its spatial resolution is far superior to that available with scintigraphy. It was for these reasons that it was evaluated as a preoperative aid in the assessment of muscle damage in electrical injuries.[16] That study compared the utility of gadolinium-enhanced MRI to triple-phase ^{99m}Tc-PYP scintigraphy in assessing muscle viability in 12 surgically evaluated limbs. Scintigraphy and MRI revealed muscle abnormalities in all patients. MRI provided superior anatomical localization of discrete regions or muscle necrosis compared to scintigraphy (Figures 30.1 to 30.4).

In eight limbs not requiring amputation, initial and "blood pool" scintigrams revealed increased or normal blood flow and no zone of absent tracer activity to promote the possibility of nonperfused tissue. In the same cases, delayed scintigrams revealed discrete volumes of muscle that had increased nuclide accumulation, consistent with necrosis. Necrotic muscle in these cases displayed edema, characterized by increased signal intensity on T_2-weighted images and little if any alteration on T_1-weighted images (Figures 30.2, 30.3), consistent with the known increase in proton T_1 and T_2 relaxation times of injured muscle.[12] Edematous muscles in these cases enhanced following gadolinium infusion on T_1-weighted images (Figures 30.2, 30.3), were found to be viable at surgery, and were variably necrotic when examined histopathologically. This was termed a type 1 edema pattern, in which edematous, necrotic muscle enhanced with gadolinium, indicating intact perfusion and therefore potential viability.

In four nonviable limbs, initial and "blood pool" scintigrams revealed a distinct zone demarcating distal, nonperfused portions of the limbs from more proximal, relatively well-perfused limbs. This transitional zone of muscle showed marked avidity for ^{99m}Tc-PYP on delayed scintigrams (Figure 30.4). Proximal to the transitional zone, MRI showed type 1 changes, as described above. At the transitional zone, MRI showed edematous muscle that did not enhance with gadolinium infusion. This type 2 edema pattern represented nonperfused and nonviable tissue at surgery. In the transitional zone, therefore, gadolinium infusion was able to distinguish between perfused (potentially viable) and nonperfused (nonviable) muscle tissue.

Distal to the zone of transition between perfused and nonperfused segments, another MRI pattern, type 3, was observed, in which little, if any, signal abnormality was apparent on T_1- or T_2-weighted images and in which gadolinium infusion failed to result in visible enhancement. Surgery, in these cases, revealed nonviable tissue necessitating amputation (Figure 30.4). It was concluded that MRI with gadolinium can distinguish zones of potential viability within radionuclide-avid tissue. However, better perfusion sensitivity was felt to be needed if MRI is to be solely depended upon to assess muscle viability after high-voltage injuries.

MRI evaluation of muscle viability following muscle–tendon grafting in humans has yet to be rigorously evaluated. However, a study in an animal model,[3] like the human study of electrical injuries,[16] found that gadolinium infusion is able to distinguish viable from nonviable muscle grafts by the fact that edematous muscle that is viable enhances upon gadolinium infusion whereas edematous muscle that is nonviable does not enhance. These principles were applied to a patient with clinical suspicion of a nonviable rectus muscle flap used to treat an open skull fracture. The rectus muscle was found to be edematous but did not enhance following gadolinium infusion, accounting for the radiologic conclusion of nonviability. Surgery confirmed that impression (Figure 30.5).

Muscle infarction is an uncommon form of severe muscle necrosis in which the viability of muscle may be an important clinical concern. Although such a finding may occur in patients with perpheral vascular disease and hypercoagulable states (such as sickle cell anemia), imaging findings in these disorders have yet to be reported. Diagnostic imaging findings in spontaneous muscle infarction have, however, been reported in patients with diabetes mellitus.

Spontaneous muscle infarction is an uncommon but distinct complication of severe diabetes mellitus characterized by a typical clinical presentation.[4–6] Abrupt onset of muscle pain, usually in the thigh, persists during rest and increases greatly with exercise. A firm and exquisitely tender mass is often palpable and biopsy demonstrates areas of infarction. This condition resembles other muscle disorders on MRI by the presence of edema, usually being isointense with normal muscle on T_1-weighted images and hyperintense on T_2-weighted or STIR images. Ultrasound and CT provide relatively less information, being limited in contrast resolution (Figure 30.6). Although the mechanism of the injury is believed to be on an ischemic basis, gadolinium infusion may result in modest enhancement of the lesion on T_1-weighted images,[4,5] implying that perfusion of tissue, although attenuated, is not totally absent. This finding may explain why patients tend to recover with only conservative management. Muscle biopsy is considered by some to be excessively invasive when given the appropriate clinical setting because the biopsy procedure itself, or vigorous stretching of the muscle before healing, may contribute to subsequent hematoma formation and further disruption of the remaining tissue.[4] Failure to recognize the syndrome has led to unnecessary and extensive surgical procedures and overenthusiastic physical therapies, including exercise protocols which prolong recovery.

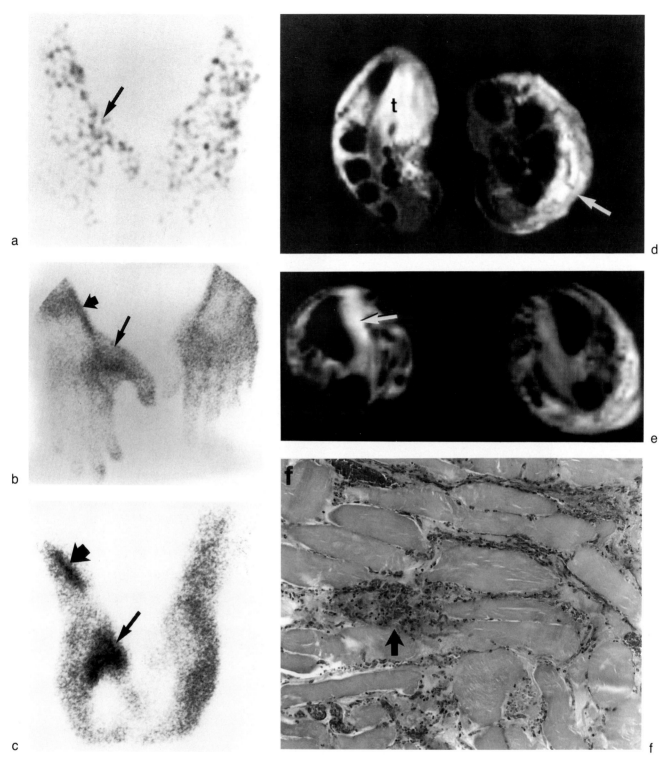

FIGURE 30.1. High-voltage, soft tissue injury of the hands as studied by triple-phase ^{99m}technetium pyrophosphate scintigraphy and unenhanced MRI. Scintigrams reveal increased tracer delivery to the right hand (arrow), as shown by subtle increased activity on 7-s (a) and more intense asymmetry on "blood pool" scintigram (b). After a 2-h delay, increased tracer activity is seen in the thenar muscles (c). Pronator quadratus abnormality was also evident on (b) and (c) as a linear area of radioactivity (arrowhead). Axial STIR image of the hands shows necrosis-related edema in the right thenar muscles (t) and the subcutaneous tissues of the left hand (arrow, 1500/ 30/95, d). Using the same sequence, signal increases are easily seen in part of the right pronator quadratus (arrow, e). A photomicrograph of longitudinally oriented skeletal muscle fibers from pronator quadratus exhibits typical features of coagulation necrosis, including a loss of fine cellular detail and absence of stainable nuclei. Extravasated erythrocytes and a scanty accumulation of neutrophils are present in the interstitium (arrow, f, hematoxylin and eosin, ×125). (Permission from Fleckenstein JL, Chason DP, Bonte FJ, et al. High-voltage electric injury: assessment of muscle viability with MR imaging and Tc-99m pyrophosphate scintigraphy. Radiology 1995;195: 205–210.)

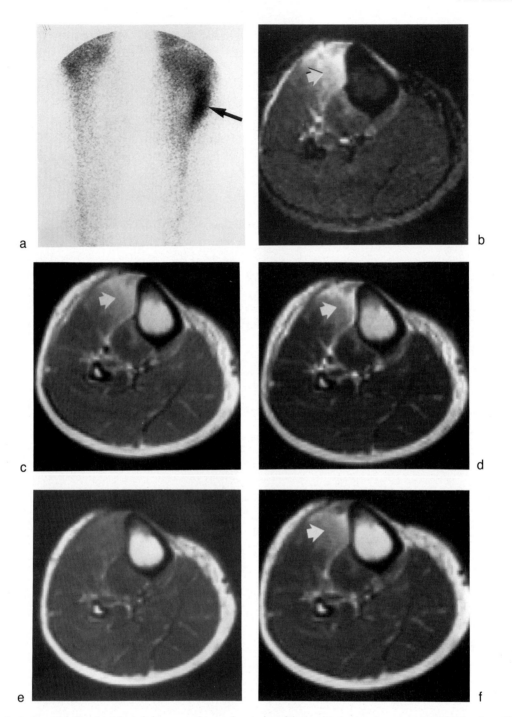

FIGURE 30.2. Anterior tibialis electrical injury as shown by
^{99m}technetium pyrophosphate and gadolinium-enhanced MRI.
Delayed phase scintigram reveals focal increased tracer
accumulation in the left leg, projected over the proximal tibia
(arrow, a). Axial edema-sensitive MRI sequences localize
necrosis-related edema to the anterior tibialis (arrowhead),
including STIR (1500/30/100, b), proton density (2000/30, c)
and T_2-weighted (2000/60, d). Using a T_1-weighted sequence,
signal intensity is nearly normal (500/30, e) until gadolinium-
DTPA is infused, after which signal is increased due to accumulation of the paramagnetic chelate in the extracellular space
and consequent shortening of the T_1 relaxation time (f).
(Permission from Fleckenstein JL, Chason DP, Bonte FJ, et al.
Highvoltage electric injury: assessment of muscle viability
with MR imaging and Tc-99m pyrophosphate scintigraphy.
Radiology 1995;195:205–210.)

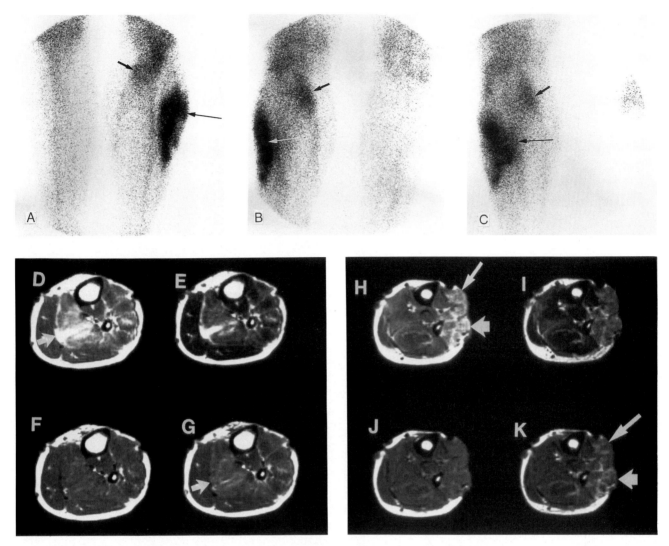

FIGURE 30.3. Superior spatial localization of muscle necrosis using MRI compared to ⁹⁹ᵐtechnetium pyrophosphate. Delayed phase scintigram of the legs 2 h after injection shows markedly increased tracer activity (long arrow) projected lateral to the proximal tibia on anterior (A) and posterior (B) views, and anterior to the tibia on the lateral (C) view. A second area of increased activity in the proximal leg (small arrow) is projected medial to the tibia on the anterior (A) and posterior views (B) and posterior to the tibia on the lateral view (C). Localization of these areas of muscle damage is more clearly demonstrated by MRI. MRI reveals that the more proximal abnormality seen on scintigraphy reflects soleus edema (arrowhead, 2000/30, D). Note that edema is also visible on a 2000/60 sequence (E) but is invisible on a T_1-weighted image (500/30, F), unless gadolinium is infused (arrowhead, 500/30, G). The more distal focus of muscle damage is shown by MRI to occur in the peroneal (arrowhead) and anterior tibialis (arrow) muscles, and is especially conspicuous on proton density (2000/30, H) and T_2-weighted images (2000/60, I). Gadolinium results in enhancement of necrotic muscles (500/30 pre-gadolinium, J; 500/30 post-gadolinium, K). (Permission from Fleckenstein JL, Chason DP, Bonte FJ, et al. High-voltage electric injury: assessment of muscle viability with MR imaging and Tc-99m pyrophosphate scintigraphy. Radiology 1995;195: 205–210.)

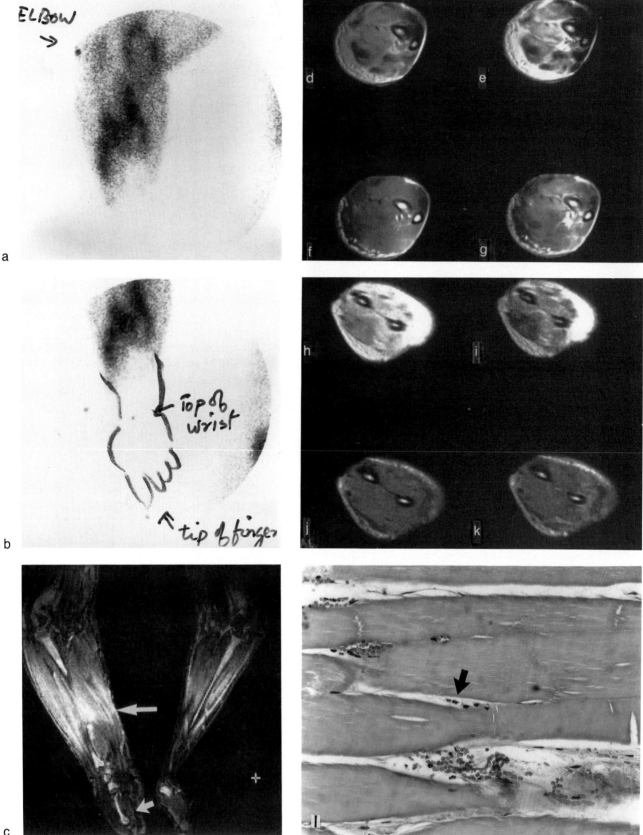

FIGURE 30.4. Tissue viability after electrical injury: limitation of MRI assessment of tissue viability. Triple-phase [99m]technetium pyrophosphate scintigrams revealed absence of tracer delivery (blood flow) to the hand and distal forearm. Delayed scintigrams of the proximal (a) and distal (b) forearm were marked by the technologist for anatomic orientation, and clinically, the hand was nonviable, requiring amputation. Gadolinium-enhanced MRI was preoperatively performed to assess necrotic muscle and tissue viability. A coronal post-gadolinium infusion T_1-weighted image shows signal intensity enhancement in the midforearm (100/20, 70°, arrow, c), corresponding to the zone of marked abnormality on scintigrams. Note that signal intensity is normal in the hand (arrowhead, c). The fact that MRI may be normal-appearing in a region of irreversibly injured muscle is further evident by comparing axial images obtained in the proximal forearm (d–g) to those obtained at the level of the hand (h–k). In the proximal forearm, striking edema is characterized by increased signal intensity on proton density (2000/30, d) and T_2-weighted (2000/60, e) but not on T_1-weighted image (500/30, f). Gadolinium infusion results in enhancement on T_1-weighted image in all muscles showing edema on 2000/30 and 2000/60 images (500/30, g). At the level of the hand, severely necrotic muscle has a nearly normal appearance on edema-sensitive images (2000/30, h; 2000/60, i), wrongly suggesting good tissue health. Lack of enhancement with gadolinium appears to support this impression (500/30, pre-gadolinium, j; 500/30, post-gadolinium, k). The case indicates the need for improved perfusion sensitivity if MRI is relied upon to determine tissue perfusion, and therefore viability, in the setting of severe ischemic injury. A photomicrograph of skeletal muscle fibers from the distal surgical amputation margin demonstrates global coagulation necrosis of skeletal muscle fibers. Scattered extravasated red blood cells and an occasional neutrophil are visible in the interstitium (arrow, l, hematoxylin and eosin, ×250). (Permission from Fleckenstein JL, Chason DP, Bonte FJ, et al. High-voltage electric injury: assessment of muscle viability with MR imaging and Tc-99m pyrophosphate scintigraphy. Radiology 1995;195:205–210.)

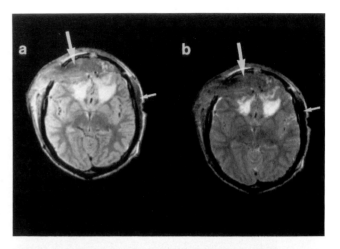

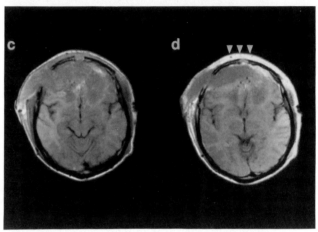

FIGURE 30.5. MRI of nonviable muscle graft. Viability of a rectus flap used for closure of an open head wound was of clinical concern. Axial SD (2000/30, a) and T_2-weighted (2000/60, b) images show mild edema, characterized by greater signal intensity in the flap (arrow) compared to temporalis (small arrow). On T_1-weighted image, signal intensity of the flap is only minimally increased prior to gadolinium infusion (500/30, c). Using the same T_1-weighted sequence, gadolinium infusion results in marked enhancement of scalp edema (500/30, arrowheads, d) but not of the edematous flap. Nonperfusion of the flap was therefore diagnosed radiologically and surgery confirmed this impression.

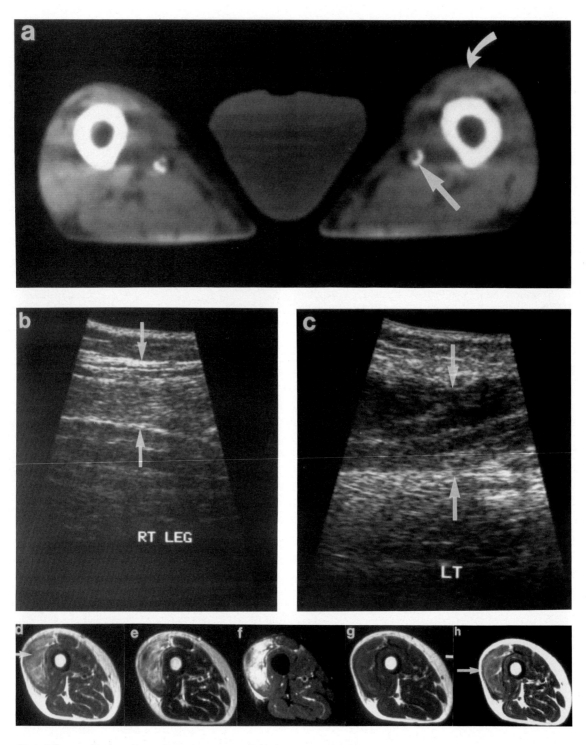

FIGURE 30.6. Diagnostic imaging of spontaneous diabetic muscle infarction in three patients. In the first patient (a), CT of the thighs reveals dense calcification of femoral arteries (arrow) and mild swelling of the infarcted left rectus femoris muscle (curved arrow). In the second patient, ultrasound longitudinal scan (7.5 mHz) of the normal right medial thigh demonstrates normal gracilis muscle echogenicity and fascial planes (between arrows, b). Longitudinal image of the contralateral gracilis reveals an oblong mass-like region of heterogeneously decreased echogenicity (arrows, c). No evidence of acoustic shadowing or through transmission/cystic change is seen. Axial MRI in third patient shows edema within the right vastus lateralis (arrow), as characterized by increased signal intensity on edema-sensitive sequences (2000/30, d; 2000/60, e; and STIR, 1500/100/30, f), and only normal signal intensity on T_1-weighted image (500/30, g). Post-gadolinium T_1-weighted image shows mild enhancement of the abnormal vastus lateralis (arrow, 500/30, h). (Permission from Chason DP, Fleckenstein JL, Burns DK, Rojas G. Diabetic muscle infaction: radiologic evaluation. Skeletal Radiology (in press 1996).)

Conclusion

When the viability of severely traumatized muscle is of clinical concern, scintigraphic localization of perfusion defects and foci of muscle necrosis is firmly established as useful. Preliminary data suggest that MRI can improve the anatomic distribution of muscle damage and, with gadolinium chelates, can further characterize muscle as edematous and perfused (potentially viable), edematous but not perfused (potentially nonviable), and non-edematous. Early limitations of MRI in identifying the most severe ischemic muscle injuries because of a peculiarly normal appearance of muscle in that condition will likely be overcome with improved availability of flow-sensitive MRI sequences.

References

1. Hunt JL, Mason AD Jr, Masterson TS, et al. The patho-physiology of acute electric injuries. J Trauma 1976;16:335–350.
2. Hunt JL, Sato RM, Baxter CR. Acute electric burns. Arch Surg 1980;115:434–438.
3. Varnell RM, Flint PW, Dalley RW, Maravilla KR, Cummings CW, Shuman WP. Myocutaneous flap failure: early detection with Gd-DTPA-enhanced MR imaging. Radiology 1989;173:755–758.
4. Chester CS, Banker EQ. Focal infarction of muscle in diabetics. Diabetes Care 1986;9:623–630.
5. Chason DP, Fleckenstein JL, Burns DK, Rojas G. Diabetic muscle infarction: radiologic evaluation. Skeletal Radiol 1996 (in press).
6. Hinton A, Heinrich SD, Craver R. Idiopathic muscular infarction: the role of ultrasound, CT, MRI and biopsy. Orthop Grand Rounds 1993;16:623–625.
7. Chang LY, Yang JY. The role of bone scans in electric burns. Burns 1991;17:250–253.
8. Hunt J, Lewis S, Parkey R, Baxter C. The use of technetium-99m stannous pyrophosphate scintigraphy to identify muscle damage in acute electric burns. Trauma 1979;19:409–413.
9. Bonte FJ, Parkey RW, Graham KD, et al. A new method for radionuclide imaging of myocardial infarcts. Radiology 1974;110:473–474.
10. Buja LM, Tofe AJ, Kulkarni PV, et al. Sites and mechanisms of localization of technetium-99m phosphorus radiopharmaceuticals in acute myocardial infarcts and other tissues. J Clin Invest 1977;60:724–740.
11. Parkey RW, Buja LM, Tofe AJ, et al. Pathophysiology of myocardial infarct scintigraphy with technetium-99m pyrophosphate, technetium-99m diphosphonate and thallium-201. Circulation 1974;50:540–546.
12. Herfkens RJ, Sievers R, Kaufman L, et al. Nuclear magnetic resonance imaging of the infarcted muscle: a rat model. Radiology 1983;147:761–764.
13. Zagoria RJ, Karstaedt N, Koubek TD. MR imaging of rhabdomyolysis. J Comput Assist Tomogr 1986;10:268–270.
14. Kurdle WA, Narayana PA, Dunsford HA. Magnetic resonance imaging of burn injury in rats. Magn Reson Imaging 1991;9:533–543.
15. Edelman RR, Mattle HP, Atkinson DJ, et al. Cerebral blood flow: assessment with dynamic contrast-enhanced T2*-weighted MR imaging at 1.5 T. Radiology 1990;176:211–220.
16. Fleckenstein J, Chason DP, Bonte FJ, et al. High-voltage electric injury: assessment of muscle viability with MR imaging and Tc-99m pyrophosphate scintigraphy. Radiology 1995;195:205–210.

31
Neoplasms and Mass Lesions Involving Muscle

Paul T. Weatherall and Gerhard E. Maale

The ability of MRI to demonstrate soft tissue lesions is unexcelled by other imaging methods as reported by many authors since 1984.[1-13] The sensitivity and discriminating ability of MRI for muscle and connective tissue pathology is shown throughout this book. The majority of this discussion will center on its use in evaluation of mass-like lesions involving muscle. The combination of clinical history and computed tomographic (CT) or plain x-ray imaging techniques has frequently provided valuable anatomic information and occasionally a specific diagnosis of lesions involving muscle.[2,14-22] Although not as anatomically precise, the utility of ultrasound and nuclear medicine techniques have been documented on many occasions[21-34] and continue to remain useful. State-of-the-art ultrasound and ionizing radiation techniques used for muscle imaging are discussed in Chapters 1 and 2. As more experience is gained in evaluating soft tissues with MRI, the distinctive patterns of injury and their variants are being recognized and the number of misdiagnoses are becoming fewer for those who have gained experience in this area of MRI. The experience gained by radiologists has allowed greater diagnostic specificity in the routine clinical settings. This is expected to continue with further usage of MRI for muscle evaluation.

The differentiation of neoplastic processes of the soft tissue and nonneoplastic pathology such as muscle contusions, hematomas, infections, and sterile inflammatory processes is not always possible. The lack of specificity of MRI signal differences in muscle diseases is partially due to the limited response of muscle and related connective tissues to various pathologic processes and injuries. Despite this, many lesions can be reliably distinguished the majority of the time using MRI. This includes several benign neoplasms and most of the nonneoplastic mass-like lesions involving muscles. The emphasis in this chapter will be the use of proper technique, avoidance of MRI misdiagnoses of soft tissue mass lesions, and description of the lesions that can usually be recognized by their MRI features. The importance of precise tumor staging and the surgical perspective on present day staging and posttreatment imaging studies will also be discussed.

Imaging Techniques

The approach for optimal imaging of musculoskeletal soft tissue neoplasms requires a combination of techniques in most cases. High-resolution imaging is required for precise definition of the internal architecture and margins of the neoplasm. Determining the presence or absence of involvement of adjacent anatomic compartments and neurovascular structures is paramount. This frequently determines whether limb-sparing surgery can be performed. Complete coverage of the involved compartment is also required when aggressive lesions are being evaluated as skip metastases may be present.

Ultrasound and CT were previously considered to be the optimal combination of imaging techniques for visualizing soft tissue tumors.[21,22] Ultrasound was shown to provide information concerning the delineation of superficial soft tissue lesions.[24] Complete evaluation of deep lesions, however, remained difficult. In most instances, ultrasound can readily discriminate between cystic and solid structures and also detect areas of liquefactive necrosis within solid neoplasms or abscesses. This allows the use of ultrasound for direct visualization during biopsy. The diagnosis and immediate drainage of abscesses also becomes relatively easy using ultrasound.

CT scanning provides much better soft tissue definition of both superficial and deep lesions when compared with plain x-ray and plain tomographic technique.[25] Its ability to detect subtle calcification or characteristic mineralization pattern remains unsurpassed. Appreciation of involvement of adjacent bone and periosteum is sometimes less obvious using CT compared to bone scintigraphy, and certain MRI techniques remain more sensitive. CT with contrast provides valuable information concerning lesion vascularity and anatomic location simultaneously, and with superior resolution compared to radionuclide techniques.

The numerous available radionuclides provide an arsenal of techniques to evaluate soft tissue masses.[25,26] Those in common use are limited to ^{67}Ga citrate for tumors[27-29] and chronic infections,[34] technetium-99 compounds for neoplasms[33] and muscle injury, and indium-111 WBC studies for acute infections.[30] PET scanners are still not common outside of research and government institutions. The advantage of most of the nuclear medicine techniques is the ease of evaluating the whole body during a single exam. High resolution, high-count technetium-99 bone scans can also be used for detecting soft tissue tumor involvement of adjacent bones.[31] Unfortunately, in the case of muscle and other soft tissue masses, there is very little specificity in the patterns of radiotracer uptake,[26,27,29,33] even when using some monoclonal antibody-labeled compounds.[32] There still remain many diagnostic needs for which radionuclide studies provide an excellent answer, with examples including metastatic and infection workups, and for specific diagnosis of lesions such as myositis ossificans.

MRI often provides an ideal assessment of the clinically important features of a soft tissue mass. Despite its high, but decreasing expense (vs. CT), it is frequently cost-effective when used as one of the initial exams following plain radiography. Avoidance of surgical or radiation therapy staging error is of the utmost importance for the patient and the health care system as a whole. MRI can provide strong clues to the specific diagnosis; however its most important contribution is usually the accurate staging of the lesion. This requires proper technique and attention to detail which often necessitates active monitoring of the exam. High-resolution images are required, usually in multiple orientations. Submillimeter in-plane spatial resolution is required for optimal evaluation of anatomic interfaces and the internal architecture of the mass, and should be obtained whenever feasible. The choice of orientation of the imaging plane is also very important. Transaxial cross-sectional techniques are the primary means of evaluating the limbs, as the compartments are oriented longitudinally. There are few exceptions to this in the extremities. Axial orientation views are also used in the torso as they are perpendicular to the vertical axis of the posterior paraspinous and psoas muscles, and the majority of the pelvic musculature. Long axis views in the sagittal and coronal planes are primarily utilized for localization which includes measurement from landmarks that are fluoroscopically identifiable. They also provide a better sense of the size and position of the lesion in a larger frame of reference. Coronal and sagittal images are also necessary when the margins of a neoplasm are near critical anatomic

structures, superiorly or inferiorly. When an aggressive lesion is suspected, the entire anatomic compartment may need to be evaluated. In the extremities, this usually requires the use of an additional separate coil, usually the transmit/receive body coil, although smaller flexible body/extremity coils can also be utilized. The head coil will frequently allow full visualization of the length of the forearm. Lesions in the upper arm are usually the most difficult to evaluate on most systems and more time may need to be allotted for these exams. There are many system-specific techniques which are invaluable for the diagnostician that are not fully known to us and cannot be included in this short discussion; attention to detail will be the guiding principle to successful imaging of these lesions.

Imaging Specificity

The ability of MRI to correctly localize and categorize soft tissue neoplasms has been described by many authors during the past 8 years, with rapidly improving diagnostic specificity both prior to and following treatment.[4,35-44] The primary advances have not resulted from evaluation of the specific T_1 and T_2 relaxation values.[45] Instead, a careful analysis of MRI signal intensity (SI) characteristics using multiple techniques, margin interfaces, and the internal architecture has yielded much greater specificity and confidence. CT and ultrasound examination remain the techniques most frequently used for evaluation of tumor matrix mineralization and detection of fluid collections, respectively.

Specific tissue diagnosis can occasionally be made using MRI signal characteristics alone. The presence of fat can be reliably discerned with T_1- and T_2-weighted (T_1W and T_2W) imaging and/or fat-suppression techniques (for exclusion of hematoma). Fibrous and/or granulation components of a lesion will commonly have an intermediate SI on T_1W and low SI on T_2W sequences. Simple and complex fluids can be differentiated from solid tissues by their very high SI on heavily T_2W (TR >2000 and TE >120 ms) and from each other on T_1W views (complex fluid has intermediate T_1 relaxation). Hyaline cartilage and myxoid components of a neoplasm will usually have a slightly higher T_1W signal, compared to muscle. Necrotic portions of a neoplasm can frequently be separated from viable components by using gadolinium-DTPA or other newer MRI contrast agents, as seen in Figure 31.1. Hypovascular portions of viable neoplasms can be distinguished from frank necrosis by their lack of increased SI after contrast injection. The pattern of growth and/or the internal architecture can be characteristic for a number of lesions including benign neurofibromas, schwannomas, aggressive fibromatosis, hemangiomas, lymphangiomas, ganglia, and well-

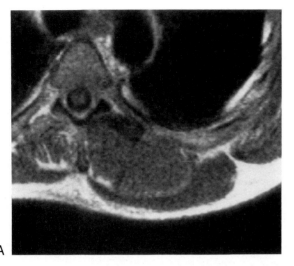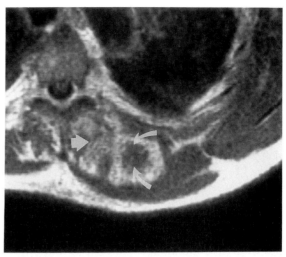

A

B

FIGURE 31.1. T_1W pre- (A) and postcontrast (B) images of synovial sarcoma involving thoracic paraspinous muscles demonstrate the ability of MRI to distinguish viable neoplasm from necrotic zones. The more medial portion of the proximal multifidus (arrow) shows heterogeneous moderate enhance-

ment whereas anterolateral well-defined zone of unenhancing erector spinae "muscle" (curved arrows) had increased signal on a T_2W sequence (not shown), suggesting a necrotic focus within the neoplasm.

differentiated cartilage lesions that will be described in more detail.

The evaluation of the tumor interface with adjacent muscle and connective tissue is informative and important but remains an area of continued difficulty in MRI evaluation of neoplasms. A well-defined, nonreactive margination of tumor is suggestive of a slowly growing process just as the infiltrative, reactive pattern of tumor interface is more suggestive of an aggressive process. These interfaces and their variants can be defined better on MRI exams than most other nonhistologic techniques at the present time. However, the fact that a tumor/parenchymal margin is well defined on MRI does not indicate a noninfiltrative lesion.[46,47] Unfortunately, there is considerable overlap in both the growth patterns and the MRI appearances of the various benign and malignant lesions and nonneoplastic processes that involve skeletal muscle.

Benign Versus Malignant Neoplasms

Despite many imaging advances the challenging clinical problem of differentiating benign and malignant processes and making specific diagnoses remains. This has been addressed by multiple investigators over the past 5 years with variable success.[7,38,41,42,48–50] Convincing features to reliably discriminate malignant from benign processes have been few in number, although several are accurate the majority of the time. Berquist et al.[48] have found a high degree of accuracy in identifying benign

lesions using criteria including well-defined margins, the lack of irregularity, homogeneity of signal, and lack of surrounding edema. However, a large percentage of his patients had cystic lesions. Wetzel and Levine[12] found characteristic features in neoplasms of the foot. One reason for their higher success rate is that only a limited number of lesions, mostly benign, commonly occur in this region and most of their patients had those diseases. These included hemangiomas, pigmented villonodular synovitis, cysts, and plantar fibromatosis, all of which have been reported to have distinctive MRI appearances. Sundaram et al.[49] and Kransdorf et al.[38] both found that the criteria used for differentiation of benign and malignant lesions were not reliable with the exception of a few distinctive lesions such as lipomas and hemangiomas. Crim et al.[47] summarized the previous authors, findings and evaluated 83 additional soft tissue lesions. They found that many of the criteria used to attempt a discrimination between benign and malignant processes were not useful. The size, degree of neurovascular encasement/displacement, peritumoral edema, inhomogeneity, and involvement of adjacent bone were not reliable features indicating malignant disease. There was generally poor accuracy in identifying malignancies, but with a greater percentage of benign lesions being correctly identified in all of the recent papers on this topic. Certain lesions do have features that are distinctive and were successfully identified by many of the authors' diagnosticians. Between 25% and 30% of the lesions were specifically diagnosed in the blinded retrospective reviews. This included lesions such as cysts and lipomas, which are almost always consistent in their appearance. Other neoplasms were noted to have a characteristic appearance but with considerable variations away from the norm. The subsequent descriptions are included so that the reader will be familiar with typical MRI, and other imaging, features of muscle masses.

Pattern recognition techniques may provide better discrimination between malignant and benign lesions, although this approach is more difficult to evaluate and teach. Specific internal architectural patterns are frequently observed in many benign lesions and are described subsequently. A reminder of the limitations of this approach is apparent in the paper by Levine et al.[51] where the lowest resolution imaging technique, ^{67}Ga-citrate, was successful in differentiating neurofibro-sarcomas from neurofibromas, unlike CT and MRI. Hermann et al.[50] described a finding that is fairly characteristic for soft tissue sarcomas. They observed that a pattern of low signal linear "septae" strongly correlated with malignancy, as it was seen in 80% of their 25 sarcomas. Only 2 of their 24 benign lesions showed a similar pattern. An additional differentiating feature may be the observation of a change in the pattern of the lesion comparing T_1 to T_2 images as they noted that 84% of the lesions that changed from homogeneous on T_1 to heterogeneous on T_2 images were malignant, whereas only 16% of benign lesions had this pattern. Our own observations confirm both of these findings (as seen in Figure 31.13), but also indicate that several benign lesions occasionally have this pattern. Hemangiomas commonly have a similar appearance, as seen in Figure 31.2. We also observed that the majority of the heterogeneous tumor volumes in most soft tissue malignancies

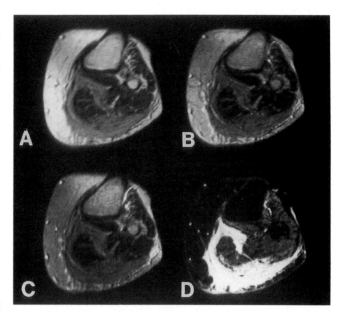

FIGURE 31.3. Diffuse lymphomatous involvement of the calf has signal intermediate between that of fat and muscle on T_1W (A), proton density (B), and T_2W (C) images. Only the STIR image (D) readily demonstrates the full extent of muscle, intermuscular, and subcutaneous involvement.

maintains an intermediate signal equal to, or less than, fat on T_2W images. This is unlike what was initially reported, but has been noted in more recent publications. It likely relates primarily to high cellular density such as reported in lymphomas[52] (Figure 31.3). Unfortunately, a few of the soft tissue sarcomas have a highly homogeneous appearance. This can rarely be seen in synovial

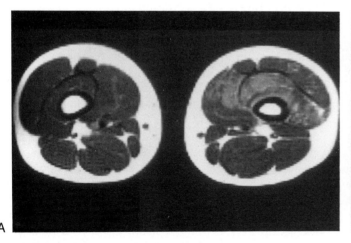

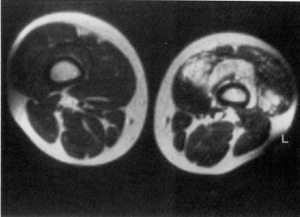

FIGURE 31.2. T_1W (A) and T_2W (B) images of intramuscular hemangioma show typical pattern and MRI signal characteristics. The hemangioma involves vastus medialis, intermedius, and lateralis, in both a diffuse and patchy pattern, with some normal muscle intervening. A lobular pattern is seen, with small focal and subtle linear areas of decreased signal being superimposed on larger zones of high signal intensity on T_2W images.

sarcoma and myxoid MFHs, and in one of the cases of rhabdomyosarcoma that we have encountered (Figure 31.12). Two confusing patterns may be seen in malignancies. The first is homogeneously low SI on T_1 and high SI on T_2 images, simulating a cyst. The less well-recognized pattern is that of homogeneous intermediate to higher signal on T_1 images with increasing signal on T_2 images, simulating a hematoma. Only a slightly higher signal relative to muscle is seen in the majority of sarcomas on T_1W exams (in 25 of 31 patients in one of our studies).[46] A smaller percentage of the soft tissue sarcomas (3 of 31) that we studied had signal that approached that of fat on the T_1W views such that they simulated hematomas.

Benign Neoplasms

Rhabdomyoma

The rhabdomyoma is exceedingly rare, as only 60 have been reported in the world literature, none of which were in the extremities, according to Enzinger and Weiss.[53] They state that, unlike most benign soft tissue neoplasms, the rhabdomyoma is much less common than the corresponding rhabdomyosarcoma; it represents only 2% of all striated muscle tumors. There is some debate as to whether they actually represent a form of hamartoma. We will not discuss this entity in detail. The true benign rhabdomyoma originating from skeletal muscle is most commonly found in the tongue or in the heart. Although there are reports of local postsurgical recurrence, there has been no documented transformation of the benign rhabdomyoma into its malignant counterpart.[53]

Neurofibromas

Peripheral neurofibromas have consistently been found to have a characteristic pattern on T_2W images.[54-57] In the great majority of cases, the central portion of the neoplasm has decreased SI and the peripheral tissue has increased SI, as shown in Figure 31.3. This was reported in 7 of 11 lesions by Burk et al.[54] and in all 14 cases we reported in 1988.[55] None of the four schwannomas had this pattern, whereas 7 of 10 neurofibromas did, in the review of 16 nerve sheath tumors by Suh et al. in 1992.[57] This pattern is related to the greater cellularity and increased percentage of collagen seen centrally, and the higher concentration of acid mucopolysaccharides (proteoglycans) that is found in the more peripheral portions of the neoplasm. This "target" pattern has also been seen in several schwannomas, as reported by Varma (Houston, Texas, personal communication) and thus cannot be used as a pathognomonic finding in a nerve tumor. The histologic correlation is demonstrated in Figure 31.4. A differing density and contrast enhancement pattern can also be seen with neurofibromas using CT, although it is less consistent and usually subtle.[17,58,59] MRI provides a greater degree of contrast between enhancing and nonenhancing tissue following IV administration of gadolinium-DTPA. The more vascular

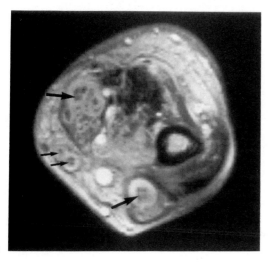
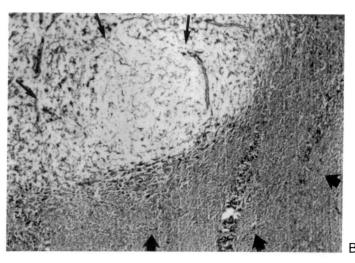

A
B

FIGURE 31.4. Multiple plexiform neurofibromas diffusely involve the arm with only a small volume of residual normal muscle. They are easily identified by their tubular configuration and characteristic MRI signal pattern on transaxial T_2W image (A). The central portions (arrows) have decreased signal relative to the high signal in the periphery in both plexiform and solitary types. The multitubular internal architecture seen here is uncommon. Trichrome stained 100× photomicrograph (B) reveals the dense cellularity and collagen content in the central volume in the lower right of the image (arrows) and the hypocellularity and abundant proteoglycan matrix in the peripheral region (arrowheads).

central region of the neurofibroma enhances early and also washes out sooner than the less vascular peripheral areas. This leaves a prominent "stain" in the peripheral portions for up to 1 h, as seen in Figure 31.5. Plexiform neurofibromas have a similar pattern but frequently show a "tubular" morphology, as demonstrated in Figure 31.4. This pattern may only be reliable when high-resolution imaging techniques are utilized, which is a likely reason for the low percentage having this pattern in some series. There are other abnormalities that have a similar pattern, including several vascular and solid

lesions that we have encountered, with hemangioma being the most common offender.

Hemangiomas

The hemangioma usually has a distinctive pattern that can easily be separated from neurofibromas and most other benign neoplasms.[60–64] They have characteristic, but not pathognomonic, MR signal features and architecture (Figure 31.2). They may remain entirely within local fascial planes, but more commonly cross tissue

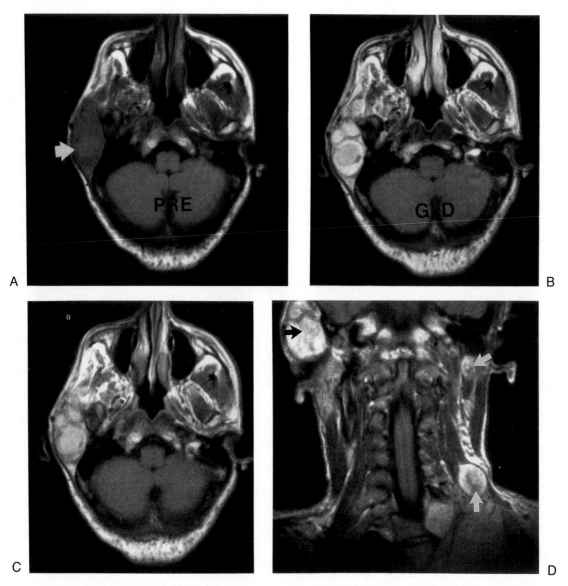

FIGURE 31.5. The larger of three neck neurofibromas shows characteristic contrast enhancement pattern. The central zone of higher cellularity (arrow) has a slightly increased signal relative to muscle on the T_1W image (A). Following intravenous administration of gadolinium DTPA, a reversal of the enhancement pattern is seen between the 3-min (B) and 20-min (C) sequences. The central vascular zone rapidly enhances and washes out early, with prolonged "staining" of the less vascular proteoglycan-containing peripheral regions. The peripheral enhancement remains in several of the neck lesions (arrows) on the 1-h delayed T_1W view (D).

planes and involve more than one compartment. On T_2W images, intramuscular hemangiomas usually have irregular and small lobular zones of decreased signal superimposed on very high signal tissue. The low signal regions histologically correspond to areas of fibrous connective tissue stroma, hemosiderin deposition, thrombus, and interposed uninvolved muscle.[60] The larger zones of markedly increased signal correspond to distended tortuous vessels. The phleboliths commonly seen by x-ray and CT exam are difficult to distinguish with MRI because their low signal blends with these other tissues. CT examination can diagnose hemangiomas based on well-defined smooth bordered, and inhomogeneous lesions that contained round calcific densities corresponding to phleboliths.[2] Both CT and MRI advantages and deficiencies are demonstrated in Figure 31.6. Hemangiomas are commonly a mixture of cavernous, venous, capillary, and even lymph vessels, and thus a specific discrimination of the subtypes is not usually possible. The malignant versions of vascular soft tissue neoplasms such as the more well-differentiated hemangioendothelioma can simulate benign hemangioma, although luckily these are quite rare. We have found that the size of the deep intramuscular hemangioma does not correlate well with any overlying involvement of the skin. Most intramuscular hemangiomas have no superficial discoloration or other physical findings and are discovered during evaluation for localized pain.[61] Obvious contrast enhancement is seen on both CT and MRI scans, but is less distinctive than seen with angiography[61] and the pattern is not specifically diagnostic.[65]

Lipoma

Lipomas are easily identified using CT on MRI cross-sectional techniques.[66] Large lipomas are readily visible as areas of low density relative to muscle on plain x-ray exams. The CT technique usually provides excellent detection and delineation of lipomas throughout the

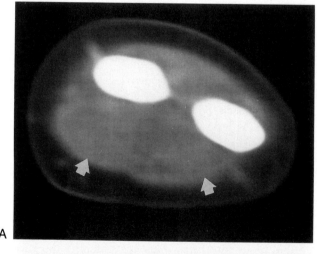

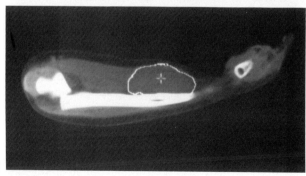

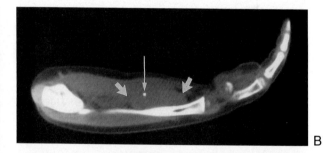

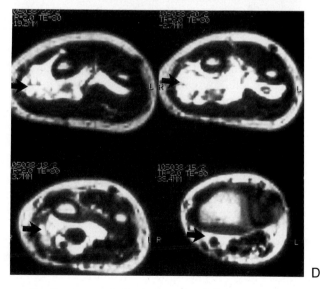

FIGURE 31.6. The diagnosis of hemangioma was made easily on the transaxial (A) and sagittal (B,C) CT exams as four rounded calcifications were identified within the mass (arrows), representing phleboliths (long arrow). Defining the extent was more difficult as the majority of the tumor was isodense with adjacent muscle; the attempt is demonstrated in (C). The extent is easily determined on the transaxial T_2W MR images (arrow, D). All of the flexor compartments were not involved, but the extension to the wrist made referring surgeons reevaluate the possibility of successful resection.

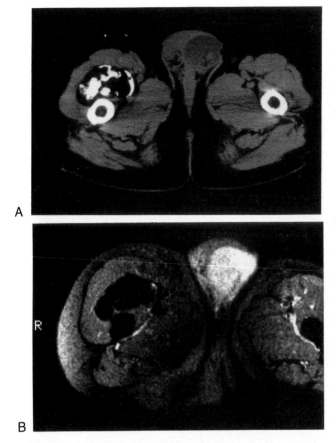

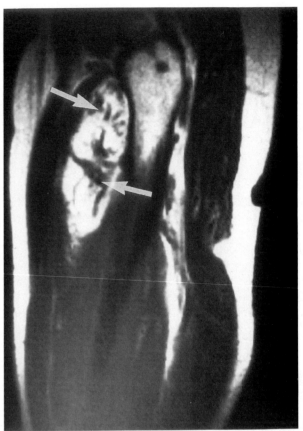

FIGURE 31.7. This lipoma of the thigh with dystrophic calcification seen on CT (A) does not show any abnormal increased signal on the highly sensitive, fat suppression STIR sequence (B). Areas of calcification (arrows) are visible on the T_1W sagittal view (C), although the presence of calcification is frequently difficult to identify on MRI exams.

body. Limitations of CT are similar to those of MRI in that lipomas frequently blend with normal subcutaneous fat and intermuscular fat, making precise discrimination of the margins impossible. CT can usually determine the presence of intermuscular and intramuscular involvement. The intramuscular variety is more common and has less well defined margins due to extensive infiltration into adjacent muscle.[67] The great majority of lipomas are primarily subcutaneous, not involving muscle.[68] Most lipomas are very homogeneous with only thin connective tissue septae around the large lobular components. However, they can have dystrophic heterogeneity, as seen in Figure 31.7. Some authors report that "atypical" lipomas have a greater number and thickness of these septae,[69] with these features being demonstrated on the CT and MRI in Figure 31.8. These variations reportedly have a higher growth rate and may border on low-grade sarcomatous histopathology, although this has been extremely difficult to confirm via standard histochemical techniques. Angiolipomas with their greater concentration of intralesional vascular elements could also have this appearance.

MRI of lipomatous lesions also provides excellent demarcation of the lesions. MRI has the theoretical and practical advantage of imaging lipomas in any orientation view with high resolution techniques. This allows use of imaging planes which are perpendicular to important tissue interfaces. This helps identify the encompassing thin capsule in difficult areas of delineation, such as in the subcutaneous fat. There is slightly superior MRI contrast between fat and the capsule compared to CT. Fat has a characteristic T_1 and T_2 appearance, being extremely high in signal on T_1W sequences and intermediate signal on T_2 images. Moderate and complete fat saturation can be achieved using several different chemical shift saturation techniques or the short TI inversion recovery (STIR) sequence. The various fat suppression techniques combined with the use of contrast enhancement may also occasionally be advantageous.

Aggressive Fibromatosis

Soft tissue fibromatosis is known by many names. The name, specific histologic subtype, treatment, and prog-

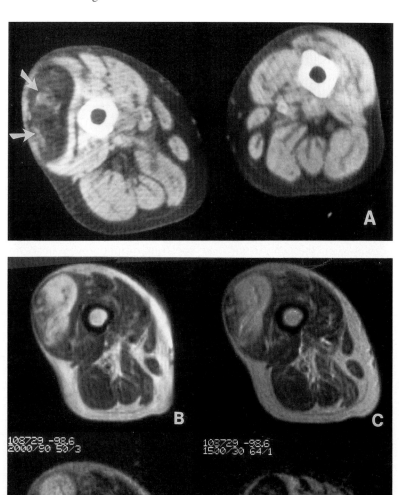

FIGURE 31.8. This large, primarily intermuscular atypical lipoma of the thigh shows multiple linear and ill-defined zones of increased density (arrows) on the CT exam (A). These areas maintain low signal on T_1W (B), spin density (C), and T_2W (D) images, relative to fat. The most significant finding is the near complete absence of increased signal on the fat-suppression STIR images (E), which essentially excludes the presence of frank sarcomatous degeneration.

nosis are partially dependent on the location of the lesion. They are also referred to as desmoid tumors or soft tissue fibromatosis. The superficial variety is usually more slowly growing, unlike the more aggressive deep musculoaponeurotic type.[70] The desmoid tumors are of uncertain specific etiology but typically involve the musculoaponeurotic interfaces and are locally invasive. They are considered to be benign, as distant metastases have not been reported. We will not discuss the features of retroperitoneal fibrosis.

The fibromatosis that involves muscle causes a serious clinical problem in that it commonly penetrates multiple anatomic compartments and is difficult to clinically localize. Examination with x-ray and nuclear medicine techniques can detect but not define the extent of these lesions.[26,71] Palpation and visual inspection of the margins at the time of surgery is also frequently misleading.[71] It readily penetrates soft tissue compartmental boundaries and can also directly involve adjacent bone. Typically, the firm central, more mature component is thought to be easily "shelled out" and cured at the time of surgical resection. Instead, gross disease is usually left behind. MRI is highly useful for pretreatment planning in that despite its variable appearance, the full extent of these lesions are identified in a great majority of cases. This allows either appropriate surgical resection of the entire lesion or appropriately directed radiation therapy to the entire area of involvement. This latter approach alone has tenatively been shown to be effective.[72,73] We have shown that follow-up MRI examination can successfully document the regression of fibromatosis and "maturation" following radiation therapy.[73] The MRI signal characteristics of soft tissue fibromatosis have been described by several authors.[74–76] The most characteristic of the several appearances is when the central portion has a persistently low signal on both T_1W and T_2W

images and also on the STIR sequence, which is the most sensitive means of delineating tumor margins. STIR is also highly sensitive to any form of reactive edema and could potentially overstate the extent, although this has not generally been a problem, judging by the rarity of reactive edema in reported cases. Exceptions to this are found when direct involvement of enthesis occurs, which has been discussed elsewhere in this chapter and in Chapter 25. The more "active" and infiltrative portion of the lesion will have intermediate signals similar to that of muscle on T_1W images and high signal on T_2W and STIR images. The overall pattern of MRI signals is highly heterogeneous, with intermediate and low signals seen on T_1W images and the entire spectrum of inhomogeneously mixed low, intermediate, and high signal patterns being present on T_2W and STIR

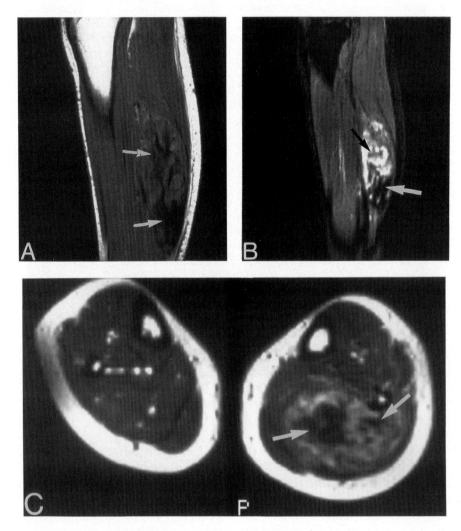

FIGURE 31.9. This patient with aggressive fibromatosis of the calf has recognizable MRI characteristics. Sagittal T_1W (A), STIR (B), and axial T_2W (C) all demonstrate a large but poorly marginated mass involving two compartments of the posterior calf, indicating an aggressive process. The irregular zones of persistently low signal (arrows) on all pulse sequences are predominantly central and rarely found in other neoplasms (and not in infections). This is a typical but not universal feature of aggressive fibromatosis.

sequences. Despite the histologic paucity of blood vessels within fibromatosis, a vascular blush and moderate contrast enhancement commonly occurs on x-ray exams.[71] The typical MRI pattern of signal is demonstrated in Figure 31.9.

Myxoma

Intramuscular myxomas are very uncommon, although they may be found more frequently with the extensive use of MRI for imaging the extremities. We have encountered eight cases in the past 5 years, which all had a similar MRI signal pattern described by Peterson et al.[77] Myxomas have a large amount of myxoid stroma and are characteristically hypovascular, which results in a homo-

geneous low signal on T_1W and extremely high signal on T_2W images, simulating the appearance of a cyst (Figure 31.10). This pattern, when seen in combination with nearby fibrous dysplasia, should allow diagnosis, as reported by Sundaram.[78] Seromas, ganglia, chronic abscesses, and sarcomas (rarely) can have a similar appearance. Abscesses are more easily differentiated by their thicker peripheral margin of fibrosis and associated reactive changes beyond it. Myxomas and ganglia have a similar appearance on MRI exams in that they can appear entirely cystic on most MRI pulse sequences and on CT exams because they are extremely homogeneous and considerably less dense than muscle. They can sometimes be more readily identified as having solid and semisolid material using ultrasound. One feature that is

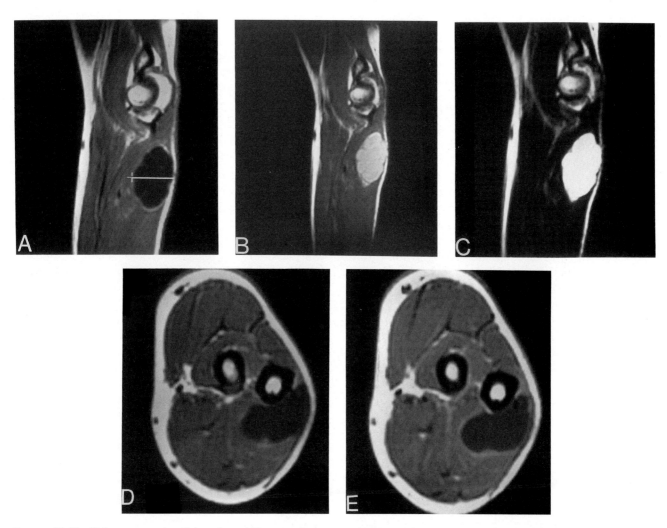

FIGURE 31.10. This myxoma involving the midforearm is extremely well defined and homogeneous on coronal T_1W (A), proton density (B), and T_2W (C) images. The very low signal on T_1W views suggests a slightly lobular cystic lesion from which it cannot be easily differentiated. Subtle diffuse inhomogeneity can sometimes be detected with wide window filming technique and is best seen in (B) in this patient. The pre- (D) and postcontrast (E) T_1W views show no enhancement, again suggestive of a ganglion or other cyst, in addition to myxoma. (Courtesy of Scott Porter, M.D., Lubbock, Texas; used with permission from Weatherall PT. Benign and malignant masses: MRI differentiation. MRI Clin North Am 1995;3(4).)

somewhat characteristic for myxomas is their extremely low signal on T_1W images, which is unlike the majority of solid neoplasms. This is more similar to a seroma than a protein-laden abscess or most ganglia. This appearance is somewhat unexpected, considering the high protein content of the myxoid material. The T_2W characteristics are as expected considering the relative hypocellularity and abundant content of mucoid material, unbound water and a paucity of collagen.[79]

Chondroma

Cartilage-containing tumors are one of the few other lesions that have recognizable features. Soft tissue chondromas can have a distinctive appearance when the cartilage growth pattern is defined on x-ray or MR images.[80–83] A prominent multilobular pattern is commonly appreciated using most MRI techniques, with small, 3- to 7-mm, individual lobules defined with high-resolution techniques.[84] The hyaline cartilage lobules usually have slightly higher signal than muscle on T_1W images and show marked increase in signal on the T_2 images. The areas of fibrosis, calcification, and ossification are less commonly seen in the soft tissue chondromas when compared with enchondromas of the bone. X-ray imaging techniques, particularly CT, can identify soft tissue cartilage tumors easily when they have the characteristic rings and arcs pattern of calcification, which are not readily visible with MRI. However, high-resolution MRI can detect the internal architecture of focal high and low signal on T_2W images in the absence of calcification in most cases. Other cartilage-containing benign neoplasms are very rare and are usually in the form of teratomas or mesenchymomas. The cartilage components may be very difficult to prospectively identify in these lesions, as seen in Figure 31.11. The ability of MRI to discriminate small amounts of fat in addition to other mesenchymal elements may occasionally allow preoperative diagnosis.[84]

Malignant Neoplasms

Malignant soft tissue neoplasms have not been shown to have features that will consistently allow their distinction by radionuclide, CT, or MRI techniques. Previous reports in both the CT and MR literature initially characterized malignant soft tissue neoplasms as having less well-defined margins and greater heterogeneity with and without contrast and on T_2W sequences.[14,48] Extra-compartmental extension of the mass was also more indicative of aggressive behavior, suggesting a malignancy. In the MRI literature, the presence of reactive peritumoral edema was initially suggested as a marker for malignancy,[85] but was later also associated with

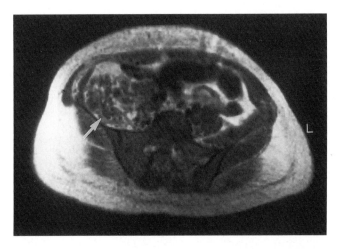

FIGURE 31.11. The large, fat-containing lesion replacing the iliacus muscle of the pelvis represents the proximal extent of a large hamartoma. The curvilinear and irregular zones of intermediate and decreased signal within the central portions of the lesion (arrow) corresponded to cartilage and connective tissue, but are similar to the appearance of plexiform neurofibromata, which can be seen in combination with hamartoma in patients with neurofibromatosis. A solitary mesenchymoma can have an appearance similar to this.

benign lesions.[86] The rapid uptake of iodine- and gadolinium-labeled contrast on CT and MRI is also used as an indicator of increased vascularity and a discriminator for malignancy.[87] The difficulty in using these and other features as a marker for malignancy is multifactorial. Some of these characteristics do correlate well with the finding of malignancy, but cannot be used as a reliable discriminator because multiple benign processes also share this same characteristic.[88] The low-grade, well-differentiated sarcomas obviously have features that are similar to their benign counterparts since the gross histology of the tissues is so close to the same. Accurate differentiation is usually impossible, or nearly so at the present time, with grade I liposarcomas and chondrosarcomas.[66,80,84,89] No reliable differentiating features of low-grade neurofibrosarcomas have been determined,[51] even though the neurofibroma has a distinct appearance. Hemangiomas, aggressive fibromatosis, myosistis ossificans, and several other less common lesions can involve multiple compartments with less well-defined margins and considerable heterogeneity. Prominent contrast enhancement can also be seen in all three of these lesions, although it is less rapid in the case of fibromatosis. Many sarcomas do not have all, or in some cases any, of these features. A few are highly homogeneous, and most, in our experience, have well-defined margins on MRI exams. This is in part due to the extremely high contrast produced between normal and abnormal soft tissues. This creates sharp demarcation of even rapidly growing malignant tissue at its interface with normal parenchyma or compartmental boundaries.[46] The common and atypical features are demonstrated in Figures 31.12 to 31.14. Most of the scintigraphic studies of soft tissue neoplasms have utilized gallium-67 citrate and technetium-99m. The number of different lesions that accumulate these radiotracers is quite broad and includes both benign and malignant neoplasms.[26] Their use is restricted to answering specific clinical questions, such as whether adjacent bone is involved by the neoplasm or reactive zone, and for detecting metastatic disease. The use of antigen-specific radiotracer as a magic bullet to attach to certain neoplasms remains a hopeful tool for the future. The combined use of MRI and superferromagnetic particulate contrast agents attached to the antigen-specific compounds is likely years away due to the low concentrations of the compounds that attach to primary or metastatic deposits. The following individual descriptions of the more common malignancies that affect muscle will include the typical MRI appearance, since MRI delineates these lesions better than other imaging techniques, almost without exception.

Rhabdomyosarcoma

Primary sarcomas of muscle are very rare. A larger percentage of malignancies previously carried this diagnosis, such as malignant fibrous histiocytomas, until the recent, more accurate histologic recognition and reclassification.[90] The subclassifications of alveolar and embryonal are associated with an unfavorable prognosis but cannot be distinguished by imaging. There are no articles specifically discussing the CT and MRI appearance of rhabdomyosarcomas, although several have evaluated them in combination with other lesions.[10,25,44,46] Most have had intermediate signal on T_1W images, slightly higher than that of muscle, and prominently increased signal on T_2W views. One of these patients had an appearance that could simulate a subacute hematoma both on T_1W and T_2W images. Unlike most sarcomas, it was highly homogeneous on both sequences and had obviously higher signal than muscle on the T_1W (500/30) view, as demonstrated in Figure 31.12.

Liposarcomas

High-grade liposarcomas usually have only small, if any, amounts of visible, well-differentiated adipose tissue on CT or MRI exams. There are a great number of subtypes that will not be discussed here. The well-differentiated grade 1 liposarcomas are almost identical in appearance to that of simple and atypical lipomas. There is some dispute among pathologists as to the criteria for specific diagnosis.[91] The inability of MRI to discriminate between benign lipomas and grade 1 liposarcomas is therefore

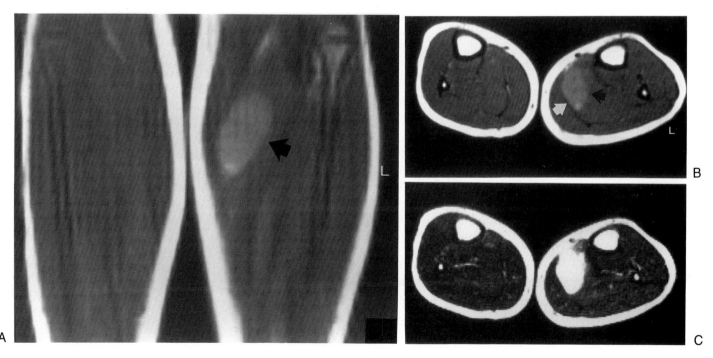

FIGURE 31.12. The rhabdomyosarcoma (arrow) has moderately high signal on the T_1W images (A and B) with extremely well defined margins and no associated reactive edema in the adjacent normal muscle, as demonstrated on T_1W coronal (A) and axial (B) images and on axial T_2W (C) image. Change "had" to "has" and "arrow" to "arrows".

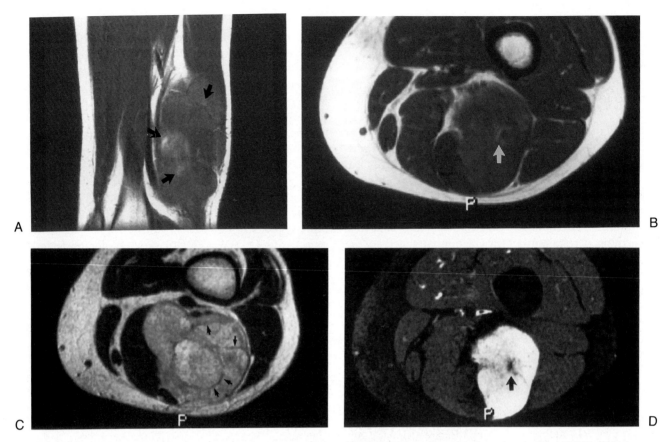

FIGURE 31.13. This large myxoid liposarcoma of the thigh shows prominent heterogeneity on both T_1 coronal (A) and transaxial T_1W (B) and T_2W (C) images. The small irregular areas of increased signal seen on T_1W images (arrows) correspond to fat and presumed hemorrhage based on low signal on STIR images through these levels. The T_2W image demonstrates one of the many thick fibrous septae (arrows). The transaxial highly sensitive STIR image (D) demonstrates no significant peritumoral edema despite the large size and aggressive behavior of the tumor.

not surprising. Frank sarcomatous degeneration is only rarely documented in relation to a previously identified simple lipoma.[67,91] One consistent appearance of liposarcomas is a large lesion with prominent heterogeneity on T_2 images within or adjacent to major muscle groups.[48,89,92,93] This is perfectly demonstrated in Figure 31.13. Heterogeneity is also usually seen on the T_1W images, although this is not usually due to simple fat within the lesion. Instead, myxoid and highly cellular undifferentiated components of other elements show a mixed pattern of low and intermediate signal on T_1W exams, which is roughly isointense to muscle. A corresponding irregular pattern of low, intermediate, and high signal on T_2W images includes a sizable component with signal only slightly higher than that of muscle.

Malignant Fibrous Histiocytoma

Malignant fibrous histiocytomas (MFH) have a similar distribution and appearance. They are frequently mildly heterogeneous on T_1W views and very inhomogeneous

on the T_2W images.[94] Their appearance can vary considerably, depending on the percentage of cell types that make up the tumor. Instead of fluid-like high signal, the larger percentage of these neoplasms have the dominant T_2 signal being intermediate, similar to that of fat. This has not been as widely reported in the literature. Our own evaluation indicated that the dominant T_2 signal was isointense or less than fat in 9 of the 15 lesions studied.

Synovial Sarcoma

Synovial sarcomas are found in the soft tissues directly adjacent to muscles and usually near the joints, rather than in the midsegments of the extremities. The small lesions may be more homogeneous than other sarcomas on both T_1 and T_2W exams.[95,96] They can occasionally simulate the appearance of a cyst, ganglion, or myxoma. This is due to the sometimes homogeneous signal seen on T_2W images and the rounded or lobular configuration that is frequently present. As expected, the larger synovial sarcomas are usually heterogeneous on T_2W

FIGURE 31.14. This plemorphic sarcoma of the adductor compartment of the thigh (arrow) has a very similar appearance to the hematoma seen in Figure 31.16. The homogeneous minimally increased signal seen on T_1W (arrow, A) and heterogeneous low and high signal seen on T_2W (B) is a common pattern seen in sarcomas although this cannot be used to definitively discriminate it from hematoma. The nodular enhancement (arrow) demonstrated on the post-contrast T_1W image (C) excludes hematoma as a diagnosis. The T_2W image shows a decreased signal in the nodule (arrow). Histologically, this corresponded to an area of increased cellularity and vascularity. (Used with permission from Weatherall PT. Benign and malignant masses: MRI differentiation. MRI Clin North Am 1995; 3(4).)

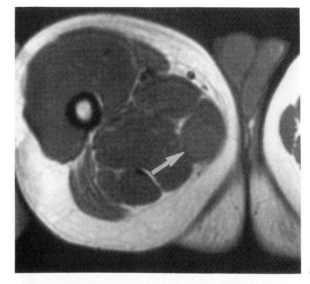

A

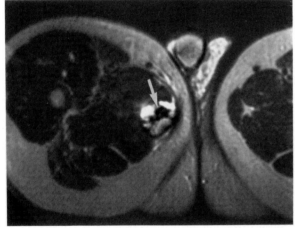

B

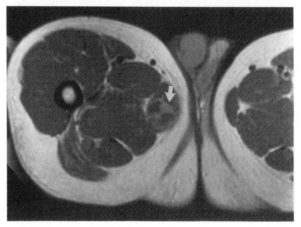

C

images, occasionally demonstrating dramatic hemorrhagic fluid–fluid levels. CT and MRI exams using intravenous contrast can help distinguish these solid vascular lesions from the cystic- and myxoid-containing tumors.

Differential Diagnosis

Common diagnostic imaging problems include the distinction of neoplasms from other pathology. Active infection and recent trauma may be difficult to distinguish from high-grade sarcoma or aggressive fibromatosis. An abscess with a thick rind may look like a necrotic neoplasm. Hematomas may occasionally simulate lipomas and soft tissue sarcomas. Unfortunately, a hematoma may be superimposed on a malignancy and produce a very confusing appearance.[97]

Hematomas

Hemorrhage can have widely varying appearances depending on the temporal relationship of the injury,

and imaging. and the technique that is used. A simple contusion with edema, mild hemorrhage, and little death will commonly be isointense relative to muscle on the T_1W images and have high SI on T_2W or STIR sequences, usually with relatively poor margination of the area affected. This injury will be visible immediately and resolve over a few weeks period. A small or large hematoma may form within a muscle or, more commonly, in intermuscular fascial planes with the appearances described being variable.[98,99] In general, the hematoma will remain relatively low in signal on T_1W images for the first week following injury. The formation of methemoglobin during the next 1 to 2 weeks results in a high MRI signal on the T_1W images and T_2W sequences progressing from peripheral to central over this time frame. An intermuscular subacute hematoma can have a signal intensity near or equal to that of fat on T_1W images, and maintains high signal on T_2W sequences, as seen in Figure 31.15. A thin, well-defined rim of decreased signal will frequently develop on T_2W images in the chronic stage relating to hemosiderin deposition at the periphery. Although these findings are distinctive,

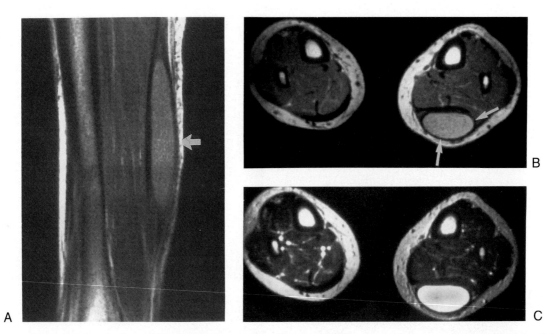

FIGURE 31.15. The large elongated posterior calf mass seen on the sagittal T_1W (arrow, A) has a common location and morphology, and typical MRI signal characteristics of a subacute phase hematoma. On the transaxial T_1W (B) image, it has much higher signal than normal muscle but much less than fat. The T_1W and T_2W (C) sequences show decreased signal from hemosiderin at the periphery (arrows) in addition to the displaced gastrocnemius aponeurosis, which also has low signal.

they can be simulated by other disease processes. When confined to the intermuscular spaces, hematomas have the more typical appearance with moderate to very high signal on T_1W images when in the subacute stage. When the hematoma is in the intramuscular compartment(s), the degree of increased T_1 relaxation and overall increase in signal is less striking and they are usually not as discrete as those involving the CNS. High-grade soft tissue sarcomas commonly have slightly increased signal relative to muscle on T_1W images,[46] and can have high, intermediate, or low signal on T_2W views, simulating a hematoma. The patient with a rhabdomyosarcoma in Figure 31.12 had recent local blunt trauma and the appearance of a hematoma, whereas the patient with the hematoma of intermediate signal in Figure 31.16 had no prior trauma or hematologic disorder. In the latter patient I.V. contrast administration demonstrated marked hypovascularity of the mass, suggesting the diagnosis of hematoma, unlike the very similar appearing sarcoma in Figure 31.14.

Infection/Abscess

The most common cause of soft tissue abscesses is the presence of a nearby infection of the bone, although in some populations penetrating trauma without osteomyelitis is a more frequent etiology. Muscle infection occurs much more commonly than has been suggested by the lack of discussion in the medical and imaging literature. This is in part due to the limited ability of previous imaging techniques to readily identify the full extent of soft tissue inflammation both in known cases of osteomyelitis and in patients with cellulitis. Erdman et al.[100] recently showed obvious muscular involvement by the active inflammatory process in 40 of 110 cases of osteomyelitis. The associated soft tissue involvement was only rarely demonstrated by their other imaging techniques.

FIGURE 31.16. The adductor compartment hematoma in this 63-year-old male closely simulated a soft tissue sarcoma. He awoke with a new onset of pain and a mass in the medial thigh with no antecedent trauma. The coronal proton density (A) and axial T_1W (B) revealed an elongated mass (arrows) with higher signal than muscle, similar to the sarcoma in Figure 31.14. The heterogeneous pattern of high, intermediate, and lower signal intensity seen on a T_2W image (C) was suggestive of a sarcoma. A T_1W precontrast (D) image 3 days later demonstrated a subtle partial rim of high signal (small arrow) indicating hemorrhage, but remained consistent with sarcoma; however, there was no appreciable postcontrast enhancement (E) except at the periphery, indicating that the vast majority, if not all, of the mass was related to hematoma only. (Used with permission from Weatherall PT. Benign and malignant masses: MRI differentiation. MRI Clin North Am 1995;3(4).)

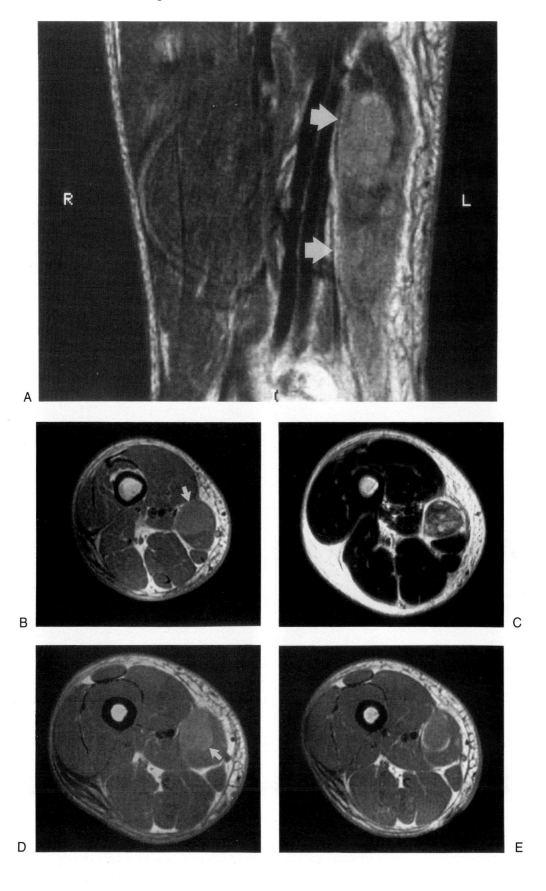

MRI is nearly ideal for demonstrating inflammatory processes of the bone and soft tissues, including the muscle. The utilization of certain MRI sequences (STIR) allows simultaneous evaluation of both, with high sensitivity, although this can occasionally cause diagnostic problems. This is due to the fact that muscle inflammation remains readily detectable long after pain from any injury has resolved and well beyond the time that a treated or untreated myositis has become sterile. It maintains the significant limitation of previous imaging techniques in its inability to discriminate between infection verses sterile inflammatory conditions. MRI techniques can provide a relatively accurate assessment of the different stages of, and tissue types in, acute and chronic infectious processes involving the bone and adjacent muscle. Acute inflammation is characterized by prominent reactive edema with high signal on T_2W images and poorly defined margins. The more chronic phase of myositis is usually characterized by the presence of a fibrous/granulation tissue partially or completely surrounding a region of residual inflammatory tissue and pus. Chronic abscesses usually have areas of intermediate signal on T_1W images and a low signal rim of fibrous tissue with central high signal on T_2W images similar to early chronic hematomas.[101] The low signal "fibrous pseudocapsule" seen on T_2W sequences is usually thicker and more irregular, as seen in Figure 31.17. This helps provide specificity,[102] although hematomas can have this appearance.[98] An unusual feature of a high signal rim on

T_1W images may help distinguish these lesions in AIDS patients when present.[102,103] Active sinus drainage tracts are commonly seen, leading from soft tissue abscesses and from the sites of osteomyelitis. A rough estimate as to the age and/or "activity level' of the inflammation may be gained by utilizing T_1, T_2, and STIR sequences together.[104] On T_1W images, collections of pus or sterile protein-laden fluids will usually have higher signal than muscle that is easily perceptible. The reactive soft tissue edema surrounding the abscess is usually isointense with muscle on these T_1W views. The suggestive finding of pus on the T_1W sections when combined with the very high signal seen in T_2W imaging usually indicates a drainable collection of infected material. More chronic abscess fluid collections will have characteristics similar to a seroma in that the fluid will have a lower signal on T_1W views. They will maintain high signal on T_2 but have a comparatively lower signal on the commonly obtained proton density-weighted sequence. A chronic sinus tract will have similar properties to the surrounding fibrous and granulation tissue adjacent to the abscess. The amount of infected material within the tract can be highly variable and, when only small amounts are present, they are difficult to visualize even utilizing high-quality T_2W images. The STIR sequence makes this much easier to identify, although during the early stages of healing a false positive diagnosis of an active sinus tract can be made because of its high sensitivity to active and chronic inflammation.

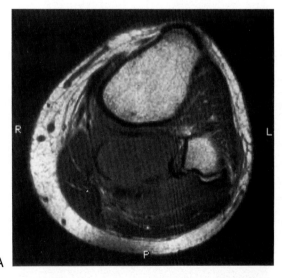
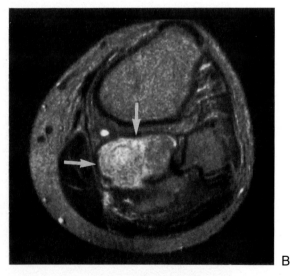

FIGURE 31.17. The T_1 (A) and T_2 (B) transaxial images through this chronic abscess of the calf demonstrate nonspecific features. The intermediate signal seen on T_1 images is higher than that of muscle, which is commonly seen in fluids with a high protein content such as pus. The well-defined rim of low signal (arrows) seen on T_2 images indicates the chronic nature of this lesion; a reactive fibrous rind is being formed. The prominent, but heterogeneous increased signal within the abscess is commonly seen and is related to internal debris, although it can simulate what has been previously described of sarcomas and other neoplasms. The peripheral rim of fibrosis argues against sarcoma, however.

Although they are also imperfect techniques, scintigraphic evaluation using ^{67}Ga citrate and ^{111}In white blood cell (WBC) studies can be valuable for detection of soft tissue infections.[105,106] The ^{111}In WBC study is the imaging technique that is the most specific for ongoing infection, although false positive results can occur, when evaluating mass-like soft tissue lesions. It is especially useful when metallic orthopedic hardware is in the vicinity, which causes artifact on CT and MRI exams. A ^{67}Ga exam is a more sensitive technique for chronic soft tissue infections, which are more likely to produce a mass. Unfortunately, ^{67}Ga uptake is also seen in a multitude of other soft tissue lesions and is thus a poor discriminator when used as the sole imaging technique.[27] As with the many other mass-like lesions of the soft tissue, a combination of clinical history and findings and imaging features from one or more studies must be utilized for the accurate diagnosis of a muscle abscess.

Muscle/Injury

A full discussion of the response of muscle to injury is included in Chapters 25 to 28, 33. Trauma to the muscle can produce a mass-like appearance, which will be discussed here. When muscle injury occurs secondary to penetrating, traction, or blunt trauma, a multiphasic response and reparative process is begun. The initial MRI appearance may be similar to that seen with a contusion, with or without associated frank hematoma formation. The patterns of muscle tear/strain are relatively characteristic, as they are located along myofacial borders and they are not usually confused with neoplasms. A problem may occur when imaging muscle after focal blunt trauma. The MRI patterns of muscle injury repair are zonal and heterogeneous, similar to that of some neoplasms. The region can maintain a moderately increased signal on the STIR sequences for up to 3 months following injury due to the increased sensitivity of this sequence to any form of chronic or active inflammatory/reparative process. One mass-like "reparative" phenomena of the muscle and soft tissues can be particularly confusing to imaging specialists, clinicians, and even the pathologists. This is when the process of myositis ossificans begins. Pseudomalignant osseous tumor, described by Stenner, is another reactive lesion that is essentially identical to this. It is distinguished from myositis ossificans because there is no antecedent history of trauma,[107] but is otherwise identical histologically and radiographically. The precise etiology of this process is not fully understood[108] but is discussed in more detail in Chapter 27. Other uncommon soft tissue lesions can ossify, including chondromas, or rarely osteomas, which are also likely posttraumatic in nature,[109] but it is most important to discern these entities from extraskeletal osteosarcoma. The reactive changes and resultant bone formation will commonly suggest and aggressive process on MRI, physical exam, and histologic study, and can be mistaken for an infection, aggressive fibromatosis, or a sarcoma. The MR images reveal a large area of involved muscle with an infiltrative pattern of reactive tissue and edema that commonly involves multiple compartments. Under these circumstances MRI may not be the best imaging technique for early evaluation of this muscle injury. In the later stages of this process, the peripheral rim of early calcification can be seen as a lower signal on T_2W images, with continued prominent heterogeneous intermediate and high signal seen both internal and external to this "rim." A technetium-99m bone scan and CT scan will detect the rim of calcification/ossification earlier than MRI, as seen in Figure 31.18. The deficiency of MRI in evaluating these lesions is related to what is usually its strength: high sensitivity to inflammatory processes.

Contrast Utilization

There will likely be many MRI contrast agents with various functions for evaluating mass-like lesions in the future. At the present time, only gadolinium-based contrast agents are being used in MRI and iodinated compounds for CT scanning. Both of these have similar properties due to the comparable molecular size and excretion characteristics. The degree of lesion vascularity can be determined with any of the contrast agents, in addition to a rough assessment of inflammatory and/or capillary permeability. The degree of contrast enhancement is usually much greater with MRI compared to CT. This allows easier detection of subtle enhancement patterns and also provides better definition of internal architecture of some lesions.

Bolus infusion techniques with corresponding rapid serial imaging have been used by multiple previous investigators to better define the degree of vascularity.[87,88,110-113] A rapid pattern of contrast enhancement has been shown to correlate with more aggressive lesions based on the greater vascularity. This does not specifically discriminate benign from malignant neoplasms, although statistically this can be useful. In 1989, Erlemann et al.[87] indicated a relationship between rapid contrast enhancement, with an enhancement slope of 30% per minute or greater with malignancy. This was seen in 84% of the 36 malignant bone and soft tissue lesions and only 28% of the 19 benign lesions. Subsequent authors reported less encouraging specificity,[87,112] with Fletcher and Hanna[88] indicating a high percentage of benign lesions (five of seven) having even more rapid contrast enhancement than the average amount found in the 27 malignant lesions. Hanna et al.[86] also reported marked differences in enhancement within different areas of nonnecrotic benign neoplasms. Differentiating tumor vascularity

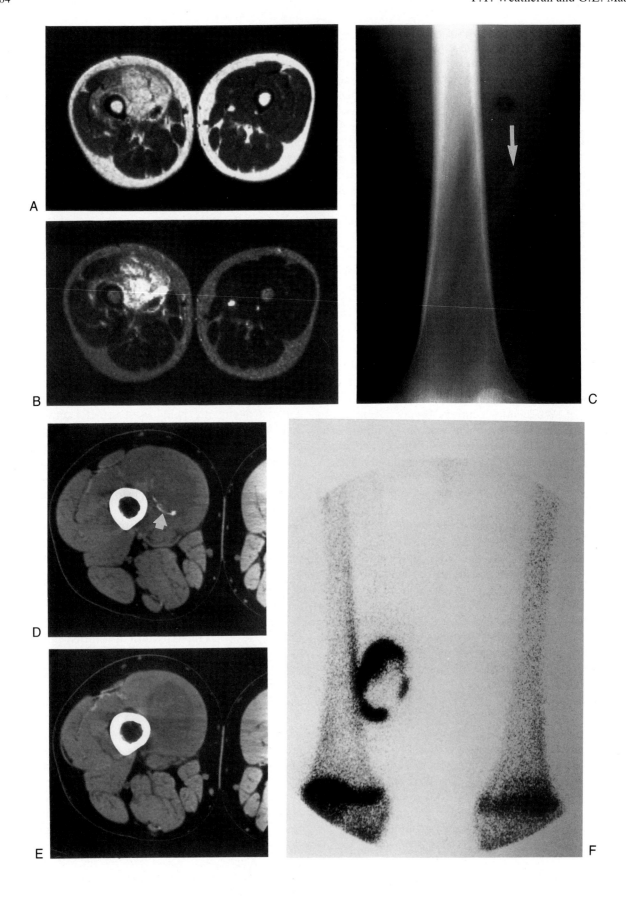

from reactive edema within muscle is possible as it has been shown to have only a delayed, mild enhancement by previous authors.[86,87] It is tempting to utilize the presence or absence of rapid contrast enhancement in the peritumoral region after IV gadolinium-DTPA as a criteria for defining the reactive zone. This would be logical in that the reactive zone is known to have an increased vascularity. Prominent edema has also been noted with benign lesions, which affects a muscle origin or insertion.[46,86] However, "massive muscle edema" has been associated with a greater incidence of metastasis, despite also being found with a few benign lesions.[86] Exceptions to these patterns likely abound and are certainly seen when skip metastasis occurs within the compartment.

The use of intravenous gadolinium-DTPA contrast can also answer more mundane questions. It is usually easier to determine whether a lesion has any significant vascular supply using contrast in combination with MRI than with CT. This can help discriminate cysts and ganglions and markedly hypovascular lesions, such as myxomas, from solid sarcomas and most other benign neoplasms. It can also demonstrate areas of avascularity within a lesion, which usually indicate areas of necrosis. This can have both diagnostic imaging value and allow avoidance of these areas when a biopsy is performed. Areas of relative avascularity also occur in zones of myxoid and cartilage tissue and abscess formation. A contrast exam can occasionally specifically identify sinus tracts, because the adjacent reactive inflammatory tissue will enhance and outline the avascular abscess and sinus. There will undoubtedly be rapid continued development of contrast agents for all of the modalities used in soft tissue imaging. Many will be directly applicable to the task of discriminating the various mass-like lesions encountered within and adjacent to muscle.

FIGURE 31.18. Myositis ossificans, involving the anterior thigh, was initially misdiagnosed as a sarcoma based in part on the MRI. The CT and bone scan obtained within 3 days of the MRI provided much better characterization of the lesion in the early stages of this process. The proton density (A) and T_2 (B) images, demonstrate multicompartmental involvement with ill-defined margination, suggesting an aggressive process. The corresponding CT demonstrates a partial rim of calcification at one level (arrow, C), but none immediately distal to this (D). This was also faintly visible on the plain x ray (arrow, E). The delayed view bone scan (F) provides the most obvious diagnostic pattern of circumferential rim of increased uptake.

Surgical Perspective

The recent technical achievements of orthopedic oncologists in limb-sparing surgical procedures makes the need for precise localization of the neoplasms and their reactive zones even more important. The compartmental approach to curative surgery introduced by Enneking[114] has become a widely accepted means for treatment of aggressive soft tissue processes. For successful treatment, a wide margin (beyond the reactive zone) must be obtained in aggressive benign and low-grade malignancies. A radical resection (removal of the entire compartment) must be performed for local eradication of high-grade lesions.

The understanding of this concept and implementation of its use in our reports is necessary for optimal patient care. Thus, the significance of peritumoral edema and its relationship to the reactive rim is of great concern. The surgical differentiation of the reactive zone involves histologic evaluation of the "cuff of tissue" at the time of surgery and no reactive tissues must remain. The reactive zone can be visualized by MRI exam, although it remains a difficult task, especially when there is prominent "reactive edema" well beyond the margins of the neoplasm; the significance of this is unknown at this time. The major neurovascular bundles must be reliably excluded from the reactive zone for optimal limb-sparing surgery.

Because of the large volume of soft tissues in the body and the numerous different types of soft tissue lesions, there is a great variety in the clinical presentations for the lesions that involve muscle. In order to successfully diagnose and treat these lesions, it is important to understand their biologic behavior. This behavior is manifested in the clinical presentations, the anatomic presurgical staging studies, and the gross and microscopic appearance of the lesions.

The two most popular staging systems at the present time are Enneking's Surgical Staging System (SSS) and that of the American Joint Commission (AJC). Because of changes taking place in the AJC system, Enneking's SSS will be presented (Table 31.1). In Enneking's SSS[115] the lesions are broken down into latent, active, and aggressive for benign tumors, low-grade malignant lesions with intra- and extracompartmental extensions, and high-grade malignant lesions with intra- and extracompartmental extensions. Stage III disease represents patients that present with metastatic sites of involvement.

It is critical for the surgeon to know which compartments are involved preoperatively and preferably prior to biopsy. Anatomic involvement is demonstrated preoperatively by diagnostic imaging studies that demonstrate size, extent, location, and tissue composition of the tumors. The compartmentalization of the lesions is determined by structures that limit tumoral growth. These

TABLE 31.1. Combined staging system for benign and malignant musculoskeletal tumors.

Stage				Characteristics
Benign stage				
1	G_0	T_0	M_0	Latent
2	G_0	T_0	M_0	Active
3	G_0	T_0	M_0	Aggressive
Malignant stage				
IA	G_1	T_1	M_0	
IB	G_1	T_2	M_0	
IIA	G_2	T_1	M_0	
IIB	G_2	T_2	M_0	
IIIA	G_{1-2}	T_1	M_1	
IIIB	G_{1-2}	T_2	M_1	

G = grade: G_0 = benign; G_1 = low-grade, malignant; G_2 = high-grade, malignant. T = site: T_0 = intracapsular; T_1 = extracapsular, intracompartmental; T_2 = extracapsular, extracompartmental. M = metastasis: M_0 = none; M_1 = regional or distant.
Reprinted with permission, William F. Enneking, M.D. Musculoskeletal tumor surgery. London: Churchill Livingstone, 1983.

structures are usually avascular tissues that act as barriers (Table 31.2). Lesions that present well with marginated capsules inside a compartment are called T-0 lesions. These lesions are usually growing slowly enough for the body to form a fibrous capsule. More active lesions may sometimes form a pseudocapsule. When they are extracapsular, but within a compartment, they are given the prefix T-1. Lesions that present with an extracompartmental extension (aggressive lesions that cross barriers) are given the prefix T-2. These lesions may be benign aggressive lesions as well as low- and high-grade malignant lesions. Difficulty arises with the idea of compartmentalization in extrafascial sites of involvement where loose alveolar tissues are found. These sites include areas like

the popliteal fossa and also the axilla, where there are no fascial structures to limit tumor growth (Table 31.2).[116-118] The metastatic categorization is irrespective of whether it is nodal, to bone or to lung parenchyma. Patients presenting without metastatic involvement are given the prefix M_0 and those with metastatic involvement, M_1.

Local recurrence is stratified by surgical margins with each surgical stage of the disease. The margins are listed as intralesional, marginal, wide, and radical (Table 31.3).[115] Intralesional procedures are those performed through a lesion that leaves gross and microscopic tumor behind. Marginal procedures are procedures performed at a level of a pseudocapsule that may leave microscopic satellite lesions behind. Wide resections are those surgical procedures that resect the tumor pseudocapsule and contain a normal cuff of tissue at the resection margins. These procedures may leave hypothetical skip lesions that occur up and down fascial planes in the faster-growing malignant lesions. Radical resections are defined as removal of all tissues of a compartment involved with the tumor. Radical resection should result in no local recurrence from even the high-grade malignant lesions. Amputation can have similar margins to a limb-sparing procedure. The chance of recurrence is determined by the margin (Table 31.3). Recent advances in the use of preoperative chemotherapy and radiation have raised new issues concerning the possibility of preserving viable extremities and not sacrificing local control. Radiation alone utilizing megavoltage has sometimes resulted in the induction of a radiation-induced rind permitting more marginal types of surgery and still allowing for high rates of local control[119] (Figures 31.19, 31.20).

TABLE 31.2. Surgical sites, anatomic setting.

Intracompartmental	Growth	Extracompartmental
Intraosseous	→	Soft tissue extension
Intra-articular	→	Soft tissue extension
Superficial to deep fascia	→	Deep fascial extension
Paraosseous	→	Intraosseous or extrafascial
Intrafascial compartments		*Extrafascial planes or spaces*
Ray of hand or foot		Mid-foot or hind foot
Posterior calf		Popliteal space
Anterolateral leg		Groin, femoral triangle
Anterolateral thigh		Intrapelvic
Medial thigh		Midhand
Posterior thigh		Antecubital fossa
Buttocks		Axilla
Volar forearm		Periclavicular
Dorsal forearm		Paraspinous
Anterior arm		Neck
Posterior arm		Retroperitoneum
Pericapsular		

Reprinted with permission, William F. Enneking, M.D. Musculoskeletal tumor surgery. London: Churchill Livingstone, 1983.

TABLE 31.3. Classification of wound margins.

Type	Plane of dissection	Result
Intracapsular	Piecemeal debulking or curettage	Leaves macroscopic disease
Marginal	Shell out en bloc through pseudocapsule or reactive zone	May leave either satellite or skips
Wide	Intracompartmental en bloc with cuff of normal tissue	May leave skips
Radical	Extracompartmental en bloc entire compartment	No residual

This table shows the types of wound margins, how they are obtained, and the result in terms of residual disease. This classification is based upon the relationship of the margin to the natural barriers to extension rather than on the physical distance between the edge of the lesion and the margin of the wound.
Reprinted with permission, William F. Enneking, M.D. Musculoskeletal tumor surgery. London: Churchill Livingstone, 1983.

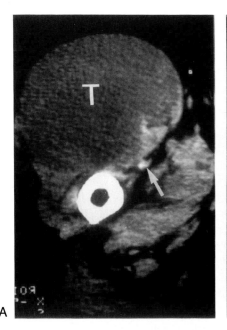
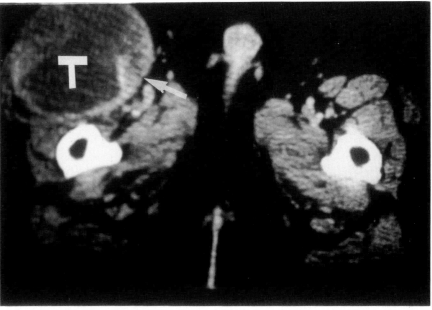

A   B

FIGURE 31.19. The (preinduction chemotherapy and radiation) CT scan (A) of a patient with a high-grade myxoid liposarcoma (T) of the proximal thigh. The arrow points to the neurovascular structures and their close proximity to the lesion on a contrast study. After treatment with doxorubicin and 2800 cGy, the postcontrast CT scan (B) shows a hypervascular tissue marginating the lesion (T) and separating it from the vessels. This area represents the radiation-induced rind (arrow).

Presurgical Staging Studies

Presurgical staging studies are usually needed to determine the anatomic boundaries of the lesion, as well as the presence or absence of metastatic disease. Plain radiographs are less useful for soft tissue lesions unless there is suspected bony involvement. Triphase bone scans are an effective means of detecting early bony involvement in adjacent bony structures and remain the best technique for evaluating the entire skeleton for bony metastases. The vascular phase images and early static "blood pool" scan demonstrate the vascularity of lesions. CT scans have been useful in deciphering the extent of lesions with high or low densities. Isodense lesions with surrounding soft tissue do not allow for discerning true anatomic extent of these lesions. With

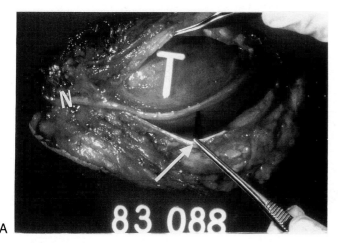
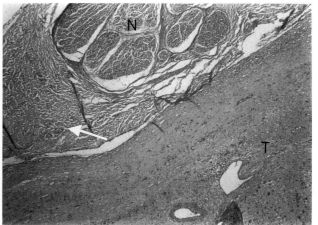

A   B

FIGURE 31.20. In the photograph of the gross specimen of a sarcoma (A), the arrow demonstrates a radiation-induced rind that acts as a capsule around the lesion. The position of the tumor (T) relative to the radial nerve (N) is evident. Photomicrograph (B) shows a segment of the mature fibrous capsule (arrow) near the radial nerve (N), partially surrounding an area of dead or dying tumor (T) cells that are embedded in fibrous tissue.

contrast studies occasionally the reactive pseudocapsule can be discerned by the increased vascularity, as seen by rim enhancement. Angiography is used less now, but may be indicated in lesions in close proximity to neuro-vascular structures or when it is necessary to discern the vascular anatomy.

The MRI scan appears to be the most accurate means of assessing anatomic sites of involvement of soft tissue tumors. Transaxial cuts seem more beneficial to the operating surgeon as most of the fascial planes are longitudinally oriented. With the exception of fibrous and highly cellular lesions, the majority of tumors demonstrate increased signal on T_2W sequence. It is important to use differential imaging techniques so that the various tissue types can be hypothesized.

Biopsy Procedures

Biopsies need to be performed as a separate surgical procedure. They need to be carefully planned so that the tracts can be excised at the time of the surgical resection. These are best performed at the institution where the definitive surgery is to be rendered.[120,121] Usually muscle-splitting incisions are required so soft tissues can be completely excised. In select incidents, the diagnosis can be obtained by histologic analysis of a frozen section so the definitive surgical procedure can be carried out at the same surgical setting.[122] It is important to recognize that these surgeries for obtaining biopsy material can be responsible for a microscopic seeding of the lesion locally. These areas need to be excised at the time of surgical resection for the tumor.

Surgical Procedure

The surgical procedure needs to be carefully planned so appropriate margins will be achieved for acceptable rates of local control.[115-118] When appropriate margins are not obtained in the resection of malignant lesions, recurrence is a rule and is associated with a 50% increase in the metastatic rate.[123,124] The surgical procedure designed preoperatively should be geared at accruing adequate margins rather than being viewed as limb salvage versus ablative surgery. Appropriate margins for acceptable rates of local control are a necessity and limb-sparing procedures are appropriate whenever good surgical margins are obtainable.

Conclusions

Appropriate margins for acceptable rates of local control are a necessity. Limb-sparing procedures are appropriate when margins associated with good local control are obtainable. Optimal clinical diagnosis and treatment of mass lesions involving the muscle will usually require the use of one or more imaging techniques. Proper selection and interpretation of imaging studies available today will usually provide differentiation between neoplastic and other soft tissue masses of the musculoskeletal system. Classic appearances for many of the benign and several of the malignant lesions have been described and provide specific diagnosis when present. MRI is frequently the most useful and anatomically accurate of these techniques, although unerring diagnostic specificity with this or any other technique remains an elusive goal. Increased experience with these tools has provided greater diagnostic confidence in many circumstances, but has also revealed the exceptions to the lesion characteristics that have been initially described. Intimate knowledge of these imaging techniques is highly desirable as they are the means by which the decisions concerning biopsy, surgery, radiation therapy, and percutaneous drainage treatments are planned and accomplished.

References

1. Reiser M, Rupp N, Heller HJ, et al. MR-tomography in the diagnosis of malignant soft-tumours. Eur J Radiol 1984;4:288–293.
2. Weekes RG, McLeod RA, Reiman HM, Pritchard DJ. CT of soft-tissue neoplasms. AJR 1985;144:355–360.
3. Petasnick JP, Turner DA, Charters JR, Gitelis S, Zacharias CE. Soft-tissue masses of the locomotor system: comparison of MRI with CT. Radiology 1986;160:125–133.
4. Totty WG. Radiographic evaluation of soft tissue sarcomas. Orthop Rev 1985;14:257–269.
5. Aisen AM, Martel W, Braunstein EM, McMillin KI, Phillips WA, Kling TF. MRI and CT evaluation of primary bone and soft-tissue tumors. AJR 1986;146:749–756.
6. Pettersson H, Gillespy T III, Hamlin DJ, et al. Primary musculoskeletal tumors: examination with MRI compared with conventional modalities. Radiology 1987;164:237–241.
7. Wetzel LH, Levine E, Murphey MD. A comparison of MRI and CT in the evaluation of musculoskeletal masses. Radiographics 1987;7:851–874.
8. Chang AE, Matory YL, Dwyer AJ. Magnetic resonance imaging versus computed tomography in the evaluation of soft tissue tumors of the extremities. Ann Surg 1987;205:340–348.
9. Sundaram M, McGuire MH, Herbold DR, Beshany SE, Fletcher JW. High signal intensity soft tissue masses on T1 weighted pulsing sequences. Skeletal Radiol 1987;16:30–36.
10. Demas BE, Heelan RT, Lane J, Marcove R, Hajdu S, Brennan MF. Soft-tisse sarcomas of the extremities: comparison of MRI and CT in determining the extent of disease. AJR 1988;150:615–620.

11. Tehranzadeh J, Mnaymneh W, Ghavam C, Morillo G, Murphy BJ. Comparison of CT and MRI in musculoskeletal neoplasms. J Comput Assist Tomogr 1989;13:466–472.

12. Wetzel LH, Levine E. Soft-tissue tumors of the foot: value of MRI for specific diagnosis. AJR 1990;155:1025–1030.

13. Reuther G, Mutschler W. Detection and local recurrent disease in musculoskeletal tumors: magnetic resonance imaging versus computed tomography. Skeletal Radiol 1990;19:85–90.

14. Egund N, Ekelund L, Sako M, Persson B. CT of soft-tissue tumors. AJR 1981;137:725–729.

15. Golding SJ, Husband JE. The role of computed tomography in the management of soft tissue sarcomas. Br J Radiol 1982;55:740–747.

16. Scally J, Garrett A. Primary extranodal lymphoma in muscle. Br J Radiol 1989;62:81.

17. Chui MC, Bird BL, Rogers J. Extracranial and extraspinal nerve sheath tumors: computed tomographic evaluation. Neuroradiology 1988;30:47–53.

18. O'Keeffe F, Lorigan JG, Wallace S. Radiological features of extraskeletal Ewing sarcoma. Br J Radiol 1990;63:456–460.

19. Herrlin K, Willén H, Rydholm A. Deep-seated soft tissue leiomyomas. Report of four patients. Skeletal Radiol 1990;19:363–365.

20. Janzen DL, Connell DG, Vaisler BJ. Calcific myonecrosis of the calf manifesting as an enlarging soft-tissue mass: imaging features. AJR 1993;160:1072–1074.

21. Yiu-Chiu VS, Chiu LC. Complementary values of ultrasound and computed tomography in the evaluation of musculoskeletal masses. Radiographics 1983;3:46–82.

22. Hermann G, Yeh HC, Schwartz I. Computed tomography of soft-tissue lesions of the extremities, pelvic and shoulder girdles: sonographic and pathological correlations. Clin Radiol 35:193–202.

23. Thijssen JM. Ultrasonic characterization: prospects of tumor diagnosis. Eur J Radiol 1984;4:312–317.

24. Fornage BD, Tassin GB. Sonographic appearances of superficial soft tissue lipomas. J Clin Ultrasound 1991;19:215–220.

25. Bernardino ME, Jing B-S, Thomas JL, Lindell MM Jr, Zornoza J. The extremity soft-tissue lesion: a comparative study of ultrasound, computed tomography, and xeroradiography. Radiology 1981;139:53–59.

26. Chew FS, Hudson TM, Enneking WF. Radionuclide imaging of soft tissue neoplasms. Semin Nucl Med 1981;11:266–276.

27. Teates CD, Bray ST, Williamson BRJ. Tumor detection with Ga67-citrate: a literature survey (1970–1978). Clin Nucl Med 1978;3:345–460.

28. Pinsky SM, Henkin RE. Gallium-67 tumor scanning. Semin Nucl Med 1976;6:397–409.

29. Kaufman JH, Cedermark BJ, Parthasarathy KL, Didolkar MS, Bakshi SP. The value of ^{67}Ga scintigraphy in soft-tissue sarcoma and chondrosarcoma. Radiology 1977;123:131–134.

30. McAfee JG, Samin A. In-111 labeled leukocytes: a review of problems in image interpretation. Radiology 1985;155:221–229.

31. Enneking WF, Chew FS, Springfield DS, Hudson TM, Spanier SS. The role of radionuclide bone-scanning in determining the resectability of soft-tissue sarcomas. J Bone Joint Surg 1981;63A:249–256.

32. Kairemo KJA, Wiklund TA, Liewendahl K, et al. Imaging of soft-tissue sarcomas with indium-111-labeled monoclonal antimyosin fab fragments. J Nucl Med 1990;31:23–31.

33. Vorne M, Saukko T. Detection of malignant soft tissue tumors in bone imaging. Eur J Nucl Med 1984;9:180–184.

34. Hayes RL. The medical use of gallium radionuclides: a brief history with some comments. Semin Nucl Med 1978;8:183–191.

35. Hudson TM, Hamlin DJ, Enneking WF, Pettersson H. Magnetic resonance imaging of bone and soft tissue tumors: early experience in 31 patients compared with computed tomography. Skeletal Radiol 1985;13:134–146.

36. Totty WG, Murphy WA, Lee JKT. Soft-tissue tumors: MRI. Radiology 1986;160:135–141.

37. Vanel D, Lacombe MJ, Couanet D, Kalifa C, Spielmann M, Genin J. Musculoskeletal tumors: follow-up with MRI after treatment with surgery and radiation therapy. Radiology 1987;164:243–245.

38. Kransdorf M, Jelinek J, Moser R, et al. Soft tissue masses: Diagnosis using MRI. AJR 1989;153:541–547.

39. Weatherall PT. Benign and malignant masses: MRI differentiation. MRI Clin North Am 1995;3(4):669–694.

40. Rubin SJ, Feldman F, Haber MM, Staron R, Alan J, Dick HM. Magnetic resonance grid analysis of soft tissue lesions. Invest Radiol 1991;26:474–478.

41. Nurenberg P, Harms SE. MRI of musculoskeletal tumors. CRC Crit Rev 1988;28(4):331–353.

42. Glazer HS, Lee JKT, Levitt RG, et al. Radiation fibrosis: differentiation from recurrent tumor by MRI. Radiology 1985;156:721–726.

43. Sanchez RB, Quinn SF, Walling A, Estrada J, Greenberg H. Musculoskeletal neoplasms after intraarterial chemotherapy: correlation of MR images with pathologic specimens. Radiology 1990;174:237–240.

44. Biondetti PR, Ehman RL. Soft-tissue sarcomas: use of textural patterns in skeletal muscle as a diagnostic feature in postoperative MRI. Radiology 1992;183:845–848.

45. Pettersson H, Stone RM, Spanier S, Gillespy T III, Fitzsimmons JR, Scott KN. Musculoskeletal tumors: T1 and T2 relaxation times. Radiology 1988;167:783–785.

46. Weatherall PT, Maale GE, Sherry CS, Fleckenstein JL, Mendelsohn DB, Pascoe R. High T1-weighted signal intensity in MRI of soft tissue sarcomas [abstract]. J Magn Reson Imaging 1991;1:194.

47. Crim JR, Seeger LL, Yao L, Chandnani V, Eckardt JJ. Diagnosis of soft-tissue masses with MRI: can benign masses be differentiated from malignant ones? Radiology 1992;185:581–586.

48. Berquist TH, Ehman RL, King BF, Hedgman CG, Ilstrup DM. Value of MRI in differentiating benign from

malignant soft-tissue masses: study of 95 lesions. AJR 1990;155:1251–1255.

49. Sundaram M, McGuire MH, Herbald DR. Magnetic resonance imaging of masses: an evaluation of fifty-three histologically proven tumors. Magn Reson Imaging 1988; 6:237–248.

50. Hermann G, Abdelwahab IF, Miller TT, Klein MJ, Lewis MM. Tumour and tumour-like conditions of the soft tissue: magnetic resonance imaging features differentiating benign from malignant masses. Br J Radiol 1992; 65:14–20.

51. Levine E, Huntrakoon M, Wetzel LH. Malignant nerve-sheath neoplasms in neurofibromatosis: distinction from benign tumors by using imaging techniques. AJR 1987; 1059–1064.

52. Stiglbauer R, Augustin I, Kramer J, et al. MRI in the diagnosis of primary lymphoma of bone: correlation with histopathology. J Comp Assist Tomogr 1992;16:248–253.

53. Enzinger FM, Weiss SW. Rhabdomyoma, Chapter 7. In: Enziner FM, Weiss SW, eds. Soft tissue tumors, 2nd ed. St. Louis: C.V. Mosby, 1988:433–447.

54. Burk DL Jr, Brunberg JA, Kanal E, Latchaw RE, Wolf GL. Spinal and paraspinal neurofibromatosis: surface coil MRI at 1.5 T1. Radiology 1987;162:797–801.

55. Weatherall PT, Mendelsohn DB, Mamourian A, et al. MRI of peripheral plexiform and solitary neurofibromas [abstract]. Magn Reson Imaging 1989;7:53.

56. Levine E, Nuntrakoon M, Wetzel LH. Malignant nerve sheath neoplasms in neurofibromatosis: distinction from benign tumors by using imaging techniques. AJR 1987; 149:1059–1064.

57. Suh JS, Abenoza P, Galloway HR, Everson LI, Griffiths HJ. Peripheral (extracranial) nerve tumors: correlation of MRI and histologic findings. Radiology 1992;183: 341–346.

58. Berlin O, Stener B, Lindahl S, Irstam L, Lodding P. Vascularization of peripheral neurilemomas: angiographic, computed tomographic, and histologic studies. Skeletal Radiol 1986;15:275–283.

59. Feldman F. Tuberous sclerosis, neurofibromatosis, and fibrous dysplasia. In: Resnick D, Niwayama G, eds. Diagnosis of bone and joint disorders. Philadelphia: W.B. Saunders, 1988:4055.

60. Cohen EK, Kressel HY, Perosio T, et al. MRI of soft-tissue hemangiomas: correlation with pathologic findings. AJR 1988;150:1079–1081.

61. Greenspan A, McGahan JP, Vogelsang P, Szabo RM. Imaging strategies in the evaluation of soft-tissue hemangiomas of the extremities: correlation of the findings of plain radiography, angiography, CT, MRI, and ultrasonography in 12 histologically proven cases. Skeletal Radiol 1992;21:11–18.

62. Kaplan PA, Williams SM. Mucocutaneous and peripheral soft-tissue hemangiomas: MRI. Radiology 1987;163: 163–166.

63. Nelson MC, Stull MA, Teitelbaum GP, et al. Magnetic resonance imaging of peripheral soft tissue hemangiomas. Skeletal Radiol 1990;19:477–482.

64. Yuh WTC, Kathol MH, Sein MA, Ehara S, Chiu L. Hemangiomas of skeletal muscle: MR findings in five patients. AJR 1987:765–768.

65. Levine F, Wetzel LH, Neff JR. MR imaging and CT of extrahepatic cavernous hemangiomas. AJR 1986;147: 1299–1304.

66. Kransdorf M, Moser R, Meis J, Neyer C. Fat containing soft-tissue masses of the extremities. Radiographics 1991; 11:81–106.

67. Madewell JE, Sweet DE. Tumors and tumor-like lesions in or about joints. In: Resnick D, Niwayama G, eds. Diagnosis of bone and joint disorders, 2nd ed. Philadelpia: W.B. Saunders, 1988:3891–3900.

68. Enzinger FM, Weiss SW. Benign lipomatous tumors. In: Soft tissue tumors, 2nd ed. St. Louis: C.V. Mosby, 1988: 304–327.

69. Bush CH, Spanier SS, Gillespy T III. Imaging of atypical lipomas of the extremities: report of three cases. Skeletal Radiol 1988;17:472–475.

70. Enzinger FM, Weiss SW. In: Enzinger FM, Weiss SW, eds. Soft tissue tumours, 2nd ed. St. Louis: C.V. Mosby, 1988:136–163.

71. Hudson TM, Vandergriend RA, Springfield DS, et al. Aggressive fibromatosis: evaluation by computed tomography and angiography. Radiology 1984;150:495–501.

72. Stockdale AD, Cassoni AM, Coe MA, et al. Radiotherapy and conservative surgery in the management of musculoaponeurotic fibromatosis. Int J Rad Oncol Biol Phys 1988;15:851–857.

73. Maale GE, Schwarz D, Weatherall PT. Results of treatment for extra-abdominal aggressvie fibromatosis utilizing megavoltage radiation for local control. Presentation at 7th International Symposium on Limb Salvage, Singapore, August 1993.

74. Sundaram M, Duffrin H, McGuire MH, Vas W. Synchronous multicentric desmoid tumors (aggressive fibromatosis) of the extremities. Skeletal Radiol 1988;17: 16–19.

75. Hawnaur JM, Jenkins JPR, Isherwood I. Magnetic resonance imaging of musculo-aponeurotic fibromatosis. Skeletal Radiol 1990;19:509–514.

76. Quinn SF, Erickson SJ, Dee PM, et al. MRI in fibromatosis: results in 26 patients with pathologic correlation. AJR 1991;156:539–542.

77. Peterson KK, Renfrew DL, Feddersen RM, Buckwalter JA, El-Khoury GY. Magnetic resonance imaging of myxoid containing tumors. Skeletal Radiol 1991;20:245–250.

78. Sundaram M, McDonald DJ, Merenda G. Intramuscular myxoma: a rare association with fibrous dysplasia of bone. AJR 1989;153:107–108.

79. Enzinger FM, Weiss SW. Benign tumors and tumorlike lesions of uncertain histogenesis. In: Enzinger FM, Weiss SW, eds. Soft tissue tumors, 2nd ed. St. Louis: C.V. Mosby, 1988:912–918.

80. Cohen E, Kressel H, Frank TS, et al. Hyaline cartilage-origin bone and soft tissue neoplasms: MRI appearance and histologic correlation. Radiology 1988;167:477–481.

81. deSantos LA, Spjut HJ. Periosteal chondroma: a radiographic spectrum. Skeletal Radiol 1981;6:15–20.

82. Zlatkin MB, Lander PH, Begin LR, Hadjipavlou A. Soft-tissue chondromas. AJR 1985;144:1263–1267.

83. Geirnaerdt MJA, Bloem JL, Eulderink F, Hogendoorn PCW, Taminiau AHM. Cartilaginous tumors: correlation of gadolinium-enhanced MRI and histopathologic findings. Radiology 1993;186:813–817.

84. Weatherall PT, Maale GE, Sherry CS, Mendelsohn DB, Erdman WA, Milchgrub S. Characteristic MRI features of low-grade cartilage lesions with histologic correlation. Scientific Exhibit, RSNA, 1992.

85. Beltran J, Simon DC, Katz W, Weis LD. Increased MRI signal intensity in skeletal muscle adjacent to malignant tumors: pathologic correlation and clinical relevance. Radiology 1987;162:251–255.

86. Hanna SL, Fletcher BD, Parham DM, Bugg MF. Muscle edema in musculoskeletal tumors: MRI characteristics and clinical significance. J Magn Reson Imaging 1991;1: 441–449.

87. Erlemann R, Reiser MF, et al. Musculoskeletal neoplasms: static and dynamic Gd-DTPA-enhanced MRI. Radiology 1989;171:767.

88. Fletcher BD, Hanna SL. Musculoskeletal neoplasms: dynamic Gd-DTPT-enhanced MRI [letter]. Radiology 1989;177:287.

89. London J, Kim EE, Wallace S, Shirkhoda A, Coan J, Evans H. MRI of liposarcomas: correlation of MRI features and histology. J Comp Assist Tomogr 1989;13: 832–835.

90. Enzinger FM, Weiss SW. Rhabdomyosarcoma. In: Enzinger FM, Weiss SW, eds. Soft tissue tumours, 2nd ed. St. Louis: C.V. Mosby, 1988:448–488.

91. Enzinger FM, Weiss SW. Lipomas. In: Enzinger FM, Weiss SW eds. Soft tissue tumors, 2nd ed. St. Louis: C.V. Mosby, 1988:351, 352, 363–366.

92. Sundaram M, Baran G, Merenda G, McDonald DJ. Myxoid liposarcoma: magnetic resonance imaging appearances with clinical and histological correlation. Skeletal Radiol 1990;19:359–362.

93. Jelinek JS, Kransdorf MJ, Shmookler BM, Aboulafia AJ, Malawer MM. Liposarcoma of the extremities: MRI and CT findings in the histologic subtypes. Radiology 1993; 186:455–459.

94. Mahajan H, Kim EE, Wallace S, Abello R, Benjamin R, Evans HL. Magnetic resonance imaging of malignant fibrous histiocytoma. Magn Reson Imaging 1989;7:283–288.

95. Morton MJ, Berquist TH, McLeod RA, Unni KK, Sim FH. MRI of synovial sarcoma. AJR 1991;156:337–340.

96. Sundaram M, McGuire MH, Fletcher J, Wolverson MK, Heiberg E. Magnetic resonance imaging of lesions of synovial origin. Skeletal Radiol 1986;15:110–116.

97. Panicek DM, Casper ES, Brennan MF, Hajdu SI, Heelan RT. Hemorrhage simulating tumor growth in malignant fibrous histiocytoma at MRI. Radiology 1991;181: 398–400.

98. Rubin JI, Gomori JM, Grossman RI, Gefter WB, Kressel HY. High-field MRI of extracranial hematomas. AJR 1987;248:813–817.

99. Sundaram M, Duffrin H, McGuire MH. In vivo and in vitro demonstration of hemorrhage in soft tissue sarcoma. Magn Reson Med 1988;6:57–60.

100. Erdman WA, Tamburro F, Jayson HT, Weatherall PT, Bond-Ferry K, Peshock RM. Osteomyelitis: characteristics and pitfalls of diagnosis with MRI. Radiology 1991; 180(2):533–539.

101. Tang JSH, Gold RH, Bassett LW, Seeger LL. Musculoskeletal infection of the extremities; evaluation with MRI. Radiology 1988;166:205–209.

102. Fleckenstein JL, Burns DK, Murphy FK, Jayson HT, Bonte FJ. Differential diagnosis of bacterial myositis in AIDS: evaluation with MRI. Radiology 1991;179: 653–658.

103. Steinbach LS, Tehranzadeh J, Fleckenstein JL, Vanarthos WJ. Human immunodeficiency virus infection: musculoskeletal manifestations. Radiology 1993;186: 833–838.

104. Weatherall PT, Maale GE, Sherry CS. Osteomyelitis, diagnosis/staging: comparison of MR imaging, CT and In^{111} white blood cell and Tc^{99m} scanning. J Magn Reson Imaging 1992;2(P):81.

105. Stakianakis GN, Al-Sheikh W, Heal A, Rodman G, Zeppa R, Serafini A. Comparisons of scintigraphy with In^{111} leukocytes and Ga^{67} in diagnosis of occult sepsis. J Nucl Med 1982;23:618–626.

106. Sayle BA, Balachandram S, Rogers CA. Indium^{111} chloride imaging in patients with suspected abscesses: concise communication. J Nucl Med 1983;24:1114–1118.

107. Angervall L, Stener B, Stener I, Ahren C. Pseudomalignant osseous tumor of soft tissue: a clinical, radiological and pathological study of five cases. J Bone Joint Surg 1969;51B:654–663.

108. Fleckenstein JL, Weatherall PT, Bertocci LA, et al. Locomotor system assessment by muscle magnetic resonance imaging. Magn Reson Q 1991;7:79–103.

109. Schweitzer ME, Greenway G, Resnick D, Haghighi P, Snoots WE. Osteoma of soft parts. Skeletal Radiol 1992; 21:177–180.

110. Pettersson H, Eliasson J, Egund N, et al. Gadolinium-DTPA enhancement of soft tissue tumors in magnetic resonance imaging—preliminary clinical experience in five patients. Skeletal Radiol 1988;17:319–323.

111. Erlemann R, Vassalo P, Bongartz G, et al. Musculoskeletal neoplasms: fast low-angle shot MRI with and without Gd-DTPA. Radiology 1990;176:489–495.

112. Herrlin K, Ling LB, Pettersson H, et al. Gadolinium-DTPA enhancement of soft tissue tumors in magnetic resonance imaging. Acta Radiol 1990;31:233.

113. Mirowitz SA, Totty WG, Lee JKT. Characterization of musculoskeletal masses using dynamic Gd-DTPA enhanced spin-echo MRI. J Comput Assist Tomogr 1992; 16:120–125.

114. Enneking WF. Staging of musculoskeletal neoplasms. Skeletal Radiol 1985;13:183–194.

115. Enneking WF, Spanier SS, Goodman MA. A system for the surgical staging of musculoskeletal sarcoma. Clin Orthop Rel Res 1980;153:106–120.

116. Enneking WF. A system of staging musculoskeletal neoplasms. Clin Orthop Rel Res 1986;204:9–24.

117. Enneking WF. Musculoskeletal tumor surgery. New York: Churchill Livingstone, 1983:69–88.

118. Enneking WF, Spanier SS, Malawer MM. The effect of anatomic setting on the results of surgical procedures for soft parts sarcomas of the thigh. Cancer 1981;47: 1005–1022.

119. Suit HD, Mankin HJ, Wood WC, Proppe KH. Radiation and surgery in the treatment of primary sarcoma of soft tissue: pre-operative, intra-operative and post-operative. Cancer 1985;55:2659–2667.

120. Mankin HJ, Lange TJ, Spanier SS. The hazards of biopsy in patients with malignant primary bone and soft-tissue tumors. J Bone Joint Surg 1982;64A:1121–1127.

121. Simon MA. Biopsy of musculoskeletal tumors. J Bone Joint Surg 1982;64A:1253–1257.

122. Dahlin DC. Seventy-five years' experience with frozen sections at the Mayo Clinic. Mayo Clin Proc 1980;55: 721–723.

123. Enneking WF, Maale GE. The effect of the tumoral contamination of wounds. Cancer 1988;62:1251–1256.

124. Bowden L, Booher RS. The principals and techniques of resection of soft parts for sarcoma. Surgery 1958;44: 963–974.

32
Muscle Edema Associated with Musculoskeletal Neoplasms and Radiation Therapy

Barry D. Fletcher and Soheil L. Hanna

The exceptional tissue contrast provided by magnetic resonance imaging (MRI) permits the observation of physiologic and pathologic changes within skeletal muscle. As described in the previous chapters, even physiologic events such as exercise may alter the signal intensity of muscle on MR images,[1] and the effects of minor trauma[2] and inflammation[3] are readily visualized. These alterations in contrast can possibly be attributed to changes in the interstitial water content of skeletal muscle and alterations in the physical state of water,[4] which modify T_1 and T_2 relaxation times.[5,6] As a result, radiologists involved in oncologic MRI are now observing muscle abnormalities that were previously undetectable by other imaging modalities. In this chapter, we will discuss the MRI findings accompanying pathophysiologic changes in muscle in patients with tumors or tumor-like lesions of the musculoskeletal system and the effects of radiation therapy.

Imaging Techniques

The muscle abnormalities described in this chapter were observed during MRI of musculoskeletal tumors using mainly spin echo techniques. Except for the images in Figures 32.1 and 32.2, which were obtained using a MRI device operating at 1.5 T, the examinations illustrated here were performed on a 1.0-T MRI device.

On T_1-weighted images made with short T_E/short T_R pulse sequences, the long T_1 relaxation time of edematous muscle may be expected to result in decreased signal intensity, compared to hypointense normal muscle, but the contrast is usually insufficient to demonstrate edema. The prolonged T_2 relaxation time associated with increased tissue hydration, however, causes edematous muscles to increase in intensity on spin density (short T_E/long T_R) images and to appear very intense on T_2-weighted (long T_E/long T_R) images.

Short inversion time inversion recovery (STIR) images permit observation of a larger volume of abnormal tissue than spin echo images and are thus useful for musculoskeletal tumor staging.[7–9] They increase the conspicuity of tumor-related edematous tissue because the signal due to the relatively short T_1 relaxation time of fatty tissues is nulled by means of an inversion pulse. The inverted spins are allowed to relax for a period of time equal to the T_1 relaxation time of fat (approximately 150 and 180 ms at 1.0 and 1.5 T, respectively). This period is followed by a 90°–180° spin echo sequence, and the signal amplitudes produced by the longer T_1 and T_2 relaxation times of water protons are added.[7] In addition to the increase in contrast of lesions on STIR images, suppression of fat signals diminishes the intensity of respiratory "ghost" artifacts in the phase encoding direction of the image and chemical shift artifacts are minimized. The major shortcoming of this sequence is lack of specificity because both tumor and adjacent edema produce strong signals, and therefore the tumor borders may be obscured by intense muscle edema, and the margins may be overestimated (see Figures 32.3A, 32.6B). STIR images also have less favorable signal-to-noise characteristics than T_2-weighted images, and are susceptible to motion and flow artifacts. Fast ("turbo") STIR imaging techniques are now available which, like fast spin echo T_2-weighted sequences, generate multiple phase-encoded echoes per T_R. They result in decreased imaging times with improved signal to noise, while permitting reduced interslice gaps and increased numbers of slices per sequence.

Another method of enhancing differences in intensity between normal and edematous muscle suppresses fat signal by utilizing a radiofrequency-selective excitation pulse and dephasing gradient followed by a spin echo sequence. By preceding a T_2-weighted sequence with a narrow band saturation pulse equal in frequency to that of the lipid protons, fat signal is suppressed. The altered dynamic range of the signal intensities of the remaining

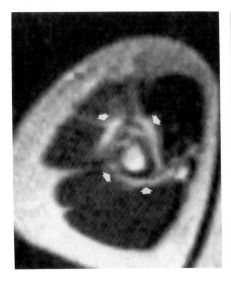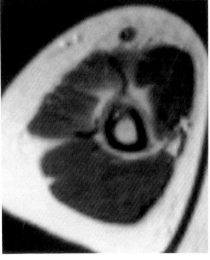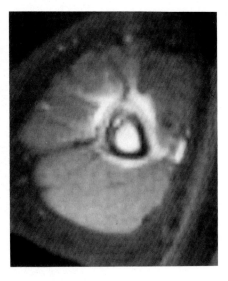

FIGURE 32.1. The proximal humerus of a patient with chronic osteomyelitis. (A) T_2-weighted (2500/80 ms, T_R/T_E); (B) gadolinium-enhanced T_1-weighted (650/15) and (C) Radiofrequency (RF) fat-suppressed, gadolinium-enhanced T_1-weighted (820/15) transverse images. The high-intensity zone of the peritumoral edema surrounding the humerus (arrows in A) is most conspicuous on the image made with fat saturation (C).

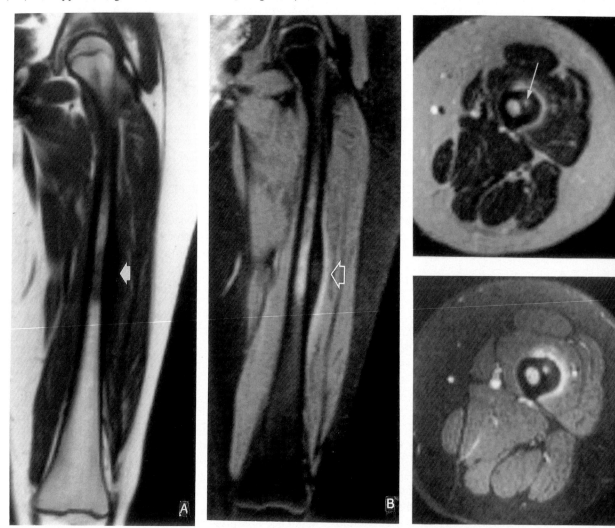

FIGURE 32.2. (A) Coronal T_1-weighted (500/15) image of the femur of a patient with an osteoid osteoma. Abnormally hypointense marrow signal is present in the midshaft and there is extensive cortical thickening laterally (arrow). Muscle intensity appears normal. (B) The coronal STIR image (2100/20/150 ms, $T_R/T_E/T_I$) shows a thin zone of edema (arrow) adjacent to the thickened cortex. The marrow edema is also hyperintense. (C) A T_2-weighted transverse image (2500/80) shows intense marrow and paratumoral edema. The nidus (arrow) is also demonstrated. (D) A transverse T_2-weighted (2205/45) image incorporating a fat-suppression RF pulse shows a more conspicuous, apparently more extensive zone of paratumoral edema with high signal in the marrow and nidus.

unsaturated nonlipid protons results in images in which hydrated tissues appear very intense (see Figure 32.2D).

Intravenous infusion of the paramagnetic contrast agent gadopentetate dimeglumine (gadolinium) enhances MR images of some muscles, particularly extraocular muscles, which are extremely well vascularized and contain prominent extravascular spaces.[10] Most normal skeletal muscle shows little gadolinium-induced change in signal intensity on T_1-weighted images. However, gadolinium has been shown to increase the signal intensity of compressed, edematous, and atrophic muscle surrounding malignant tumors.[11] The abundant extravascular spaces of these muscles are well perfused by gadolinium. The resultant increased T_1 relaxation rate of portons produces an increased signal on short T_R/T_E images (see Figure 32.1B). Fat-suppressed, T_1-weighted, gadolinium-enhanced images[12] further increase the conspicuity of muscle edema (see Figure 32.1C). However, because tumor signal is also increased on static contrast-enhanced MR images, neoplastic involvement of contiguous muscle cannot be differentiated from edema by this means.[13] In this situation, the use of dynamic MRI may help differentiate the two, because the rate of gadolinium enhancement of edematous, but otherwise normal, muscle is slower than that in tumors.[14,15]

Muscle Edema Associated with Muculoskeletal Lesions

Imaging Characteristics

Edema adjacent to benign and malignant musculoskeletal tumors and inflammatory lesions has been described by several authors,[14–17] and is characterized by a zone of increased signal intensity with ill-defined, feathery, or radiating borders. On transverse MR images, the edema frequently forms a concentric ring around the lesion, in

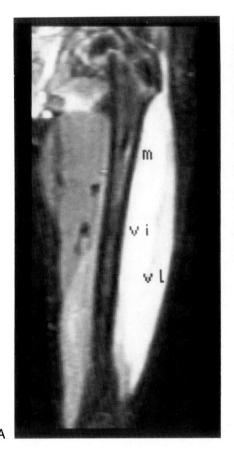

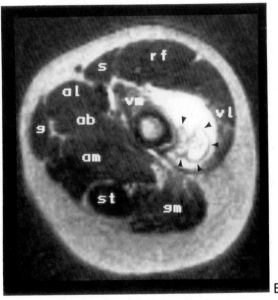

FIGURE 32.3. (A) Coronal STIR (2500/22/150) image showing massive edema involving the vastus lateralis (vl) and vastus intermedius (vi), adjacent to poorly defined myositis ossificans (m) of the thigh. (B) A transverse T_2-weighted image (2500/90) shows the margins of the mass (arrowheads) and the extent of edema. The adductor brevis (ab), adductor longus (al), adductor magnus (am), gracilis (g), gluteus maximus (gm), rectus femoris (rf), sartorius (s), and semitendinosus (st) are not edematous. (Reprinted from Hanna SL, et al. Muscle edema in musculoskeletal tumors: MRI characteristics and clinical significance. J Magn Reson Imaging 1991;1: 441–449.)

which case it is termed "peritumoral" (Figure 32.1). Peritumoral edema is nonselective in its distribution, involving portions of several muscles contiguous to the lesion regardless of bony attachments. Less frequently, the edema does not encircle the entire neoplasm and is therefore "paratumoral" (Figure 32.2). In the majority of cases, peri- or paratumoral edema (PTE) extends no more than two centimeters beyond the margins of the lesion, although the intense signal occasionally extends further peripherally into the subcutaneous tissues.

We have also identified another pattern in which the edema is distributed throughout at least one contiguous muscle in the vicinity of the tumor, rather than being confined to portions of the muscles in the immediate environment.[15] This is referred to as "massive edema" (Figure 32.3). In patients with bone tumors, massive edema selectively affects the mucles that are disrupted at their bony attachments by the tumor (Figure 32.4). In the case of soft tissue masses, the edematous muscles are generally those that contain the neoplasm (Figure 32.5).

On T_2-weighted images, edema associated with a bone tumor is usually separated from the neoplasm itself by a thin, low signal intensity rim composed of dense collagen fibers[17] or reactive bone. In the absence of this boundary the tumor margins may be obscured by the high signal intensity of the edema, especially on STIR images (Figure 32.6). Edematous muscle can be distinguished from a mass of similar intensity if on the accompanying T_1-weighted images, normal architecture, and "texture" of the muscle in question is noted to be preserved (Figure 32.6C).[18]

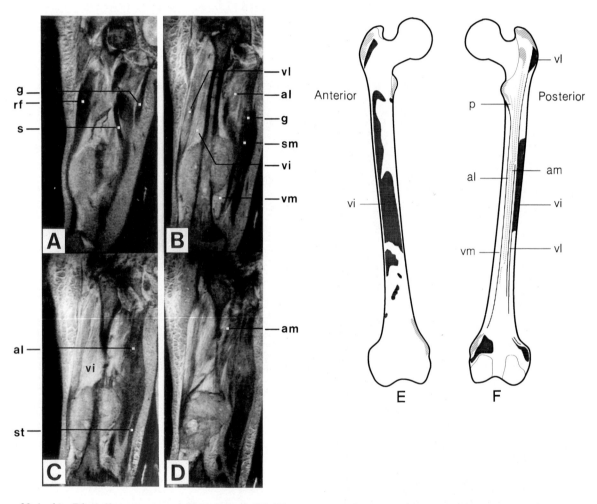

FIGURE 32.4. (A–D) Adjacent coronal T_2-weighted (T_R/T_E: 2500/90) images show a large circumferential Ewing sarcoma involving the lower half of the right femoral shaft (A: most anterior image). (E,F) Diagram showing osseous attachments of the affected muscles. (E: anterior aspect, F: posterior aspect). The tumor has disrupted the origin of the vastus intermedius (vi) anteriorly, and the muscular attachments to the linea aspera posteriorly, including the vastus medialis (vm), vastus lateralis (vl), adductor magnus (am), and adductor longus (al) muscles. Note that all muscles disrupted at their bony attachments by the large tumor mass are edematous. g: gracilis, rf: rectus femoris, p: psoas, s: sartorius, sm: semimembranous, st: semitendinous.

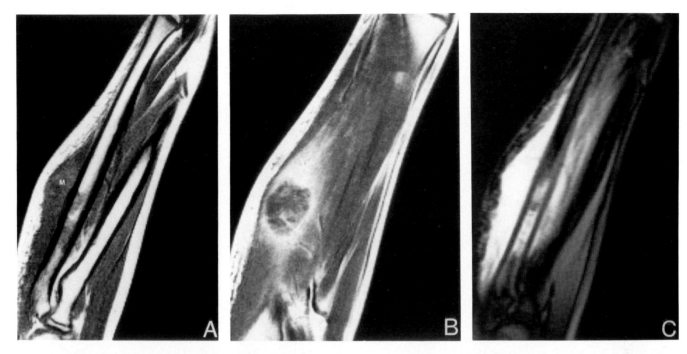

FIGURE 32.5. Longitudinal images of the forearm of a patient with epithelioid sarcoma involving the soft tissue adjacent to dorsum of the radius. (A) T_1-weighted image (600/15) shows an ill-defined intramuscular mass (M) with slightly more intense signal than muscle. There is also secondary involvement of the medullary cavity. (B) Gadolinium-enhanced T_1-weighted image (600/15) shows an ill-defined zone of enhancement surrounding the unenhanced soft tissue tumor. (C) STIR image (2500/22/150) shows more extensive muscle edema.

Clinical Relevance

Muscle edema has also been described with a variety of nonneoplastic lesions of the musculoskeletal system including inflammation, infection, hematoma, and infarction.[15,16,19] Indeed, in one study[19] edema was found to be more extensive in the muscles adjacent to nonneoplastic processes than in those affected by neoplasms.

Reports of the incidence of muscle edema with primary benign and malignant musculoskeletal neoplasms differ. In one series, an edematous reaction was noted with 27 of 33 high-grade malignant tumors, and the investigators felt that the presence of edema made the diagnosis of a benign tumor unlikely.[20] Edema was also reported to accompany 16 of 17 untreated primary osteogenic sarcomas,[17] and it may also accompany skeletal metastases (Figure 32.7). Beltran[16] described increased signal intensity adjacent to 13 of 25 primary and secondary soft tissue malignancies studied, and noted that, in the absence of previous radiation, it was a useful sign of malignancy. Crim et al.[21] observed peritumoral edema more often in association with malignant than with benign soft tissue lesions but concluded that its presence did not contribute to the differential diagnosis. Indeed, only 4 of the 27 soft tissue malignancies studied by Kransdorf[22] were surrounded by edema; none of these were primary tumors.

A variety of benign neoplasms, including osteoid osteoma, chondroblastoma, and eosinophilic granuloma, have been described in which soft tissue edema is a prominent feature.[23,24] Thus, although edema adjacent to a lesion lends it an aggressive appearance, its presence should not be considered indicative of malignant disease.

We analyzed the relative incidence of PTE and massive edema in consecutive patients presenting to St. Jude Children's Research Hospital with benign (nine cases) or primary malignant (27 cases) bone or soft tissue lesions.[15] The incidences of PTE (67%) and massive edema (22%) were identical in these two groups. When massive edema occurred in the presence of a malignant tumor, it was highly correlated with large tumor size, poor response to chemotherapy, and metastatic disease at diagnosis. Also, in all 13 patients whose tumors responded to chemotherapy, and two of five with stable tumors, muscle edema decreased. In another series,[25] a reduction in edema was seen in 82% of responders and 50% of nonresponders, and this change alone could therefore not be relied on as an indicator of response.

Histologic Correlations

On gross examination, edematous muscles can be identified at the periphery of resected tumor specimens by

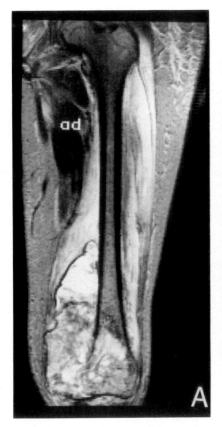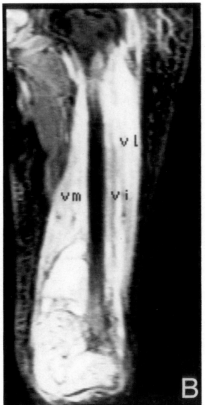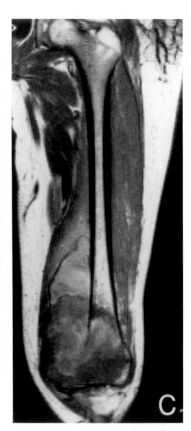

FIGURE 32.6. (A) Coronal T_2-weighted (2500/90) and (B) STIR (2500/22/150) images of the thigh of a patient with "massive" edema associated with a large distal femoral osteosarcoma. The edema involves the entire vastus group of muscles. The adductors are spared. The tumor margins are better defined on the T_2-weighted image than on the STIR image. Note also the extensive high signal of subcutaneous edema. ad: adductor magnus, vm: vastus medius, vi: vastus intermedius, vl: vastus lateralis. (C) On the coronal T_1-weighted image, "texture" of the edematous muscles is normal. The high signal intensity within the tumor is presumably due to hemorrhage. (Reprinted from Hanna SL, et al. Muscle edema in musculoskeletal tumors: MRI characteristics and clinical significance. J Magn Reson Imaging 1991;1:441–449.)

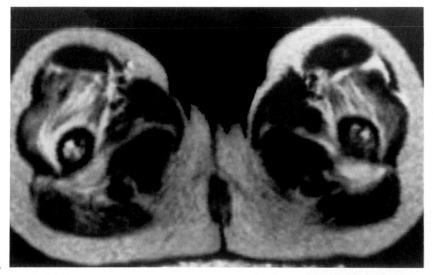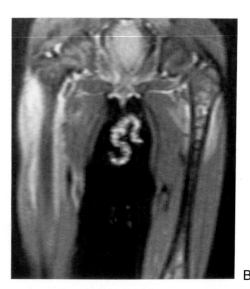

FIGURE 32.7. (A) T_2-weighted transverse (2500/90) and (B) coronal STIR (2500/22/150) images of the proximal thighs of a 7-year-old patient with metastatic neuroblastoma. Note abnormal signal in the medullary cavity of the proximal femurs. There is extensive bilateral peritumoral edema. Radiographs showed demineralization without cortical abnormalities or periosteal reaction.

their pale color. Histologically, the edematous muscle fibers are smaller than those of their nonedematous counterparts, and there is an increase in interstitial fluid in the widened intercellular spaces (Figure 32.8). In our series,[15] periostitis with periosteal lymphocytic infiltration and perivascular cuffing was another frequent finding, the importance of which is yet to be determined.

Unfortunately, MR images cannot detect microscopic collections of malignant cells, and even macroscopic involvement of muscle adjacent to musculoskeletal tumors may be obscured by edema. In the case of malignant soft tissue tumors, direct invasion of the edematous zone can be predicted when the involved muscle is thickened and the tumor and edema are poorly demarcated on MR studies.[16] In the case of bone tumors, malignant infiltration of edematous muscles appears to be uncommon.[15,26] In our study, malignant cells were present in edematous muscle in only 1 of 16 malignant specimens (an osteosarcoma), although several had benign lymphocytic infiltration. In Beltran's series of malignant soft tissue neoplasms, tumor cells were found in adjacent muscle in two of the nine patients with increased signal intensity adjacent to the tumor.[16] Although this has a bearing on the surgical resectability of soft tissue tumors, in the case of malignant bone lesions, the presence of cancer cells in tissues adjacent to the main body of the tumor may have less clinical significance, because most oncologic surgical procedures are wide resections that include abundant normal tissue beyond the tumor margins.[27] However, this issue is assuming more importance with the growing use of limb-sparing procedures in which

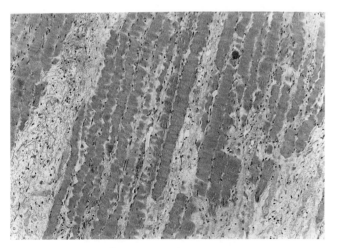

FIGURE 32.8. A photomicrograph of edematous muscle adjacent to an osteosarcoma. The interstitial spaces between groups of muscle fibers are widened, and some fibers are smaller than normal (hematoxylin and eosin ×450). (Reprinted from Hanna SL, et al. Muscle edema in musculoskeletal tumors: MRI characteristics and clinical significance. J Magn Reson Imaging 1991;1:441–449.

it is necessary to preserve major nerves and blood vessels which may be in close proximity to the tumor.

Pathogenesis

The mechanism that produces muscle edema in the vicinity of musculoskeletal tumors is unknown. Analysis of the anatomic features of massive edema in our study[15] ruled out mere compression by a tumor as a cause. However, muscles subjected to continuous tension by lesions that disrupted their origin or insertion were frequently edematous. We postulated that the increased functional demand on these muscles leads to increased vascularity and expansion of the interstitial fluid volume. Another possible contributing factor pertaining to bone tumors is periosteal reaction,[28] which was present in most of our cases with edema. Either of these changes would be expected to produce increased signal on T_2-weighted, STIR and gadolinium-enhanced T_1-weighted MR images.

Muscle Edema Associated with Radiation Therapy

Therapeutic radiation may cause significant cellular injury to normal tissues. The normal anatomic structures most obviously affected by external beam irradiation include the skin, gastrointestinal tract, bladder and bone marrow.[29]

An increase in the signal intensity of normal bone marrow has been observed on T_2-weighted and STIR images in the first days and weeks after radiation therapy.[30,31] Irradiated bone tumors also show increased signal intensity on T_2-weighted images.[32] These changes have been attributed to edema and inflammation. It is not surprising that normal muscles within the radiation field are subject to similar radiation changes. We have identified increased signal intensity on T_2-weighted, STIR, and gadolinium-enhanced T_1-weighted images in the musculature adjacent to irradiated Ewing sarcomas and malignant soft tissue neoplasms[33] (Figure 32.9). These tumors were treated with a combination of chemotherapy and radiation therapy consisting of conventional (once daily) or hyperfractionated (twice daily) radiation to total doses of 55 to 60 Gy.

Like bone marrow edema, these muscle abnormalities appear to be an acute or subacute reaction to radiation. In our retrospective study[33] of 10 children who received hyperfractionated radiation therapy, the earliest change was noted 6 weeks after completion of radiation therapy and persisted for more than a year. In the one patient

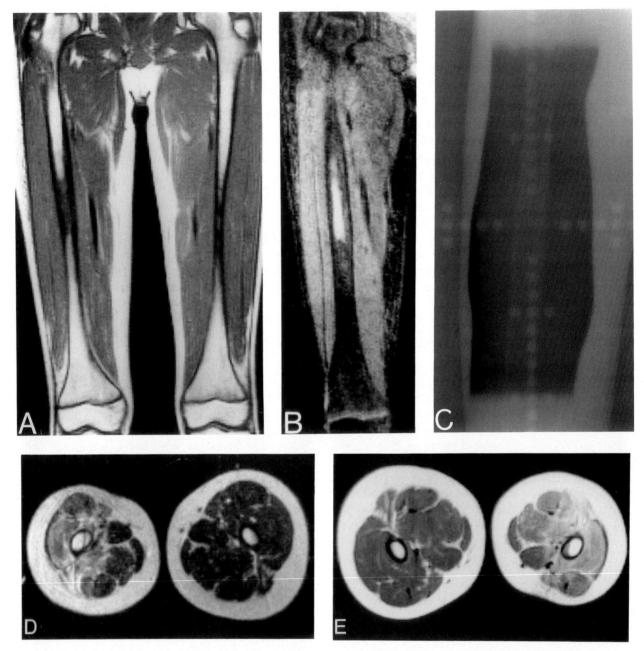

FIGURE 32.9. (A) A T_1-weighted (600/15) coronal image of the thighs of a patient with Ewing sarcoma treated with hyperfractionated radiation 4 months earlier. Focal residual marrow hypointensity is seen. The right thigh muscles are mildly atrophic, but are normal in intensity. (B) The coronal STIR (2500/22/150) image of the right thigh shows a large hyperintense area that corresponds to the irradiated field shown in the port film (C). (D) Transverse T_2-weighted (2500/90) and (E) gadolinium-enhanced T_1-weighted (760/15) images also show increased signal intensity of the affected muscles. The linear medial border of the radiation field is well defined. [(B,C,D,E) reprinted from Fletcher BD, et al. Changes in MRI signal intensity and contrast enhancement of therapeutically irradiated soft tissue. Magn Reson Imag 1990;8:771–777.]

treated with conventional radiation fractions, increased signal intensity of involved muscle was first observed on an MRI exam performed during the sixth week of radiation therapy. However, a prospective study is needed to clarify the timing of these events in relation to the dose and treatment schedule.

Imaging Characteristics

Radiation-related changes in muscle signal intensity are not apparent on T_1-weighted images, and the muscle architecture remains normal. However, changes manifested by linear strands of edema or fibrosis can be

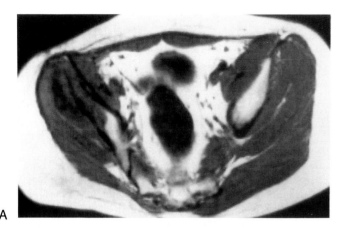

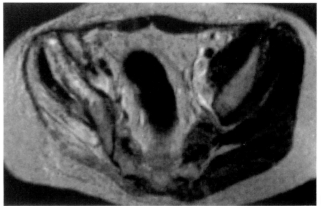

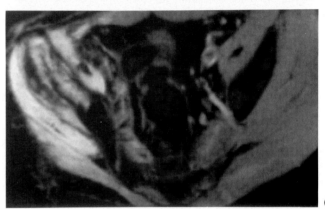

FIGURE 32.10. Transverse MR images of the pelvis of a patient 6 months postradiation therapy for Ewing sarcoma of the right ilium. (A) The T_1-weighted image (760/15) shows residual hypointense iliac tumor and marked atrophy of the right gluteal muscles. (B) A T_2-weighted image (2500/90) shows increased signal in the right pelvic muscles due to radiation therapy. (C) On a STIR image (2500/22/150), the margins of the residual tumor are partially obscured by the equally intense muscle edema.

visualized within irradiated subcutaneous fat on T_1- as well as T_2-weighted images. Atrophy of the irradiated muscles can also be seen on transverse images as early as 6 weeks after completion of radiation therapy.

Abnormally high signal intensity of the irradiated muscles appears on T_2-weighted and STIR images, and on T_1-weighted images there is local muscle enhancement with gadolinium. These changes can be readily related to radiation therapy, because the abnormally intense muscle is contained within a geometrically shaped region, the margins of which correspond precisely with those of the irradiated volume as shown on simulator and port films or dosimetric displays (Figure 32.9). On T_2-weighted images, the muscle is usually somewhat less intense than the irradiated tumor it surrounds, but on STIR images the similar intensities of muscle and neoplasm may partially obscure the tumor margins (Figure 32.10). The intense radiation changes may even mask recurrent primary malignancy.

Clinical Relevance and Pathophysiology

No symptoms can be directly attributed to the radiation-induced muscle abnormalities observed on MR images, but involvement of other in-field structures may result in clinically important findings that include bladder wall thickening with hematuria, small bowel reaction, proctitis, subcutaneous edema, and fibrosis.

We have not performed histologic examinations of irradiated muscle of any of our patients, so the exact mechanisms of high MRI signal production are unknown. The long-term results of radiation on the muscle of experimental animals is a reduction in the percentage of muscle fibers and capillaries relative to that of connective tissue suggesting that radiation may have caused injury to the supporting vasculature.[34] We speculate that the imaging findings in our patients probably reflect increased extracellular fluid volume and total water content of the affected muscle[5,35] associated with reduced fiber size.[6]

Summary

Edema in muscles adjacent to bone tumors and non-neoplastic lesions or encompassing neoplastic and non-neoplastic soft tissue lesions is best demonstrated on STIR sequences and those sensitive to T_2-weighted contrast. These sequences also optimally reveal the "massive edema" that involves entire muscles in extremities containing large tumors. Muscle edema enhances with gadolinium. The presence of edema is not predictive of malignancy and does not necessarily indicate peritumoral infiltration of malignant cells. The pathophysiology of edema is not clear. However, in the presence of known malignancy, the finding of massive edema suggests an aggressive tumor that will respond poorly to initial chemotherapy.

In patients who have received radiation therapy for musculoskeletal malignancies, an asymptomatic increase in signal intensity has been observed on T_2-weighted, STIR, and gadolinium-enhanced T_1-weighted images in the surrounding muscle. The therapy-induced changes can be differentiated from widespread tumor by recognition of the geometric borders of the region of increased signal intensity that conform to the margins of the radiation field. These findings, which are probably caused by increased interstitial water content of the muscles, may obscure a recurrent primary tumor of similar signal intensity.

In the near future one may look forward to better delineation of tumor and adjacent muscle edema using dynamic contrast-enhanced MRI, perfusion-weighted MRI, ^{31}P-MR spectroscopy, or positron emission tomography. On a more fundamental level, the relationship between edema and tumor perfusion begs investigation. If, as in the brain, increased interstitial fluid pressure in growing tumors leads to inadequate tumor perfusion,[36] we may speculate that another effect of increased intratumoral pressure would be to promote the accumulation of fluid within the tissues surrounding the tumor. This possibility would be consistent with our finding of massive edema associated with bulky tumors that respond poorly to chemotherapy.[15]

Acknowledgments. We thank Karen Dame for editorial assistance. Supported in part by the National Cancer Institute, Cancer Center Support (CORE) grant P30 CA-21765 and by the American Lebanese Syrian Associated Charities.

References

1. Fleckenstein JL, Canby RC, Parkey RW, Peshock RM. Acute effects of exercise on MRI of skeletal muscle in normal volunteers. AJR 1988;151:231–237.

2. Huber DJ, Sumers E, Klein M. Soft tissue pseudotumor following intramuscular injection of "DPT": a pitfall in magnetic resonance imaging. Skeletal Radiol 1987;16:469–473.

3. Fleckenstein JL, Burns DK, Murphy FR, Jayson HT, Bonte FJ. Differential diagnosis of bacterial myositis in AIDS: evaluation with MRI. Radiology 1991;179:653–658.

4. Mitchell DG, Burk DL Jr, Vinitski S, Rifkin MD. The biophysical basis of tissue contrast in extracranial MRI. AJR 1987;149:831–837.

5. Polak JF, Jolesz FA, Adams DF. NMR of skeletal muscle differences in relaxation parameters related to extracellular/intracellular fluid spaces. Invest Radiol 1988;23:107–112.

6. Polak JF, Jolesz FA, Adams DF. Magnetic resonance imaging of skeletal muscle prolongation of T1 and T2 subsequent to denervation. Invest Radiol 1988;23:365–369.

7. Dwyer AJ, Frank JA, Sank VJ, Reinig JW, Hickey AM, Doppman JL. Short-TI inversion-recovery pulse sequence: analysis and initial experience in cancer imaging. Radiology 1988;168:827–836.

8. Golfieri R, Baddeley H, Pringle JS, Souhami R. The role of the STIR sequence in magnetic resonance imaging examination of bone tumours. Br J Radiol 1990;63:251–256.

9. Shuman WP, Patten RM, Baron RL, Liddell RM, Conrad EU, Richardson ML. Comparison of STIR and spin-echo MRI at 1.5 T in 45 suspected extremity tumors: lesion conspicuity and extent. Radiology 1991;179:247–252.

10. Kaissar G, Kim JH, Bravo S, Sze G. Histologic basis for increased extraocular muscle enhancement in gadolinium-enhanced MRI. Radiology 1991;179:541–542.

11. Pettersson H, Eliasson J, Egund N, et al. Gadolinium-DTPA enhancement of soft tissue tumors in magnetic resonance imaging—preliminary clinical experience in five patients. Skeletal Radiol 1988;17:319–323.

12. Tien RD. Fat-suppression MR imaging in neuroradiology: techniques and clinical application. AJR 1992;158:369–379.

13. Seeger LL, Widoff BE, Bassett LW, Rosen G, Eckardt JJ. Preoperative evaluation of osteosarcoma: value of gadopentetate dimeglumine-enhanced MRI. AJR 1991;157:347–351.

14. Erlemann R, Reiser MF, Peters PE, et al. Musculoskeletal neoplasms: static and dynamic Gd-DTPA-enhanced MRI. Radiology 1989;171:767–773.

15. Hanna SL, Fletcher BD, Parham DM, Bugg MF. Muscle edema in musculoskeletal tumors: MRI characteristics and clinical significance. J Magn Reson Imaging 1991;1:441–449.

16. Beltran J, Simon DC, Katz W, Weis LD. Increased MRI signal intensity in skeletal muscle adjacent to malignant tumors: pathologic correlation and clinical relevance. Radiology 1987;162:251–255.

17. Pan G, Raymond AK, Carrasco CH, et al. Osteosarcoma: MRI after preoperative chemotherapy. Radiology 1990;174:517–526.

18. Biondetti PR, Ehman RL. Soft-tissue sarcomas: use of textural patterns in skeletal muscle as a diagnostic feature in postoperative MRI. Radiology 1992;183:845–848.

19. Harkens KL, Yuh WTC, Kathol MH, et al. Differentiating musculoskeletal neoplasm from nonneoplastic process: value of MRI and Gd-DTPA. Society of Magnetic Resonance in Medicine. 8th Annual Meeting, Book of Abstracts, Vol. 1, 1989:21.

20. Bohndorf K, Reiser M, Lochner B, de Lacroix WF, Steinbrich W. Magnetic resonance imaging of primary tumours and tumour-like lesions of bone. Skeletal Radiol 1986;15:511–517.

21. Crim JR, Seeger LL, Yao L, Chandnani V, Eckardt JJ. Diagnosis of soft-tissue masses with MRI: can benign masses be differentiated from malignant ones? Radiology 1992;185:581–586.

22. Kransdorf MJ, Jelinek JS, Moser RP Jr, et al. Soft-tissue masses: diagnosis using MRI. AJR 1989;153:541–547.

23. Hayes CW, Conway WF, Sundaram M. Misleading aggressive MRI appearance of some benign musculoskeletal lesions. RadioGraphics 1992;12:1119–1134.

24. Biebuyck J-C, Katz LD, McCauley T. Soft tissue edema in osteoid osteoma. Skeletal Radiol 1993;22:37–41.

25. Erlemann R, Sciuk J, Bosse A, et al. Response of osteosarcoma and Ewing sarcoma to preoperative chemotherapy: assessment with dynamic and static MRI and skeletal scintigraphy. Radiology 1990;175:791–796.

26. Liddell RM, Shuman WP, Weinberger E, Conrad EU, Lazerte GG. Prospective anatomic and histologic correlation of increased MRI signal intensity in skeletal muscle adjacent to tumor. Abstr Radiol 1989;173(P):397.

27. Sundaram M, McLeod RA. MRI of tumor and tumorlike lesions of bone and soft tissue. AJR 1990;155:817–824.

28. Moore SG, Sebag GH, Dawson KL. MRI evaluation of cortical bone and periosteal reaction in bone lesions: pathologic and radiographic correlation. Society of Magnetic Resonance in Medicine, 8th Annual Meeting, Book of Abstracts, Vol. 1, 1989:19.

29. Bloomer WD, Hellman S. Normal tissue responses to radiation therapy. N Engl J Med 1975;293:80–83.

30. Stevens SK, Moore SG, Kaplan ID. Early and late bone-marrow changes after irradiation: MRI evaluation. AJR 1990;154:745–750.

31. Remedios PA, Colletti PM, Raval JK, et al. MRI of bone after radiation. Magn Reson Imaging 1988;6:301–304.

32. Vanel D, Lacombe M-J, Couanet D, Kalifa C, Speilmann M, Genin J. Musculoskeletal tumors: follow-up with MRI after treatment with surgery and radiation therapy. Radiology 1987;164:243–245.

33. Fletcher BD, Hanna SL, Kun LE. Changes in MRI signal intensity and contrast enhancement of therapeutically irradiated soft tissue. Magn Reson Imaging 1990;8:771–777.

34. Herfkens RJ, Sievers R, Kaufman L, et al. Nuclear magnetic resonance imaging of infarcted muscle: a rat model. Radiology 1983;147:761–764.

35. Powers BE, Gillette EL, McChesney Gillette SL, LeCouteur RA, Withrow SJ. Muscle injury following experimental intraoperative irradiation. Int J Radiation Oncology Biol Phys 1990;20:463–471.

36. Steen RG. Edema and tumor perfusion: characterization by quantitative ^{1}H MRI. AJR 1992;158:259–264.

33
Miscellaneous Muscle Lesions

Michael T. McNamara and Alina Greco

The role of magnetic resonance (MRI) in the assessment of muscle pain has become an important one for both athletes and nonathletes.[1-14] Although professional and other elite athletes continue to seek new standards of excellence, amateur athletes also continue to further their level of fitness and skill in traditional and more recent and innovative sporting activities, all resulting in a concomitant rise in the number of muscle and locomotor injuries.[15-29] Physicians involved in the diagnosis and treatment of such injuries are thus faced with the ever-increasing task of providing rapid and efficacious medical care to the patient in order to allow rapid recovery and to insure a minimum of physical sequelae. The clinical problem of muscle pain in nonathletes has also benefitted from MRI in order to determine the cause and severity of the lesions.

Prior to the advent of MRI, radiologists and sports medicine specialists relied upon plain radiographs, computed tomography (CT), sonography, and scintigraphy for imaging diagnosis of most muscle lesions.[11,30-40] These imaging techniques each have their own relative strengths and weaknesses. None, however, provide the combined sensitivity and specificity of MRI for the evaluation of muscle pathology.[1-14,41]

Technical Considerations

Present indications for MRI of muscle lesions include muscle strain,[3-6,8,11,12] hemorrhage,[8,13,41] edema,[42,43] contusion,[2] infection,[44-47] tumor,[48-51] and fibrosis.[8,52] As detailed in Chapter 3, the benefit of MRI in imaging the various muscle lesions is derived from the innate relaxivity of normal skeletal muscle and from the altered relaxation times and proton spin density that occur with pathologic states. Because the T_2 relaxation time of skeletal muscle is short (35 ms at 1.5 T field strength[13,53-55]), it is readily apparent that even modest changes in T_2 will produce obvious alterations in MRI

signal intensity. The intermediate to long T_1 of muscle also contributes to its intermediate to low signal intensity.

Although these signal changes have been demonstrated on long T_R, long T_E spin echo T_2-weighted sequences, the short tau inversion recovery sequence (STIR) provides a most powerful technique for depicting muscle pathology.[56-59] This sequence takes advantage of pathologic prolongation of T_1 and T_2, both of which are common in acute muscle trauma.[2,8,60] STIR images significantly reduce the contribution of fat to image intensity, depicting most traumatic muscle lesions as hyperintense compared to the intermediate signal intensity of normal muscle tissue. A relative drawback to the STIR sequence has been the limited number of image sections and long image acquisition time. This was significantly improved by the creation of fast STIR imaging, which permits reasonable acquisition times and more slices with better spatial resolution than was previously feasible in clinical practice.[58,59]

Spin echo imaging has also been improved by spectral radiofrequency fat presaturation and by fast spin echo (FSE) imaging.[12] We use both FSE with fat presaturation (FSE/FS) and fast STIR imaging sequences with fairly equal frequency for the study of the musculoskeletal system (Figures 33.1, 33.2). Smaller or more discrete muscle lesions tend to be more easily seen on STIR images, due to their slightly superior homogeneity.

Acute muscle trauma produces edema and/or intramuscular hemorrhage, which are manifested by corresponding signal alterations on MR images (Figure 33.3). These changes reflect prolonged T_2 relaxation time, indeed a common denominator for most acute traumatic muscle lesions. Our imaging protocol in this clinical setting calls for an initial axial STIR sequence centered on the region of muscle pain, followed by a longitudinal STIR or FSE/FS sequence. The second sequence (Figures 33.4, 33.5) provides valuable infor-

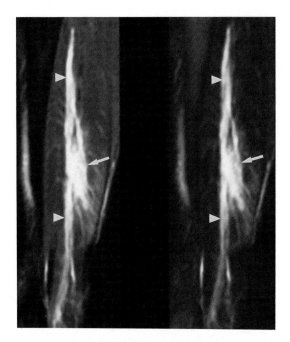

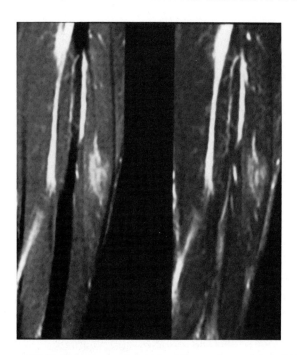

FIGURE 33.1. Soleus contusion. This 28-year-old male professional soccer player with painful ambulation was kicked in the calf 6 days prior to the MRI exam. Sagittal fast STIR (4000/30/140, left) image and sagittal fast spin echo image with fat presaturation (4200/114, right) reveal intramuscular edema-like change in the soleus muscle (arrows). Note the anterior perimuscular fluid in a linear configuration (arrowheads) and the high signal within the anterior subcutaneous tissue. The muscle findings are readily identified on both the STIR and fast spin echo images.

FIGURE 33.2. Soleus muscle strain: Comparison of fast STIR (4000/30/1400) image on left and fast spin echo (4200/114) image with fat presaturation on right. Diffuse hazy signal is seen in the soleus muscle of this athlete who experienced pain after a short sprint. The size and contour of the strain are virtually identical on the two images.

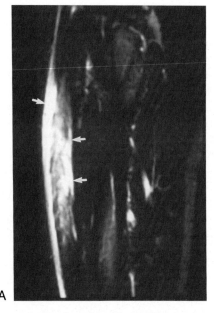

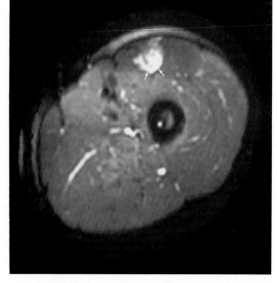

A   B

FIGURE 33.3. Rectus femoris strain. This 21-year-old male professional soccer player experienced sudden excruciating anterior thigh pain during a sprinting exercise 2 weeks earlier. This pain reoccurred 4 days later while jogging. (A) Sagittal fast spin echo (4000/19) image with fat presaturation demon-strates extensive high signal intensity in the rectus femoris muscle with presumed hemorrhage surrounding the muscle (arrows). (B) Axial fast STIR (3000/26/150) image shows hyperintense intramuscular and intermuscular (arrows) fluid/hemorrhage.

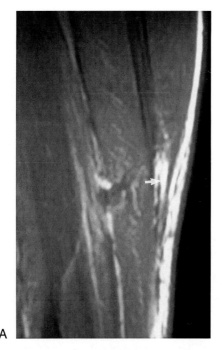

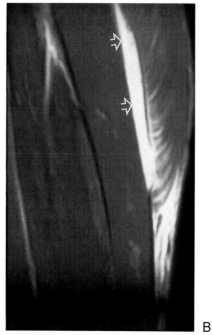

A   B

FIGURE 33.4. Gastrocnemius strain involving musculotendinous junction. Soccer player developed pain while running during a match 3 weeks prior to this study. The patient described a history of muscle contusion at the same level 2 years earlier. (A) Sagittal T_1-weighted (400/14) image reveals thinned distal tendon and musculotendinous junction without avulsion. Note the presence of hyperintense paramagnetic methemoglobin within the hemorrhage (arrow) surrounding the musculo-tendinous junction. (B) Sagittal fast STIR (3000/30/150) image at the same location as image (A) demonstrates cephalad extent of intermuscular fluid (open arrows) and diffuse linear intramuscular edema-like change.

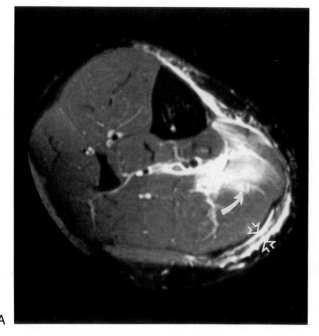

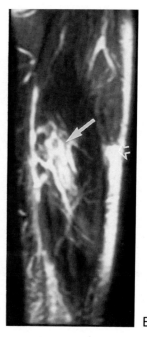

A   B

FIGURE 33.5. Tennis leg: gastrocnemius and soleus strains. This 29-year-old male patient experienced sudden pain in the posterior calf while playing tennis 10 days before the MRI examination. (A) Axial fast STIR (3000/28/150) image shows high signal intensity surrounding the distal medial gastroc-nemius musculotendinous junction (open arrows). The soleus muscle strain appears as a zone of hazy increased signal inten-sity (curved arrow). (B) Sagittal fast spin echo (4000/119) image with fat presaturation demonstrates high signal intensity in the distal portion of the medial gastrocnemius muscle (open arrow) and diffuse hyperintensity of the proximal muscle. The soleus strain is well seen in the anterior portion of the muscle, appearing as a region of hazy ill-defined increased signal (closed arrow).

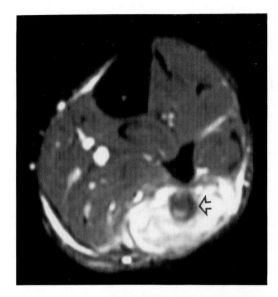

FIGURE 33.6. Acute gastrocnemius hematoma. This young man fell off a ladder just prior to the MRI study. He experienced immediate pain in the posterior calf. The axial fast STIR (3000/26/150) image shows a low signal intensity hematoma (open arrow) in the anterolateral aspect of the soleus muscle. Some higher signal intensity is also seen within the hematoma. There is diffuse muscular hyperintense signal change, consistent with extensive associated muscle edema.

mation about the size and extent of the injury and displays to better advantage the musculotendinous junction in order to rule out musculotendinous avulsion. The

longitudinal sequence should be oriented parallel to the longitudinal axis of the muscles being evaluated, either in the coronal, sagittal, or longitudinal oblique plane of section.

The choice between a FSE/FS T_2-weighted sequence and a STIR sequence for the second sequence of the study may be made after inspection of the characteristics and severity of the muscle lesion(s), if possible. An uncomplicated muscle strain with significant associated intramuscular or intermuscular hematoma formation may be evaluated with either a FSE or STIR sequence. However, acute hematoma may exhibit signal changes that reflect a short T_2 component.[61,62] This may appear hypointense to isointense to normal muscle on T_2-weighted spin echo images. The T_1 and T_2 alterations are additive on STIR images and hyperacute hematomas may also appear hypointense with this technique. However, the signal changes due to edema adjacent to the hematoma are usually readily demonstrated with STIR, thus providing excellent contrast between the hematoma and surrounding muscle (Figure 33.6). The STIR sequence is not specific for differentiating between hemorrhage and fluid.

In selected cases a T_1-weighted spin echo sequence may be performed to exhibit certain characteristics of hematomas. In particular, authors have shown that subacute to chronic intramuscular and intermuscular hematomas may contain paramagnetic extracellular methemoglobin, which appears hyperintense on T_1-weighted images (Figures 33.7 to 33.12). In clinical

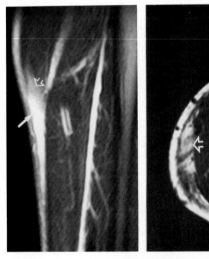

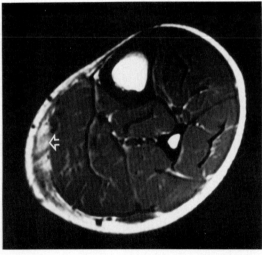

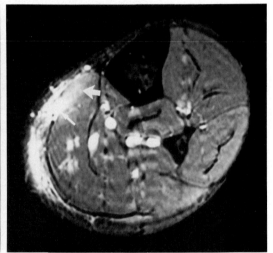

A   B   C

FIGURE 33.7. Hemorrhagic gastrocnemius strain. Calf pain occurred suddenly during exertion in this 32-year-old soccer player 1 week prior to the MRI exam. (A) Sagittal fast spin echo (4000/105) image with fat presaturation reveals distal medial gastrocnemius muscle strain (open arrow) and blood collection (closed arrow). (B) Axial T_1-weighted (700/12) image demonstrates high signal intensity of gastrocnemius hemorrhage (open arrow) consistent with methemoglobin content. (C) Axial STIR (3200/30/140) image displays hyperintense gastrocnemius strain, intermuscular hematoma (thin arrow), and soleus muscle strain (thick arrow).

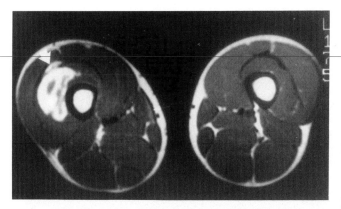

FIGURE 33.8. Subacute vastus intermedius muscle hematoma. The axial T_1-weighted (600/20) image reveals a predominantly hyperintense hemorrhagic collection (arrow). The high signal intensity reflects the oxidative degradation of blood, resulting in the production of paramagnetic methemoglobin.

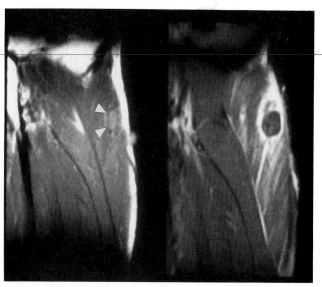

FIGURE 33.9. Subacute soleus hematoma. MRI examination performed 4 days following direct blow to the upper calf. Coronal T_1-weighted (500/11) image (left) demonstrates methemoglobin as high signal intensity (arrowheads). Coronal fast STIR (3000/26/150) image (right) reveals low signal intensity of hematoma, reflecting intracellular methemoglobin and deoxyhemoglobin. Surrounding muscle edema and hemorrhage are hyperintense.

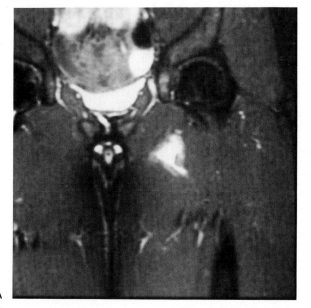

A

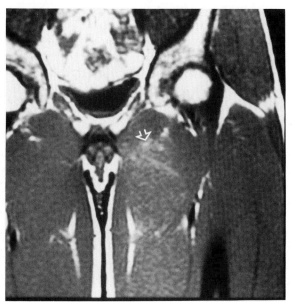

B

FIGURE 33.10. Subacute adductor magnus hemorrhagic strain. This young male professional soccer player suffered sudden left thigh pain during exertion 11 days prior to the MRI study. (A) The coronal fast STIR (3000/26/150) image exhibits a triangular focus of hyperintense blood in the superior adductor compartment. (B) Patchy high signal intensity on the coronal T_1-weighted image (400/11) supports the presence of paramagnetic methemoglobin (open arrow).

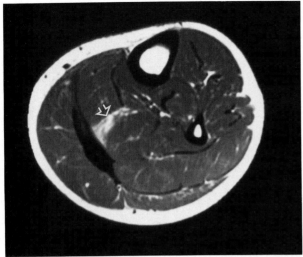

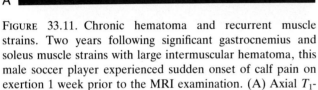

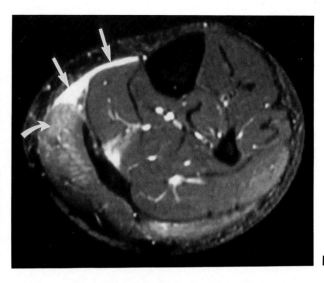

FIGURE 33.11. Chronic hematoma and recurrent muscle strains. Two years following significant gastrocnemius and soleus muscle strains with large intermuscular hematoma, this male soccer player experienced sudden onset of calf pain on exertion 1 week prior to the MRI examination. (A) Axial T_1-weighted (690/12) image shows hypointense residua of intermuscular hematoma as well as hyperintense hemorrhagic soleus muscle strain (arrow). (B) Axial fast STIR (3000/34/140) image reveals gastrocnemius (curved arrow) and soleus strains and anterior perimuscular fluid (straight arrows).

practice this is usually not necessary because such hematomas are usually readily detected on T_2-weighted or STIR images. Clinical correlation with the images usually leaves no doubt as to the nature of the fluid collection. In the case of hemorrhagic muscle reinjury, the T_1-weighted acquisition may provide insight into differentiating acute hemorrhage from older hematoma.

A relatively uncommon use for T_1-weighted images at our institution is for anatomic localization of lesions. This may seem unnecessary for an accurate tomographic technique such as MRI. In our practice we often evaluate elite athletes with significant leg muscle hypertrophy that renders distinction between muscle and fascia difficult. In addition, fat suppression techniques will often eliminate the little intermuscular fat that is present and thus it may be difficult to accurately localize certain muscle strains and their sequelae, particularly in small muscles and in the periphery of certain muscle bellies. T_1-weighted images in corroboration with STIR or T_2-weighted images may facilitate precise localization of such lesions. Gradient recalled echo images with fat presaturation are equally satisfactory for this indication, in our experience. (Figure 33.13).

Muscle Abnormalities

The utility of MRI for the detection of acute muscle strain has been well documented in Chapter 25 and in the medical literature.[4-8,12] In this chapter we will attempt to focus primarily on miscellaneous aspects of muscle injuries and their sequelae as well as non-traumatic causes of muscle pain.

Muscle Overuse Syndrome

Muscle lesions of this nature may occur in response to occupational overuse and in athletes. Such injuries do not result from a single traumatic event but rather are related to a single repetitive action or activity. Most often the activity produces muscle strain or musculo-tendinous injury. Some of the more common overuse

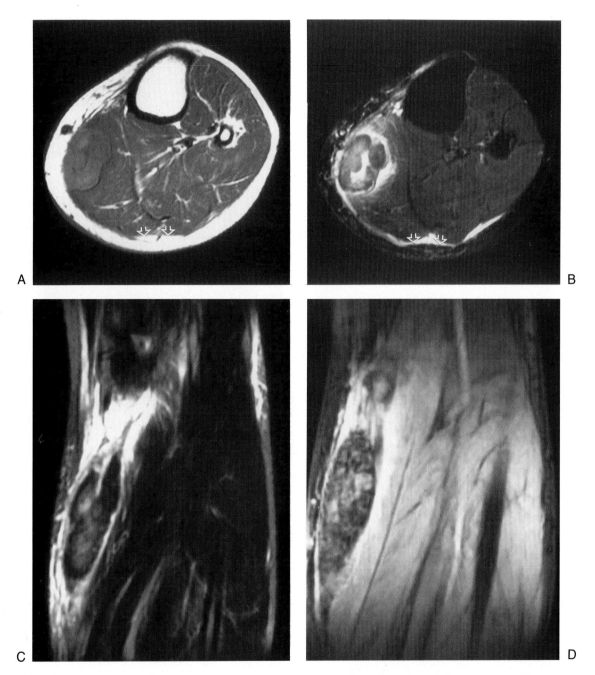

FIGURE 33.12. Chronic gastrocnemius hematoma. This patient was examined by MRI 25 days following direct muscle trauma. (A) Axial T_1-weighted (600/12) image shows hematoma that is slightly hyperintense to adjacent muscle tissue. Posterior perimuscular blood is hyperintense, reflecting methemoglobin content (open arrows). (B) Axial STIR (3000/28/150) image shows the hematoma to be primarily hypointense, whereas surrounding edema is very hyperintense. Note that posterior blood is suppressed due to its short T_1 time (open arrows). (C) Coronal fast T_2-weighted (4000/104) image with fat presaturation shows full craniocaudal dimension of the hematoma and surrounding muscle injury. (D) Coronal gradient echo (500/15/30 degrees) image with fat presaturation displays low signal intensity of hematoma.

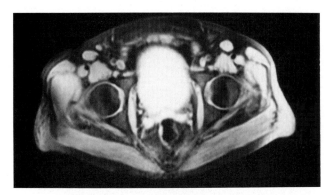

FIGURE 33.13. Gradient echo image (640/15/35 degrees) with fat presaturation. Note excellent depiction of pelvic musculature and fascial planes, aided by the suppression of pelvic fat signal intensity. The peripheral high signal intensity of fat is a pitfall of presaturation techniques, however.

syndromes involve the lower extremities, particularly in cases such as so-called "tennis leg," in which the distal medial gastrocnemius myotendinous junction is involved

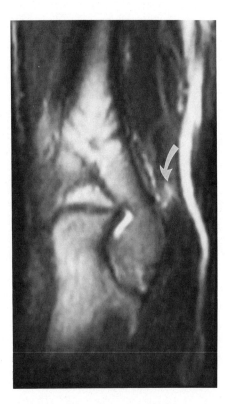

FIGURE 33.14. Pronator teres strain. This 36-year-old male laborer felt sudden elbow pain while lifting a heavy object. The pain recurred during exertion related to lifting. Coronal fast T_2-weighted (3000/95) image with fat presaturation demonstrates edema-like change within the pronator teres muscle (curved arrow).

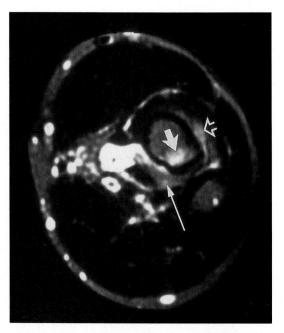

FIGURE 33.15. Overuse syndrome. This 73-year-old female patient experienced chronic shoulder and elbow pain following repetitive exercise rehabilitation of the upper extremity. Axial fast T_2-weighted (3000/98) image with fat presaturation shows high signal intensity within the supinator muscle, compatible with muscle strain (open arrow). Hyperintense liquid in the vicinity of the biceps tendon and increased signal intensity within the tendon (thin arrow) suggested chronic tenosynovitis and/or microtear. There is also bright signal within the radial tuberosity at the biceps tendon insertion (thick arrow), compatible with partial avulsion.

(Figure 33.5). Other sites include the shoulder and the elbow (Figures 33.14, 33.15), often in the epicondylar region such as in tennis elbow or golf elbow (Figure 33.16), or in the olecranon region involving the triceps muscle and tendon (Figure 33.17). In athletes we often see such muscle lesions in the myotendinous junction of the lower extremities (Figures 33.4, 33.18). MRI may play an important role in the diagnosis of such muscle lesions because of its good sensitivity for detection of abnormal signal on STIR or T_2-weighted images, and also because of the lack of other modalities for diagnosis of overuse syndrome.[63–72] When the lesion involves a myotendinous junction, persistent bright signal on STIR images may occur in proximity to fibrous scar[8] resulting from previous muscle injury (Figure 33.19). In our experience such signal changes correlate well with incomplete or ongoing repair, and clinicians usually allow return to full-level activity only after MRI documentation of lack of abnormal hyperintense signal as well as resolution of pain.

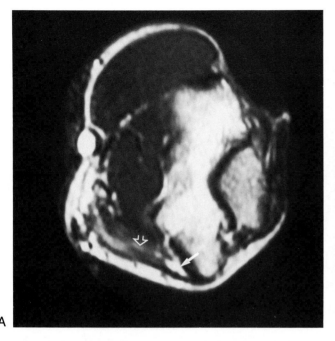

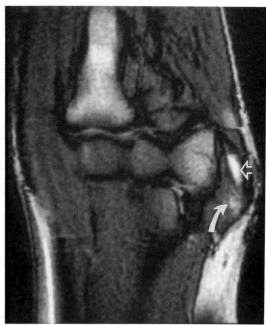

A

B

FIGURE 33.16. Golf elbow. For 6 months, this middle-aged avid golfer has experienced significant pain in the medial elbow, with tenderness of the medial epicondyle. (A) Axial T_2-weighted (2000/80) image of the elbow reveals diffuse high signal within the pronator teres muscle (open arrow) and particularly at the level of the common flexor tendon (thin arrow). (B) Coronal STIR (1800/31/170) image demonstrates high signal intensity within the pronator teres muscle (curved arrow) and common flexor tendon (open arrow). Note that fat is poorly suppressed due to an excessively long TI.

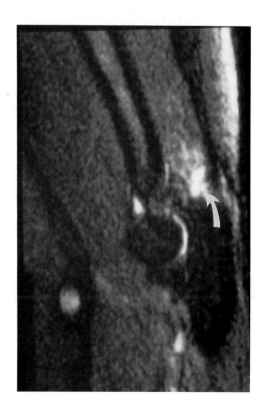

FIGURE 33.17. Overuse syndrome: triceps muscle strain. This 30-year-old female sanitation worker had a history of direct trauma with olecranon fracture 4 years earlier. She complains of painful extension that is particularly exacerbated by her repetitive activity of mopping floors. The sagittal fast STIR (4000/34/140) image reveals patchy high signal intensity in the distal triceps muscle (curved arrow), surrounding the tendon. No evidence of avulsion is apparent in the olecranon.

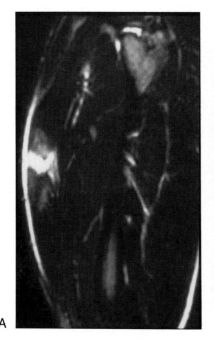

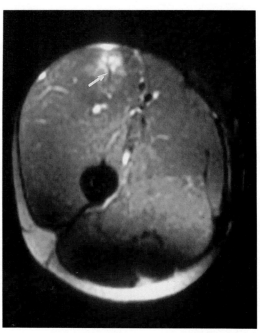

A   B

FIGURE 33.18. Rectus femoris strain involving musculotendinous junction. This young male professional soccer player strained his rectus femoris muscle 4 weeks ago. Upon return to activity 5 days ago he felt a sharp pain in the same region of the thigh as he did previously. Muscle strength was felt to be mildly diminished at this time. (A) The sagittal fast T_2-weighted (4000/102) image with fat presaturation demonstrates edema within a tear that traverses the full thickness of the muscle. Note the diffuse intramuscular signal change reflecting acute recurrent muscle strain. (B) Axial fast STIR (4000/34/140) image shows diffuse hyperintense muscle edema that surrounds the muscle tendon (arrow).

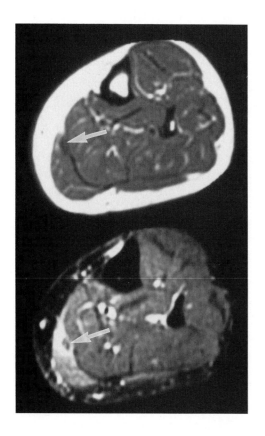

FIGURE 33.19. Medial gastrocnemius fibrosis and recurrent strain. This middle-aged woman strained the medial head of the gastrocnemius muscle 7 weeks earlier. Pain recurred recently during exertion in the same calf. Axial T_1-weighted (500/19, top) image and fast T_2-weighted (4000/96, bottom) image with fat presaturation demonstrate focal low signal intensity fibrous scar (arrows) that is more easily appreciated on the T_2-weighted image. Note the high signal intensity inflammatory signal surrounding the scar on the fast T_2-weighted image, consistent with mild recurrent strain in this clinical setting.

Muscle Contusion and Muscle Hematoma

Muscle contusion is easily visualized on MRI due to signal changes reflecting the presence of increased extracellular water and hemorrhage. Often forces are transmitted to the deep muscle layers with significantly less involvement of the overlying superficial muscle layer. We see this most often in soccer players (Figures 33.20, 33.21). The goal of the MRI study is to rule out significant disruption of muscle fiber bundles. The appearance of muscle contusion in most cases is virtually indistinguishable from that of muscle strain. Both lesions may produce intramuscular as well as intermuscular hemorrhage and edema (Figure 33.20). Contusion often produces muscle lesions that are deep in the muscle belly and are therefore less symptomatic than muscle strain, which tend to localize more peripherally in the muscle.

Although the prognosis for hematoma and tearing of muscle fibers resulting from muscle strain and muscle contusion is similar, the often less painful deep muscle contusion may encourage a more rapid return to activity, which increases the risk of recurrent muscle injury or of increasing the severity of the incompletely healed lesion. The MRI appearances of muscle reinjury

following muscle strain and muscle contusion may be identical (Figure 33.18). Thus, the primary goal of MRI in the clinical setting of acute muscle contusion at our institution is to determine the degree of muscle damage. In some cases, the clinician may elect to percutaneously drain large intramuscular hematomas in order to promote apposition of muscle fibers and subsequent healing.

Acute hematomas may appear isointense to hyperintense to normal muscle tissue on T_2-weighted images and hypointense to isointense on T_1-weighted images. Acute blood collections tend to have variable signal intensity on STIR images and thus we have seen both hyperintense and hypointense appearances (Figure 33.6).

Subacute to chronic hematomas are most often readily identified as high signal intensity collections on STIR and T_2-weighted sequences.[8,41] They contain varying amounts of paramagnetic extracellular methemoglobin that produces high signal intensity on T_1-weighted images due to T_1 shortening.[8,41,61,62] In some cases, however, such blood collections may appear markedly hypointense on STIR and T_2-weighted images (Figures 33.9, 33.12), reflecting different states of oxidative degradation of hemoglobin.

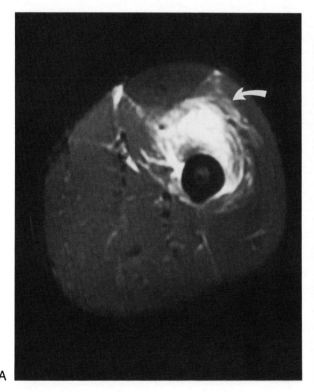
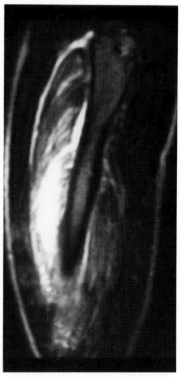

FIGURE 33.20. Acute vastus intermedius contusion. During a match played 6 days prior to the MRI study, this young male soccer player was kicked in the anterior thigh. He since experienced significant pain in the thigh during exertion. (A) Significant hyperintense signal is seen within the vastus intermedius muscle on the axial fast STIR (3000/26/150) image.

Note the relative paucity of signal change within the more superficial vastus lateralis muscle (curved arrow). (B) Sagittal fast T_2-weighted (4000/19) image with fat presaturation displays the hemorrhagic vastus intermedius signal and deep perimuscular hemorrhage.

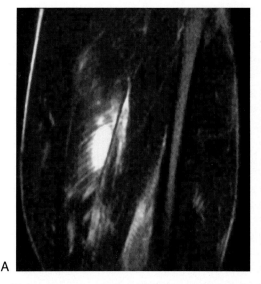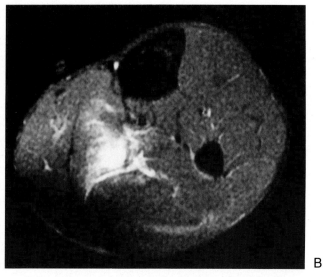

FIGURE 33.21. Soleus contusion. This 26-year-old professional soccer player received a direct blow to the calf 6 days prior to the MRI examination and experienced persistent pain while walking since that time. (A) Coronal fast spin echo (4000/104) image with fat presaturation demonstrates soleus muscle edema as a collection of hyperintense homogeneous signal, surrounded by diffuse hazy signal change. (B) Axial fast STIR (3000/28/150) image displays the presumed hemorrhage and surrounding posttraumatic hyperintense signal. Note the absence of visible superficial gastrocnemius muscle injury.

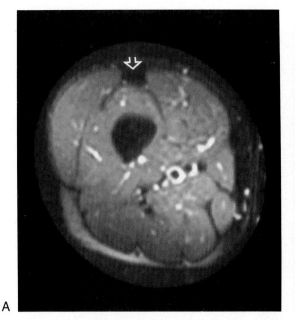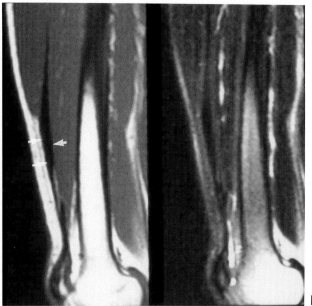

FIGURE 33.22. Distal rectus femoris fibrosis. This 35-year-old athlete suffered a strain of the rectus femoris muscle while kicking a soccer ball 17 months earlier. Following a prolonged recovery period he was noted to have a physically deformed anterior thigh and reduced muscle strength. (A) Axial fast STIR (3000/26/150) image shows anteromedial low signal intensity fibrous scar that occupies a gap between the vastus medialis and vastus lateralis muscles (open arrow). (B) Sagittal T_1-weighted (500/10, left) image demonstrates distal rectus femoris retraction and hypointense fibrous tissue (arrows). Fibrous tissue also has low signal intensity on fast T_2-weighted (4000/91, right) image with fat presaturation.

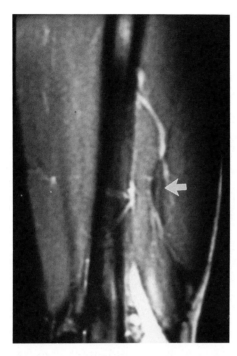

FIGURE 33.23. Biceps femoris fibrosis. This 17-year-old male professional soccer player presented for MRI examination due to persistent discomfort during mild exertion, 8 weeks after experiencing biceps femoris muscle strain. Sagittal STIR (3000/26/150) image reveals elongated low signal intensity fibrous scar within the short head of the biceps femoris muscle (arrow). The central portion of the scar has higher signal intensity than the peripheral region.

Fibrosis

A clinically important indication for MRI in muscle trauma is the assessment of the presence and severity of muscle scar. Skeletal muscle injury may result in fibroblast proliferation and fibrosis.[8,52,73] It is felt that muscle scar formation may predispose skeletal muscle to recurrent muscle strain.[8,74] Scar consists of fibrous tissue that appears hypointense on nearly all MRI sequences, particularly on T_2-weighted images (Figures 33.22 to 33.25). This appearance reflects the relatively short T_2 relaxation time of fibrous tissue compared to normal tissue.[74] Depending upon the age of the lesion and the degree of muscle healing, the low signal intensity of the fibrous scar may be initially heterogeneous (Figure 33.16), becoming more homogeneous as maturity increases.

Because many traumatic muscle injuries occur at the musculotendinous junction,[28] difficulty may arise in separating scar tissue from tendon, because tendon is also characteristically hypointense due to its short T_2 relaxation time and low proton density.[75,76] The MRI findings usually consist of a thickened tendon at the site of previously documented muscle strain (Figures 33.22, 33.24). Subtle scar may be detected by comparison with the contralateral extremity. Recurrent injury is diagnosed in the clinical setting of recurrent pain with hyperintense signal intensity at the site of muscle scar on STIR or T_2-weighted images (Figures 33.19, 33.24, 33.25).

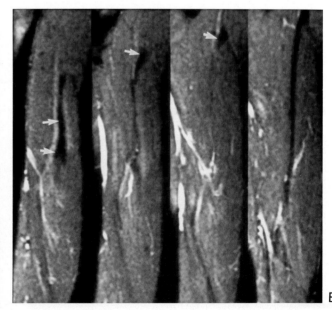

FIGURE 33.24. Semitendinosus fibrosis. This male professional soccer player suffered a muscle strain of the hamstring muscles 10 months prior to this MRI examination. He recently experienced mild pain while running. (A) Axial STIR (3200/30/140) image demonstrates hypointense fibrous scar of the semitendinosus muscle (curved arrow). Mild high signal medial to the scar likely represents recurrent muscle injury. There is also a hyperintense strain of the long head of the biceps muscle (open arrow). (B) Sagittal fast STIR (3000/26/150) images. These four adjacent sections depict the muscle scar that involves the superior tendinous portion of the muscle (arrows).

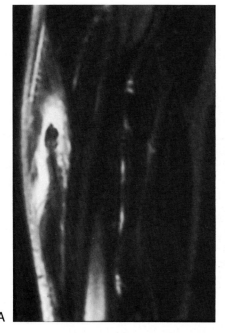
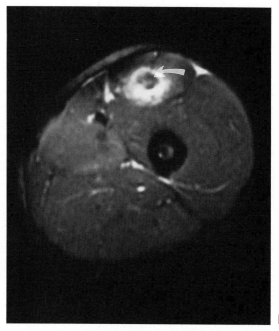

FIGURE 33.25. Rectus femoris fibrosis and recurrent strain. This 16-year-old soccer player has a long history of multiple rectus femoris muscle strains, resulting in significant reduction in leg strength with reduced physical capacity for exertion and increased thigh muscle fragility during exercise. The most recent episode of sudden sharp pain during exercise occurred 1 week earlier. (A) Sagittal fast T_2-weighted (4000/119) image with fat presaturation demonstrates extensive intramuscular edema surrounding a low intensity, retracted fibrous scar. (B) Muscle fibrosis (curved arrow) and surrounding hemorrhage and edema are also obvious on the axial fast STIR (3000/26/150) image.

Myositis Ossificans

Myositis ossificans is a benign solitary self-limiting sequela of muscle injury for which the exact mechanism is unknown.[77] A history of trauma may be absent in some cases. This lesion consists of muscle swelling with pain and loss of muscle function, which typically does not subside over time. Histologic examination reveals fibroblastic reaction that subsequently organizes and produces peripheral new bone formation at 6 to 8 weeks.[78] At 6 months the lesion will mature into peripheral compact bone with a central core of lamellar bone.[79-81] This condition is detailed in Chapter 27.

The MRI findings of myositis ossificans consist of nonspecific high-intensity lesions on STIR or T_2-weighted images in the early phase.[82] Fluid–fluid levels have been described. In the subacute phase, low-intensity peripheral, curvilinear or irregular ossification may be

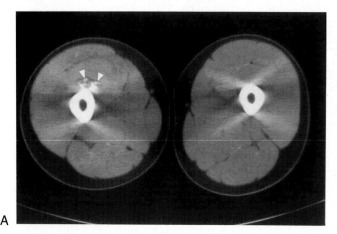
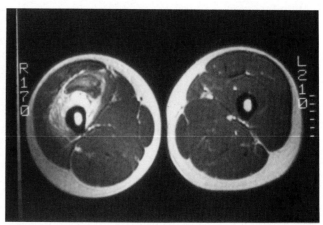

FIGURE 33.26. Myositis ossificans. (A) Axial CT scan reveals vastus intermedius calcified mass (arrowheads). (B) Axial T_2-weighted (2000/60) image. The calcified portion of the mass is hypointense whereas the remainder of the vastus intermedius displays edema-like change. (Images courtesy of Richard L. Ehman, M.D., Rochester, MN.)

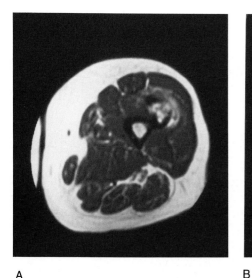
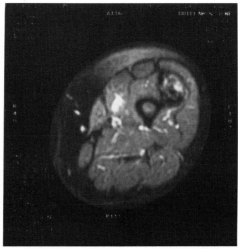
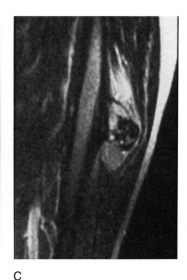

A   B   C

FIGURE 33.27. Chronic mature myositis ossificans. This 68-year-old patient noted the gradual appearance of a tender soft tissue swelling in the anterior thigh. (A) Axial T_1-weighted (540/19) image shows vastus intermedius mass that is hyperintense centrally due to fatty marrow within bone trabeculae. The peripheral mineralized portion of the mass has high intensity and low intensity elements. (B) Axial fast STIR (3000/26/150) image displays the calcified portions of the mass as low signal intensity, with fluid-like signal intensity elsewhere within the lesion. (C) Sagittal fast spin echo (4000/119) with fat presaturation demonstrates the peripheral and central low intensity mass calcifications. The periphery of the mass is hyperintense to adjacent muscle.

seen, appearing with characteristic low signal intensity. (Figure 33.26). Persistent soft tissue hyperintensity is noted in this phase. Bone marrow edema may also be seen adjacent to the muscle lesions.

Chronic mature myositis ossificans is typically hypointense and inhomogeneous on most sequences, corresponding with cortical bone and fibrosis (Figure 33.27). A feature of myositis ossificans is the peripheral and central muscle ossification and fibrosis, which may be readily identified on MR images as low signal intensity. Fatty marrow within bone trabeculae may appear isointense to fatty tissue elsewhere on the image, and therefore hyperintense on T_1-weighted images (Figure 33.27A).

Calcific Myonecrosis

This muscle lesion is associated with peripheral nerve damage, typically producing fusiform mass-like swelling of a single muscle. Central muscle liquefaction appears hyperintense on STIR images (Figure 33.28). There are plaque-like *peripheral* calcifications (Figures 33.28E 33.28F) replacing muscle that may be distinguished from ossification associated with myositis ossificans, which progress *centrally* within the lesion over time. Central involvement with calcification is not a feature of calcific myonecrosis.

Authors have suggested that the underlying cause of calcific myonecrosis is compartment syndrome and

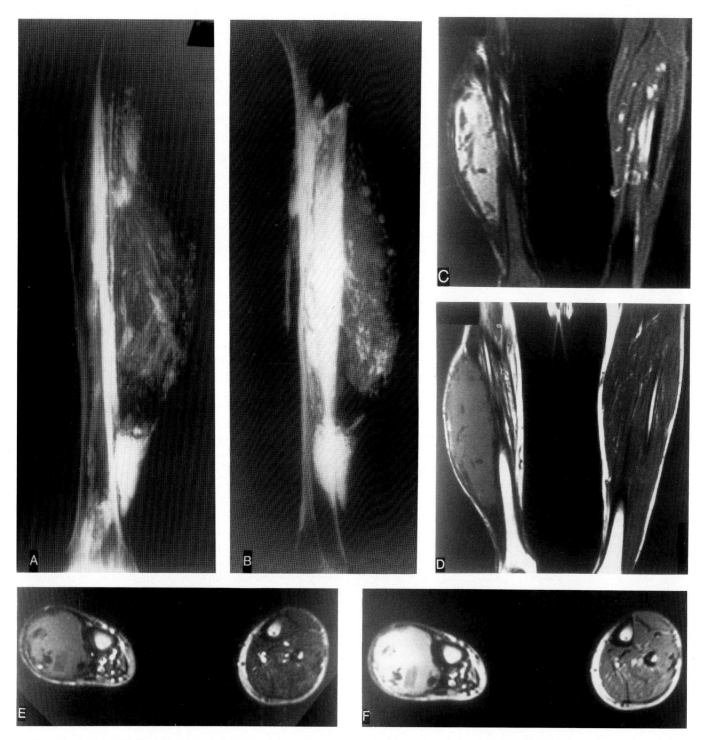

FIGURE 33.28. Calcific myonecrosis. This adult male complained of slowly progressing mass lesion in the calf and a remote history of trauma. The anteroposterior (A) and lateral (B) radiographs demonstrate fusiform soft tissue enlargement and calcification. The bones are normal in appearance. The lesion is primarily hyperintense on the coronal STIR (2200/20/ 180, C) image. The calcifications are hypointense on the STIR image and on the coronal T_1-weighted (510/15, D) image. The low intensity peripheral calcifications are also readily identified on the axial spin density (2645/20, E) and T_2-weighted (2645/ 90, F) images. (Images courtesy of James L. Fleckenstein, M.D., Dallas, TX.)

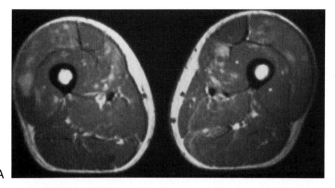
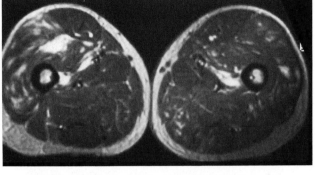

FIGURE 33.29. Acute bilateral myonecrosis. Spin density (A) and T_2 (B) weighted images at slightly different levels show multiple foci of edema in both thighs as a result of bicycle overtraining. (Images courtesy of Richard L. Ehman, M.D., Rochester, MN.)

ischemia.[83,84] All previously reported cases have been associated with trauma. The calf is a frequent site of involvement, often with associated fracture. Injury to the common peroneal nerve has been implicated as a factor in cases of calf calcific myonecrosis.[85] Myonecrosis may also occur as a result of excessive strenuous exercise (see Chapter 26 and Figure 33.29).

Compartment Syndrome

Muscle trauma or injury may produce edema and hemorrhage within fascial boundaries, which produce abnormally elevated intracompartmental pressure.[26,86] Muscle volume may increase by 20% during exercise due to increased capillary filtration, which is not compensated for by removal of excess fluid.[86] Tissue pressures may attain 40 to 60 mmHg, which impairs blood flow,[87] capillary perfusion and oxygen supply. As described in Chapter 28, this results in pain, decreased function, and sensory deficits. Compartment syndrome occurs most often in the lower leg and arm but has been reported in the posterior thigh[6,86–90] (Figure 33.30).

MRI findings include muscle swelling and increased signal intensity on STIR and T_2-weighted images[88]

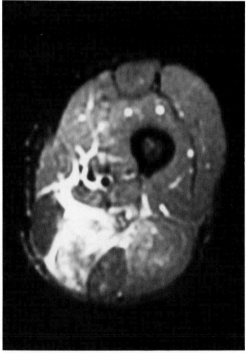
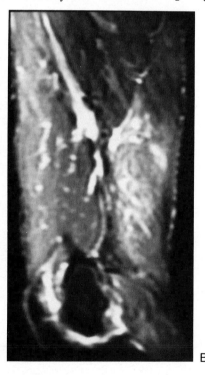

FIGURE 33.30. Compartment syndrome. This 54-year-old male patient fell from a height of 5 m several months earlier, resulting in extensive posterior thigh muscle hemorrhage. Following prolonged rest to allow resorption of the hemorrhage the patient continued to complain of pain with exertion and decreased function. Axial (A) and sagittal (B) STIR (3000/ 26/150) images show diffuse and heterogeneous increased signal intensity within the posterior thigh, primarily within the semimembranosus muscle (axial and sagittal images), and to a lesser extent within the long head of the biceps femoris (axial image only).

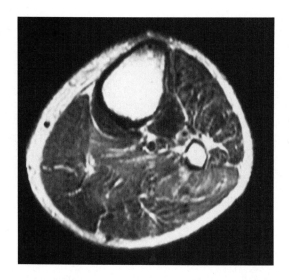

FIGURE 33.31. Chronic compartment syndrome. The axial T_2-weighted (2000/80) image of the calf demonstrates diffuse, mild posterior compartment edema-like change. The patient had a history of medial gastrocnemius strain several months earlier and still complains of pain with exertion.

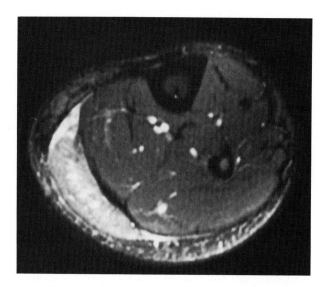

FIGURE 33.33. Chronic compartment syndrome. Male adult patient with a history of gastrocnemius muscle strain 2 years ago but with continued calf pain during physical activity. Axial fast STIR (3000/34/140) image reveals diffuse hyperintensity of medial gastrocnemius muscle.

(Figures 33.31 to 33.34). This pattern is nonspecific and clinical correlation is important.[6,88] The patient history should include pain with exercise.

Neoplasm

Although other symptoms such as swelling and mass effect may predominate, muscle tumors may occasionally present solely with muscle pain. Muscle tumors may be primary or metastatic. As detailed in Chapter 31, MRI findings are those of infiltration of muscle by hyperintense, often heterogeneous signal on STIR or T_2-weighted images, often with variable necrosis, hemorrhage, and calcification. Benign lesions tend to be homo-

geneous and sharply circumscribed (Figure 33.35), whereas malignant tumors are often more heterogeneous and less well marginated (Figure 33.36). Metastatic muscle masses are readily detected on STIR and T_2-weighted sequences due to their prominent but nonspecific high signal intensity (Figure 33.37). Differentiation between benign and malignant muscle tumors with MRI is not at present considered to be absolutely reliable.[48–51,91–94]

Intravenous gadolinium chelates may produce moderate tumor enhancement but we often find that the pattern of enhancement or lack of enhancement does not add significantly to the findings on STIR or T_2-weighted images alone.

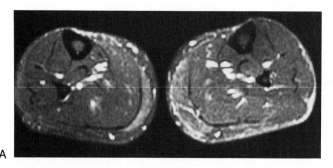

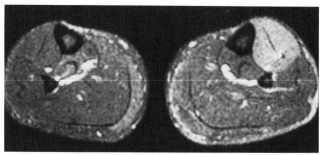

A   B

FIGURE 33.32. Subacute compartment syndrome. (A) Preexercise axial STIR image shows questionable swelling of left tibialis anterior muscle and extensor hallucis longus muscle. (B) Postexercise STIR image demonstrates prolonged and exaggerated signal intensity increase in anterior muscle compartment. (Images courtesy of Richard L. Ehman, M.D., Rochester, MN.)

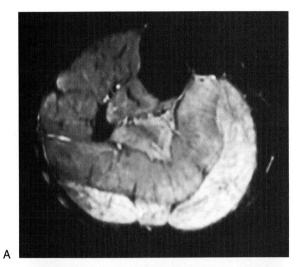

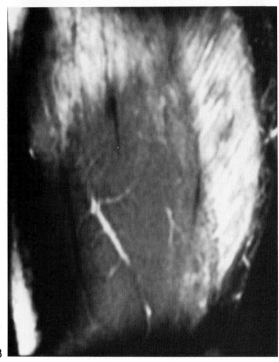

FIGURE 33.34. Compartment syndrome. This 21-year-old male was involved in an automobile accident that produced a direct blow to the calf 1 month prior to the MRI study. He continued to experience calf pain while walking. (A) Axial fast STIR (3000/26/150) image shows diffuse high signal intensity of the medial and lateral gastrocnemius muscles and to a lesser extent of the soleus muscle. (B) Coronal fast STIR (4000/26/140) image. High signal intensity is depicted within both of the gastrocnemius muscles, reflecting edema.

Abscess

Muscle abscesses may have specific MRI features that differentiate them from other muscle lesions.[44–47] They are usually fairly well defined with an irregular thick capsule. T_2-weighted or STIR images often reveal

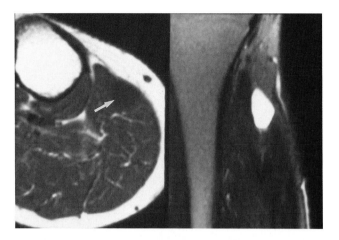

FIGURE 33.35. Soleus cyst. This patient has noted the gradual appearance of a focal painless posterior calf swelling. He reported no history of trauma or symptomatic knee derangement. The T_1-weighted (540/19, left) and fast T_2-weighted (4000/102, right) image with fat presaturation reveal a homogeneous sharply defined cystic lesion (arrow). The signal intensity characteristics are typical for a liquid-containing lesion.

hyperintense muscle edema surrounding the abscess (Figure 33.38). The contents of the abscess demonstrate fluid-like signal intensity characteristics, except that they tend to be less homogeneous. The capsule enhances following intravenous administration of gadolinium chelates, as does the surrounding tissue inflammation (Figures 33.39, 33.40). Lack of enhancement of the central portion of the abscess may help to distinguish this lesion from muscle tumor, which generally enhances throughout to a variable degree.

Miscellaneous

Intramuscular injection may produce acute muscular inflammation with resultant signal changes on STIR and T_2-weighted images.[95] Unless complications such as hemorrhage or infection ensue, these lesions usually do not require MRI. However, when localization of specific muscle lesions[96] is required the examination may be facilitated by the injection of paramagnetic gadolinium chelate contrast media (Figure 33.41). The most readily appreciable MRI findings are those of T_1 shortening on T_1-weighted images producing high signal intensity compared to adjacent muscle tissue. Spectral presaturation of fatty tissue further enhances the signal altering effect of gadolinium (Figure 33.41B). Gadolinium chelates shorten both T_1 and T_2, and when full concentration chelate solution is injected into the muscle, the T_2 shortening effect will reduce the signal intensity at the injection site, particularly on T_2-weighted images (Figures 33.41C, 33.41D).

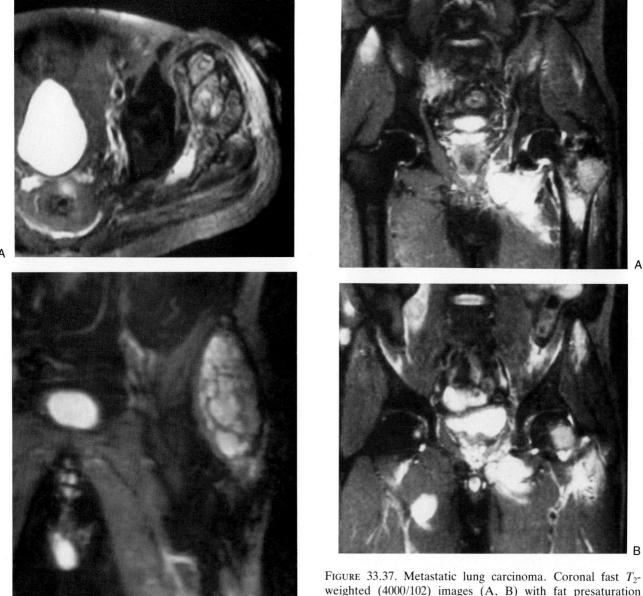

FIGURE 33.36. Gluteus medius undifferentiated sarcoma. The (A) axial fast T_2-weighted (4000/91) image with fat presaturation and (B) coronal STIR (3000/26/150) image display a high signal intensity heterogeneous, septated, and poorly defined mass. The lesion is confined to the muscle and does not involve the iliac bone.

FIGURE 33.37. Metastatic lung carcinoma. Coronal fast T_2-weighted (4000/102) images (A, B) with fat presaturation demonstrate metastases in both iliacus muscles, right psoas, left obturator internus and obturator externus, and both adductor magnus muscles. Note the right sacral and left femoral bone metastases.

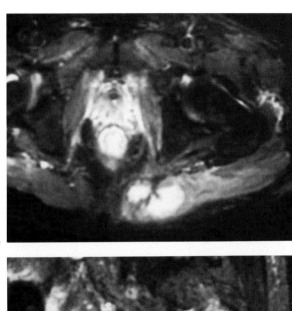

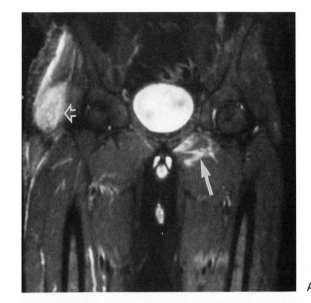

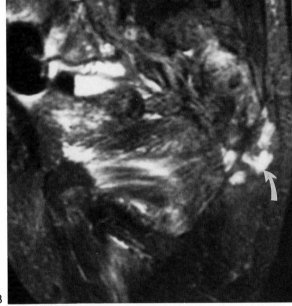

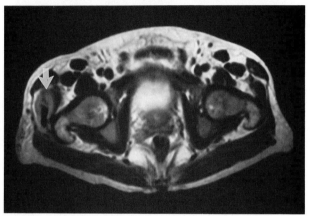

FIGURE 33.38. Gluteus maximus abscess. This 85-year-old patient was operated twice for colon cancer resection and colostomy and underwent resection of a rectal pyogenic abscess 3 months earlier. The (A) axial STIR (3000/32/150) image and the (B) sagittal fast T_2-weighted (4200/102) image with fat presaturation show a multiloculated fluid-like lesion (curved arrow) with thick irregular walls and high intensity muscle edema adjacent to the abscess.

FIGURE 33.39. Staphylococcus gluteus medius and obturator externus muscle abscesses. This adult male patient undergoing vincristine chemotherapy for non-Hodgkin's lymphoma has fever and right hip and buttock pain. (A) Coronal fast STIR (3000/26/150) image demonstrates right gluteus medius muscle abscess (open arrow) and lateral perimuscular high intensity. Note also the left obturator internus and adductor infectious lesion (long arrow). (B) Axial T_1-weighted (600/12) image following intravenous infusion of gadolinium chelate. There is strong enhancement of the peripheral portion of the gluteus abscess (arrow) with absence of enhancement of the central portion.

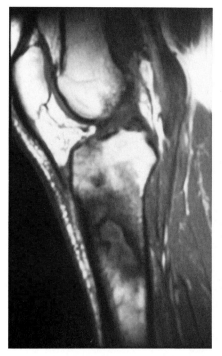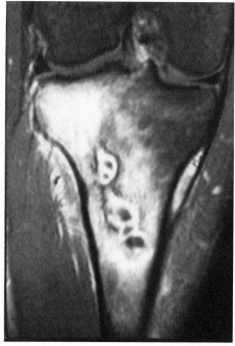

FIGURE 33.40. Staphylococcus osteomyelitis and myositis. (A) Sagittal preinjection image and (B) coronal T_1-weighted image (600/12) with fat presaturation following intravenous administration of gadolinium chelate. There is significant bone and surrounding soft tissue enhancement. Note the multiple bone abscesses.

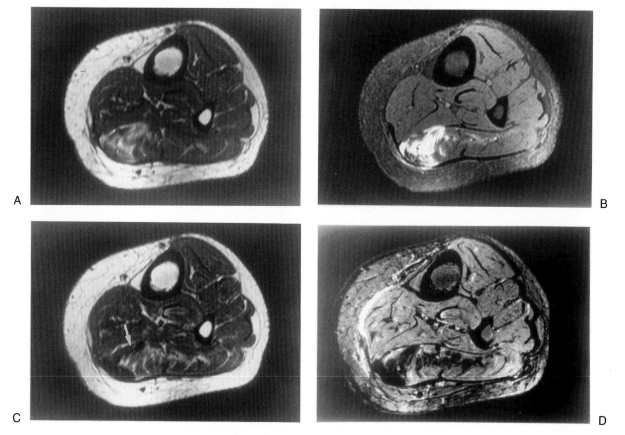

A

B

C

D

FIGURE 33.41. Intramuscular injection of 5 mM gadolinium-DTPA (0.5 ml), marking a muscle biopsy site. Gadolinium results in T_1 shortening as evidenced by high signal intensity on T_1-weighted (600/12, A) image and on moderately T_1-weighted (961/20 with spectral presaturation inversion recovery resulting in fat suppression, B) image. T_2 shortening of full-strength gadolinium chelate produces low signal intensity (arrow) on T_2-weighted (2100/80, C) image. The effect of T_2 shortening is most obvious on gradient echo sequence with T_2^* weighting (300/30, 30 degrees, D). (Images courtesy James L. Fleckenstein, M.D., Dallas, TX.)

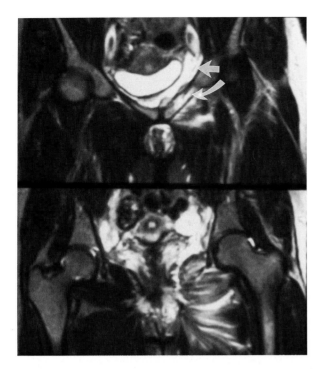

FIGURE 33.42. Pubic ramus fracture and multiple tears. The coronal fast T_2-weighted (4400/91) images with fat presaturation images display a 24-h-old left pubic fracture (curved arrow) and left pelvic hematoma that displaces the inferolateral bladder wall (thick arrow). Diffuse posttraumatic high signal intensity is present within the obturator internus, obturator externus, muscle, and adductor muscles (bottom image).

Another frequent indication for MRI at our institution is the evaluation of acute pelvic trauma, particularly to rule out radiographically occult pelvic ring or hip fractures and to diagnose pelvic hematoma. In virtually all such cases where MRI demonstrates osseous lesions we have detected associated posttraumatic increased signal lesions within the pelvic musculature (Figure 33.42). Such lesions are rarely suspected clinically due to significant bone or joint pain, which may mask the muscle injury, and due to the stationary position of the bedridden patient.

Summary

MRI is highly sensitive to alterations in the composition of skeletal muscle that occur in nearly all muscle lesions. Hemorrhage, edema, necrosis, inflammation, calcification, ossification, and fibrosis each have characteristic but not necessarily specific appearances with the various MRI pulse sequences. MRI provides early and accurate diagnosis that is not possible with any other single imaging modality or diagnostic technique. MRI often plays a crucial role in determining if treatment is conservative or surgical, possibly preventing or reducing the severity of sequelae: pain, fibrosis, atrophy, muscle shortening, and reduced strength. When considering the potentially severe and debilitating nature of the sequelae of muscle injuries and lesions, the information provided by MRI should prove to be cost-effective.

References

1. Berquist TH, Ehman RL. Musculoskeletal trauma. In: Berquist TH, Ehman RL, Richardson ML, editors. Magnetic resonance imaging of the musculoskeletal system. New York: Raven Press, 1987:127–163.
2. Ehman RL, Berquist TH. Magnetic resonance imaging of musculoskeletal trauma. Radiol Clin North Am 1986;24: 291–319.
3. Deutsch AL, Mink JH. Magnetic resonance imaging of musculoskeletal injuries. Radiol Clin North Am 1989;27: 983–1002.
4. Fleckenstein JL, Weatherall PT, Parkey RW, Payne JA, Peshock RM. Sports related muscle injuries: evaluation with MRI. Radiology 1989;172:793–798.
5. DeSmet AA, Fisher DR, Heiner JP, Keene JS. Magnetic resonance imaging of muscle tears. Skeletal Radiol 1990; 19:283–286.
6. Fleckenstein JL, Shellock FG. Exertional muscle injuries: magnetic resonance imaging evaluation. Top Magn Reson Imaging 1991;3:50–70.
7. Fleckenstein JL, Weatherall PT, Bertocci LA, et al. Locomotor system assessment by muscle magnetic resonance imaging. Magn Res Q 1991;7(2):79–103.
8. Greco A, McNamara MT, Escher MB, Trifilio G, Parienti J. Spin-echo and STIR MRI of sports-related muscle injuries at 1.5 T. J Comput Assist Tomogr 1991;15: 994–999.
9. Moon KL, Genant HK, Helms CA, Chafetz NI, Crooks LE, Kaufman L. Musculoskeletal applications of nuclear magnetic resonance. Radiology 1983;147:161–171.
10. Scott JA, Rosenthal DI, Brady T. The evaluation of musculoskeletal diseases with magnetic resonance imaging. Radiol Clin North Am 1984;22:917–924.
11. Speer KP, Lohnes H, Garrett WE. Radiographic imaging of muscle strain injury. Am J Sports Med 1993;21:89–95.
12. Hiroshi Y, Anno I, Niitsu M, Takahashi H, Matsumoto K, Itai Y. MRI of muscle strain injuries. J Comput Assist Tomogr 1994;18:454–460.
13. Fisher MR, Dooms GC, Hricak H, et al. Magnetic resonance imaging of the normal and pathologic muscular system. Magn Reson Imaging 1986;4:491–496.
14. Whitehouse GH. Magnetic resonance imaging in the diagnosis of muscle and tendon injuries. Imaging 1992;4: 95–105.
15. Muckle DS. Injuries in professional football. Br J Sports Med 1981;15:77–79.
16. Garrett WE. Basic science of musculotendinous injuries. In: Nicholas JA, Hershman EB, editors. The lower extremity and spine in sports medicine. St. Louis, MO: Mosby, 1986:42–58.

17. Garrett WE. Injuries to the muscle tendon unit. Instr Course Lect 1988;37:275–282.

18. Jackson DW, Feagin JA. Quadriceps contusions in young adults: relationship of severity of injury to treatment and prognosis. J Bone Joint Surg Am 1973;55:95–105.

19. Zarins B, Ciullo JV. Acute muscle and tendon injuries in athletes. Clin Sports Med 1983;2:167–182.

20. Anzel SH, Covey KW, Weiner AD, et al. Disruption of muscles and tendons: an analysis of 1014 cases. Surgery 1959;45:406–414.

21. Garrett WE. Muscle strain injuries: clinical and basic aspects. Med Sci Sports Exerc 1990;22:436–443.

22. Glick JM. Muscle strains: prevention and treatment. Physician Sports Med 1980;8:73–77.

23. Kibler WB. Clinical aspects of muscle injury. Med Sci Sports Med 1990;22:450–452.

24. O'Donoghue DH. Principles in the management of specific injuries. In: O'Donoghue, DH, editor. Treatment of injuries to athletes. 4th ed. Philadelphia, PA: Saunders, 1984:39–91.

25. Ryan AJ. Quadriceps strain: rupture and charley horse. Med Sci Sports 1969;1:106–111.

26. Baker BE. Current concepts in diagnosis and treatment of musculotendinous injuries. Med Sci Sports Exerc 1984;16:323–327.

27. Cooney WP. Sports injuries to the upper extremity. How to recognize and deal with some common problems. Postgrad Med 1984;76:45–50.

28. Orava S, Sorasto A, Aalto K, Kvist H. Total rupture of the pectoralis major muscle in athletes. Int J Sports Med 1984;5:272–274.

29. Noonan TJ, Garrett WEJ. Injuries of the myotendinous junction. Clin Sports Med 1992;11:783–806.

30. Berquist TH, editor. Imaging of orthopedic trauma and surgery. Philadelphia: WB Saunders, 1985.

31. Berquist TH. Imaging techniques in the acutely injured patient. Baltimore: Urban and Schwarzenberg, 1985.

32. Bowerman JW. Radiology of injury in sports. New York: Appleton-Century-Crofts, 1977.

33. Middleton WD, Edelstein G, Reinus WR, Melson GL, Totty WG, Murphy WA. Sonographic detection of rotator cuff tears. AJR 1985;144:349–353.

34. Allard JC, Bancroft J, Porter G. Imaging of plantaris muscle rupture. Clin Imaging 1992;16:55–58.

35. Garrett WE, Rich FR, Nikolaou PK, et al. Computed tomography of hamstring muscle strains. Med Sci Sports Exerc 1989;21:506–514.

36. Matin P. Basic principles of nuclear medicine techniques for detection and evaluation of trauma and sports medicine injuries. Semin Nucl Med 1988;18:90–112.

37. Matin P, Lang G, Garretta R, et al. Scintigraphic evaluation of muscle damage following extreme exercise: concise communication. J Nucl Med 1983;24:308–311.

38. Shirkoda A, Mauro MA, Staab EV, Blatt PM. Soft-tissue hemorrhage in hemophiliac patients: computed tomography and ultrasound study. Radiology 1983;147:811–814.

39. Termote J, Baert A, Crolla D, Palmers Y, Bulcke JA. Computed tomography of the normal and pathologic muscular system. Radiology 1980;137:439–444.

40. Valk P. Muscle localization of Tc-99 m MDP after exertion. Clin Nucl Med 1983;24:308–311.

41. Dooms GC, Fisher MR, Hricak H, Higgins CB. MRI of intramuscular hemorrhage. J Comput Assist Tomogr 1985;9:908–913.

42. Fleckenstein JL, Canby RC, Parkey RW, Peshock RM. Acute effects of exercise on MRI of skeletal muscle in normal volunteers. AJR 1988;15:231–237.

43. Herfkens RJ, Sievers R, Kaufman L, et al. Nuclear magnetic resonance imaging of the infarcted muscle: a rat model. Radiology 1983;147:761–764.

44. Fleckenstein JL, Burns DK, Murphy FK, Jayson HT, Bonte FJ. Differential diagnosis of bacterial myositis in AIDS: evaluation with MRI. Radiology 1991;179:653–658.

45. Hernandez RJ, Keim DR, Chenevert TL, Sullivan DB, Aisen AM. Fat-suppressed MRI of myositis. Radiology 1992;182(1):217–219.

46. Berquist TH, Brown ML, Fitzgerald RH Jr, May GR. Magnetic resonance imaging: application in musculoskeletal injection. Magn Reson Imaging 1985;3:219–230.

47. Berquist TH. Musculoskeletal infection. In: Magnetic resonance imaging of the musculoskeletal system. New York: Raven Press, 1987:109–126.

48. Hanna SL, Fletcher BD, Parham DM, Bugg MF. Muscle edema in musculoskeletal tumors: MRI characteristics and clinical significance. J Magn Reson Imaging 1991;1(4):441–449.

49. Biondetti PR, Ehman RL. Soft-tissue sarcomas: use of textural patterns in skeletal muscle as a diagnostic feature in postoperative MRI. Radiology 1992;183:845–848.

50. Crim JR, Seeger LL, Yao L, Chandnani V, Eckardt JJ. Diagnosis of soft-tissue masses with MRI: can benign masses be differentiated from malignant ones? Radiology 1992;185:581–586.

51. Berquist TH, Ehman RL, King BF, Hodgman CG, Iistrup DM. Value of MRI in differentiating benign from malignant soft-tissue masses: study of 95 lesions. AJR 1990;155:1251–1255.

52. Whyte AM, Lufkin RB, Bredenkamp J, Hoover L. Sternocleidomastoid fibrosis in congenital muscular torticollis: MRI appearance. J Comput Assist Tomogr 1989;13:163–166.

53. Bernardino ME, Chaloupka JC, Malko JA, Chezmar JL, Nelson RC. Are hepatic and muscle T2 values different at 0.5 and 1.5 Tesla? Magnetic Resonance Imaging 1989;7(4):363–367.

54. Kuno S-y, Katsuta S, Inouye T, Anno I, Matsumoto K, Akisada M. Relationship between relaxation times and muscle fiber composition. Radiology 1988;169:567–568.

55. Polak JF, Jolesz FA, Adams DF. NMR of skeletal muscle differences in relaxation parameters related to extracellular/intracellular fluid spaces. Invest Radiol 1988;23:107–111.

56. Dwyer AJ, Frank JA, Sank VJ, Reinig JW, Hickey AM, Doppman JL. Short-TI inversion recovery pulse sequence: analysis and initial experience in cancer imaging. Radiology 1988;168:827–836.

57. Bydder GM, Young IR. MRI: clinical use of the inversion recovery sequence. J Comput Assist Tomogr 1985;9:659–675.

58. Fleckenstein JL, Archer BT, Barker BA, Vaughan JT, Parkey RW, Peshock RM. Fast short-tau inversion-recovery imaging. Radiology 1991;179:499–504.

59. Fleckenstein JL, Archer BT, Barker BA, Vaughan JT, Parkey RW, Peshock RM. Fast, short tau inversion recovery (FASTIR) imaging [abstract]. Magn Reson Imaging 1989;7:87.

60. Fisher MJ, Meyer RA, Adams GR, Foley JM, Potchen EJ. Direct relationship between proton T2 and exercise intensity in skeletal muscle MR images. Invest Radiol 1990;25:480–485.

61. Rubin JI, Gomori JM, Grossman RI, Gefter WB, Kressel HY. High-field MRI of extracranial hematomas. AJR 1987;248:813–817.

62. Unger EC, Glazer HS, Lee JKT, et al. MRI of extracranial hematomas: preliminary observations. AJR 1986; 146:403–407.

63. McKeag DB. The concept of overuse: the primary care aspects of overuse syndromes in sports. Primary Care 1984;11:43–59.

64. Stern PJ. Tendinitis, overuse syndromes, and tendon injuries. Hand Clin 1990;6:467–476.

65. Dennett X, Fry HJ. Overuse syndrome: a muscle biopsy study. Lancet 1988;1:905–908.

66. Frymoyer JW, Mooney V. Occupational orthopaedics. J Bone Joint Surg Am 1986;68:469–474.

67. Repetition strain injury [editorial]. Lancet 1987;2:316.

68. Ireland DC. Repetitive strain injury. Austr Fam Physician 1986;15:415–418.

69. Lockwood AH. Medical problems of musicians. N Engl J Med 1989;320:221–227.

70. Larsson SE, Bengtsson A, Bodegard L, Hendricksson KG, Larsson J. Muscle changes in work-related chronic myalgia. Acta Orthop Scand 1988;59:552–556.

71. Simons D. Muscle pain syndromes. I. Am J Phys Med 1975;54:289–311.

72. Simons D. Muscle pain syndromes. II. Am J Phys Med 1976;55:15–42.

73. Fleckenstein JL. Skeletal muscle disorders: the emerging role of MRI. In: Kressel HY, Modic MT, Murphy WA, editors. Syllabus: a special course in MRI 1990. Oak Brook, IL: Radiological Society of North America, 1990: 197–206.

74. Sundaram M, McGuire MH, Schajowicz F. Soft-tissue masses: histologic basis for decreased signal (short T2) on T2-weighted MR images. AJR 1987;148:1247–1250.

75. Fullerton GD, Cameron IL, Ord VA. Orientation of tendons in the magnetic field and its effect on T2 relaxation times. Radiology 1985;155:433–435.

76. Beltran J, Noto AM, Herman LJ, Lubbers LM. Tendons: High-field-strength, surface coil MRI. Radiology 1987; 162:735–740.

77. Booth DW, Westers BM. The management of athletes with myositis ossificans traumatica. Can J Sport Sci 1986; 14:10–16.

78. Johnson LC. Histogenesis of myositis ossificans. Am J Pathol 1948;24:681–682.

79. Hudson TM. Radiologic-pathologic correlation of musculoskeletal lesions. Williams & Wilkins, Baltimore, 1987: 589–604.

80. Amendola MA, Glazer GM, Agha FP, Francis IR, Weatherbee L, Martel W. Myositis ossificans circumscripta: computed tomographic diagnosis. Radiology 1983;149:775–779.

81. Zeanah WR, Hudson TM. Myositis ossificans: radiologic evaluation of two cases with diagnostic computed tomograms. Clin Orthop 1982;168:187–192.

82. Kransdorf MJ, Meis JM, Jelinek JS. Myositis ossificans: MRI appearance with radiologic-pathologic correlation. AJR 1991;157:1243–1248.

83. Malisano LP, Hunter GA. Liquefaction and calcification of a chronic compartment syndrome of the lower limb. J Orthop Trauma 1992;6:245–247.

84. Viau MR, Pederson HE, Salciccioli GG, Manoli A. Ectopic calcification as a late sequela of compartment syndrome. Clin Orthop 1983;176:178–180.

85. Janzen DL, Connell DG, Vaisler BJ. Calcific myonecrosis of the calf manifesting as an enlarging soft tissue mass: imaging features. AJR 1993;160:1072–1074.

86. Raether PM, Luther LD. Recurrent compartment syndrome in the posterior thigh. Report of a case. Am J Sports Med 1982;10:40–43.

87. Whitesides TE, Haney TC, Moremoto K. Tissue pressure measurements as a determinator for need for fasciotomy. Clin Orthop 1975;113:43–51.

88. Amendola A, Rorabeck CH, Vellett D, Vezina W, Rutt B, Nott L. The use of magnetic resonance imaging in exertional compartment syndromes. Am J Sports Med 1990;18:29–34.

89. Fleckenstein JL, Bertocci LA, Nunnally RL, Parkey RW, Peshock RM. Exercise-enhanced MRI of variations in forearm muscle anatomy and use: importance in MRI spectroscopy. AJR 1989;153:693–698.

90. Wolfort FG, Modelvang LC, Filtzer HS. Anterior tibial compartment syndrome following muscle hernia repair. Arch Surg 1973;106:97–99.

91. Binkovitz LA, Berquist TH, McLeod RA. Masses of the hand and wrist: Detection and characterization with MRI. AJR 1990;154:323–326.

92. Wetzel LH, Levine E. Soft-tissue tumors of the foot: Value of MRI for specific diagnosis. AJR 1990;155: 1025–1030.

93. Morton MJ, Berquist TH, McLeod RA, Unni KK, Sim FH. Pictorial essay. MRI of synovial sarcoma. AJR 1991; 156:337–340.

94. Murphy WD, Hurst GC, Duerk JL, Feiglin DH, Christopher M, Bellon EM. Atypical appearance of lipomatous tumors on MR images: High signal intensity with fat-suppression STIR sequences. JMRI 1991;1(4):477–480.

95. Resendes M, Helms CA, Fritz RC, Genant HK. MRI appearance of intramuscular injections. AJR 1992;158: 1293–1294.

96. Nurenberg P, Giddings CJ, Stray-Gundersen J, Fleckenstein JL, Gonyea WJ, Peshock RM. MRI-guided muscle biopsy for correlation of increased signal intensity with ultrastructural change and delayed-onset muscle soreness after exercise. Radiology 1992;184:865–869.

Index